Renal Cancer

John A. Libertino • Jason R. Gee
Editors

Renal Cancer

Contemporary Management

Third Edition

Springer

Editors
John A. Libertino, MD
Professor of Urology
Tufts University School of Medicine
Department of Urology
Tufts University Medical Center
Boston, MA, USA

Jason R. Gee, MD
Associate Professor of Urology
Tufts University School of Medicine
Department of Urology
Tufts University Medical Center
Boston, MA, USA

Department of Urology
MGH Cancer Center
Emerson Hospital
Concord, MA, USA

ISBN 978-3-031-97598-1 ISBN 978-3-031-97599-8 (eBook)
https://doi.org/10.1007/978-3-031-97599-8

This Springer imprint is published by the registered company Springer Nature Switzerland AG
The registered company address is: Gewerbestrasse 11, 6330 Cham, Switzerland

TO OUR WIVES WHO SACRIFICED MUCH TIME OVER MANY YEARS AND OUR COLLEAGUES WHO HAVE MADE THIS TEXTBOOK A REALITY.

Preface

In 2024, renal cell carcinoma accounted for approximately 15,000 deaths in the United States, and the worldwide mortality rate was 179,368 deaths in 2022.

With considerable effort over the past decade, much has been learned about the pathogenesis of renal cancer and its treatment, but we have much farther to go.

This the third edition of *Renal Cancer: Contemporary Management*, which provides us with a current view of the etiology and the management of patients who have renal cancer. In editing this textbook, we have included the authors who have been responsible for many of the most significant advances made in the diagnosis and treatment of renal cancer.

This textbook provides the most contemporary, up to date, summary of the advances made in the field and will hopefully be of great benefit to urologists engaged in the care of patients with kidney cancer.

Boston, MA, USA — John A. Libertino
Boston, MA, USA — Jason R. Gee

Contents

1 **Epidemiology, Screening, and Clinical Staging** 1
Benjamin I. Joffe, Christopher R. Haas, and James M. McKiernan

2 **Molecular Genetics of Renal Cell Carcinoma** 25
Jonathan S. Kim and Louis S. Liou

3 **Familial and Hereditary Syndromes in Renal Cell Cancer** 35
Mark W. Ball, Jaskirat Saini, and Peter A. Pinto

4 **Pathology of Renal Cell Carcinoma** 51
Ming Zhou

5 **Imaging of Renal Cancer** 77
Jalil Afnan, Rose-Anna Voog, and Christoph Wald

6 **Molecular Imaging for Renal Cell Carcinoma**. 103
Brandon Koo, Yamin Dou, and Eric Dietsche

7 **Interventional Radiology and Angioinfarction Transcatheter Embolization of Renal Tumors** 127
Sebastian Flacke

8 **Natural History, Diagnostic Evaluation, and Active Surveillance of Small Renal Masses** 141
Robert S. Wang, Andres F. Correa, Robert G. Uzzo, David Y. T. Chen, and Benjamin T. Ristau

9 **Rationale for Partial Nephrectomy, Current Practice Patterns** 169
Jesse B. Persily and William C. Huang

10 **Objectifying Complexity of Kidney Cancers: Relationship of Tumor Anatomy and Outcomes** 201
Jason R. Gee, Alexander Kutikov, Joseph Izes, and John A. Libertino

11 **History of Renal Surgery for Cancer** 215
Samuel Donnenfeld and Brendan M. Browne

12 **The Surgical Approaches to Renal Masses and Their Impact on Postoperative Renal Function** 221
John A. Libertino

13 **Open Partial Nephrectomy** 239
Marianne M. Casilla-Lennon, Patrick A. Kenney, Matthew Wszolek, and John A. Libertino

14 **Minimally Invasive Partial Nephrectomy and Ablative Procedures for Small Renal Masses** 263
Tony Luongo

15 **Surgery for Renal Cell Carcinoma with Thrombus Extension into the Vena Cava** 281
John A. Libertino, Chad Wotkowicz, and Jason R. Gee

16 **Role of Lymphadenectomy in Renal Cell Cancer** 311
Jacqueline Bultiauw, Mattias van Hattem, Maarten Albersen, Hendrik Van Poppel, and Eduard Roussel

17 **Role of Surgery in Locally Recurrent and Metastatic Renal Cancer** 333
Katiana Vazquez-Rivera, Marc Ganz, and A. Ari Hakimi

18 **Management of Renal Cell Carcinoma of Variant Histology** . . . 349
Kevin Kayvan Zarrabi, Mehmet Asim Bilen, Nizar M. Tannir, and Pedro C. Barata

19 **Surgical Management for Transitional Cell Carcinoma of the Upper Tract** 365
Jason R. Gee

20 **Postoperative Surveillance Protocols for Renal Cell Carcinoma** 391
Elizabeth E. Ellis, Brittney H. Cotta, Megan M. Merrill, and Jose A. Karam

21 **Role of Radiation Therapy in Renal Cancer** 419
Andrea McKee, Arul Mahadevan, and Chad Tang

22 **Systemic Therapies for the Treatment of Renal Cell Carcinoma** 435
Sonia Gowda and Paul Mathew

23 **Unified Approaches to Surgery and Systemic Therapy for Renal Cell Carcinoma** 447
Shayan Smani, Soum D. Lokeshwar, Alejandro Abello, and Patrick A. Kenney

24 **CAR-T Therapy for Kidney Cancer** 475
Jonathan Yeshwanth Daniel, Sheron Raja, S. Iswarya, V. Yohitha, Meenu Soorajj, Zulfiqur Ali, Alex Khariton, Merrel Holley, and Vinoth-Kumar Lakshmanan

Correction to: Systemic Therapies for the Treatment of Renal Cell Carcinoma C1
Sonia Gowda and Paul Mathew

Index 489

List of Contributors

Alejandro Abello Department of Urology, Beth Israel Deaconess Medical Center, Boston, MA, USA

Jalil Afnan Department of Radiology, Lahey Hospital & Medical Center, Burlington, MA, USA

Maarten Albersen Department of Urology, University Hospitals Leuven, Leuven, Belgium

Zulfiqur Ali Teesside University, Middlesbrough, England, UK

Mark W. Ball Urologic Oncology Branch, Center for Cancer Research, National Cancer Institute, National Institutes of Health Clinical Center, Bethesda, MD, USA

Pedro C. Barata Division of Solid Tumor Oncology, University Hospitals Seidman Cancer Center, Case Western Reserve University, Cleveland, OH, USA

Mehmet Asim Bilen Department of Hematology and Medical Oncology, Emory University School of Medicine, Atlanta, GA, USA

Brendan M. Browne Department of Urology, Emory University School of Medicine, Atlanta, GA, USA

Jacqueline Bultiauw Department of Urology, University Hospitals Leuven, Leuven, Belgium

Marianne M. Casilla-Lennon Department of Urology, Yale New Haven Health, New Haven, CT, USA

David Y. T. Chen Department of Urology, Fox Chase Cancer Center – Temple University Health System, Philadelphia, PA, USA

Andres F. Correa Department of Urology, Fox Chase Cancer Center – Temple University Health System, Philadelphia, PA, USA

Brittney H. Cotta Department of Urology, The University of Texas MD Anderson Cancer Center, Houston, TX, USA

Jonathan Yeshwanth Daniel Prostate Cancer Biomarker Laboratory, Faculty of Clinical Research, Sri Ramachandra Institute of Higher Education & Research, Chennai, India

Eric Dietsche Department of Radiology, Rhode Island Hospital, Warren Alpert Medical School of Brown University, Providence, RI, USA

Samuel Donnenfeld Department of Urology, Brown University, Providence, RI, USA

Yamin Dou Nuclear Medicine, Department of Radiology, Veterans Affairs Boston Healthcare System, West Roxbury, MA, USA

Elizabeth E. Ellis Department of Urology, The University of Texas MD Anderson Cancer Center, Houston, TX, USA

Sebastian Flacke, MD, PhD, FACR Department of Radiology at UMass Chan-Lahey, Lahey Hospital and Medical Center, Burlington, MA, USA

Marc Ganz Department of Urology, SUNY Downstate Health Sciences University, Brooklyn, NY, USA

Jason R. Gee, MD Associate Professor of Urology, Tufts University School of Medicine, Department of Urology, Tufts University Medical Center, Boston, MA, USA
Department of Urology, MGH Cancer Center, Emerson Hospital, Concord, MA, USA

Sonia Gowda Division of Hematology-Oncology, Tufts Medical Center, Boston, MA, USA

Christopher R. Haas Department of Urology, New York-Presbyterian, Columbia University Irving Medical Center, Herbert Irving Pavilion, New York, NY, USA

A. Ari Hakimi Department of Surgery, Urology Service, Memorial Sloan Kettering Cancer Center, New York, NY, USA

Mattias van Hattem Department of Urology, University Hospitals Leuven, Leuven, Belgium

Merrel Holley International Hyperbaric Medical Foundation, Morgan City, LA, USA

William C. Huang Division of Urologic Oncology, Department of Urology, NYU Langone Medical Center, New York, NY, USA

S. Iswarya Prostate Cancer Biomarker Laboratory, Faculty of Clinical Research, Sri Ramachandra Institute of Higher Education & Research, Chennai, India

Joseph Izes Department of Urology, Thomas Jefferson University Hospital, Philadelphia, PA, USA

Benjamin I. Joffe Department of Urology, New York-Presbyterian, Columbia University Irving Medical Center, Herbert Irving Pavilion, New York, NY, USA

Jose A. Karam Department of Urology, The University of Texas MD Anderson Cancer Center, Houston, TX, USA

Patrick A. Kenney Department of Urology, Yale School of Medicine, Yale New Haven Hospital, New Haven, CT, USA

Alex Khariton Sidney Kimmel Comprehensive Cancer Center, Philadelphia, PA, USA

Jonathan S. Kim Drexel University College of Medicine, Philadelphia, PA, USA

Brandon Koo Department of Radiology, Rhode Island Hospital, Warren Alpert Medical School of Brown University, Providence, RI, USA

Alexander Kutikov Division of Urology and Urologic Oncology, Department of Surgery, Fox Chase Cancer Center, Temple University School of Medicine, Philadelphia, PA, USA

Vinoth-Kumar Lakshmanan Prostate Cancer Biomarker Laboratory, Faculty of Clinical Research, Sri Ramachandra Institute of Higher Education & Research, Chennai, India

John A. Libertino, MD Professor of Urology, Tufts University School of Medicine, Department of Urology Tufts University Medical Center, Boston, MA, USA

Louis S. Liou Department of Urology, Emerson Hospital, Concord, MA, USA
Tufts University School of Medicine, Boston, MA, USA

Soum D. Lokeshwar Department of Urology, Yale School of Medicine, Yale New Haven Hospital, New Haven, CT, USA

Tony Luongo Department of Urology, Tufts Medicine, Tufts University School of Medicine, Boston, MA, USA

Arul Mahadevan Department of Radiation Oncology, Massachusetts General Cancer Center at Wentworth Douglass Hospital, Dover, NH, USA

Paul Mathew Division of Hematology-Oncology, Tufts Medical Center, Boston, MA, USA

Andrea McKee Department of Radiation Oncology, Massachusetts General Cancer Center at Wentworth Douglass Hospital, Dover, NH, USA

James M. McKiernan Department of Urology, New York-Presbyterian, Columbia University Irving Medical Center, Herbert Irving Pavilion, New York, NY, USA

Megan M. Merrill Department of Urology, Kaiser Permanente South Sacramento, Sacramento, CA, USA

Jesse B. Persily Department of Urology, NYU Langone Medical Center, New York, NY, USA

Peter A. Pinto Urologic Oncology Branch, Center for Cancer Research, National Cancer Institute, National Institutes of Health Clinical Center, Bethesda, MD, USA

Hendrik Van Poppel Department of Urology, University Hospitals Leuven, Leuven, Belgium

Sheron Raja Prostate Cancer Biomarker Laboratory, Faculty of Clinical Research, Sri Ramachandra Institute of Higher Education & Research, Chennai, India

Benjamin T. Ristau Department of Surgery/Division of Urology, UConn Health, Farmington, CT, USA

Eduard Roussel Department of Urology, University Hospitals Leuven, Leuven, Belgium

Jaskirat Saini Urologic Oncology Branch, Center for Cancer Research, National Cancer Institute, National Institutes of Health Clinical Center, Bethesda, MD, USA

Shayan Smani Department of Urology, Yale School of Medicine, Yale New Haven Hospital, New Haven, CT, USA

Meenu Soorajj Prostate Cancer Biomarker Laboratory, Faculty of Clinical Research, Sri Ramachandra Institute of Higher Education & Research, Chennai, India

Chad Tang Department of Genitourinary Radiation Oncology, MD Anderson Cancer Center, Houston, TX, USA

Nizar M. Tannir Genitourinary Medical Oncology, UT MD Anderson Cancer Center, Houston, TX, USA

Robert G. Uzzo Department of Urology, Fox Chase Cancer Center – Temple University Health System, Philadelphia, PA, USA

Katiana Vazquez-Rivera Department of Urology, Maimonides Health, Brooklyn, NY, USA

Rose-Anna Voog Department of Radiology, Lahey Hospital & Medical Center, Burlington, MA, USA

Christoph Wald Department of Radiology, Lahey Hospital & Medical Center, Burlington, MA, USA

Robert S. Wang Department of Urology, Massachusetts General Hospital – Mass General Brigham, Boston, MA, USA

Chad Wotkowicz Midcoast Hospital, Brunswick, ME, USA

Matthew Wszolek Department of Urology, Massachusetts General Hospital, Boston, MA, USA

V. Yohitha Prostate Cancer Biomarker Laboratory, Faculty of Clinical Research, Sri Ramachandra Institute of Higher Education & Research, Chennai, India

Kevin Kayvan Zarrabi Department of Medical Oncology, Sidney Kimmel Cancer Center, Thomas Jefferson University, Philadelphia, PA, USA

Ming Zhou Department of Pathology, Molecular and Cell-based Medicine, Icahn School of Medicine at Mount Sinai, New York, NY, USA

Epidemiology, Screening, and Clinical Staging

1

Benjamin I. Joffe, Christopher R. Haas, and James M. McKiernan

Introduction to Epidemiology

Kidney cancer among adults includes malignant tumors arising from the renal parenchyma and renal pelvis, but the differential of a renal mass should also include benign tumors and inflammatory causes as summarized in Table 1.1. Tumors arising from the renal pelvis are mostly of the urothelial cell type and comprise less than 10% of kidney carcinomas. Renal cell carcinoma (RCC), also known as renal cell adenocarcinoma, accounts for 90% of kidney carcinomas and is much more common than benign tumors or other malignant cancers [1]. Renal cell carcinoma is divided into a variety of histologic subtypes, which may differ in clinical features and prognosis. The most common form of RCC is the clear cell type, comprising 75% of new cases; this is followed by the papillary, chromophobe, medullary, and collecting duct subtypes which make up 10%, 5%, 1%, and 1%, respectively [2].

Kidney cancer is the fourteenth most common cancer worldwide, with over 430,000 new cases in 2022 and almost 460,000 new cases predicted in 2025. It is the tenth most commonly occurring cancer in men and the thirteenth most commonly occurring cancer in women [3]. The highest incidence rates can be found in Northern and Eastern Europe, as well as North America [3, 4]. In the United States, kidney cancer ranks as the seventh most commonly diagnosed cancer, with 1.8% of men and women diagnosed with kidney or renal pelvis cancer at some point in their lifetime [5]. According to the Surveillance, Epidemiology, and End Results (SEER) program, the prevalence of kidney and renal pelvis cancer in 2021 was estimated to be 646,960 in the United States. The National Cancer Institute (NCI) reports that within the United States, there have been an estimated 81,610 new cases in 2024 with a male-to-female predominance of about 2:1 and almost 15,000 deaths due to kidney and renal pelvis cancers. As a result, kidney cancers account for 4.1% of all new cancer cases and 2.4% of all cancer deaths, and remain the twelfth leading cause of cancer death. Among all new diagnoses of kidney cancer in the United States, 5-year survival is 78.1% [5, 6].

B. I. Joffe (✉) · C. R. Haas · J. M. McKiernan
Department of Urology, New York-Presbyterian, Columbia University Irving Medical Center, Herbert Irving Pavilion, New York, NY, USA
e-mail: bij2106@cumc.columbia.edu; haas1@tuftsmedicalcenter.org; jmm23@cumc.columbia.edu

J. A. Libertino, J. R. Gee (eds.), *Renal Cancer*, https://doi.org/10.1007/978-3-031-97599-8_1

Table 1.1 Differential diagnosis of a renal mass

Malignant	Benign	Inflammatory
Renal cell carcinoma	Simple cyst	Abscess
Clear cell	Angiomyolipoma	Focal pyelonephritis
Papillary	Oncocytoma	Xanthogranulomatous pyelonephritis
Chromophobe	Renal adenoma	Infected renal cyst
Collecting duct carcinoma	Metanephric adenoma	Tuberculosis
Urothelium derived	Cystic nephroma	Rheumatic granuloma
Urothelial cell carcinoma	Mixed epithelial/stromal tumor	
Squamous cell carcinoma	Reninoma	
Adenocarcinoma	Leiomyoma	
Sarcoma	Fibroma	
Leiomyosarcoma	Hemangioma	
Liposarcoma	Vascular malformation	
Angiosarcoma	Pseudotumor	
Hemangiopericytoma		
Malignant fibroid histiocytoma		
Synovial sarcoma		
Osteogenic sarcoma		
Clear cell sarcoma		
Rhabdomyosarcoma		
Wilms tumor		
Primitive neuroectodermal tumor		
Carcinoid		
Lymphoma		
Metastasis		
Invasion by an adjacent neoplasm		

Incidence and Mortality Rates over Time

From 1992 to 2015, the incidence of kidney cancer in the United States increased at 2.4%/year; however, this increase has slowed to a near plateau from 2008 to 2015 [7]. This increase in RCC incidence was most notable in localized and regional disease rather than metastatic RCC in which the overall incidence has been stable [8] . Incidence-based mortality rates increased from 1992 and peaked in 2001, but then started to decline with the sharpest decline in recent years of 32% from 2013 to 2015, likely in the setting of improved treatments for advanced RCC such as the introduction of various immunotherapies [7, 9, 10]. Over 2004 to 2015, 5-year overall survival rates have improved with gains in advanced RCC while localized RCC rates have remained stable [8].

In the last decade, 18 countries experienced increased incidence rates for both men and women, with sharper increases occurring in Latin America, Brazil, Thailand, and Bulgaria [4]. Reporting bias, advancement in health record systems, and accessibility to healthcare providers should also be considered in comparing rates accurately between regions. Increasing incidence and a decreasing mortality-to-incidence ratio have been found to be correlated with increasing human development index levels and gross domestic product per capita [11]. One explanation for the rising incidence in developed nations is the higher prevalence of risk factors for RCC (such as smoking, obesity, physical inactivity, and hypertension) present in developed countries. Increased access to care and availability of advanced therapeutics have been postulated to account for the decreased mortality-to-incidence ratio [7, 9].

Another likely explanation for the higher incidence of kidney cancer observed in developed countries is the greater availability and more liberal use of abdominal computed tomography imaging techniques resulting in more incidental findings of renal masses [12–15]. Within the United States Medicare population, 43% of patients receive a CT of the chest or abdomen over a 5-year period [16]. Tandem with the detection of more incidental renal masses is the increased diagnosis of small renal masses <4 cm, which now account for 48–66% of new RCC diagnosis [8, 11]. Tumor size has extensively been shown to be correlated with aggressive malignant histology, with likelihood of malignancy increasing 33% per centimeter and specifically aggressive histology increasing from 6% for tumors <1 cm to 52% for tumors >10 cm [17, 18]. The risk of metastasis rises as well, with a 25% increased odds of metastasis with each centimeter increase in tumor diameter [19]. In patients with tumor diameter < 3 cm, the risk of metastasis is remote with several active surveillance cohorts reporting 0–1.1% metastatic events occurring in tumors <3 cm [20–22]. In addition to improvements made in local and systemic therapies for RCC, the decreasing mortality rates from RCC can also partly be attributed to the lead-time bias from earlier diagnosis and treatment of small renal masses [7]. In states and developed nations that have aimed to curtail advanced radiologic testing, there has been recent data to suggest that the incidence of renal cancer has plateaued [23].

Demographic Factors in Renal Cell Carcinoma

Renal cancer is twice as common in males as females, and the rate of incidence has continued to rise twice as rapidly in males compared to females [24, 25]. A 2008 study looking at retrospective data of 39,434 patients from 1988 to 2004 in the California Cancer Registry determined that overall, females showed a higher percentage of localized cancer than males, which may be responsible for a higher relative survival rate in females [26] . Potential explanations for differences in survival rates also include biological differences in the tumor, more extensive use of the healthcare system by females, higher rates of smoking in males, and a higher prevalence of hypertension in males [24, 26].

With a median age at RCC diagnosis of 75 years old worldwide and 65 years old in the United States, RCC is primarily a malignancy of the elderly [6, 27]. In fact, 55.9% of patients are diagnosed between the ages of 55 and 74, while less than 10% are diagnosed at less than 45 years of age in the United States [6]. However, recent studies note that rates of RCC in young patients have increased up to 5% annually [28]. As mortality rates continue to decrease in the United States and overall RCC incidence rises, the incidence of RCC in the elderly will also likely continue to rise. Of note, adolescents and young adults more commonly present with rare histologic subtypes such as translocation carcinoma or renal medullary carcinoma. Though RCC in younger patients is still rare, translocation carcinomas account for up to 50% of all RCC in patients under the age of 40 [29].

Along with sex and age, ethnicity is an important factor in the epidemiology of RCC. Within the United States, SEER data show that Native American patients have a higher incidence rate than all other ethnicities, while Asian and Pacific Islander patients have the lowest incidence rates. Caucasians had an incidence of 18.1 per 100,000 person-years in 2021 in comparison to 33.8 per 100,000 person-years in the Native American population [6, 30]. Mortality rates also vary greatly with ethnicity, despite being diagnosed at a younger age with more localized disease, black RCC patients had a significantly lower survival rate than all other ethnicities [26]. The disparity in survival rates between black patients and other ethnicities is unknown, but can be partially explained by stressors associated with socioeconomic status, comorbidities such as hypertension, and lower likelihood of undergoing nephrectomy or receiving systemic therapies for metastatic disease [31, 32].

RCC tumor subtype also varies among ethnic groups. Looking at 18 US population-based registries of the SEER program in 2011, a study found that among 84,255 RCC patients, clear cell RCC is more common in white populations than black populations (50% vs. 31%), and the papillary subtype presents more often in people of African or Caribbean descent than Caucasian descent (23% vs. 9%). These authors also found that compared to whites, blacks were four times more likely to have papillary RCC than clear cell RCC, while Asian or Pacific Islanders were less likely to have papillary or chromophobe RCC than white patients [33]. Other rare and aggressive subtypes of RCC, such as collecting duct carcinoma and renal medullary carcinoma, have been linked to African American heritage, with renal medullary carcinoma seen almost exclusively with sickle cell trait [34, 35].

Risk Factors in the Development of RCC

Risk factors for renal cell carcinoma include male gender, age, smoking, diet, obesity, hypertension, renal disease, family history, certain medication use, and environmental exposures. In addition, there is a significant contribution by various genomic mutations. While some components such as gender and age have been discussed under demographics, current literature regarding the remaining factors is described below.

Smoking

According to the International Agency for Research on Cancer (IARC) and the US Surgeon General, smoking is a well-established causal risk factor for RCC [36]. A 2019 meta-analysis of 56 studies shows that the overall RR for developing RCC in someone who has ever smoked a cigarette was 1.39 (95% CI = 1.28–1.51). Furthermore, these data reported a dose–response relationship of increasing RR with more exposure to cigarette smoke, both in terms of the number of cigarettes smoked per day as well as years spent smoking. The RR for patients who smoked 30 cigarettes/day was 1.72 compared with an RR of 1.18 for those who smoked 5 cigarettes/day. Similarly, the RR for patients who smoked for 25 years was 1.70 compared to 1.24 for those who smoked for 10 years. A promising finding from the study indicated that a greater length of abstinence from smoking actually reduced the RR, as low as 0.82 for those who abstained for 30 years compared to current smokers, but never to the level of never smokers [37].

Compared to nonsmokers, current smokers with RCC were shown to be at an increased risk for death with an HR of 1.7 (95% CI = 1.2–2.5) [38]. A recent study found that all smokers, including those who have quit, have a higher mortality risk with an RR of 1.23 (95% CI = 1.08–1.40) [39]. Smokers were seen to have a higher likelihood of increased stage or even metastases at diagnosis [40]. Similarly to chronic obstructive pulmonary disease (COPD), the pathogenesis of cigarette smoking in RCC is linked to carbon monoxide exposure and chronic tissue hypoxia. Smokers with RCC were also shown to have increased DNA damage and mutations within peripheral blood lymphocytes due to N-nitrosamine and benzo[α]pyrene diol exposure compared to a control group [41, 42].

Diet

Many different foods and substances have been researched to look for an increased risk of RCC. Most notably, consumption of fruits and vegetables was shown to be inversely related to the development of RCC in a meta-analysis reviewing 13 prospective studies [43]. In addition, vitamin C may have a protective role as well, but data are limited for protective dietary factors in general [44]. The role of high fat and protein consumption is more controversial because while it has been considered a risk factor in the past, a large multicenter European cohort study revealed that there is no significant association between the development of RCC and these nutrients [45].

There is a large literature on the risk of alcohol consumption as a carcinogen [46]. However, like fruits and vegetables, alcohol has been inversely associated with renal cancer risk; this includes beer, wine, and liquor. A dose-dependent risk reduction was discovered in a pooled analysis of 12 prospective studies, showing a 28% lower risk in those who drank more than 15 grams per day. Interestingly, no association was found between total fluid intakes from other beverages, such as water, juice, milk, tea, coffee, or soda, implying that alcohol itself is a modifying factor [47]. Another meta-analysis of 22 studies looked at the association between alcohol and all malignancies, finding lower risk for RCC with an RR of 0.92 (95% CI 0.86–0.99) and 0.79 (95% CI 0.72–0.86) for light and moderate consumption, respectively [48].

Obesity

Obesity was first shown to be associated with RCC as early as 1984 when McLaughlin et al. conducted a case–control analysis that suggested body mass index (BMI) and RCC in women were related [49]. Since then, much more literature has been published regarding the relationship between waist-to-hip ratios, weight gain during adulthood, and the mechanisms of its influence on kidney cancer [50–52]. The World Cancer Research Fund reports that since the 1980s, obesity has continued to increase in both resource-rich countries as well as low- and middle-income countries [53]. Between genders, there is an estimated 24% increased risk in men and 34% increased risk in women for every 5 kg/m increase in BMI [54]. One study found that up to 20% of RCCs are directly related to patient obesity [51]. However, it is important to note that despite the link between obesity and increased incidence of RCC, there is a paradoxical protective effect on RCC outcomes. Multiple studies have shown improved cancer-specific survival among overweight and obese patients, with a meta-analysis including 34 studies showing HR 0.85 (95% CI 0.79–0.93) and HR 0.68 (95% CI 0.59–0.78), respectively, compared to normal BMI [55]. This effect was also seen in the metastatic RCC population for overall survival [56].

Proposed mechanisms for the development of RCC include insulin resistance, sex hormone dysregulation, inflammatory responses, and oxidative stress [30, 57]. In particular, insulin resistance may cause abnormalities in the insulin-like growth factor pathway involving IGF-1 and IGF-2, whose receptors have been shown to be overexpressed in RCC [58, 59]. Therefore, overexpression of this pathway may spur potential tumor growth via cell cycle dysregulation [60]. This, in combination with the oxidative stress pathway, creates a tumor-promoting microenvironment that may explain the risk of RCC development.

Given this relationship between RCC and obesity, it is also important to consider that obesity is a modifiable risk factor. In particular, various studies have shown that the addition of medications that treat metabolic syndrome, such as metformin or statins, can reduce the risk of RCC up to 30% [61, 62].

Hypertension

According to the Centers for Disease Control and Prevention, about 48% of American adults had high blood pressure from 2021 to 2023. This translates into 1 in 2 adults having a chronic condition that increases risk for several diseases, such as heart disease, renal failure, and stroke [63]. While chronic hypertension is a leading cause for the development of chronic kidney disease, several studies have shown that hypertension is an independent risk factor for developing RCC. In a meta-analysis of 13 case–control studies from 1966 to 2000, hypertensive patients were found to have a pooled odds ratio of 1.75 for having RCC [64]. A more recent meta-analysis of 18 studies, including 10 with longitudinal follow-up confirmed that hypertension is a severely harmful risk factor [65]. Independent dose-dependent and time-dependent effects of hypertension were further elucidated in a 2017 meta-analysis that showed every increase of 10 mm Hg in systolic and diastolic blood pressure was associated with a 10% and 22% increased risk of RCC, respectively [66]. Further, a Swedish cohort study found an association with decreased RCC risk after a reduction in blood pressure, suggesting that effective hypertension control may lower risk [50]. Like the association with obesity and RCC, the findings relating blood pressure to increased cancer risk also present an opportunity to enact preventative measures.

Chronic Renal Disease

Patients with end-stage renal disease (ESRD) who undergo renal transplantation after long-term hemodialysis or with acquired cystic disease have all been shown to have an increased risk for multiple forms of malignancy, ranging from immune deficiency-related malignancy to urinary tract tumors [67, 68] . Post-transplant kidney cancer is particularly seen in native kidneys of transplanted patients with acquired cystic kidney disease (ACKD). ACKD is present in 40% of graft recipients at the time of transplant and appears in another 16% of patients after transplant [69]. This inflammatory environment from epithelial cell hypertrophy, chronic ischemia, and uremia is thought to be oncogenic, especially when combined with immunosuppression in the post-transplant population [70]. A retrospective study looking at the outcomes of RCC in native kidneys of transplant patients determined that the median interval between transplantation and RCC occurrence was 5.6 years and that ACKD was present in 83% of these transplanted patients [71]. The 2022 European Association of Urology guidelines reinforce the risk of RCC in patients with ESRD, stating that the risk is at least ten times higher than in the general population [72]. There is mixed data, however, on the histologic predominance of RCC in patients with ESRD, with some studies showing notably less aggressive tumors, while other studies show a similar profile as the non-ESRD population [73–76]. However, these data are generally retrospective analyses of small samples, thus further investigation must be done.

In addition, there is also evidence for increased risk for RCC even among patients with milder renal dysfunction. In a large-scale retrospective study of over 1,000,000 patients, Lowrance et al. examined the relationship between estimated glomerular filtration rate (eGFR) and risk of incident RCC, finding risk even for mild CKD. They reported HR 1.39 (95% CI = 1.22–1.58) for eGFR 45–59, HR 1.81 (95% CI = 1.51–2.17) for eGFR 30–44, and HR 2.28 (95% CI = 1.78–2.92) for eGFR <30 [77] .

Family History

While there are several inheritable conditions that portend an increased risk of RCC that will be discussed, the vast majority of RCC occurs sporadically. The question of whether there is an association between family history and sporadic RCC was explored by a study at the University of Texas MD Anderson Cancer Center. Using several analytic strategies, the authors were able to establish a significant association between a family history of kidney cancer and sporadic RCC. Furthermore, a higher risk of developing RCC was found in patients who had an affected sibling rather than a parent or child with an RR of 3.52 (95% CI = 1.70–3.04) found on meta-analysis [78]. Another study in Sweden looked at over 9000 patients with similar findings, showing an OR of 1.9 (95% CI = 1.65–2.16) for developing RCC with one affected first-degree relative and an OR of 6 (95% CI = 2.37–15.5) for two or more affected first-degree relatives [79]. These findings stress that while dominant familial RCC syndromes such as VHL, hereditary papillary renal cancer, and Birt-Hogg-Dubé disease exist, there is a role for recessive effects in the inheritance of sporadic RCC.

Medications

Researchers have studied a variety of antihypertensive medications, including diuretics, calcium channel blockers, and beta-blockers, to explore an association with RCC independent of hypertension. Results have remained inconsistent, with some showing doubled risk for RCC with long-term diuretic use, while others have presented data that was not statistically significant [80]. A 2017 study published by Colt et al. found that while there was no relationship between any antihypertensive drug class and overall RCC, there was some significant data regarding specific histologic subtypes. The authors found that long-term use of diuretics (OR = 3.1, 95% CI = 1.4–6.7) and having ever used calcium channel blockers (OR = 2.8, 95% CI = 1.1–7.4) were associated with papillary RCC, but associations with clear cell RCC were weak or not significant [81]. Possible mechanisms for the carcinogenic effects of antihypertensive medications include conversion of diuretics to nitroso derivatives in the stomach, chemical effects on renal tubular epithelium over long periods of time, and calcium channel blockers inhibiting apoptosis to facilitate division of malignant cells [82, 83] .

Similar to studies on antihypertensive medications, individual studies examining analgesic's association with RCC have largely been inconsistent. Among the most commonly used analgesics, acetaminophen has been implicated in RCC risk. A large case–control analysis of the US Kidney Cancer Study showed a positive trend for developing RCC with increasing duration of over-the-counter use of acetaminophen, with a twofold risk observed for those who took acetaminophen ≥10 years [84]. However, the effect size was diluted to an odds ratio of 1.5 when prescription use of acetaminophen was included. A meta-analysis of four cohort and nine case–control studies supported this finding with a summarized odds ratio of 1.25 (95% CI = 1.1–1.4) [85]. A potential biological explanation for acetaminophen's effects is the depletion of glutathione at higher doses and the subsequent rise in N-acetyl-p-benzoquinone imine (NAPQI). NAPQI is able to disrupt homeostasis in both kidney and liver cells by binding covalently to DNA [85].

Nonsteroidal anti-inflammatory drugs (NSAIDs) have also been examined for potentially increasing RCC risk. A large prospective study showed an increased risk of RCC with long-term NSAID use, with an RR of 2.92 (95% CI = 1.71–5.01) for >10 years of NSAID use [86]. Similarly, a large meta-analysis identifying 20 studies found increased risk of RCC with non-aspirin NSAID use (RR = 1.25, 95% CI = 1.06–1.46), but no relationship between aspirin use and RCC [87]. Other meta-analytic reviews have not shown a positive association between RCC and NSAID use, including the US Kidney Cancer Study, which looked at NSAID use and aspirin use in heart regimens and the CONFIRM case–control study [85, 88]. Theories for NSAID-mediated RCC carcinogenesis reference the inhibition of prostaglandin synthesis, leading to chronic subacute renal injuries; these in turn could cause DNA damage and uncontrolled cell proliferation.

Environmental Exposure

Exposure to agents classically considered carcinogenic, including cadmium, uranium, arsenic, nitrate, and radon, has not been established as a risk factor for RCC but is being explored [1]. The most extensively examined substance is trichloroethylene (TCE), a degreaser used for metal cleaning that is also present in adhesives, paint removers, typewriter correction fluids, and spot removers. The US Environmental Protection Agency 2001 draft TCE health risk assessment concluded that epidemiologic studies do show an increased risk of kidney cancer in association with TCE [89]. TCE is considered a Group 2A "probably" human carcinogen by the International Agency for Research on Cancer (IARC). A retrospective analysis of 292 patients exposed to TCE via groundwater showed an elevated risk of developing RCC with OR 1.78 (95% CI = 1.05–3.03) [90].

Aristolochic acid (AA) has also been associated with RCC development and is found in some herbal products that include *Aristolochia* plants. A large population-based case-control study found that ingestion of a cumulative 250 mg of AA increased the risk of RCC by 25% (OR 1.25, 95% CI 1.00–1.55). In addition, authors were able to find mutational signatures associated with AA consumption during whole-exome sequencing [91]. In a real-world example, the rates of various urologic malignancies, including RCC, appeared to decrease after a 2000 ban of AA-containing herbal products in Taiwan [92].

With the growing awareness of microplastics and their effects on long-term health, these exposures have also become targets for cancer and renal dysfunction research. A recent study in rat models showed that microplastics and nanoplastics cause nephrotoxic changes including oxidative stress, inflammation, and loss of cellular architecture [93]. Further research must be done to assess association with the development of RCC.

Screening for RCC

Although 30% of patients present with metastatic disease, the remainder are diagnosed with localized RCC and may be candidates for definitive treatment [94]. Screening programs for earlier detection and treatment have the potential to improve survival outcomes if the ideal screening regimen is identified. The Wilson and Jungner criteria for suitable screening include the following: the condition should be a significant health problem, there should be a recognizable latent or early symptomatic stage, and there should be an accepted treatment for patients with recognized disease [95]. In regard to RCC, well-established treatments with minimal risk are available for localized tumors. In addition, there is likely an ample preclinical window—estimated at about 3.7–5.8 years—where patients are developing RCC without clinical manifestations when a screening program may be able to detect tumors [96]. There is currently no recommendation for screening for RCC, but several techniques and regimens have been explored.

Cost-effective techniques that have been explored for the early detection of RCC include urine dipsticks and biomarkers. Identifying hematuria on dipsticks has not been reliable for RCC due to a stronger association with bladder cancer, low diagnostic yield, as well as poor sensitivity and specificity. When comparing incidence of all hematuria in patients with RCC to hematuria in patients with urothelial carcinoma, the rates are 35% versus 94%, respectively [97]. A Korean study that performed 56,632 dipsticks as part of a checkup on individuals over the age of 20 found hematuria in 3517 patients, but only three cases of RCC were detected among these patients [98]. This is most likely because microscopic hematuria is a common finding and less likely to indicate cancer than other causes, such as infection or kidney stones in a younger, low-risk population.

There is a growing investigation into urinary biomarkers to monitor for the development of RCC. These include multiple proteins such as Aquaporin-1 (AQP1) and Perilipin-2 (PLIN2), as well as others still in development. AQP1 is a transmembrane protein that is expressed throughout the human body, but its urinary secretion is restricted to disease states and localized to the proximal convoluted tubules—a site associated with clear cell and papillary RCC variants [99]. It has been demonstrated to be elevated in the urine samples of RCC patients [100]. Initial studies have been promising, reporting 100% sensitivity and specificity [99–101]. However, subsequent studies have shown conflicting information, with RCC patients having decreased AQP1 instead [102, 103]. Similar to AQP1, PLIN2 is a perilipin protein in adipocytes that is found to be overexpressed in clear cell RCC and has been shown to differentiate RCC versus control patients with 100% sensitivity and specificity [99–101]. A prospective cohort study was done by Morrissey et al. to evaluate the use of both AQP1 and PLIN2 for the diagnosis of RCC in patients who were undergoing screening with abdominal imaging. Among 19 patients with known RCC compared to 80 healthy patients, the combination of AQP1 and PLIN2 was significantly higher with area under receiver operating curve (AUROC) 0.990, 95% sensitivity, and 91% specificity [104]. It is important to note that these biomarkers are specific to clear cell and papillary histologic subtypes, implying that they would produce false-negative results in patients with variant histology [105]. Further prospective studies are required to investigate these potential biomarkers, as well as further scientific research into other novel biomarkers, such as CAIX, KIM-1, NMP-22, and RKIP [99].

Computed tomography (CT) scanning is currently used to screen for a wide variety of malignancies in middle-aged Americans. These screening practices include but are not limited to abdominal CTs for the detection of aortic aneurysms, CT colonography, CT angiography, and chest CTs for lung cancer. In an era where many patients are receiving CT imaging, researchers have attempted to detect solid abdominal organ malignancies simultaneously. One study screened 4543 healthy patients over 40 years old who had received an abdominal CT, but solid organ malignancy prevalence was only found to be 0.1%, and therefore, the method was deemed ineffective [106]. The US Preventive Services Task Force recognizes that despite the not infrequent detection of extracolonic incidental lesions on CT, only 3% require definitive treatment [107]. Recently, a UK-based group studied the addition of RCC screening to those patients receiving CT scans for lung cancer. Using a biobank cohort with over 400,000 patients, they found that lung cancer screening methods had an AUROC between 0.6 and 0.66. However, the authors note that more RCCs occur in never-smokers than lung cancer; thus, it would miss many tumors [108]. As a result of the overall low incidence of malignant renal masses detected on screening CT with increased costs and burdens to the patient and healthcare system, CT has not been found to be a cost-effective screening strategy for RCC.

Compared to CT, ultrasound has the benefit of using benign sound waves instead of ionizing radiation while also being less expensive. The kidneys are able to be completely visualized in 97.4% of cases, with a sensitivity of 82–83% and specificity of 98–99% in detecting RCC [96]. A cost-benefit analysis for sonographic screening shows that at $36 US dollars per ultrasound, the opportunity to prevent metastatic RCC is worth considering [109]. A recent decision analysis found that a single ultrasound screening event at 60 years old in men may be cost-effective for identifying RCC and maximizing quality-adjusted life years [110] . However, ultrasound is less accurate in detecting renal masses than CT, especially with less sensitivity in detecting lesions under 3 cm in size or in obese patients who are known to have higher rates of RCC [111, 112]. There is also a lack of randomized trials to support the use of ultrasound screening for RCC. Rossi et al. identified ten observational studies that were completed, nine of which were published before 2004 [105]. Of these trials, a 1999 Japanese study screened 219,640 patients (ages 29–70 years) over 13 years and detected 193 cases of RCC. These patients were followed to show a 97.4% cumulative survival rate after 5 years and 94.6% at 10 years [113].

Other screening considerations include the psychological impact on patients and over-diagnosis of small renal masses that may never become clinically significant. A false-positive screening result may result in a similar degree of patient harm as a false-negative result. Studies have shown that 15–30% of small renal masses are found to be benign after surgical excision, and those that are malignant are unlikely to progress and become metastatic [18, 21, 114]. As a result, clinicians must contemplate the psychological and emotional impact of delivering an incorrect diagnosis and the potential harm from more unnecessary testing or invasive procedures. Large-scale randomized controlled trials for screening would help determine the exact benefit of screening to help inform these conversations.

Genomic Risk Factors and Screening of Targeted Populations

With the establishment of known risk factors and understanding of inheritable conditions, high-risk populations do exist, and screening has been evaluated for these patients. In 2005, the European Association of Urology guidelines had recommended annual ultrasounds of native kidneys in patients who have received transplants due to their higher risk for developing RCC [115]. However, a more recent meta-analysis by the American Society of Transplantation found that ultrasound screening for RCC in transplant recipients was not cost-effective and recommended against the practice [116]. Examining other risk factors, Starke et al. identified 925 patients as high-risk individuals for bladder cancer based on age ≥ 50, smoking with ≥ 10 pack-year history, and occupational carcinogen exposure of ≥15 years. After following these patients for 6.5 years, ten of the patients were diagnosed with RCC, indicating a prevalence of RCC in these patients that is roughly ten times higher than the general population [117]. Since then, algorithms for early screening and management have been proposed for asymptomatic high-risk patients [109]. These targeted screening methods may be endorsed in the future, even if screening of the general population is not.

Incidence of von Hippel-Lindau disease is 1 in 36,000 live births, with a penetrance of over 90% by the age of 65, making it the most common hereditary renal cancer syndrome [118]. The von Hippel-Lindau gene, *VHL*, is a tumor suppressor gene on the short arm of chromosome 3 (3p25.3). The gene encodes a protein that is part of the VCB-CUL2 ubiquitin ligase complex, which is responsible for the degradation of hypoxia-inducible factor 1 (HIF-1) and insulin-like growth factor 1 (IGF-1). Loss of *VHL* activity leads to cell growth and angiogenesis due to downstream enhanced expression of factors such as VEGF, PDGFB, EPO, and TGF-α. CNS hemangioblastomas, clear cell renal carcinomas, pheochromocytomas, and pancreatic tumors have all been described as part of the phenotypical classifications of VHL. As patients with VHL have a 70% lifetime risk of developing RCC with a mean age of clinical diagnosis at age 40, screening with annual abdominal MRIs from the age of 16 is recommended [119]. MRI is preferred over CT to avoid the substantial cumulative radiation exposure that annual CT scans would incur. Pathologic examination of nephrectomy specimens from patients with VHL has revealed that nearly all complex cysts contain RCC [120]. Even normal-appearing parenchyma on CT may harbor large numbers of microscopic tumor foci, explaining the high risk of multiple and bilateral RCC in VHL [121]. Patients with VHL require complex decision-making analysis of tumors found during screening as they are likely to have extensive tumor burden requiring multiple surgeries over the course of their lives, making nephron-sparing surgery important; this will be discussed in a further section.

Other autosomal dominant disorders that increase a patient's risk for RCC include hereditary papillary renal carcinoma, Birt-Hogg-Dubé (BHD) syndrome, Cowden syndrome, tuberous sclerosis, *BAP1* tumor predisposition syndrome, and hereditary leiomyomatosis and renal cell carcinoma (HLRCC). These conditions generally require screening in the form of germline mutation testing rather than biomarkers. Patients with hereditary papillary renal carcinoma are caused by an activating mutation in the *MET* proto-oncogene that confers a 90% chance of developing RCC by age 80, but no extrarenal manifestations, with screening via annual MRI starting at age 30 [122, 123]. In BHD families or patients who present with cutaneous fibrofolliculomas, familial pneumothorax, or oncocytic RCC pathology, germline *FLCN* testing should begin at age 21, and patients should undergo biannual MRI screening beginning at age 20 [124]. Cowden syndrome is caused by a mutation in the *PTEN* tumor suppressor gene that leads to the development of hamartomas and malignancies throughout the body, as well as clear cell and papillary RCC with a lifetime risk of about 34% requiring biannual ultrasound beginning at age 40 [125, 126]. Tuberous sclerosis is characterized by the development of hamarrtomas, seizures, and developmental delay, and is associated with a loss of function mutation in *TSC1* or *TSC2* gene. Although many of the tumors that develop are angiomyolipomas, patients with tuberous sclerosis may develop malignant RCCs at a young age—mean age as young as 30 to 42 years old—and should begin in childhood with MRI every 1–3 years [127, 128]. *BAP1* tumor predisposition syndrome stems from a mutation in the *BAP1* tumor suppressor gene that leads to the development of high-grade, aggressive RCC. Given these aggressive and often advanced presentations, patients are recommended to have yearly MRIs [124, 128]. HLRCC, now also known as fumarate hydrogenase tumor predisposition syndrome, involves a germline mutation of *fumarate hydratase* (*FH*), which is a gene that encodes an enzyme in the TCA cycle. HLRCC-associated kidney cancer has the potential to be lethal, and therefore, testing in suspected patients begins as early as 8 years old. Patients who are affected with HLRCC should subsequently have annual abdominal MRIs to screen for kidney tumors [129].

The American Urological Association states that genetic counseling should be strongly recommended for patients suspected of having familial RCC [130]. Although not specifically a strategy for screening for RCC, screening for genetic syndromes or genomic alterations associated with RCC can help with eventual diagnosis and avoidance of later disease progression. A recent consensus statement suggested that patients who develop bilateral or multifocal RCC or specific rare histologies like papillary type 1 RCC should undergo screening, or any patient with significant family history [131]. Urologists and primary care physicians alike should also be aware that many genetic syndromes that confer risk for RCC may initially present with extrarenal symptoms.

Clinical Staging

Clinical staging systems are developed to classify malignant diseases in a uniform manner with prognostic capability. They are used to guide treatment and planning decisions and manage expected outcomes by stratifying the risk of cancer progression. Ultimately, uniform staging systems allow for the comparison of patient outcomes worldwide [132]. Flocks and Kadesky proposed one of the earliest kidney cancer staging systems in 1958, including organ-confined, locally invasive, locally metastatic, and distant metastatic disease [133]. The predominant TNM staging system used currently (tumor, nodes, metastases) was developed in 1974 by the American Joint Committee on Cancer (AJCC) and the *Union Internationale Contre le Cancer*, renamed the Union for International Cancer Control (UICC) [134]. This TNM staging system has had several major revisions to improve prognostic accuracy, with the most recent update, Version 9, published in 2024 after a structured review process with input from several professional groups (Tables 1.2 and 1.3) [135].

In 1987, T1 and T2 renal lesions were divided at 2.5 cm in largest dimension by imaging, which did not differentiate well between survivals for these groups [136]. In 1997, T2 disease started at 7 cm for greater differentiation from T1 [137]. The 2002 AJCC update further subdivided T1 disease, T1a ≤4 cm and T1b 4–7 cm [138]. Work done by the Cleveland Clinic contributed to this development [139]. They described 485 patients who underwent partial nephrectomy prior to 1997, finding that 5-year cancer-specific survival was better with tumor diameter ≤ 4 cm compared to 4–7 cm and > 7 cm (Fig. 1.1). This was confirmed in a multi-institutional study of more than 2200 patients, showing a difference in disease-free survival (DFS) at 5 and 10 years between T1a (95.3% and 91.4%), T1b (91.4% and 83.4%), and T2 (81.6% and 75.2%) tumors [140]. This outcome difference has been further substantiated irrespective of the form of surgery performed. Oncologic outcomes among tumors with a diameter greater than 4 cm were worse than tumors less than 4 cm, regardless if radical or partial nephrectomy was performed [141].

Several groups have attempted to further reclassify T1 and T2 disease. Investigators at the Mayo Clinic proposed a cutoff of 5 cm for better postoperative DFS prediction [142]. In a similar study, a group at UCLA suggested that disease-specific patient survival was more accurate if T2 started at 4.5 cm [143]. Ficarra and colleagues reported that a cut point of 5.5 cm improved cancer-related outcome stratification [144]. These same groups examined T2 patients with tumors >7 cm to gain better prognostic ability. This was supported by work from an international collaboration finding that for T2 disease, tumors larger than 11 cm have worse DFS [145]. Frank and colleagues studied an additional 544 T2 patients and proposed a 10-cm cutoff point to sub-classify patients [146]. This was eventually codified in the seventh edition TNM staging update with subdivision of the T2 category into 7–10 cm and > 10 cm (Fig. 1.2) [147]. Most recently, the EAU guidelines panel has proposed distinguishing T1a and T1b disease as greater or less than 3 cm rather than 4 cm [148]. This is based on extensive active surveillance data suggesting that long-term cancer-specific mortality changes drastically above this size [149]. The collective evidence from the multitude of these retrospective studies indicates that primary tumor size plays an important role in predicting survival.

Table 1.2 AJCC TNM classification for RCC

Classification	Definition
Tumor (T)	
TX	Primary tumor cannot be assessed
T0	No evidence of primary tumor
T1	Tumor ≤7 cm in greatest dimension, limited to the kidney
T1a	Tumor ≤4 cm in greatest dimension, limited to the kidney
T1b	Tumor >4 cm but ≤7 cm in greatest dimension, limited to the kidney
T2	Tumor >7 cm in greatest dimension, limited to the kidney
T2a	Tumor >7 cm but ≤10 cm in greatest dimension, limited to the kidney
T2b	Tumor >10 cm, limited to the kidney
T3	Tumor extends into major veins or perinephric tissues, but not into the ipsilateral adrenal gland and not beyond Gerota's fascia
T3a	Tumor extends into the renal vein or its segmental branches, or invades the pelvicalyceal system, or invades perirenal and/or renal sinus fat but not beyond Gerota's fascia
T3b	Tumor extends into the vena cava below the diaphragm
T3c	Tumor extends into the vena cava above the diaphragm or invades the wall of the vena cava
T4	Tumor invades beyond Gerota's fascia (including contiguous extension into the ipsilateral adrenal gland)
Node (N)	
NX	Regional lymph nodes cannot be assessed
N0	No regional lymph node metastasis
N1	Metastasis in regional lymph node(s)
Metastasis (M)	
M0	No distant metastasis
M1	Distant metastasis

Table 1.3 Stages of RCC

Stage	TNM classifications
Stage I	T1, N0, M0
Stage II	T2, N0, M0
Stage III	T1 or T2, N1, M0 T3, N0 or N1, M0
Stage IV	T4, any N, M0 Any T, any N, M1

The T3 category was changed significantly in the 2009 seventh edition TNM staging update. T3 had previously included invasion of perinephric fat, adrenal gland, renal vein, or different levels of the IVC [138]. Direct adrenal gland invasion is now classified as T4 and will be discussed subsequently. Invasion of perinephric fat has been shown to have a minimal impact on prognosis. Murphy and colleagues reported on their series of 717 patients at Columbia University Medical Center and found that the absolute size of T2 tumors was more predictive of DFS than the presence of renal capsular invasion, implying that some T3 tumors may not fare as poorly as larger T2 tumors [150]. Similarly, Lam et al. describe dividing patients with fat invasion only (2002 TNM T3a disease) into greater than 7 cm or ≤ 7 cm and found that smaller tumors behaved more like T2 tumors and that larger tumors were similar to those with renal vein involvement (2002 TNM T3b) [151]. Seimer et al. reviewed nearly 1800 cases and found that perinephric fat invasion did not play an independent prognostic role, though tumor size did [152]. This may be because studies have shown that likelihood of extrarenal invasion, including into perinephric fat, varied directly according to tumor size [153].

Other studies have found that the location or type of fat invasion does play a prognostic role. Renal sinus fat invasion has been shown to have worse 5-year cancer-specific survival compared to perinephric fat invasion (71% vs. 45%) [154, 155]. The Mayo Clinic group also describes a group of patients with 2002 TNM classification T3 or T4 disease that were reclassified based on the presence of perinephric fat invasion and level of tumor thrombus. Patients with perinephric fat

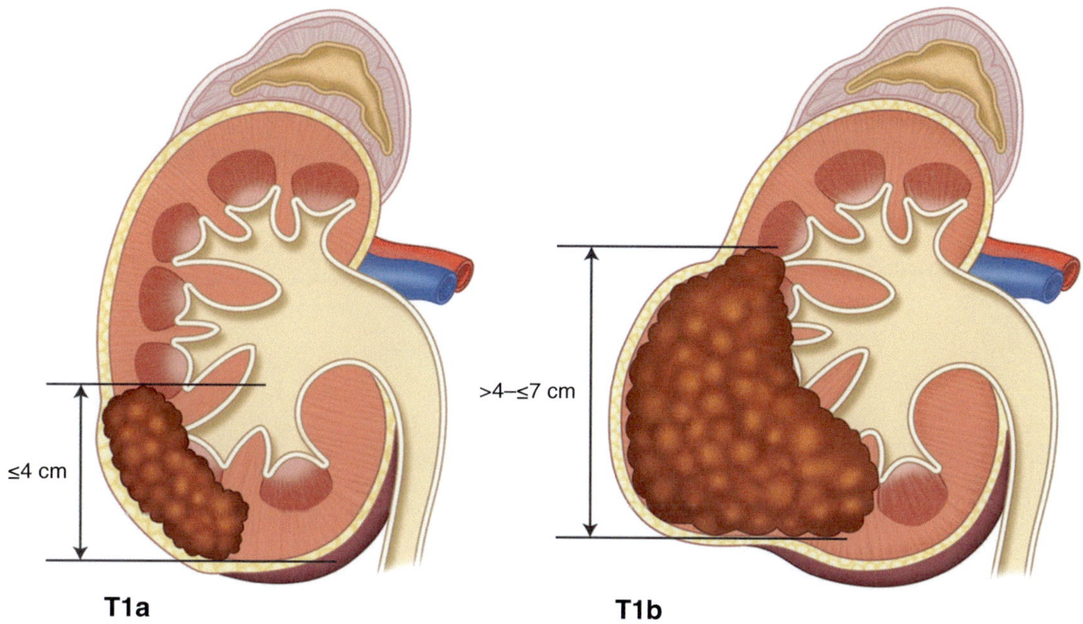

Fig. 1.1 Stage T1a—limited to kidney and ≤ 4 cm; T1b tumors (4–7 cm)

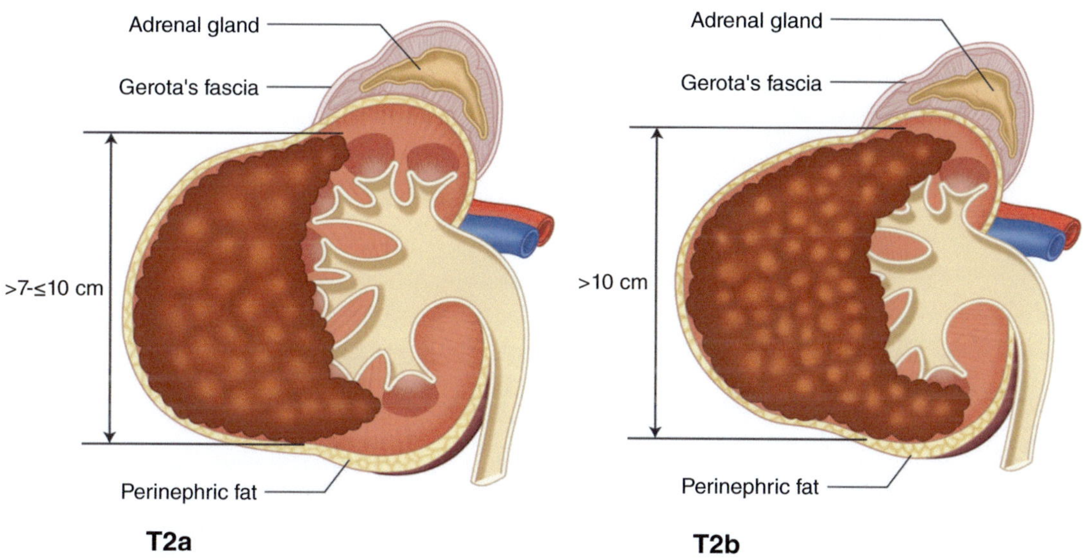

Fig. 1.2 Stage T2a—limited to kidney and 7–10 cm; T2b tumors (>10 cm)

invasion alone were more likely to die of disease than patients with renal vein thrombus alone [156]. In a slightly less complex system, the group from MD Anderson reported on a cohort of patients with pT3N0/NxM0 disease and found that the presence but not the extent of venous thrombus correlated with survival. Unlike the Mayo Clinic findings, they reported that patients with extra-renal extension into fat, regardless of location, had similar DFS as those with any amount of venous thrombus alone. Subjects with both were at greater risk of death from RCC [157]. This was confirmed by da Costa and colleagues in Brazil, which also found equivalent

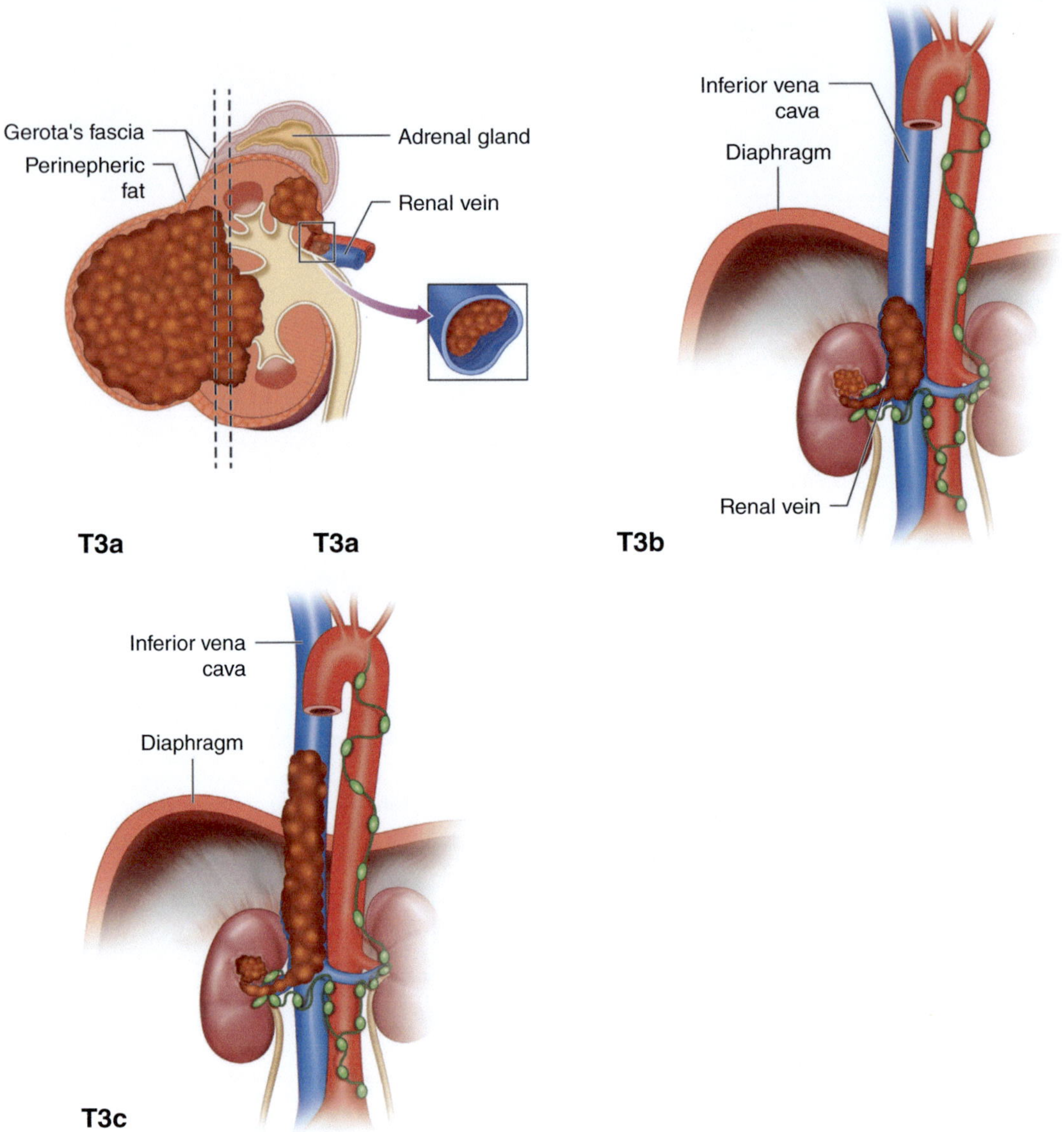

Fig. 1.3 Stage T3a—tumor thrombus extends into renal vein or invades perirenal and/or renal sinus fat. Stage T3b—extends into IVC below the diaphragm. Stage T3c—extends into IVC above the diaphragm or invades wall of IVC

disease-specific survival for fat invasion or renal vein thrombus alone [158]. A recent study also supports this, showing no difference between perinephric fat, renal sinus, and renal invasion, but that having multiple types of invasion conferred a worse prognosis [159].

As of this time, the most recent Version 9 does not provide updates to the staging of RCC. In the eighth edition TNM staging update published in 2017, changes in kidney cancer staging were minimal and focused on clarifying T3a disease classification (Fig. 1.3). In the seventh edition, the term "grossly" was used to describe renal vein and segmental branch invasion. Because it is common to have tumor involvement that is missed within the vasculature, this term was removed from the new edition. A 2007 study examined the venous systems of 54 pT3b clear cell tumors and compared them with ten normal renal kidneys. The investigators found that intravenous tumor extension is the first step in extrarenal spread, with renal sinus fat invasion usually occurring secondarily, and that tumor within the sinus fat usually represents venous involvement when confirmed histologically [160]. Therefore, it is evident that grossly examining a tumor for venous invasion would not be a reliable method of staging. Furthermore, the update has clarified invasion of the pelvicalyceal system as T3a because this part of the collecting system is contained within the hilum [161].

Renal Vein and IVC Involvement

The extent of tumor thrombus in the inferior vena cava (IVC) has long been used in the TNM system and occurs in 5–10% of patients with RCC [162]. It is well established that IVC tumor thrombus (T3b–c) carries a worse prognosis than renal vein thrombus (T3a). Moinzadeh and Libertino compared long-term outcomes of patients with renal vein involvement versus thrombus extending only as far as the subhepatic IVC and found a significant difference in 10-year cancer-specific survival rate (66% vs. 29%, $p = 0.0001$) [163]. A multi-institutional European cohort of 1192 patients clearly demonstrated that disease-free survival is significantly different between renal vein invasion versus IVC invasion. Dividing the cohort into T3a, T3b, and T3c, median survival times were 52.0, 25.8, and 18 months, respectively. The survival difference between T3a and T3b/T3c was significant ($p < 0.001$), whereas the difference between infradiaphragmatic and supradiaphragmatic IVC thrombus did not reach significance ($p = 0.613$ (120)) [164]. The role of renal vascular invasion is important to distinguish from microscopic vascular invasion, which varies widely in both its proportion reported in pathologic specimens as well as its prognostic significance [153].

There has been a long-standing controversy with regard to the prognostic value of the extent of tumor thrombus in the IVC. Examining the SEER database from 2000 to 2007, Whitson et al. demonstrated that tumor thrombus extension above the diaphragm did not correlate with survival [162]. Similarly, neither renal vein nor IVC extension was found to be an independent predictor of worse prognosis when considering other factors such as tumor size, histology, and nodal status in a cohort of 1082 patients from Memorial Sloan Kettering Cancer Center [165]. A large population-based analysis of the SEER database showed that tumor size, adverse histology, positive lymph nodes, and/or metastasis held more prognostic value than the extent of IVC thrombus extension [162]. Similarly, one of the most recent studies in this space was a large multinational study of 228 that showed no effect on recurrence-free or overall survival based on the extent of IVC involvement [166]. In contrast to the aforementioned studies, several studies have shown survival differences dependent on the degree of IVC tumor thrombus extension. In a series of 222 nephrectomy and tumor thrombectomy patients, Kim et al. reported that patients with a thrombus in the renal vein or infradiaphragmatic IVC fared better than those with supradiaphragmatic IVC thrombi (3-year disease = specific survival of 35% vs. 12%) [167]. A German group also confirmed this in their series of 111 patients with a median survival of 25.1 months versus 13.2 months ($p = 0.032$) [168]. A recent large multinational study of 636 nonmetastatic RCC patients with tumor thrombus found thrombus level above the hepatic veins to be an independent predictor of recurrence in a nomogram model including six patient and tumor characteristics [169]. As many studies demonstrate survival differences between infra- and supradiaphragmatic IVC extension, this criterion continues to play a role in stratification of risk in the current TNM system despite conflicting data.

T4

Previous versions of the TNM system treated ipsilateral adrenal gland involvement similarly to other T3a features. However, direct adrenal gland invasion is rare, occurring only in about 2.5% of cases [170]. When compared to perinephric or renal sinus fat invasion, direct adrenal gland invasion has a worse 5-year cancer-specific survival

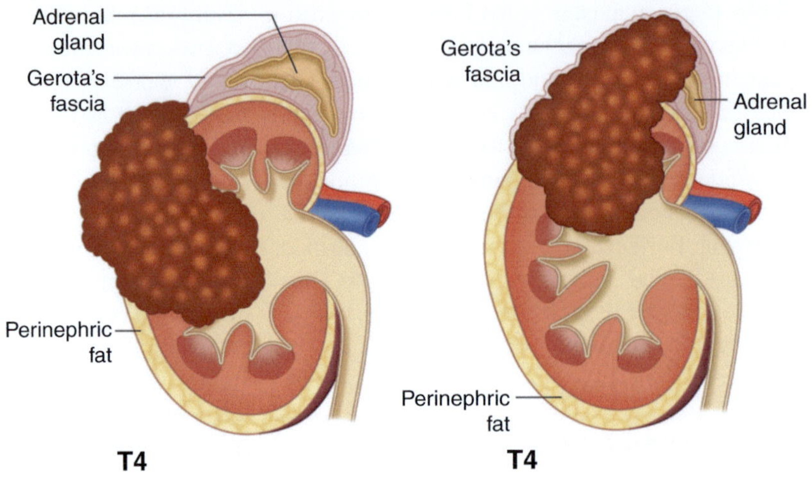

Fig. 1.4 Stage T4 tumor extends beyond Gerota's fascia or contiguously into the ipsilateral adrenal gland. (Used with the permission of the American Joint Committee on Cancer (AJCC), Chicago, Illinois. The original source for this material is the AJCC Cancer Staging Manual, Seventh Edition (2010), published by Springer-Verlag New York, www.springer.com)

(36% vs. 0%) [170]. Siemer et al. analyzed the prognostic significance of direct adrenal gland invasion, controlling for tumor size, and found worse cancer-specific survival in this group, leading them to propose reclassifying direct adrenal gland invasion as T4 (Fig. 1.4) [152]. Similarly, Thompson et al. found that T3a or T3b tumor with direct adrenal extension had similar 5-year cancer-specific survival to patients with extension beyond Gerota's fascia at 20% and 14%, respectively. These patients were significantly more likely to die from RCC (HR 2.11, $p = 0.004$) [171] .

Nodal Status

Prior versions of the TNM system included both size and number of lymph nodes involved to stratify lymph node disease in patients with renal cell carcinoma. The seventh and eighth editions simplify nodal involvement into a binary system, disease absence, or presence in any regional lymph nodes. Terrone et al. from Torino, Italy, reviewed 618 cases that had regional lymphadenectomy at the time of nephrectomy and found a node-positive rate of 14%. Patients were stratified by the 2002 TNM node criteria (number of nodes involved), and no difference was found between 1 positive node and more than 1 positive node [172]. In a similar study, 2000 patients with RCC were reviewed, and survival for the 69 with nodal involvement was similar regardless of the number of lymph nodes involved [173]. These authors also suggest that poorer survival was associated with extranodal extension of disease. The prognosis for patients with lymph node involvement may be similar to those with metastatic disease, though their effect may be additive, as having both nodal and distant metastases confers worse survival [174] .

In nodal staging, it is important to also consider the relationship between clinical staging based on radiographic evidence and pathologic staging, especially since templated lymphadenectomy is not recommended as standard during surgery. There is a high rate of false-positive lymphadenopathies, with a recent study finding that only 28.8% of clinically positive nodes ended up being pathologically positive [175]. Establishing the nodal status of patients is important for management, given previously discussed studies. A recent study from MD Anderson Cancer Center even suggests that those patients with nodal disease have a high likelihood of micrometastatic disease, given similar outcomes between node-positive and metastatic patients [176].

Metastatic Disease

Patients with metastatic disease have uniformly worse survival than localized RCC [177]. Memorial Sloan Kettering developed a widely used risk stratification criteria for metastatic

RCC patients (the Motzer criteria), with each of the following parameters receiving 1 point: Karnofsky performance status (<80%), high lactate dehydrogenase (>1.5 times upper limit of normal), low serum Hb, high corrected serum calcium (>10 mg/dL), and time from diagnosis to systemic treatment <1 year. Favorable-risk patients have no risk factors, intermediate-risk one or two risk factors, and poor-risk three or more risk factors. Median survival for favorable-, intermediate-, and poor-risk groups is 20, 10, and 4 months, respectively [178]. As the management of metastatic RCC has been rapidly evolving with improved targeted therapies and now immunotherapy, the median survival of patients with metastatic RCC is improving across all risk groups.

With the advancement in therapies for metastatic RCC, there have been multiple randomized controlled trials examining the present role of surgery for these patients. Both CARMENA and SURTIME studies showed that systemic therapy followed by surgery was noninferior and perhaps superior to upfront cytoreductive nephrectomy [179–181]. However, upfront cytoreductive nephrectomy still has a place in many patients' management and is included in recent EAU guidelines [72]. This has led to a recent proposal for the M1 stage to be subdivided, with the creation of M1a being those with a single metastasis in a single organ who may still be amenable to cytoreductive nephrectomy. The authors propose M1b as more than one metastasis in a single organ and M1c as multiple organs with metastases, with the latter being an indication for medical treatment alone, while the former may warrant multidisciplinary discussion [148].

Improving the TNM Staging System

Staging systems like the TNM system should be continuously reviewed and updated as necessary. Though the AJCC seventh and eighth editions improve upon the 2002 edition and version 9 will be coming soon, there may already be areas for improvement. In a large collaboration from Italy, authors found continued support for using primary tumor size to stratify 5339 renal tumors. Some groups, such as T2b and T3a or T3c and T4, had similar disease-specific outcomes. Analyzing only the 4848 N0/NxM0 patients, there were no differences in survival between T1a and T1b, T2b and T3a, and T3c and T4 [177]. Furthermore, a group of investigators from Korea compared the prognostic ability of the sixth and seventh TNM editions in 1691 patients. They found a similar concordance index in both schemas (0.906 and 0.904 for version 6 and 7, respectively). A concordance index this high suggests that both do an excellent job separating patients with different outcomes, though the seventh edition of the AJCC TNM system does not offer improvement over the sixth edition [182].

In an effort to further enhance staging, several academic centers also advocate for adding more patient-related features to the TNM system. Using symptoms at presentation of none, local, or systemic symptoms, Patard et al. found that symptom grading correlated with the TNM stage and that when included in a model with TNM, age, ECOG performance status, and other features, symptom grade was independently related to cancer-specific survival [183]. An integrated system was also proposed at UCLA. This system includes TNM, grade, and ECOG performance status and was superior to the 1997 TNM system alone and has been externally validated [184]. The stage, size, grade, and necrosis model have also been suggested and may offer improved prognostic ability of the UCLA model [185]. Though it may be augmented, the TNM staging system remains the basis for most prognostic systems. It will continue to undergo periodic updates and refinements, so that it can best serve the needs of patients and physicians.

References

1. Chow W, Dong L, Devesa S. Epidemiology and risk factors for kidney cancer. Nat Rev Urol. 2010;7:245–57.
2. Shuch B, Amin A, Armstrong AJ. Understanding pathologic variants of renal cell carcinoma: distilling therapeutic opportunities from biologic complexity. Eur Urol. 2015;67:85–97.

3. Bray F, Laversanne M, Sung H, et al. Global cancer statistics 2022: GLOBOCAN estimates of incidence and mortality worldwide for 36 cancers in 185 countries. CA: A Cancer J Clin. 2024;74:229–63. https://doi.org/10.3322/caac.21834.
4. Wong M, Goggins W, Yip B, et al. Incidence and mortality of kidney cancer: temporal patterns and global trends in 39 countries. Sci Rep. 2017;7:15698.
5. Siegel RL, Giaquinto AN, Jemal A. Cancer statistics, 2024. CA: A Cancer J Clin. 2024;74:12–49. https://doi.org/10.3322/caac.21820.
6. Anon. SEER Cancer Stat Facts: Kidney and Renal Pelvis Cancer. Bethesda, MD: National Cancer Institute; 2024.
7. Saad AM, Gad MM, Al-Husseini MJ, et al. Trends in renal-cell carcinoma incidence and mortality in the United States in the last 2 decades: a SEER-based study. Clin Genitourin Cancer. 2019;17:46–57.e5. https://doi.org/10.1016/j.clgc.2018.10.002.
8. Patel HD, Gupta M, Joice GA, et al. Clinical stage migration and survival for renal cell carcinoma in the United States. Eur Urol Oncol. 2019;2:343–8. https://doi.org/10.1016/j.euo.2018.08.023.
9. Sung W-W, Ko P-Y, Chen W-J, et al. Trends in the kidney cancer mortality-to-incidence ratios according to health care expenditures of 56 countries. Sci Rep. 2021;11:1479. https://doi.org/10.1038/s41598-020-79367-y.
10. Motzer RJ, Hutson TE, Piotr T, et al. Sunitinib versus Interferon Alfa in Metastatic Renal-Cell Carcinoma. N Engl J Med. 2007;356:115–24. https://doi.org/10.1056/nejmoa065044.
11. Patel A, Prasad S, Shih Y, Eggener S. The association of the human development index with global kidney cancer incidence and mortality. J Urol. 2012;187:1978–83.
12. Sánchez-Martín F, Millán-Rodríguez F, Urdaneta-Pignalosa G, et al. Small renal masses: incidental diagnosis, clinical symptoms, and prognostic factors. Adv Urol. 2008;2008:1–6.
13. Turner RM, Morgan TM, Jacobs BL. Epidemiology of the small renal mass and the treatment disconnect phenomenon. Urol Clin North Am. 2017;44:147–54. https://doi.org/10.1016/j.ucl.2016.12.001.
14. Hollingsworth JM, Miller DC, Daignault S, Hollenbeck BK. Rising incidence of small renal masses: a need to reassess treatment effect. J Natl Cancer Inst. 2006;98:1331–4. https://doi.org/10.1093/jnci/djj362.
15. Vasudev NS, Wilson M, Stewart GD, et al. Challenges of early renal cancer detection: symptom patterns and incidental diagnosis rate in a multicentre prospective UK cohort of patients presenting with suspected renal cancer. BMJ Open. 2020;10:e035938. https://doi.org/10.1136/bmjopen-2019-035938.
16. Welch H, Skinner J, Schroeck F, et al. Regional variation of computed tomographic imaging in the United States and the risk of nephrectomy. JAMA Intern Med. 2018;178:178.
17. Bhindi B, Thompson RH, Lohse CM, et al. The probability of aggressive versus indolent histology based on renal tumor size: implications for surveillance and treatment. Eur Urol. 2018;74:489–97. https://doi.org/10.1016/j.eururo.2018.06.003.
18. Pierorazio PM, Patel HD, Johnson MH, et al. Distinguishing malignant and benign renal masses with composite models and nomograms: a systematic review and meta-analysis of clinically localized renal masses suspicious for malignancy. Cancer. 2016;122:3267–76. https://doi.org/10.1002/cncr.30268.
19. Thompson RH, Hill J, Babayev Y. Risk of metastatic renal cell carcinoma according to tumor size. J Urol. 2009;182:41–5.
20. Ristau BT, Kutikov A, Uzzo RG, Mladone MC. Active surveillance for small renal masses: when less is more. Eur Urol Focus. 2016;2:660–8.
21. Smaldone MC, Kutikov A, Egleston BL, et al. Small renal masses progressing to metastases under active surveillance. Cancer. 2012;118:997–1006. https://doi.org/10.1002/cncr.26369.
22. Pierorazio PM, Hyams ES, Mullins JK, Allaf ME. Active surveillance for small renal masses. Rev Urol. 2012;14:13–9.
23. Morris CR, Lara PN, Parikh-Patel A, Kizer KW. Kidney cancer incidence in California: end of the trend? Kidney Cancer. 2017;1:71–81.
24. Scelo G, Larose TL. Epidemiology and risk factors for kidney cancer. J Clin Oncol. 2018;36:3574–81. https://doi.org/10.1200/jco.2018.79.1905.
25. Scelo G, Li P, Chanudet E, Muller DC. Variability of sex disparities in cancer incidence over 30 years: the striking case of kidney cancer. Eur Urol Focus. 2018;4:586–90. https://doi.org/10.1016/j.euf.2017.01.006.
26. Stafford H, Saltzstein S, Shimasaki S, et al. Racial/ethnic and gender disparities in renal cell carcinoma incidence and survival. J Urol. 2008;179:1704–8.
27. Znaor A, Lortet-Tieulent J, Laversanne M, et al. International variations and trends in renal cell carcinoma incidence and mortality. Eur Urol. 2015;67:519–30. https://doi.org/10.1016/j.eururo.2014.10.002.
28. Palumbo C, Pecoraro A, Rosiello G, et al. Renal cell carcinoma incidence rates and trends in young adults aged 20-39 years. Cancer Epidemiol. 2020;67:101762. https://doi.org/10.1016/j.canep.2020.101762.
29. Matrana M, Dreisin A. Kidney cancers in adolescents & young adults. Oncol Times. 2016;38:9–10.
30. Bukavina L, Bensalah K, Bray F, et al. Epidemiology of renal cell carcinoma: 2022 update. Eur Urol. 2022;82:529–42. https://doi.org/10.1016/j.eururo.2022.08.019.
31. Berndt S, Carter H, Schoenberg M, Newschaffer C. Disparities in treatment and outcome for renal cell cancer among older black and white patients. J Clin Oncol. 2007;25:3589–95.

32. Siagal CS, Deibert CM, Lai J, Schonlau M. Disparities in treatment of patients with IL-2 for metastatic renal cell carcinoma. Urol Oncol Semin Orig Invest. 2010;28:308–13.
33. Olshan A, Kuo T, Meyer A, et al. Racial difference in histologic subtype of renal cell carcinoma. Cancer Med. 2013;2:744–9.
34. Dason S, Allard C, Sheridan-Jonah A. Management of renal collecting duct carcinoma: a systematic review and the McMaster experience. Curr Oncol. 2013;20:223.
35. Shetty A, Matrana MR. Renal medullary carcinoma: a case report and brief review of the literature. Ochsner J. 2014;14:270–5.
36. Benjamin EJ, Blaha MJ, Chiuve SE, et al. Heart disease and stroke statistics—2017 update. Circulation. 2017;135:e146–603. https://doi.org/10.1161/cir.0000000000000485.
37. Liu X, Peveri G, Bosetti C, et al. Dose-response relationships between cigarette smoking and kidney cancer: a systematic review and meta-analysis. Crit Rev Oncol Hematol. 2019;142:86–93. https://doi.org/10.1016/j.critrevonc.2019.07.019.
38. Levi F, Ferlay J, Galeone C, et al. The changing pattern of kidney cancer incidence and mortality in Europe. BJU Int. 2008;101:949–58.
39. Cumberbatch MG, Rota M, Catto JWF, Vecchia CL. The role of tobacco smoke in bladder and kidney carcinogenesis: a comparison of exposures and meta-analysis of incidence and mortality risks. Eur Urol. 2016;70:458–66. https://doi.org/10.1016/j.eururo.2015.06.042.
40. Ehdaie B, Furberg H, Zabor EC, et al. Comprehensive assessment of the impact of cigarette smoking on survival of clear cell kidney cancer. J Urol. 2014;191:597–602. https://doi.org/10.1016/j.juro.2013.08.081.
41. Clague J, Shao L, Lin J, et al. Sensitivity to NNKOAc is associated with renal cancer risk. Carcinogenesis. 2009;30:706–10. https://doi.org/10.1093/carcin/bgp045.
42. Zhu Y, Horikawa Y, Yang H, et al. BPDE induced lymphocytic chromosome 3p deletions may predict renal cell carcinoma risk. J Urol. 2008;179:2416–21.
43. Lee J, Mannisto S, Spiegelman D, et al. Intakes of fruit, vegetables, and carotenoids and renal cell cancer risk: a pooled analysis of 13 prospective studies. Cancer Epidemiol Biomarkers Prev. 2009;18:1730–9.
44. Liao Z, Fang Z, Gou S, et al. The role of diet in renal cell carcinoma incidence: an umbrella review of meta-analyses of observational studies. BMC Med. 2022;20:39. https://doi.org/10.1186/s12916-021-02229-5.
45. Lee J, Spiegelman D, Hunter D, et al. Fat, protein, and meat consumption and renal cell cancer risk: a pooled analysis of 13 prospective studies. J Natl Cancer Inst. 2008;100:1695–706.
46. Klein WMP, Jacobsen PB, Helzlsouer KJ. Alcohol and cancer risk. JAMA. 2020;323:23–4. https://doi.org/10.1001/jama.2019.19133.
47. Lee J, Hunter D, Spiegelman D, et al. Alcohol intake and renal cell cancer in a pooled analysis of 12 prospective studies. J Natl Cancer Inst. 2007;99:801–10.
48. Bagnardi V, Rota M, Botteri E, et al. Alcohol consumption and site-specific cancer risk: a comprehensive dose–response meta-analysis. Br J Cancer. 2015;112:580–93. https://doi.org/10.1038/bjc.2014.579.
49. McLaughlin JK, Hrubec Z, Heineman EF, et al. A population based case control study of renal cell carcinoma. J Natl Cancer Inst. 1984;72:275–84.
50. Chow W, Gridley G, Fraumeni J, Järvholm B. Obesity, hypertension, and the risk of kidney cancer in men. N Engl J Med. 2000;343:1305–11.
51. Bhaskaran K, Douglas I, Forbes H, et al. Body-mass index and risk of 22 specific cancers: a population-based cohort study of 5·24 million UK adults. Lancet. 2014;384:755–65. https://doi.org/10.1016/s0140-6736(14)60892-8.
52. Lauby-Secretan B, Scoccianti C, Loomis D, et al. Body fatness and cancer—viewpoint of the IARC working group. N Engl J Med. 2016;375:794–8. https://doi.org/10.1056/nejmsr1606602.
53. World Cancer Research Fund. Kidney cancer statistics. online. 2018
54. Renehan A, Tyson M, Egger M, et al. Body-mass index and incidence of cancer: a systematic review and meta-analysis of prospective observational studies. Lancet. 2008;371:569–78.
55. Kim LH, Doan P, He Y, et al. A systematic review and meta-analysis of the significance of body mass index on kidney cancer outcomes. J Urol. 2021;205:346–55. https://doi.org/10.1097/ju.0000000000001377.
56. Albiges L, Hakimi AA, Xie W, et al. Body mass index and metastatic renal cell carcinoma: clinical and biological correlations. J Clin Oncol. 2016;34:3655–63. https://doi.org/10.1200/jco.2016.66.7311.
57. Klinghoffer Z, Yang B, Kapoor A, Pinthus J. Obesity and renal cell carcinoma: epidemiology, underlying mechanisms and management considerations. Expert Rev Anticancer Ther. 2009;9:975–87.
58. Solarek W, Koper M, Lewicki S, et al. Insulin and insulin-like growth factors act as renal cell cancer intratumoral regulators. J Cell Commun Signal. 2019;13:381–94. https://doi.org/10.1007/s12079-019-00512-y.
59. Tracz AF, Szczylik C, Porta C, Czarnecka AM. Insulin-like growth factor-1 signaling in renal cell carcinoma. BMC Cancer. 2016;16:453. https://doi.org/10.1186/s12885-016-2437-4.
60. Moschos SJ, Mantzoros CS. The role of the IGF system in cancer: from basic to clinical studies and clinical applications. Oncology. 2002;63:317–32. https://doi.org/10.1159/000066230.

61. DeCensi A, Puntoni M, Goodwin P, et al. Metformin and cancer risk in diabetic patients: a systematic review and meta-analysis. Cancer Prev Res. 2010;3:1451–61. https://doi.org/10.1158/1940-6207.capr-10-0157.
62. Gandini S, Puntoni M, Heckman-Stoddard BM, et al. Metformin and cancer risk and mortality: a systematic review and meta-analysis taking into account biases and confounders. Cancer Prev Res. 2014;7:867–85. https://doi.org/10.1158/1940-6207.capr-13-0424.
63. Fryar CD, Kit B, Carroll MD, Afful J. Hypertension prevalence, awareness, treatment, and control among adults age 18 and older: United States, august 2021–august 2023. National Center for Health Statistics; 2024.
64. Grossman E, Messerli FH, Boyko V, Goldbourt U. Is there an association between hypertension and cancer mortality? Am J Med. 2002;112:479–86.
65. Al-Bayati O, Hasan A, Pruthi D, et al. Systematic review of modifiable risk factors for kidney cancer. Urol Oncol: Semin Orig Investig. 2019;37:359–71. https://doi.org/10.1016/j.urolonc.2018.12.008.
66. Hidayat K, Du X, Zou S-Y, Shi B-M. Blood pressure and kidney cancer risk. J Hypertens. 2017;35:1333–44. https://doi.org/10.1097/hjh.0000000000001286.
67. Au EH, Chapman JR, Craig JC, et al. Overall and site-specific cancer mortality in patients on dialysis and after kidney transplant. J Am Soc Nephrol. 2019;30:471–80. https://doi.org/10.1681/asn.2018090906.
68. Serkies K, Dębska-Ślizień A, Kowalczyk A, et al. Malignancies in adult kidney transplant candidates and recipients: current status. Nephrol Dial Transplant. 2022;38:1591–602. https://doi.org/10.1093/ndt/gfac239.
69. Stewart J, Vajdic C, Leeuwen M, et al. The pattern of excess cancer in dialysis and transplantation. Nephrol Dial Transplant. 2009;24:3225–31.
70. Shirazian S, Starakiewicz P, Latcha S. Cancer screening in end-stage kidney disease. Adv Chronic Kidney Dis. 2021;28:502–508.e1. https://doi.org/10.1053/j.ackd.2021.09.006.
71. Goh A, Vathsala A. Native renal cysts and dialysis duration are risk factors for renal cell carcinoma in renal transplant recipients. Am J Transpl. 2011;11:86–92.
72. Ljungberg B, Albiges L, Abu-Ghanem Y, et al. European Association of Urology guidelines on renal cell carcinoma: the 2022 update. Eur Urol. 2022;82:399–410. https://doi.org/10.1016/j.eururo.2022.03.006.
73. Klatte T, Seitz C, Waldert M, et al. Features and outcomes of renal cell carcinoma of native kidneys in renal transplant recipients. BJU Int. 2010;105:1260–5.
74. Gigante M, Neuzillet Y, Patard J-J, et al. Renal cell carcinoma (RCC) arising in native kidneys of dialyzed and transplant patients: are they different entities? BJU Int. 2012;110:E570–3. https://doi.org/10.1111/j.1464-410x.2012.11273.x.
75. Breda A, Lucarelli G, Luccarelli G, et al. Clinical and pathological outcomes of renal cell carcinoma (RCC) in native kidneys of patients with end-stage renal disease: a long-term comparative retrospective study with RCC diagnosed in the general population. World J Urol. 2015;33:1–7. https://doi.org/10.1007/s00345-014-1248-y.
76. Joffe BI, Martina LP, Stillman M, et al. Tumor characteristics in immunosuppressed and renal dysfunction populations. Urol Oncol: Semin Orig Investig. 2024;42:453.e9–453.e14. https://doi.org/10.1016/j.urolonc.2024.09.011.
77. Lowrance WT, Ordoñez J, Udaltsova N, et al. CKD and the risk of incident cancer. J Am Soc Nephrol. 2014;25:2327–34. https://doi.org/10.1681/asn.2013060604.
78. Clague J, Lin J, Cassidy A, et al. Family history and risk of renal cell carcinoma: results from a case-control study and systematic meta-analysis. Cancer Epidemiol Biomarkers Prev. 2009;18:801–7.
79. Jakobsson RG, Nasic S, Bratt O, et al. Family history and risk of renal cell carcinoma: a National multi-register case-control study. J Urol. 2024;211:71–9. https://doi.org/10.1097/ju.0000000000003765.
80. McLaughlin J, Chow W, Mandel J, et al. International renal-cell cancer study. VIII. Role of diuretics, other anti-hypertensive medications and hypertension. Int J Cancer. 1995;63:216–21.
81. Colt J, Hofmann J, Schwartz K, et al. Antihypertensive medication use and risk of renal cell carcinoma. Cancer Causes Control. 2017;28:289–97.
82. Gold B, Mirvish S. N-Nitroso derivatives of hydrochlorothiazide, niridazole, and tolbutamide. Toxicol Appl Pharmacol. 1977;40:131–6.
83. Pahor M, Guralnik J, Ferrucci L, et al. Calcium-channel blockade and incidence of cancer in aged populations. Lancet. 1996;348:493–7.
84. Karami S, Daughtery SE, Schwartz K, Davis FG. Analgesic use and risk of renal cell carcinoma: a case-control, cohort and meta-analytic assessment. Int J Cancer. 2016;139:584–92.
85. Bessems J, Vermeulen N. Paracetamol (acetaminophen)-induced toxicity: molecular and biochemical mechanisms, analogues and protective approaches. Crit Rev Toxicol. 2001;31:55–138.
86. Cho E, Curhan G, Hankinson SE, et al. Prospective evaluation of analgesic use and risk of renal cell cancer. Arch Intern Med. 2011;171:1487–93. https://doi.org/10.1001/archinternmed.2011.356.
87. Choueiri T, Je Y, Cho E. Analgesic use and the risk of kidney cancer: a meta-analysis of epidemiologic studies. Int J Cancer. 2013;134:384–96.
88. Bruinsma FJ, Jordan S, Bassett JK, et al. Analgesic use and the risk of renal cell carcinoma—findings from the consortium for the investigation of renal malignancies (CONFIRM) study. Cancer Epidemiol. 2021;75:102036. https://doi.org/10.1016/j.canep.2021.102036.

89. Scott C, Chiu W. Trichloroethylene cancer epidemiology: a consideration of select issues. Environ Health Perspect. 2006;114:1471–8.
90. Andrew AS, Li M, Shi X, et al. Kidney cancer risk associated with historic groundwater trichloroethylene contamination. Int J Environ Res Public Heal. 2022;19:618. https://doi.org/10.3390/ijerph19020618.
91. Hoang ML, Chen C-H, Chen P-C, et al. Aristolochic acid in the etiology of renal cell carcinoma. Cancer Epidemiol Prev Biomark. 2016;25:1600–8. https://doi.org/10.1158/1055-9965.epi-16-0219.
92. Jhuang J-R, Chiang C-J, Su S-Y, et al. Reduction in the incidence of urological cancers after the ban on Chinese herbal products containing Aristolochic acid: an interrupted time-series analysis. Sci Rep. 2019;9:19860. https://doi.org/10.1038/s41598-019-56394-y.
93. Ahmed YH, El-Naggar ME, Rashad MM, et al. Screening for polystyrene nanoparticle toxicity on kidneys of adult male albino rats using histopathological, biochemical, and molecular examination results. Cell Tissue Res. 2022;388:149–65. https://doi.org/10.1007/s00441-022-03581-5.
94. Gong J, Maia M, Dizman N, et al. Metastasis in renal cell carcinoma: biology and implications for therapy. Asian J Urol. 2016;3:286–92.
95. Wilson JM, Jungner YG. Principles and practice of mass screening for disease. Bol Oficina Sanit Panam. 1968;65:281–393.
96. Usher-Smith J, Simmons RK, Rossi SH, Stewart GD. Current evidence on screening for renal cancer. Nat Rev Urol. 2020;17:637–42. https://doi.org/10.1038/s41585-020-0363-3.
97. Sugimura K, Ikemoto SI, Kawashima H, et al. Microscopic hematuria as a screening marker for urinary tract malignancies. Int J Urol. 2001;8:1–5.
98. Kang M, Lee S, Jeong SJ, et al. Characteristics and significant predictors of detecting underlying diseases in adults with asymptomatic microscopic hematuria: a large case series of a Korean population. Int J Urol. 2015;22:389–93.
99. Flitcroft JG, Verheyen J, Vemulkar T, et al. Early detection of kidney cancer using urinary proteins: a truly non-invasive strategy. BJU Int. 2022;129:290–303. https://doi.org/10.1111/bju.15601.
100. Morrissey JJ, Kharasch ED. The specificity of urinary aquaporin 1 and Perilipin 2 to screen for renal cell carcinoma. J Urol. 2013;189:1913–20. https://doi.org/10.1016/j.juro.2012.11.034.
101. Morrissey JJ, London AN, Luo J, Kharasch ED. Urinary biomarkers for the early diagnosis of kidney cancer. Mayo Clin Proc. 2010;85:413–21. https://doi.org/10.4065/mcp.2009.0709.
102. Raimondo F, Morosi L, Corbetta S, et al. Differential protein profiling of renal cell carcinoma urinary exosomes. Mol BioSyst. 2013;9:1220–33. https://doi.org/10.1039/c3mb25582d.
103. Mijušković M, Stanojević I, Milović N, et al. Urinary KIM-1 and AQP-1 in patients with clear renal cell carcinoma: potential noninvasive biomarkers. Vojn Pregl. 2016;73:266–72. https://doi.org/10.2298/vsp150124006m.
104. Morrissey JJ, Mellnick VM, Luo J, et al. Evaluation of urine Aquaporin-1 and Perilipin-2 concentrations as biomarkers to screen for renal cell carcinoma: a prospective cohort study. JAMA Oncol. 2015;1:204–12. https://doi.org/10.1001/jamaoncol.2015.0213.
105. Rossi S, Klatte T, Usher-Smith J, Stewart G. Epidemiology and screening for renal cancer. World J Urol. 2018;36:1341–53.
106. Ishikawa S, Aoki J, Ohwada S, et al. Mass screening of multiple abdominal solid organs using mobile helical computed tomography scanner–a preliminary report. Asian J Surg. 2007;30:118–21.
107. USPSTF B-DK, Grossman D, Curry S, Davidson K. Screening for colorectal cancer: US preventive services task force recommendation statement. JAMA. 2016;315:2564–75.
108. Harrison H, Wood A, Pennells L, et al. Estimating the effectiveness of kidney cancer screening within lung cancer screening Programmes: a validation in UK biobank. Eur Urol Oncol. 2023;6:351–3. https://doi.org/10.1016/j.euo.2023.02.012.
109. Shea M. A proposal for a targeted screening program for renal cancer. Front Oncologia. 2013;3:207.
110. Rossi SH, Klatte T, Usher-Smith JA, et al. A decision analysis evaluating screening for kidney cancer using focused renal ultrasound. Eur Urol Focus. 2021;7:407–19. https://doi.org/10.1016/j.euf.2019.09.002.
111. Jamis-Dow CA, Choyke PL, Jennings SB, et al. Small (< or = 3-cm) renal masses: detection with CT versus US and pathologic correlation. Radiology. 1996;198:785–8.
112. Uppot RN. Technical challenges of imaging & image-guided interventions in obese patients. Br J Radiol. 2018;91:20170931. https://doi.org/10.1259/bjr.20170931.
113. Mihara S, Kuroda K, Yoshioka R, Koyama W. Early detection of renal cell carcinoma by ultrasonographic screening–based on the results of 13 years screening in Japan. Ultrasound Med Biol. 1999;25:1033–9.
114. Corcoran AT, Russo P, Lowrance WT, et al. A review of contemporary data on surgically resected renal masses–benign or malignant? Urology. 2013;81:707–13.
115. Kalble T, Lucan M, Nicita G, et al. EAU guidelines on renal transplantation. Eur Urol. 2005;47:156–66.
116. Acuna SA, Huang JW, Scott AL, et al. Cancer screening recommendations for solid organ transplant recipients: a systematic review of clinical practice guidelines. Am J Transplant. 2017;17:103–14. https://doi.org/10.1111/ajt.13978.
117. Starke N, Singla N, Haddad A, Lotan Y. Long-term outcomes in a high-risk bladder cancer screening cohort. BJU Int. 2016;117:611–7.

118. Richard S, Graff J, Lindau J, Resche F. Von Hippel-Lindau disease. Lancet. 2004;363:1231–4.
119. Mahler ER, Neumann HP, Richard S. Von-Hippel-Lindau disease: a clinical and scientific review. Eur J Hum Genet. 2011;19:617–23.
120. Choyke PL, Glenn GM, Walther MM, et al. The natural history of renal lesions in von Hippel-Lindau disease: a serial CT study in 28 patients. AJR Am J Roentgenol. 1992;159:1229–34.
121. Mandriota SJ, Turner KJ, Davies DR. HIF activation identifies early lesions in VHL kidneys: evidence for site-specific tumor suppressor function in the nephron. Cancer Cell. 2002;1:459–68.
122. Al-Obaidy KI, Alruwaii ZI, Williamson SR, Cheng L. The pathological and molecular genetic landscape of the hereditary renal cancer predisposition syndromes. Histopathology. 2022;81:15–31. https://doi.org/10.1111/his.14641.
123. Freifeld Y, Ananthakrishnan L, Margulis V. Imaging for screening and surveillance of patients with hereditary forms of renal cell carcinoma. Curr Urol Rep. 2018;19:82. https://doi.org/10.1007/s11934-018-0829-5.
124. Yanus GA, Kuligina ES, Imyanitov EN. Hereditary renal cancer syndromes. Méd Sci. 2024;12:12. https://doi.org/10.3390/medsci12010012.
125. Tan M-H, Mester JL, Ngeow J, et al. Lifetime cancer risks in individuals with germline PTEN mutations. Clin Cancer Res. 2012;18:400–7. https://doi.org/10.1158/1078-0432.ccr-11-2283.
126. Tischkowitz M, Colas C, Pouwels S, et al. Cancer surveillance guideline for individuals with PTEN hamartoma tumour syndrome. Eur J Hum Genet. 2020;28:1387–93. https://doi.org/10.1038/s41431-020-0651-7.
127. Northrup H, Aronow ME, Bebin EM, et al. Updated international tuberous sclerosis complex diagnostic criteria and surveillance and management recommendations. Pediatr Neurol. 2021;123:50–66. https://doi.org/10.1016/j.pediatrneurol.2021.07.011.
128. Cicchetti R, Basconi M, Litterio G, et al. Advances in molecular mechanisms of kidney disease: integrating renal tumorigenesis of hereditary cancer syndrome. Int J Mol Sci. 2024;25:9060. https://doi.org/10.3390/ijms25169060.
129. Linehan W. Evaluation and screening for hereditary renal cell cancers. Can Urol Assoc J. 2013;7:324.
130. Campbell SC, Uzzo RG, Karam JA, et al. Renal mass and localized renal cancer: evaluation, management, and follow-up: AUA guideline (2021). J Urol. 2021;206:209–18. https://doi.org/10.1097/ju.0000000000001912.
131. Bratslavsky G, Mendhiratta N, Daneshvar M, et al. Genetic risk assessment for hereditary renal cell carcinoma: clinical consensus statement. Cancer. 2021;127:3957–66. https://doi.org/10.1002/cncr.33679.
132. Gospodarowicz MK, Miller D, Groome PA. The process for continuous improvement of the TNM classification. Cancer. 2004;100:1–5.
133. Flocks RH, Kadesky MC. Malignant neoplasms of the kidney: an analysis of 353 patients followed five years or more. J Urol. 1958;79:196–201.
134. Harmer M. NM classification of malignant tumors. 3rd ed. Geneva: International Union Against Cancer.
135. Goodman KA. AJCC cancer staging system, version 9. American College of Surgeons; 2024.
136. Howard GE, Wood CG. Staging refinements in renal cell carcinoma. Curr Opin Urol. 2006;165:317–20.
137. Ficarra V, Novara G, Galfano A, Artibani W. Neoplasm staging and organ-confined renal cell carcinoma: a systematic review. Eur Urol. 2004;46:559–64.
138. Greene FL. AJCC cancer staging manual. 6th ed. Chicago: Springer; 2002.
139. Hafez KS, Gergany AF, Novick AC. Nephron sparing surgery for localized renal cell carcinoma: impact of tumor size on patient survival, tumor recurrence and TNM staging. J Urol. 1999;162:1930–3.
140. Ficarra V, Schips L, Guille F. Multi-institutional European validation of the 2002 TNM staging system in conventional and papillary localized renal cell carcinoma. Cancer. 2005;104:968–74.
141. Mitchell RE, Gilbert SM, Murphy AM, et al. Partial nephrectomy and radical nephrectomy offer similar cancer outcomes in renal cortical tumors 4 cm or larger. J Urol. 2006;67:260–4.
142. Cheville JC, Blute ML, Zincke H, et al. Stage pT1 conventional (clear cell) renal cell carcinoma: pathological features associated with cancer specific survival. J Urol. 2001;166:453–6.
143. Zisman A, Pantuck AJ, Chao D. Reevaluation of the 1997 TNM classification for renal cell carcinoma: T1 and T2 cutoff point at 4.5cm rather than 7cm better correlates with clinical outcome. J Urol. 2001;166:54–8.
144. Ficarra V, Guille F, Schips L. Proposal for revision of the RNM classification system for renal cell carcinoma. Cancer. 2005;104:2116–23.
145. Klatte T, Patard JJ, Goel RH, Kleid MD. Prognostic impact of tumor size on pT2 renal cell carcinoma: an international multicenter experience. J Urol. 2007;178:35–40.
146. Frank I, Blute ML, Leibovich BC, Cheville JC. pT2 classification for renal cell carcinoma: can its accuracy be improved? J Urol. 2005;173:380–4.
147. Edge SB. AJCC cancer staging manual. 7th ed. Chicago: Springer; 2010.
148. Capitanio U, Bedke J, Albiges L, et al. A renewal of the TNM staging system for patients with renal cancer to comply with current decision-making: proposal from the European Association of Urology guidelines panel. Eur Urol. 2023;83:3–5. https://doi.org/10.1016/j.eururo.2022.09.026.
149. Tang Y, Liu F, Mao X, et al. The impact of tumor size on the survival of patients with small renal masses: a population–based study. Cancer Med. 2022;11:2377–85. https://doi.org/10.1002/cam4.4595.

150. Murphy AM, Gilbert SM, Katz AE, Goluboff ET. Re-evaluation of the tumour-node-metastasis staging of locally advanced renal cortical tumours: absolute size (T2) is more significant than renal capsular invasion (T3a). BJU Int. 2005;95:27–30.
151. Lam JS, Klatte T, Patard JJ, et al. Prognostic relevance of tumour size in T3a renal cell carcinoma: a multicentre experience. Eur Urol. 2007;52:155–62.
152. Simer S, Lehmann J, Loch A, Becker F. Current TNM classification of renal cell carcinoma: revising stage T3a. J Urol. 2005;173:33–7.
153. Delahunt B, Eble JN, Samaratunga H, et al. Staging of renal cell carcinoma: current progress and potential advances. Pathology. 2021;53:120–8. https://doi.org/10.1016/j.pathol.2020.08.007.
154. Bertini R, Roscigno M, Freschi M, Strada E. Renal sinus fat invasion in pT3a clear cell renal cell carcinoma affects outcomes of patients without nodal involvement or distant metastases. J Urol. 2009;181.2027–32.
155. Thompson RH, Leibovich BC, Cheville JC, Webster WS. Is renal sinus fat invasion the same as perinephric fat invasion for pT3a renal cell carcinoma? J Urol. 2005;174:1218–21.
156. Thompson RH, Cheville JC, Lohse CM, Webster ES. Reclassification of patients with pT3 and pT4 renal cell carcinoma improves prognostic accuracy. Cancer. 2005;104:53–60.
157. Margulis V, Tamboli P, Matin SF, et al. Redefining pT3 renal cell carcinoma in the modern era: a proposal for a revision of the current TNM primary tumor classification system. Cancer. 2007;109:2439–44.
158. Costa W, Moniz R, Cunha I, Fonseca F. Impact of renal vein invasion and fat invasion in pT3a renal cell carcinoma. BJU Int. 2012;109:544–8.
159. Shah PH, Lyon TD, Lohse CM, et al. Prognostic evaluation of perinephric fat, renal sinus fat, and renal vein invasion for patients with pathological stage T3a clear-cell renal cell carcinoma. BJU Int. 2019;123:270–6. https://doi.org/10.1111/bju.14523.
160. Bonsib S. Renal veins and venous extension in clear cell renal cell carcinoma. Mod Pathol. 2006;20:44–53.
161. Paner G, Stadler W, Hansel D, et al. Updates in the eighth edition of the tumor-node-metastasis staging classification for urologic cancers. Eur Urol. 2018;73:560–9.
162. Whitson JM, Reese AC, Meng MV. Population based analysis of survival in patients with renal cell carcinoma and venous tumor thrombus. Urol Oncol. 2013;31:259–63.
163. Moinzadeh A, Libertino JA. Prognostic significance of tumor thrombus level in patients with renal cell carcinoma and venous tumor thrombus extension: is all T3b the same? J Urol. 2004;171:598–601.
164. Wagner B, Patard J, Mejean A, et al. Prognostic value of renal vein and inferior vena cava involvement in renal cell carcinoma. Eur Urol. 2009;55:452–9.
165. Rabbani D, Hakimian P, Reuter VE, et al. Renal vein or inferior vena caval extension in patients with renal cortical tumors: impact of tumor histology. J Urol. 2004;171:1057–61.
166. Shiff B, Breau RH, Mallick R, et al. Prognostic significance of extent of venous tumor thrombus in patients with non-metastatic renal cell carcinoma: results from a Canadian multi-institutional collaborative. Urol Oncol: Semin Orig Investig. 2021;39:836.e19–27. https://doi.org/10.1016/j.urolonc.2021.08.016.
167. Kim HL, Zisman A, Han KR, et al. Prognostic significance of venous thrombus in renal cell carcinoma. Are renal vein and inferior vena cava involvement different? J Urol. 2004;171:588–91.
168. Haferkamp A, Bastian PJ, Jakobi H, et al. Renal cell carcinoma with tumor thrombus extension into the vena cava: prospective long-term follow-up. J Urol. 2007;177:1703–8.
169. Abel EJ, Masterson TA, Karam JA, Master VA. Predictive nomogram for recurrence following surgery for nonmetastatic renal cell cancer with tumor thrombus. J Urol. 2017;198:810–6.
170. Han KR, Bui MH, Pantuck AJ, Freitas DG. TNM T3a renal cell carcinoma: adrenal gland involvement is not the same as renal fat invasion. J Urol. 2003;169:899–903.
171. Thompson RH, Leibovich BC, Cheville JC, et al. Should direct ipsilateral adrenal invasion from renal cell carcinoma be classified as pT3a? J Urol. 2005;173:918–21.
172. Terrone C, Cracco C, Porpiglia F, Bollito E. Reassessing the current TNM lymph node staging for renal cell carcinoma. Eur Urol. 2006;49:324–31.
173. Dimashkieh HH, Lohse CM, Blute ML, Kwon ED. Extranodal extension in regional lymph nodes is associated with outcome in patients with renal cell carcinoma. J Urol. 2006;176:1978–82.
174. Pantuck AJ, Zisman A, Dorey F, Chao DH. Renal cell carcinoma with retroperitoneal lymph nodes: role of lymph node dissection. J Urol. 2003;169:2076–83.
175. Capitanio U, Deho' F, Dell' Oglio P, et al. Lymphadenopathies in patients with renal cell carcinoma: clinical and pathological predictors of pathologically confirmed lymph node invasion. World J Urol. 2016;34:1139–45. https://doi.org/10.1007/s00345-015-1747-5.
176. Yu K, Keskin SK, Meissner MA, et al. Renal cell carcinoma and pathologic nodal disease: implications for American joint committee on cancer staging. Cancer. 2018;124:4023–31. https://doi.org/10.1002/cncr.31661.
177. Novara G, Ficarra V, Antonelli A, Artibani W. Validation of the 2009 TNM version in a large multi-institutional cohort of patients treated for renal cell carcinoma: are further improvements needed? Eur Urol. 2010;58:588–95.
178. Motzer RJ, Mazumdar M, Bacik J, Berg W. Survival and prognostic stratification of 670 patients with advanced renal cell carcinoma. J Clin Oncol. 1999;17:2530–40.

179. Bex A, Mulders P, Jewett M, et al. Comparison of immediate vs deferred Cytoreductive nephrectomy in patients with synchronous metastatic renal cell carcinoma receiving Sunitinib. JAMA Oncol. 2019;5:164–70. https://doi.org/10.1001/jamaoncol.2018.5543.
180. Méjean A, Ravaud A, Thezenas S, et al. Sunitinib alone or after nephrectomy in metastatic renal-cell carcinoma. N Engl J Med. 2018;379:417–27. https://doi.org/10.1056/nejmoa1803675.
181. De Bruijn R, Wimalasingham A, Szabados B, et al. Deferred Cytoreductive nephrectomy following Presurgical vascular endothelial growth factor receptor–targeted therapy in patients with primary metastatic clear cell renal cell carcinoma: a pooled analysis of prospective trial data. Eur Urol Oncol. 2020;3:168–73. https://doi.org/10.1016/j.euo.2019.12.004.
182. Lee C, You D, Park J, Jeong IG. Validation of the 2009 TNM classification for renal cell carcinoma: comparison with the 2002 TNM classification by concordance index. Korean J Urol. 2011;52:524–30.
183. Patard JJ, Leray E, Cindolo L, Fiacrra V. Multi-institutional validation of a symptom based classification for renal cell carcinoma. J Urol. 2004;172:858–62.
184. Patard JJ, Kim HL, Lam JS, Dorey FJ. Use of the University of California Los Angeles integrated staging system to predict survival in renal cell carcinoma: an international multicenter study. J Clin Oncol. 2004;22:3316–22.
185. Ficarra V, Novara G, Galfano A, et al. The 'stage, size, grade and necrosis' score is more accurate than the University of California Los Angeles Integrated Staging System for predicting cancer-specific survival in patients with clear cell renal cell carcinoma. BJU Int. 2009;103:165–70. https://doi.org/10.1111/j.1464-410x.2008.07901.x.

2 Molecular Genetics of Renal Cell Carcinoma

Jonathan S. Kim and Louis S. Liou

Introduction

Renal cell carcinomas (RCC) represent approximately 3% of all malignancies in the United States and is the most common subtype of renal malignancy [1]. RCC comprises many different forms of histopathological entities as described in the 2016 World Health Organization classification. The clear cell histotype (ccRCC) is the most common, while other histotypes are grouped as non-clear cell renal cell carcinoma (e.g., papillary renal cell carcinoma and chromophobe renal cell carcinoma).

The classic clinical presentation of RCC includes the triad of hematuria, flank pain, and palpable abdominal mass. However, only 10% of patients present with this constellation of symptoms [1, 2]. Approximately 20% of RCC cases are associated with paraneoplastic manifestations and present with laboratory abnormalities that cannot be directly attributed to the primary tumor itself, including hypercalcemia, erythrocytosis, and nonmetastatic hepatic dysfunction (i.e., Stauffer syndrome) [1, 3]. The diagnostic work-up for RCC involves imaging studies to enable characterization of tumor size, extent, and vascular involvement. Contrast-enhanced CT scans have become the preferred imaging procedure, and ultrasonography can be useful in cases where CT imaging is inconclusive [1]. The evolution of imaging techniques has allowed for the detection of smaller tumors at earlier stages, often before patients become symptomatic. Emerging genomic screening modalities have the potential for enhancing early detection and risk stratification, and their clinical utility in RCC is currently still under investigation.

Standard treatment for localized RCC typically includes nephrectomy, ablation, or active radiographic surveillance [4]. Approximately 25-30% of patients with RCC present with metastatic disease when diagnosed, and 30% of patients with initially localized RCC eventually develop recurrence or metastasis [4, 5]. For metastatic RCC, current treatment options include target therapies (e.g., tyrosine kinase inhibitors, VEGF inhibitors) and immunotherapies (interferon-α, IL-2, and nivolumab) [4]. Despite these advancements, treatment response in metastatic RCC is highly variable, pointing to the tumor's heterogeneity in its molecular biology and genetics [4–6].

This chapter aims to describe the genetic and epigenetic factors that drive RCC progression as well as explore these insights in the context of therapeutic strategies.

J. S. Kim
Drexel University College of Medicine, Philadelphia, PA, USA

L. S. Liou (✉)
Department of Urology, Emerson Hospital, Concord, MA, USA

Tufts University School of Medicine, Boston, MA, USA

J. A. Libertino, J. R. Gee (eds.), *Renal Cancer*, https://doi.org/10.1007/978-3-031-97599-8_2

VHL-HIF Axis and Tumor Metabolism

The discovery of the von-Hippel-Lindau (VHL) gene represents a cornerstone in the current understanding of the molecular biology of RCC. The clinical phenotype was first described by ophthalmologist Eugen von Hippel in 1904 and later expanded by pathologist Arvid Lindau in 1927, who described them as vascular tumors in the retina and central nervous system. It was not until decades later that genetic studies identified the VHL gene on chromosome 3p25 [7, 8].

In normal healthy cells, VHL ensures proper degradation of hypoxia-inducible transcription factors (HIF-1a; HIF-2a) under normal oxygen levels. HIF-1a and HIF-2a are tagged for destruction via ubiquitination through prolyl hydroxylation. In ccRCC, mutations in the VHL gene disrupt this mechanism, leading to the stabilization and abnormal accumulation of HIF proteins even in normoxic conditions, and this overexpression leads to downstream upregulation of gene factors that promote angiogenesis, proliferation, invasion, and progression of RCC, such as VEGF, EGF, and TGF-a. This molecular signature is a defining feature of ccRCC and is fundamental to the current understanding of its pathophysiology [9, 10].

The VHL gene is inactivated in up to 90% of cases through the loss of one copy of the gene (i.e., loss of heterozygosity). Germline mutation in one copy of the VHL gene predisposes individuals if the second copy is later lost or mutated, consistent with the one-hit hypothesis. However, sporadic ccRCC occurs in 60–80% of cases, whereby both copies of the gene are affected through mutation or deletions, consistent with the two-hit hypothesis [9] (Fig. 2.1).

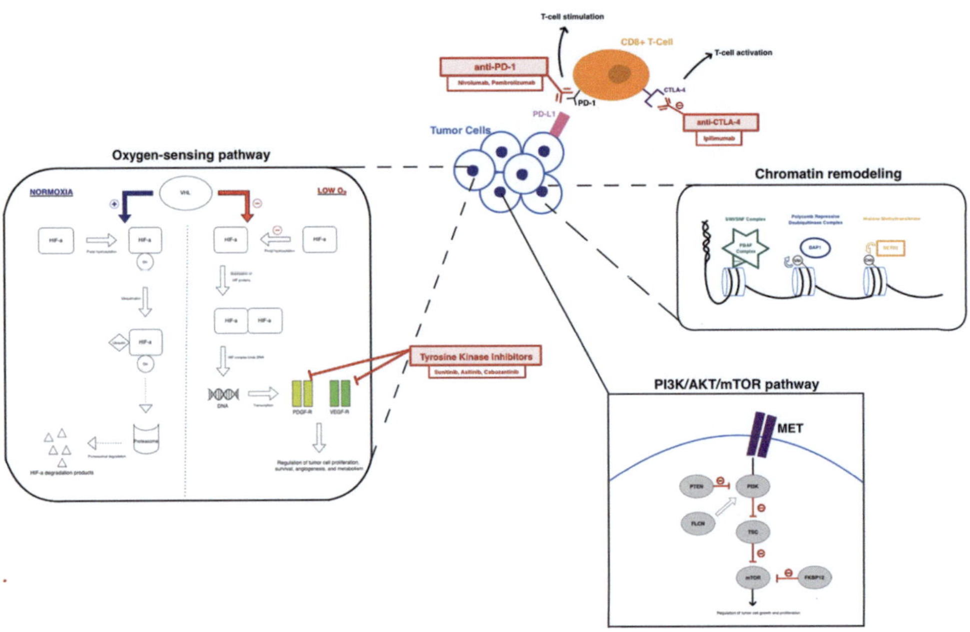

Fig. 2.1 Molecular pathways involved in the genetic basis of ccRCC. (1) Oxygen-sensing pathway: Mutation in VHL and hypoxia exposure will result in failure of HIF to undergo ubiquitin-mediated degradation and accumulation. HIF multimers bind DNA to increase transcription of tumorigenic elements (VEGF, PDGF, among others). (2) Chromatin remodeling: Main chromatin remodeling systems involved in RCC tumorigenesis. SWI/SNF is a complex that alters nucleosome positioning. The polycomb repressive deubiquitinase complex involves BAP1 and acts by deubiquitinating histones. Methyltransferases, such as SETD2, add methyl groups to histones to alter gene expression. (3) PI3K/AKT/mTOR pathway: This pathway is a key signaling cascade that promotes tumor growth and proliferation by transducing signals from growth factors and cellular stress. It is often dysregulated by the loss of tumor suppressors such as PTEN and FLCN, as well as mutations in TSC, with mTOR activity modulated by FKBP12, an mTOR inhibitor binding partner. *VHL* von Hippel-Lindau, *HIF* hypoxia-inducible factor, *VEGF* vascular endothelial growth factor, *PDGF* platelet-derived growth factor, *SWI/SNF* switch/sucrose nonfermentable, *BAP* BRCA-associated protein, *SETD* SET domain containing, *PTEN* phosphatase and tensin homolog, *FLCN* folliculin, *TSC* tuberous sclerosis complex, *mTOR* mechanistic target of rapamycin, *FKBP* FK506-binding protein

Clear Cell Renal Cell Carcinoma

Clear cell renal cell carcinoma (ccRCC) is the most common subtype of renal cell carcinoma, which originates from the epithelial cells of the renal proximal tubules. It is characterized by its distinct histological appearance with tumor cells demonstrating a clear cytoplasm due to their high glycogen and lipid content. The disease course is known to be widely variable, ranging from localized and slow-growing tumors to rapidly progressing metastatic disease. Notably, ccRCC has a high propensity for hematogenous spread. Growing advances in genomic profiling have revealed novel mutations involved in ccRCC, contributing to its heterogeneity and overall prognosis of the disease [4–6, 9, 10].

Chromatin-Remodeling Tumor Suppressor Genes

Chromatin remodeling is an epigenetic mechanism whose mutations are observed in ccRCC and may have potential prognostic significance. Three of these genes—polybromo 1 (PBRM1), BRCA1-associated protein-1 (BAP1), and SET domain-containing protein 2 (SETD2)—are tumor suppressors that are frequently inactivated in ccRCC due to their location close to the VHL gene. and thus, are altered as a consequence of 3p chromosome loss [11]. These genes typically follow the two-hit hypothesis for inactivation; therefore, both alleles must be affected for functional loss [11, 12].

PBRM1 is a protein that is involved in the PBAF complex and plays a role as a tumor suppressor. PBAF is a complex that acts by regulating cellular proliferation and differentiation. Alterations in PBRM1, a component of the SWI/SNF chromatin-remodeling complex, are present in approximately 41% of ccRCC cases [13]. PBRM1 mutations are inconsistently linked to survival outcomes. Specifically, one study suggests an improved overall survival (OS) [14]. Other studies report no significant effect on cancer-specific survival (CSS) [15–17]. Notably, PBRM1 mutations have been linked to the advanced tumor stage at presentation [11, 16, 17].

BAP1 is a tumor suppressor with histone deubiquitinase activity and is a component of the polycomb repressive complex (PR-DUB), which is involved in chromatin rearrangement [11, 18]. BAP1 is mutated in 5–15% of ccRCC cases and is associated with worse CSS and OS [11, 18, 19]. Truncating mutations in BAP1 are associated with significantly poorer outcomes compared to other mutation types. Studies have shown that patients without BAP1 protein expression exhibit markedly worse disease-specific survival (DSS) even after accounting for tumor stage and grade [19]. BAP-1 negative tumors in patients with otherwise low-risk disease demonstrate a threefold increase in disease-specific mortality [19]. The relationship between BAP1 mutations and PBRM1 mutations has previously been studied. Notably, BAP1 and PBRM1 are found to occur almost always mutually exclusively. However, in a small percentage of ccRCC patients, BAP1 and PBRM1 mutations were found to coexist, and the neoplasm exhibited rhabdoid features [20]. Further, in tumors where PBRM1 and BAP1 mutations coexist, patients have been shown to exhibit significantly poorer CSS [19].

The role of SETD2 in ccRCC prognosis is less well defined. SETD2 is a histone methyltransferase responsible for H3K36 trimethylation that plays a role in transcription regulation and alternative splicing, and mutations in this gene are seen in about 8–30% of tumors [11]. One study by Hakimi et al. demonstrated that SETD2 mutations are associated with decreased CSS in a Cancer Genome Atlas cohort [16]. However, a subsequent study by Gulati et al. failed to confirm these findings [14]. These inconsistent findings suggest that further research is needed to clarify the impact of SETD2 mutations on ccRCC outcomes [11, 16].

Hypoxia-Induced Genes in Clear Cell Renal Cell Carcinoma

Additional hypoxia-responsive genes have been implicated in the pathogenesis of ccRCC. EGLN3 is paradoxically upregulated 12.5-fold in RCC. Despite its usual role in tagging HIF-1a for degradation, EGLN3 appears to be ineffective due to VHL dysfunction, thus allowing HIF-1a to persist and activate downstream target genes [21].

Among these downstream targets are specific genes that have been shown to enhance tumor aggression and adaptability. ANGPTL4 is overexpressed 24.2-fold and is known to regulate vascular remodeling and angiogenesis, thus promoting the metastatic potential of the tumor. Similarly, PLOD2 plays a role in extracellular matrix remodeling and facilitates invasive growth potential by stabilizing collagen. RTP801 is upregulated 4.2-fold in RCC, and as a stress response gene, it plays a protective role against hypoxia-induced apoptosis and aids tumor survival in low-oxygen states. The identification of ANGPTL4, PLOD2, and RTP801 expands the current understanding of the pathogenesis of ccRCC beyond angiogenesis [21].

The prognostic significance of VHL mutations remains uncertain. Some studies suggest that these mutations are associated with earlier-stage disease and improved outcomes, including longer progression-free survival (PFS), CSS, and OSS [22–25]. However, other research indicates that certain types of VHL mutations, such as those causing a loss of function, are linked to worse PFS, CSS, and OS [26]. A recent large-scale analysis using data from The Cancer Genome Atlas (TCGA) found no consistent relationship between VHL mutations and CSS [27]. Further investigation into how these genetic changes influence patient outcomes is warranted.

Carbonic Anhydrase IX

Carbonic anhydrase IX (CAIX) is a hypoxia-inducible transmembrane protein that plays a critical role in regulating pH in renal tumors via the catalyzation of the reversible conversion of carbon dioxide to bicarbonate and protons. It is commonly overexpressed in ccRCC as a downstream effect of the inactivation of the VHL gene. In ccRCC, the hallmark loss of VHL stabilizes HIF-1a, leading to its accumulation and subsequent increased downstream transcription of hypoxia-inducible genes, which include CAIX [28, 29].

CAIX's expression correlates with tumor grade and has been explored as a diagnostic and prognostic marker. Low CAIX expression on tissue immunostaining has been linked to worse DSS in both metastatic and nonmetastatic ccRCC cases [28]. A meta-analysis of 15 studies also confirmed that low CAIX expression is associated with worse DSS, OS, and PFS [29]. Additionally, low CAIX expression has been correlated with more aggressive disease features, including higher tumor grade, deeper invasion, lymph node involvement, and distant metastasis [29]. Studies specifically focused on nonmetastatic ccRCC reported conflicting results. Zerati et al. found no relationship between CAIX expression and OS or adverse pathologic features in a cohort of 95 patients [30]. Chamie et al. observed an association between low CAIX expression and poor disease-free survival (DFS) and OS in a larger cohort of 831 high-risk patients [31]. Thus, CAIX expression may be used to stratify ccRCC disease severity and may potentially guide therapeutic strategies.

The potential of CAIX as a predictor of treatment response remains undetermined. Stillebroer et al. confirmed that high CAIX expression has been considered a predictor of response to interleukin-2 immunotherapy; however, its ability to predict response to treatment with angiogenesis inhibitors was inconclusive [32]. Other studies have confirmed the correlation between high CAIX expression with better clinical outcomes after treatment with interleukin-2 therapy. However, a more recent prospective, nonrandomized study did not confirm these observations [33]. CAIX expression status was found to be neither predictive nor prognostic in treatment with sorafenib, a receptor tyrosine kinase inhibitor that targets multiple pathways involved in tumor growth and angiogenesis [34].

Epigenetic Alterations

DNA methylation is an epigenetic mechanism in which methyl groups are added to cytosine bases of DNA to regulate gene activity, silence unnecessary genes, and maintain cellular stability. In

7% of ccRCC cases, VHL inactivation has been linked to hypermethylation, occurring independently of VHL mutations. Additionally, over 280 other genes exhibit epigenetic silencing in 5% of tumors. Notably, the tumor suppressor UQCRH is hypermethylated in 36% of tumors, with its promoter methylation correlating with more advanced stages and higher tumor grades. Mutations in SETD2 were associated with reduced methylation in nonpromoter regions, demonstrating its role in maintaining chromatin structure and heterochromatin stability [35–37].

mRNA editing is a post-transcriptional modification process that leads to RNA sequence diversity and influences gene expression and protein function. Abnormalities in mRNA editing have been implicated in the development and progression of ccRCC. APOBEC3 is a member of the large apolipoprotein B mRNA editing enzyme catalytic polypeptide-like (APOBEC) family. While recognized for its unique role in antiviral immunity, these enzymes have been shown to be dysregulated in various malignancies as they can introduce mutations in genomic DNA. Elevated levels of APOBEC3G have been associated with poor prognosis and high tumor grade [38]. Further, this protein has been shown to upregulate immune checkpoints (e.g., PD-L1, CTLA4, and PD-1) to facilitate an immunosuppressive environment for tumor progression [38, 39]. Xu et al. found that high APOBEC3B expression is an independent predictor of cancer recurrence in patients with ccRCC and has positive prognostic value in those with low-risk disease [39].

Papillary Renal Cell Carcinoma

Papillary renal cell carcinoma (pRCC) is the second most common subtype of renal cell carcinoma and is characterized by distinct genetic and molecular features (Table 2.1). pRCC is a heterogeneous disease consisting of two main subtypes that vary in disease progression and patient outcomes. Type 1 pRCC is characterized by papillae and tubular structures surrounded by small cells containing basophilic cytoplasm and small nuclei. Genetically, type 1 pRCC often involves mutations in the MET proto-oncogene located on chromosome 7q31. MET mutations promote dysregulation of the MET tyrosine kinase receptor, leading to the abnormal activation of downstream pathways, including the PI3K/AKT/mTOR pathway, which drives tumor growth and survival [40, 41] (Table 2.2).

Type 2 pRCC is more heterogeneous and is characterized by large cells containing eosinophilic cytoplasm and large spherical nuclei. A significant subset of type 2 pRCC is associated with alterations in the fumarate hydratase (FH) gene and the NRF2-ARE pathway, and has been associated with more aggressive behavior and poorer outcomes. Loss of FH function leads to the accumulation of fumarate, which subsequently causes the activation of HIF pathways. Type 2 pRCC has also been associated with mutations in chromatin remodeling genes, namely SETD2 and CDKN2A. Currently, very little is known about the genetic basis of pRCC, and there are currently no effective forms of

Table 2.1 Genetic changes and pathways involved in renal cell carcinoma subtypes

Subtype	Common genetic changes	Distinctive features
Clear cell RCC (ccRCC)	VHL, PBRM1, BAP1, SETD2	High HIF1a activity, angiogenesis-driven
Papillary RCC (pRCC) type 1	MET mutation	MET pathway activation, less aggressive
Papillary RCC (pRCC) type 2	FH mutation, CDKN2A, SETD2, NRF2-ARE pathway alterations	HIF pathway activation, more aggressive
Chromophobe RCC (ChRCC)	FLCN mutation, TP53 mutation, PTEN mutation	Loss of multiple chromosomes, favorable prognosis

VHL von Hippel-Lindau, *HIF* hypoxia-inducible factor, *PBRM* protein polybromo, *BAP* BRCA-associated protein, *SETD* SET domain containing, *MET* mesenchymal–epithelial transition, *FH* fumarate hydratase, *CDKN* cyclin-dependent kinase inhibitor, *NRF* nuclear factor erythroid-related factor, *ARE* antioxidant responsive element, *FLCN* folliculin, *TP53* tumor protein 53, *PTEN* phosphatase and tensin homolog

Table 2.2 Role of key genetic changes and pathways affected in progression of clear cell renal cell carcinoma

Genetic change	Pathway	Role in metastasis
VHL mutation	VHL-HIF1a pathway	Stabilizes HIF1a, upregulates angiogenesis, and tumor progression
PBRM1 mutation	Chromatin remodeling (SWI/SNF complex)	Modulates cellular proliferation, associated with advanced tumor stages
BAP1 mutation	Chromatin remodeling (PR-DUB complex)	Linked to poor cancer-specific survival and aggressive disease
SETD2 mutation	Epigenetic regulation (histone H3 methylation)	Impacts chromatin stability and transcription regulation
MET mutation	MET tyrosine kinase receptor pathway	Promotes tumor growth via dysregulation of downstream signaling
FH mutation	Krebs cycle/HIF1a pathway	Drives HIF1a activation through fumarate accumulation

VHL von Hippel-Lindau, *HIF* hypoxia-inducible factor, *SWI/SNF* switch/sucrose nonfermentable *PR-DUB* polycomb repressive deubiquitinase, *MET* mesenchymal–epithelial transition

treatment for patients with advanced disease. Despite advances in understanding the molecular mechanisms underlying pRCC, there remains the need for further research to determine how these molecular alterations can be targeted therapeutically to improve patient outcomes [40–43].

Chromophobe Renal Cell Carcinoma

Chromophobe RCC (ChRCC) is a less common subtype that arises from the intercalated cells of the renal collecting duct and is characterized histologically by large polygonal cells with eosinophilic cytoplasm often forming solid sheets [44]. Clinically, ChRCC is often diagnosed as a localized disease and carries a relatively favorable prognosis, although metastatic disease can occur [44]. Genetically, ChRCC is distinguished from other types of RCC by loss of entire chromosomes or large segments of chromosomes 1, 2, 6, 10, 17, and 21 [11, 44]. ChRCC can occur sporadically but is associated with several hereditary syndromes. It occurs with germline mutation of the FLCN gene in Birt-Hogg-Dubé syndrome, where the inactivation of the FLCN gene results in the upregulation of the mTOR pathway. FLCN-related CRCC typically display less aggressive behaviors and thus intervention is not indicated for tumors sized below 3 cm [45]. ChRCC has also been linked to tuberous sclerosis complex involving mutations in the TSC1 and TSC2 genes. Mutations in the TP53 and PTEN genes have also been commonly observed [45–47]. ChRCC has a distinct metabolic profile as it retains oxidative phosphorylation as its primary energy source. Recent research reveals that alterations in mitochondrial DNA, particularly those affecting the electron transport chain, may contribute to this unique characteristic [45, 48].

Clinical Applications of Renal Cell Carcinoma Genomic Characterization

Tyrosine Kinase Inhibitors

Insights into the genomic characterization of RCC have revolutionized the treatment landscape for RCC and enabled more precise targeting of molecular pathways. The advent of sunitinib (Sutent) was a landmark discovery as it introduced targeted therapy for cases of advanced RCC. Sunitinib is a tyrosine kinase inhibitor (TKI), targeting VEGF and PDGF pathways. As such, sunitinib effectively disrupts tumor angiogenesis and growth by inhibiting these key pathways [49]. Phase III clinical trials demonstrated its efficacy in improving progression-free survival and overall survival in metastatic RCC, as well as a higher response rate compared to interferon-a [49]. This effectiveness, coupled with its favorable toxicity profile, has solidified sunitinib's role as a cornerstone in RCC therapy. However, treatment resistance to sunitinib presents a major challenge, typically occurring within 6–15 months of treatment [49]. The mechanism behind resistance involves the upregulation of compensatory angiogenic pathways, changes in the tumor microenvironment, and genetic mutations in the VEGFR or PDGFR signaling pathways [49, 50]. As one of the earliest targeted therapies approved for RCC, sunitinib remains the best-characterized treatment in terms of its mechanism of action and treatment resistance, and importantly, it has laid the foundation for ongoing RCC therapy advancements [49–51].

Immune Checkpoint Inhibitors

The integration of immune checkpoint inhibitors (ICIs) as a treatment option for RCC has also emerged as another key treatment strategy. Tumors evade immune destruction by exploiting immune checkpoint pathways, such as the PD-1/PD-L1 and CTLA-4 axes. By blocking these pathways, immune checkpoint inhibitors restore T-cell activity and promote an antitumor immune response. Nivolumab, an anti-PD-1 agent, and ipilimumab, an anti-CTLA-4 agent, have demonstrated clinical efficacy. In treating ccRCC, a combination regimen of nivolumab and Ipilimumab has shown improved overall survival and objective response rates compared to sunitinib [50]. Dual combinations of ICIs and TKIs have also been evaluated in various clinical trials and demonstrated superior outcomes compared to monotherapy. Pembrolizumab (anti-PD-1) combined with axitinib (TKI) showed improved progression-free survival and overall survival compared to sunitinib monotherapy [50, 51]. The combination of nivolumab and cabozantinib (TKI) demonstrated a significant overall survival benefit with responses observed even in poor-risk patients. This regimen was also associated with a more favorable toxicity profile [50, 51].

Advances in Molecular Profiling

Circulating tumor DNA (ctDNA) represents an emerging biomarker in RCC that offers a novel method of managing RCC through real-time, noninvasive molecular profiling. ctDNA is a fragment of DNA released into the bloodstream from tumor cells that are typically shed as a result of tumor cell death. ctDNA has been shown to have high sensitivity in detecting mutations frequently altered in RCC, such as VHL, PBRM1, and TP53. In addition to detecting genetic mutations, ctDNA also has the ability to detect epigenetic modifications and has the potential to serve as biomarkers for early detection and prognosis. Specifically, ctDNA assays have been shown to be effective in detecting RCC-specific methylation patterns in early-stage disease. Unlike traditional biopsies, ctDNA reflects real-time changes, which may be utilized to track tumor response to therapy and detect the development of resistance during treatment [50, 52].

The current understanding of the molecular diversity of RCC can be further enhanced by consideration of population-specific genetic variations. Patients of African ancestry are found to have a lower frequency of VHL and PBRM1 mutations, hallmark alterations in clear cell RCC (ccRCC) but exhibit a higher prevalence of BAP1 mutations, which are typically associated with more aggressive disease. Patients of European ancestry have higher frequencies of VHL mutations and chromosome 3p loss. These molecular differences are reflected in clinical presentations, with patients of African ancestry more likely to exhibit non-clear cell RCC histologies and higher-risk disease profiles at the time of diagnosis [53].

Conclusion

RCC is a heterogeneous cancer with diverse histologic subtypes, genetics, and molecular alterations that influence disease behavior and treatment responses. Molecular profiling has significantly enhanced our understanding of RCC and contributed to more targeted and effective therapeutic strategies. Due to its complexity and heterogeneity, RCC remains an active area of investigation with an increasing number of reported ongoing clinical trials aimed at developing and refining treatment options, which has been largely driven by the field of medical oncology. This underscores the need for broader multidisciplinary engagement within urology and knowledge of recent genomic advances to optimize patient outcomes in RCC.

References

1. Bahadoram S, Davoodi M, Hassanzadeh S, Bahadoram M, Barahman M, Mafakher L. Renal cell carcinoma: an overview of the epidemiology, diagnosis, and treatment. G Ital Nefrol. 2022;39(3):2022-vol3.
2. Padala SA, Barsouk A, Thandra KC, et al. Epidemiology of renal cell carcinoma. World J Oncol. 2020;11(3):79–87. https://doi.org/10.14740/wjon1279.
3. Ikuerowo S, Ojewuyi O, Omisanjo O, Abolarinwa A, Bioku M, Doherty A. Paraneoplastic syndromes and oncological outcomes in renal cancer. Niger J Clin Pract. 2019;22(9):1271. https://doi.org/10.4103/njcp.njcp_35_19.
4. Hsieh JJ, Purdue MP, Signoretti S, et al. Renal cell carcinoma. Nat Rev Dis Primers. 2017;3(1):17009. https://doi.org/10.1038/nrdp.2017.9.
5. Vankayala H, Shi D, Vaishampayan U. Renal cell carcinoma: clinical presentation, staging, and prognostic factors. In: Lara Jr P, Jonasch E, editors. Kidney cancer. Berlin: Springer; 2012. https://doi.org/10.1007/978-3-642-21858-35.
6. Hsieh JJ, Manley BJ, Khan N, Gao J, Carlo MI, Cheng EH. Overcome tumor heterogeneity-imposed therapeutic barriers through convergent genomic biomarker discovery: a braided cancer river model of kidney cancer. Semin Cell Dev Biol. 2016;64:98–106. https://doi.org/10.1016/j.semcdb.2016.09.002.
7. Clark PE, Cookson MS. The von Hippel-Lindau gene. Cancer. 2008;113(S7):1768–78. https://doi.org/10.1002/cncr.23645.
8. Büscheck F, Fraune C, Simon R, Kluth M, Hube-Magg C, Möller-Koop C, Sarper I, Ketterer K, Henke T, Eichelberg C, Dahlem R, Wilczak W, Sauter G, Fisch M, Eichenauer T, Rink M. Prevalence and clinical significance of VHL mutations and 3p25 deletions in renal tumor subtypes. Oncotarget. 2020;11(3):237–49. https://doi.org/10.18632/oncotarget.27428.
9. Zbar B, Brauch H, Talmadge C, Linehan M. Loss of alleles of loci on the short arm of chromosome 3 in renal cell carcinoma. Nature. 1987;327(6124):721–4.
10. Klatte T, Pantuck AJ. Molecular biology of renal cortical tumors. Urol Clin N Am. 2008;35(4):573–80. https://doi.org/10.1016/j.ucl.2008.07.006.
11. Huang JJ, Hsieh JJ. The pan-omics landscape of renal cell carcinoma and its implication on future clinical practice. Kidney Cancer. 2020;4(3):121–9. https://doi.org/10.3233/kca-200085.
12. Brugarolas J. Molecular genetics of clear-cell renal cell carcinoma. J Clin Oncol. 2014;32(18):1968–76. https://doi.org/10.1200/jco.2012.45.2003.
13. Varela I, Tarpey P, Raine K, et al. Exome sequencing identifies frequent mutation of the SWI/SNF complex gene PBRM1 in renal carcinoma. Nature. 2011;469(7331):539–42.
14. Gulati S, Martinez P, Joshi T, Birkbak NJ, Santos CR, Rowan AJ, Pickering L, Gore M, Larkin J, Szallasi Z, Bates PA, Swanton C, Gerlinger M. Systematic evaluation of the prognostic impact and intra tumour heterogeneity of clear cell renal cell carcinoma biomarkers. Eur Urol. 2014;66(5):936–48. https://doi.org/10.1016/j.eururo.2014.06.053.
15. Kapur P, Peña-Llopis S, Christie A, Zhrebker L, Pavía-Jiménez A, Rathmell WK, Xie XJ, Brugarolas J. Effects on survival of BAP1 and PBRM1 mutations in sporadic clear-cell renal-cell carcinoma: a retrospective analysis with independent validation. Lancet Oncol. 2013;14(2):159–67. https://doi.org/10.1016/s1470-2045(12)70584-3.
16. Hakimi AA, Ostrovnaya I, Reva B, Schultz N, Chen YB, Gonen M, Liu H, Takeda S, Voss MH, Tickoo SK, Reuter VE, Russo P, Cheng EH, Sander C, Motzer RJ, Hsieh JJ. Adverse outcomes in clear cell renal cell carcinoma with mutations of 3p21 epigenetic regulators BAP1 and SETD2: a report by MSKCC and the KIRC TCGA research network. Clin Cancer Res. 2013;19(12):3259–67. https://doi.org/10.1158/1078-0432.ccr-12-3886.
17. Da Costa WH, Rezende M, Carneiro FC, Rocha RM, Da Cunha IW, Carraro DM, Guimaraes GC, De Cassio ZS. Polybromo-1 (PBRM1), a SWI/SNF complex subunit is a prognostic marker in clear cell renal cell carcinoma. BJU Int. 2013;113(5b):E157. https://doi.org/10.1111/bju.12426.
18. Sato Y, Yoshizato T, Shiraishi Y, Maekawa S, Okuno Y, Kamura T, Shimamura T, Sato-Otsubo A, Nagae G, Suzuki H, Nagata Y, Yoshida K, Kon A, Suzuki Y, Chiba K, Tanaka H, Niida A, Fujimoto A, Tsunoda T, Morikawa T, Maeda D, Kume H, Sugano S, Fukayama M, Aburatani H, Sanada M, Miyano S, Homma Y, Ogawa S. Integrated molecular analysis of clear-cell renal cell carcinoma. Nat Genet. 2013;45(8):860–7. https://doi.org/10.1038/ng.2699.
19. Joseph RW, Kapur P, Serie DJ, et al. Loss of BAP1 protein expression is an independent marker of poor prognosis in patients with low-risk clear cell renal cell carcinoma. Cancer. 2014;120(7):1059–67.
20. Peña-Llopis S, Vega-Rubín-De-Celis S, Liao A, Leng N, Pavía-Jiménez A, Wang S, Yamasaki T, Zhrebker L, Sivanand S, Spence P, Kinch L, Hambuch T, Jain S, Lotan Y, Margulis V, Sagalowsky AI, Summerour PB,

Kabbani W, Wong SWW, Grishin N, Laurent M, Xie XJ, Haudenschild CD, Ross MT, Bentley DR, Kapur P, Brugarolas J. BAP1 loss defines a new class of renal cell carcinoma. Nat Genet. 2012;44(7):751–9. https://doi.org/10.1038/ng.2323.
21. Lenburg ME, Liou LS, Gerry NP, Frampton GM, Cohen HT, Christman MF. Previously unidentified changes in renal cell carcinoma gene expression identified by parametric analysis of microarray data. BMC Cancer. 2003;31(3):1112.
22. Kim JH, Jung CW, Cho YH, et al. Somatic VHL alteration and its impact on prognosis in patients with clear cell renal cell carcinoma. Oncol Rep. 2005;13(5):859–64.
23. Patard J-J, Fergelot P, Karakiewicz PI, et al. Low CAIX expression and absence of VHL gene mutation are associated with tumor aggressiveness and poor survival of clear cell renal cell carcinoma. Int J Cancer. 2008;123(2):395–400.
24. Klatte T, Rao PN, de Martino M, et al. Cytogenetic profile predicts prognosis of patients with clear cell renal cell carcinoma. J Clin Oncol. 2009;27(5):746–53.
25. Kroeger N, Klatte T, Chamie K, et al. Deletions of chromosomes 3p and 14q molecularly subclassify clear cell renal cell carcinoma. Cancer. 2013;119(8):1547–54.
26. Schraml P, Struckmann K, Hatz F, et al. VHL mutations and their correlation with tumour cell proliferation, microvessel density, and patient prognosis in clear cell renal cell carcinoma. J Pathol. 2002;196(2):186–93.
27. Gulati S, Martinez P, Joshi T, et al. Systematic evaluation of the prognostic impact and intratumour heterogeneity of clear cell renal cell carcinoma biomarkers. Eur Urol. 2014;66(5):936–48.
28. Bui MHT, Seligson D, Han K-R, et al. Carbonic anhydrase IX is an independent predictor of survival in advanced renal clear cell carcinoma: implications for prognosis and therapy. Clin Cancer Res. 2003;9(2):802–11.
29. Zhao Z, Liao G, Li Y, Zhou S, Zou H, Fernando S. Prognostic value of carbonic anhydrase IX immunohistochemical expression in renal cell carcinoma: a meta-analysis of the literature. PLoS One. 2014;9(11):e114096.
30. Zerati M, Leite KRM, Pontes-Junior J, et al. Carbonic anhydrase IX is not a predictor of outcomes in non-metastatic clear cell renal cell carcinoma—a digital analysis of tissue microarray. Int Braz J Urol. 2010;39(4):484–92.
31. Chamie K, Klöpfer P, Bevan P, et al. Carbonic anhydrase-IX score is a novel biomarker that predicts recurrence and survival for high-risk, nonmetastatic renal cell carcinoma: data from the phase III ARISER clinical trial. Urol Oncol. 2015;33(5):204.e25–33.
32. Stillebroer AB, Mulders PFA, Boerman OC, Oyen WJG, Oosterwijk E. Carbonic anhydrase IX in renal cell carcinoma: implications for prognosis, diagnosis, and therapy. Eur Urol. 2010;58(1):75–83. https://doi.org/10.1016/j.eururo.2010.03.015.
33. McDermott DF, Cheng S-C, Signoretti S, et al. The high-dose aldesleukin "select" trial: a trial to prospectively validate predictive models of response to treatment in patients with metastatic renal cell carcinoma. Clin Cancer Res. 2015;21(3):561–8.
34. Choueiri TK, Cheng S, Qu AQ, Pastorek J, Atkins MB, Signoretti S. Carbonic anhydrase IX as a potential biomarker of efficacy in metastatic clear-cell renal cell carcinoma patients receiving sorafenib or placebo: analysis from the treatment approaches in renal cancer global evaluation trial (TARGET). Urol Oncol. 2013;31(8):1788–93.
35. Herman JG, Latif F, Weng Y, et al. Silencing of the VHL tumor-suppressor gene by DNA methylation in renal carcinoma. Proc Natl Acad Sci USA. 1994;91(21):9700–4.
36. Modena P, Testi MA, Facchinetti F, et al. UQCRH gene encoding mitochondrial Hinge protein is interrupted by a translocation in a soft-tissue sarcoma and epigenetically inactivated in some cancer cell lines. Oncogene. 2003;22(29):4586–93.
37. Wagner EJ, Carpenter PB. Understanding the language of Lys36 methylation at histone H3. Nat Rev Mol Cell Biol. 2012;13(2):115–26.
38. Peng T, Liu B, Lin S, et al. APOBEC3G expression correlates with unfavorable prognosis and immune infiltration in kidney renal clear cell carcinoma. Heliyon. 2022;8(12):e12191. https://doi.org/10.1016/j.heliyon.2022.e12191.
39. Xu L, Chang Y, An H, Zhu Y, Yang Y, Xu J. High apobec3b expression is a predictor of recurrence in patients with low-risk clear cell renal cell carcinoma. Urol Oncol Sem Orig Invest. 2015;33(8):340.e1–8. https://doi.org/10.1016/j.urolonc.2015.05.009.
40. Delahunt B, Eble JN. Papillary renal cell carcinoma: a clinicopathologic and immunohistochemical study of 105 tumors. Mod Pathol. 1997;10(6):537–44.
41. Cancer Genome Atlas Research Network WM, Linehan WM, Spellman PT, et al. Comprehensive molecular characterization of papillary renal-cell carcinoma. N Engl J Med. 2016;374(2):135–45.
42. Zbar B, Tory K, Merino M, et al. Hereditary papillary renal cell carcinoma. J Urol. 1994;151(3):561–6.
43. Durinck S, Stawiski EW, Pavia-Jimenez A, et al. Spectrum of diverse genomic alterations define non-clear cell renal carcinoma subtypes. Nat Genet. 2015;47(1):13–21.
44. Pezzicoli G, Musci V, Ciciriello F, Salonne F, Cafforio P, Lionetti N, Ragno A, Rizzo M. Genomic profiling and molecular characterization of non-clear cell renal cell carcinoma: a narrative review from a clinical perspective. Ther Adv Med Oncol. 2024;16:17588359241298500. https://doi.org/10.1177/17588359241298500.
45. Yanus GA, Kuligina ES, Imyanitov EN. Hereditary renal cancer syndromes. Med Sci. 2024;12(1):12. https://doi.org/10.3390/medsci12010012.
46. Habib SL, Al-Obaidi NY, Nowacki M, Pietkun K, Zegarska B, Kloskowski T, Zegarski W, Drewa T, Medina EA, Zhao Z, Liang S. Is MTOR inhibi-

tor good enough for treatment all tumors in TSC patients? J Cancer. 2016;7(12):1621–31. https://doi.org/10.7150/jca.14747.
47. Rathmell KW, Chen F, Creighton CJ. Genomics of chromophobe renal cell carcinoma: implications from a rare tumor for pan-cancer studies. Oncoscience. 2015;2(2):81–90. https://doi.org/10.18632/oncoscience.130.
48. Garje R, Elhag D, Yasin HA, Acharya L, Vaena D, Dahmoush L. Comprehensive review of chromophobe renal cell carcinoma. Crit Rev Oncol Hematol. 2021;160:103287. https://doi.org/10.1016/j.critrevonc.2021.103287.
49. Jin J, Xie Y, Zhang JS, Wang JQ, Dai SJ, He WF, Li SY, Ashby CR, Chen ZS, He Q. Sunitinib resistance in renal cell carcinoma: from molecular mechanisms to predictive biomarkers. Drug Resist Updat. 2023;67:100929. https://doi.org/10.1016/j.drup.2023.100929.
50. Srivastava A, Doppalapudi SK, Patel HV, Srinivasan R, Singer EA. The roaring 2020s: a new decade of systemic therapy for renal cell carcinoma. Curr Opin Oncol. 2022;34(3):234–42. https://doi.org/10.1097/cco.0000000000000831.
51. Huang JJ, Hsieh JJ. The therapeutic landscape of renal cell carcinoma: from the dark age to the Golden age. Semin Nephrol. 2020;40(1):28–41. https://doi.org/10.1016/j.semnephrol.2019.12.004.
52. Gerke MB, Jansen CS, Bilen MA. Circulating tumor DNA in genitourinary cancers: detection, prognostics, and therapeutic implications. Cancers. 2024;16(12):2280. https://doi.org/10.3390/cancers16122280.
53. Kotecha RR, Knezevic A, Arora K, Bandlamudi C, Kuo F, Carlo MI, Fitzgerald KN, Feldman DR, Shah NJ, Reznik E, Hakimi AA, Carrot-Zhang J, Mandelker D, Berger M, Lee C, Motzer RJ, Voss MH. Genomic ancestry in kidney cancer: correlations with clinical and molecular features. Cancer. 2023;130(5):692–701. https://doi.org/10.1002/cncr.35074.

Familial and Hereditary Syndromes in Renal Cell Cancer

3

Mark W. Ball, Jaskirat Saini, and Peter A. Pinto

Introduction

Kidney cancer—Familial and hereditary syndromes is a heterogeneous group of diseases that are clinically, genetically, and morphologically distinct. Currently, the World Health Organization recognizes 16 subtypes of renal cell carcinoma (RCC) [1], and up to 12 hereditary conditions have been identified with increased lifetime risk of developing renal tumors [2]. Together, the different forms of RCC will be diagnosed in almost 74,000 persons and lead to 15,000 deaths in the United States in 2019 [3].

Hereditary kidney cancer is thought to represent around 5% of kidney cancer cases [2]; however, the true incidence may be higher due in part to limitations in understanding the role of cancer susceptibility genes in RCC. Upward of 25% of kidney cancer cases have multifocal tumor involvement [4, 5]. Furthermore, a multigenerational study of Icelandic people indicated that 58% of RCC cases thought to be sporadic occur in patients with one or more family members with RCC, supporting the notion that far more cases of seemingly sporadic RCC are actually hereditary in origin [6].

Clinicians treating patients must recognize the hereditary syndromes, as their management strategies can differ from one another as well as differ from sporadic kidney cancer treatment paradigms. Specific management strategies have been developed to provide oncologic control and maximize kidney function in this population. It is not uncommon that patients with a hereditary syndrome are not recognized either due to unfamiliarity, incomplete penetrance, poor family history, or the development of de novo mutations—any of which can mislead clinicians with limited experience with these patients. Recognizing these syndromes and understanding their genetics directly translates in how patients are managed both in terms of local disease management with surgery [7] and advanced disease management with systemic therapy [8].

Clinical Features of Hereditary RCC and Genetic Testing

All physicians involved in the treatment of patients with cancer have the responsibility to consider if a patient may benefit from genetic counseling and initiate the referral process. Some individuals may present with a known family history of a hereditary syndrome, which may simplify the genetic workup. These individuals still benefit from appropriate counseling to ensure they are appropriately diagnosed. A provider cannot assume that a cancer in an affected organ

M. W. Ball (✉) · J. Saini · P. A. Pinto
Urologic Oncology Branch, Center for Cancer Research, National Cancer Institute, National Institutes of Health Clinical Center, Bethesda, MD, USA
e-mail: mark.ball@nih.gov; jaskirat.saini@nih.gov; pintop@mail.nih.gov

J. A. Libertino, J. R. Gee (eds.), *Renal Cancer*, https://doi.org/10.1007/978-3-031-97599-8_3

means that an individual is affected. For these individuals, knowledge of the family mutation can greatly limit the costs of genetic testing. Rather than test multiple genes and do whole exome sequencing, a genetic counselor can perform an analysis of the region of interest.

Many patients may present with a previously undiagnosed hereditary RCC syndrome. While they may represent a de novo mutation, other factors may have limited prior diagnosis in affected first-degree relatives, including poor family history, incomplete penetrance, and unrecognized features. Specific features should raise the suspicion of a clinician for hereditary syndrome (Table 3.1). Bilateral, multifocal tumors that occur at an early age of onset are key features of hereditary RCC syndromes. Dermatologic manifestations are common to

Table 3.1 Hereditary kidney cancer syndromes

Name	Gene	RCC histology	Non-renal manifestations	Preferred surgical approach	Surveillance
Von Hippel-Lindau (VHL)	*VHL* (3p25)	Clear cell RCC, cystic RCC	CNS hemangioblastomas, retinal angiomas, pancreatic neuroendocrine tumors and cysts, epididymal/broad ligament cyst adenomas, pheochromocytoma	Enucleation	Until largest tumor reaches 3 cm
Hereditary papillary renal carcinoma (HPRC)	*MET* (7q34)	Type 1 papillary RCC	None	Enucleation	Until largest tumor reaches 3 cm
Birt-Hogg-Dube (BHD)	*FLCN* (17p11.2)	Chromophobe RCC, oncocytoma, hybrid oncocytic tumors	Cutaneous fibrofolliculomas, lung cysts, spontaneous pneumothorax	Enucleation	Until largest tumor reaches 3 cm
Hereditary leiomyomatosis and renal cell carcinoma	*FH* (1q42)	Type 2 papillary RCC	Cutaneous leiomyomas Uterine leiomyomas	Partial nephrectomy with wide excision; consider lymphadenectomy	No surveillance
Succinate dehydrogenase-deficient RCC	*SDHB (1p36), SDHC (1q21), SDHD (11q23)*	SDHB: Oncocytic RCC SDHC/D: Clear cell RCC	Pheochromocytomas, paragangliomas, gastrointestinal stromal tumors	Partial nephrectomy with wide excision; consider lymphadenectomy	No surveillance
BAP1-associated RCC	*BAP1* (3p21)	Clear cell RCC	Benign melanocytic tumors, malignant uveal and cutaneous melanoma, and malignant mesothelioma	Partial nephrectomy with wide excision	No surveillance
MITF family translocation RCC	*TFE3 (Xp11), TFEB (6p21), MITF (3p13)*	Various RCC histologies	MITF: Melanoma	Partial nephrectomy with wide excision.	No surveillance
Tuberous sclerosis complex (TSC)	*TSC1* (9q34) *TSC2* (16p13)	Angiomyolipomas, RCC, renal cysts	Facial angiofibromas, ungual/periungual fibroma, shagreen patch, retinal hamartomas, subependymal nodule, cortical hamartoma	Enucleation	RCC: Until the largest tumor reaches 3 cm. AML: Surveillance until 4 cm or symptomatic
Familial translocation RCC	Chromosome 3 translocation	Clear cell RCC	None	Enucleation	Until largest tumor reaches 3 cm

several of the cancer syndromes. Evaluation by an experienced dermatologist can often aid genetic testing. Detailed family history on both the maternal and paternal sides should note which family members had a history of RCC and denote the age of onset. Prior personal and family past medical history should note the presence of benign and malignant tumors in organs such as the brain, spine, pancreas, small and large bowel, adrenal, uterus, breast, and eyes. A perceptive clinician with knowledge of the various hereditary conditions can be critical to a successful diagnosis. Besides assisting with the case of the individual patient, a family diagnosis can help all members of that lineage.

Description of Hereditary Syndromes

Von Hippel-Lindau

VHL is an autosomal dominant inherited multisystem disorder that affects 1:35,000 individuals. Affected patients are predisposed to develop kidney tumors, kidney cysts, pheochromocytomas and paragangliomas, pancreatic neuroendocrine tumors, pancreatic cysts and islet cell tumors, hemangioblastomas of the central nervous system and retina, endolymphatic sac tumors, and cystadenomas of the epididymis and broad ligament (Fig. 3.1) [9]. Linkage analysis of families

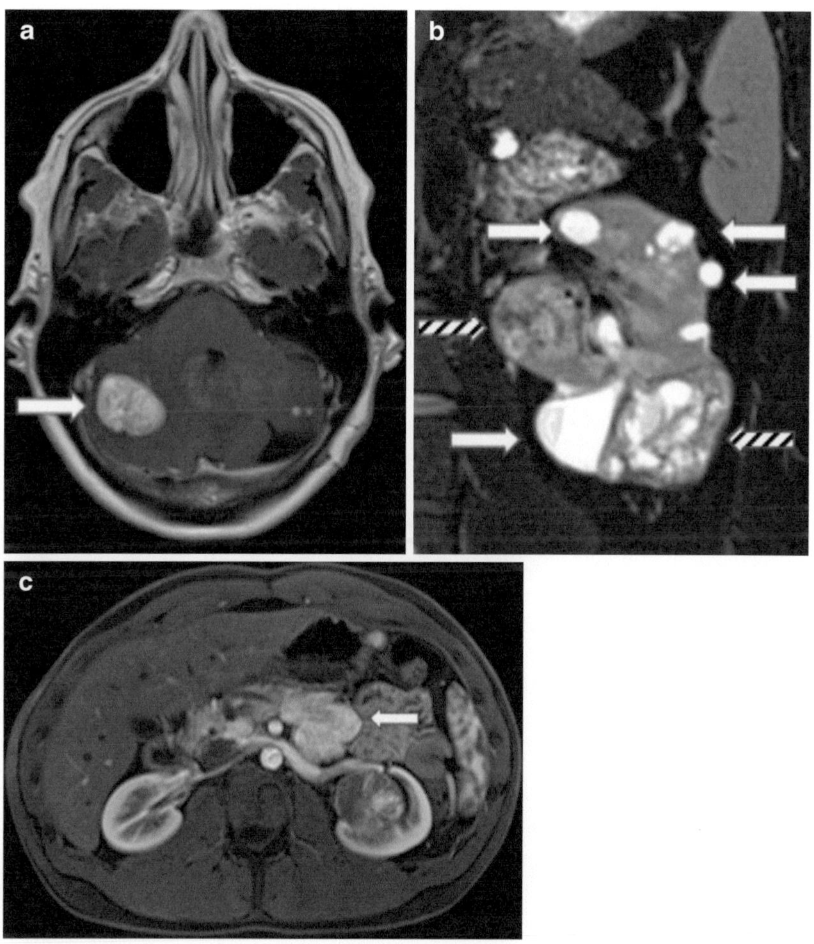

Fig. 3.1 VHL-associated lesions: (**a**) cerebellar hemangioblastoma, (**b**) multifocal kidney tumors (striped arrows) and cysts (white arrows), and (**c**) pancreatic neuroendocrine tumor

with VHL identified a novel gene at chromosome 3p25 [10]. *VHL* was identified as a tumor suppressor gene in which both copies of the gene are inactivated to drive tumorigenesis. Nearly all VHL-associated renal tumors demonstrate loss of chromosome 3p or somatic "second hit" *VHL* mutations [11, 12]. VHL patients inherit one mutant copy of the gene, and then the second, functional copy is damaged or lost, leading to tumorigenesis. As a result of improved mutation detection methods enabling a nearly 100% detection rate, germline *VHL* mutations have been identified in over 900 families worldwide who present with >200 different mutations [9, 13, 14].

Approximately 25–60% of patients with VHL develop bilateral, multifocal renal lesions consisting of cysts and clear cell RCC [15]. While cysts are considered benign in sporadically occurring patients, they are often lined with malignant tissue in patients with VHL and should be removed at the time of surgery [16]. Prior to the current management recommendations, a third of patients died of metastatic RCC [15, 17]. With proper screening, recommended with ultrasounds beginning in childhood, renal lesions are identified early, and treatment can prevent the development of metastatic disease [15]. The historic management of those with multifocal RCC included bilateral radical nephrectomy with hemodialysis. The past two decades have seen the emergence of patients having been managed with repeat partial nephrectomy.

Management of VHL-associated renal tumors is focused on preventing metastasis while preserving the renal function. To that end, our institutional practice has been to perform active surveillance when tumors are less than 3 cm in diameter and resecting all ipsilateral tumors with a nephron-sparing approach once the largest tumor has reached 3 cm [18]. Considering the multiple small tumors and the need to preserve normal renal parenchyma, enucleation of the tumors is used and has been demonstrated to be a safe surgical technique [19]. In general, the overarching goal of the surgeon is to "reset the clock," meaning to remove as many lesions as possible in one surgery in an attempt to prolong the interval between ipsilateral renal surgeries. Toward that end, all solid and complex lesions are removed with frequent intraoperative ultrasound being utilized to localize and ensure complete removal of all tumors.

Hereditary Papillary Renal Cell

Hereditary papillary renal carcinoma (HPRC) is a rare, autosomal dominant inherited disorder in which affected individuals are at risk to develop bilateral, multifocal type 1 papillary renal carcinoma [20]. Germline mutations in the *MET* proto-oncogene located at 7q31 were identified in the germline of individuals affected with HPRC by linkage analysis [21–23].

HPRC-associated renal tumors are characterized by "incipient lesions" in the apparently "normal" surrounding kidney parenchyma, with an estimation of >3000 of these microscopic papillary tumors in a single kidney that suggest multiple, independent, early events [24, 25]. HPRC patients are at risk of developing renal tumors during the fifth and sixth decades of life [22, 26]; however, early-onset HPRC families have also been reported [27]. Age-dependent penetrance has been estimated at 67% by the age of 60 years, with complete penetrance by 80 years of age [22]. Fewer than 40 families with HPRC have been reported to date, underscoring the rarity of this inherited renal cancer syndrome.

HPRC lesions are often hypoechoic to renal parenchyma and may be poorly enhancing. Hypoenhancing CT lesions can be confused with hyperdense cysts. MRI may be more useful than CT scans for detecting and monitoring HPRC renal lesions. Similar to the approach with patients affected with VHL, active surveillance until the largest renal tumor reaches the 3-cm threshold is recommended for management of patients affected with HPRC. Nephron-sparing surgical approaches are recommended for HPRC-associated renal tumors, as HPRC renal tumors tend to be bilateral and multifocal, and numerous surgical procedures may be required to treat recurrent tumors.

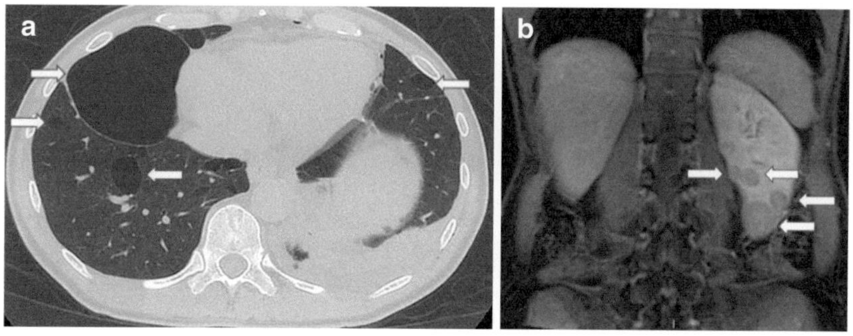

Fig. 3.2 BHD-associated lesions: (**a**) lung cysts, (**b**) multifocal renal masses

Birt-Hogg-Dubé

Birt-Hogg-Dubé (BHD) is an autosomal dominant inherited cancer syndrome in which patients are at risk for developing benign hair follicle hamartomas (fibrofolliculomas), multiple and bilateral pulmonary cysts, spontaneous pneumothorax, and renal tumors (Fig. 3.2) [28, 29]. The most common manifestations of BHD, fibrofolliculomas, and lung cysts occur in >83% of affected individuals and tend to develop after puberty [29–31]. Approximately 24–38% of BHD-affected individuals will experience at least one spontaneous pneumothorax event during their lifetime with a median age of occurrence of 38 years [29–31]. BHD-affected individuals have a 6.9-fold greater risk for developing renal tumors compared to unaffected family members [29]. Bilateral, multifocal renal tumors have been reported to develop in 29–34% of BHD-affected patients [30, 31], but this rate may reflect ascertainment bias since the frequency of renal tumors was considerably lower in other BHD cohorts [32]. The median age of renal tumor diagnosis is 48–51 years [29, 30]. BHD-associated renal tumors may present with variable histologies, including hybrid oncocytic tumors (50%) that contain features of chromophobe renal cancer and oncocytoma, chromophobe renal carcinoma (34%), clear cell renal carcinoma (9%), and oncocytoma (5%) [33]. Renal tumors with different histologies can arise even in a single kidney of a BHD patient. Microscopic oncocytic lesions ("oncocytosis") can be seen scattered throughout the "normal" renal parenchyma of most patients and may represent precursors of BHD-associated renal tumors [33].

Patients with BHD often have imaging of their kidneys starting from the age of 20–25 years [34]. Abdominal imaging every 3 years is recommended for affected individuals with no renal masses. In recommending the frequency of imaging for individuals with renal masses, the urologic oncologic surgeon takes into consideration the tumor size, location, and growth rate. Renal ultrasound is not recommended as the sole modality for screening. As with VHL and HPRC, it is recommended that BHD-associated tumors be monitored until the largest tumor reaches the 3-cm threshold, at which time surgical intervention is recommended [7, 34]. As BHD patients are at risk for the development of bilateral, multifocal tumors, partial nephrectomy is recommended whenever possible.

Hereditary Leiomyomatosis and Renal Cell

Hereditary leiomyomatosis and renal cell carcinoma (HLRCC) is a familial cancer syndrome associated with cutaneous leiomyomas, uterine leiomyomas, macronodular adrenal hyperplasia, and type II papillary kidney cancer [35–38] (Fig. 3.3). Cutaneous leiomyoma is a common clinical feature that can occur on the arms or trunk. Kidney cancer, which presents in approximately 10–15% of HLRCC patients, may be soli-

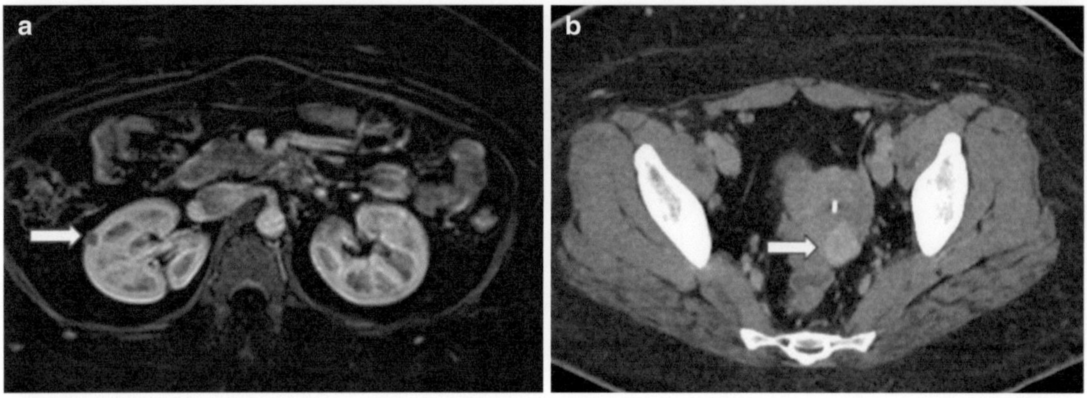

Fig. 3.3 HLRCC-associated lesions: (**a**) small papillary type 2 tumor, (**b**) uterine leiomyoma

tary, multifocal, and/or bilateral. These tumors have the potential to spread, even when tumors are small (0.5–2 cm) [36, 39, 40]. These type 2 papillary tumors demonstrate a distinct histologic staining pattern that is characterized by cells with abundant eosinophilic cytoplasm and a large nucleus containing prominent inclusion-like eosinophilic nucleoli surrounded by perinucleolar halos [36].

HLRCC is characterized by an autosomal dominant inheritance pattern and is associated with germline mutation of the *FH* gene at chromosome 1p42.1 gene which encodes the Krebs cycle enzyme, fumarate hydratase [39–41]. Somatic loss of the remaining functional "wild-type" copy of *FH* is observed within HLRCC renal tumors resulting in biallelic loss of fumarate hydratase activity. Inactivation of this enzyme leads to a metabolic shift to aerobic glycolysis with decreased oxidative phosphorylation.

The initial experience with these tumors was much different than the other hereditary RCC syndromes with patients having an extremely aggressive disease. Over half of the patients in the initial series demonstrated regional or distant disease even when associated with small renal primaries [37]. Peripheral renal cysts or lesions too small to characterize are common in these patients. When not monitored closely, we have observed individuals develop disseminated disease.

It is recommended that HLRCC patients undergo annual abdominal screening by contrast-enhanced CT or MRI. Our practice is to recommend lifelong annual imaging beginning at age 8. Because patients affected with HLRCC are at risk for the development of bilateral renal tumors over their lifetime, nephron-sparing approaches are recommended when possible. HLRCC-associated renal tumors have an invasive growth pattern and an open surgical procedure with intraoperative ultrasound and a wide surgical margin and ipsilateral hilar lymphadenectomy is recommended. In contradistinction to the recommended management, approach for many VHL-, HPRC-, and BHD-associated renal tumors, active surveillance is not recommended for HLRCC-associated renal tumors [34, 42].

Succinate Dehydrogenase-Deficient Kidney Cancer

Succinate dehydrogenase-deficient kidney cancer is associated with and seen as a part of familial paraganglioma/pheochromocytoma. It is an inherited cancer syndrome associated with an increased risk for pheochromocytoma, paraganglioma, gastrointestinal stromal tumor, and renal cell carcinoma. This syndrome demonstrates an autosomal dominant inheritance pattern and is associated with germline mutations within one of four succinate dehydrogenase complex subunit genes: *SDHA*, *SDHB*, *SDHC*, and *SDHD* or a succinate dehydrogenase complex assembly factor, *SDHAF2* [43]. Germline mutation in all five genes has been associated with the development of bilateral or multifocal pheochromocytomas or paragangliomas, while succinate dehydrogenase-deficient renal cell carcinoma (SDH-RCC) has been associated with germline mutation of SDHB, SDHC, and SDHD. SDH-RCC can be aggressive and patients have demonstrated locally advanced or disseminated disease when tumors are still relatively small (1–2 cm) [43]. These tumors demonstrate a variety of histologic staining patterns including clear cell and oncocytic neoplastic patterns [43, 44].

The current clinical practice at the National Cancer Institute involves annual imaging with enhanced CT or MRI. These patients are monitored and managed in a similar fashion as the HLRCC patients since even small renal SDH-RCC masses have been known to metastasize [43]. As these tumors are considered aggressive, active surveillance is not recommended. Nephron-sparing approaches, with wide surgical margin, are recommended when possible [7, 34].

BAP1-Associated RCC

BAP1-associated RCC is seen as a part of *BRCA1-associated protein-1 (BAP1)*-associated tumor predisposition syndrome. It is an autosomal dominant inherited disorder in which patients are at risk for the development of benign melanocytic tumors, malignant uveal and cutaneous melanoma, malignant mesothelioma, and RCC. RCC can develop in ~10% of *BAP1* mutation carriers and is associated with an aggressive clear cell RCC [45]. Several families with *BAP1* germline mutations have been reported in which renal cell carcinoma is the only manifestation [46, 47].

The potentially aggressive nature of BAP1-associated tumors requires individualized management. It is recommended that patients with germline BAP1 alteration have annual abdominal imaging to evaluate for the presence of renal tumors. Because of the potential aggressive nature of these tumors and the lack of long-term outcomes in these patients, active surveillance is not currently recommended. Nephron-sparing surgery, depending on the tumor size and location, is recommended when possible. Patients affected by germline mutation of the *BAP1* gene are at risk for the development of bilateral, multifocal, and recurrent renal tumors, and preservation of renal function is recommended whenever possible [7, 34, 48].

MITF Family Translocation RCC

The microphthalmia-associated transcription factor (MiTF) family of genes includes TFE3, TFEB, and MITF. Members of this transcription factor family share similar protein structures and drive the transcription of similar genes. TFE3 and TFEB RCCs are caused by somatic chromosomal translocations, while MITF RCC is caused by a germline mutation, and together RCC that develops as a result of these alterations is referred to as MITF family translocation RCC. Translocation RCCs are defined as a histologically variable subtype of sporadic RCCs and make up approximately 1–5% of RCC tumors [49].

TFE3 is on the X chromosome at Xp11, and TFE3 RCC is said to account for 20–45% of renal tumors in children and young adults [50]. Xp11 translocation tumors can show a wide spectrum of morphology. Histologically, tumors frequently display a papillary architecture formed by clear cells with granular eosinophilic cytoplasm. TFE3 RCC can spread when the tumors are small (2 cm) and, like HLRCC- and SDH-associated RCC, active surveillance is not recommended for TFE3 or TFEB translocation RCC. TFE3-fusion RCCs have been seen with late-onset metastasis, which makes a long clinical follow-up necessary [50].

TFEB-translocation RCC is less common than TFE3 RCC and involves chromosome 6p21. Histologically, TFEB-fusion RCCs typically present with a biphasic microscopic architecture, characterized by large, epithelioid cells with clear and eosinophilic cytoplasm (mimicking ccRCC) and small, eosinophilic cells with hyperchromatic nuclei forming rosette-like structures [50].

MITF RCC is associated with a germline missense mutation of MITF (p.E318K). Affected patients have a more than fivefold increased risk to develop RCC and co-occurrence of RCC and melanoma [51]. The p.E318K mutant MITF protein is affected by impaired sumoylation, differentially regulates DNA binding, and drives enhanced transcriptional activity of genes involved in cell growth, proliferation, and inflammation. This may explain the oncogenic role of the MITF p.E318K mutation [51].

Because TFE3 and TFEB alterations are not hereditary, associated RCCs are often not recognized until the time of surgery. Partial nephrectomy is acceptable in this population [52], although the safety of enucleation for these tumors is unknown. Management of germline MITF-altered RCC is currently unknown, but we do not currently advocate active surveillance in this population.

Tuberous Sclerosis Complex

Tuberous sclerosis complex (TSC) is a multisystem, autosomal dominant inherited hamartomatous disorder affecting both adults and children. Affected individuals are predisposed to develop a variety of skin lesions, including facial angiofibromas, hypopigmented macules, shagreen patches, and ungual fibromas that are detected in more than 90% of affected individuals. Pulmonary lymphangioleiomyomatosis characterized by proliferation of abnormal smooth muscle cells and cystic changes in the lung affects adolescent girls and women with TSC. Cerebral cortex tubers develop in >80% of TSC patients and can lead to a number of neurologic manifestations, including epilepsy, cognitive disability, and neuro-behavioral abnormalities. Bilateral, multifocal renal angiomyolipomas, which are benign tumors of the kidney consisting of abnormal vessels, immature smooth muscle cells, and fat cells, develop in an estimated 55–75% of TSC patients occurring as early as 10 years of age [53]. Additionally, renal cell carcinomas with a variety of histologies may develop in TSC-affected individuals. Although the lifetime risk is similar to the general population (2–3%), the age of onset of renal tumor in TSC patients is younger, an average age of 36 years in one study [53, 54]. In addition to AMLs, patients with TSC are also at an increased risk to develop RCC.

Renal management of TSC is aimed at renal function preservation. AMLs greater than 4 cm may be at risk for spontaneous bleeding, although some studies suggest a bleeding risk for 3-cm lesions [55]. Historically embolization has been used; however, recent advances in microwave ablation have also shown successful treatment of AMLs with this method [56]. Renal AMLs may be seen in up to 75% of patients with TSC and can develop in patients as young as 10 years old. The main differential for solid lesions in this population includes fat-poor AML and RCC.

Intense effort is underway to develop a systemic therapeutic approach for patients with TSC-associated renal masses. In 2008, a clinical trial of sirolimus in patients with TSC-associated AML showed encouraging results, and this area remains very promising for future research [57].

Chromosome 3 Translocation Kidney Cancer

The identification of a family with recurrent multifocal clear cell kidney cancer without VHL identified a different genetic alteration involving chromosome 3: a balanced germline translocation t(3;8)(p14;q24) [58]. Subsequently, germline chromosome 3 translocations have been identified involving chromosomes 1, 2, 4, 6, and 8 [59, 60]. Histologically, familial translocation tumors are similar to VHL-associated RCC tumors, and patients are at risk for the development of bilateral and multifocal RCC. The average age of onset is later than in VHL, in the fourth–fifth decade of life. Some clear cell kidney tumors in patients affected with chromosome 3 translocations have been shown to have loss of the 3p derivative chromosome and mutation in the *VHL* gene. These findings led to the proposition of a "three-hit" hypothesis for the carcinogenesis of these tumors where the first hit is inheritance of the germline chromosome 3 translocation, the second hit is loss of the derivative chromosome, and the third hit is somatic mutation of the remaining allele of a chromosome 3p (i.e., *VHL* or others) [61].

The diagnosis of a chromosome 3 translocation is made on germline karyotype. Patients should undergo regular cross-sectional imaging to identify kidney tumors that require surgical resection. Management is similar to VHL, with active surveillance until tumors reach 3 cm followed by nephron-sparing surgery.

Management of Hereditary Cancer Syndromes

Active Surveillance

Patients with hereditary kidney cancer syndromes such as HPRC and VHL may never be completely disease-free, as their kidneys can contain hundreds if not thousands of incipient lesions. Patients treated with radical nephrectomy may cure the individual of cancer, but this places patients at risk to the complications of renal insufficiency. Partial nephrectomy in patients with hereditary cancer syndromes was first advocated in patients with VHL [62]. While over half of patients frequently had disease recurrence, almost all patients demonstrated excellent cancer-specific survival [62]. As patients are predisposed to tumors throughout their lives, it is not feasible to remove all lesions at the first sign of emergence. Such an approach would lead to cumulative renal damage from frequent surgery. Our institution was the first to assess a strict cut point for renal intervention in patients with VHL and HPRC. Prior to tumors reaching 3 cm, all patients were closely observed. With this approach, no patients developed metastatic disease, and all patients were able to avoid end-stage renal disease [63]. When tumors approached this size threshold, patients would undergo partial nephrectomy and removal of all solid lesions when feasible. Besides VHL and HPRC, other hereditary cancer syndromes such as BHD and FRC have been managed successfully with close surveillance of small renal masses and intervention with a 3-cm rule [64].

Surveillance is not recommended for individuals with HLRCC as small lesions have shown the propensity for locoregional and distant spread [37]. As SDH and HLRCC share similar biology, we also do not recommend surveillance for this patient population. Other syndromes such as TSC can also be associated with aggressive malignancy, and observation should be cautioned in these individuals [65, 66]. More clinical experience is needed to evaluate the aggressiveness of kidney cancer associated with BAP1 or MITF prior to recommending a surveillance strategy.

Surgical Management

Multifocality occurs in both hereditary and sporadic cases. Multifocality refers to having more than one tumor in a single kidney, while bilaterality refers to at least one tumor in each kidney. Multifocality and bilaterality are commonly encountered together, with nearly nine of 10 patients with multifocal RCC also having bilateral tumors [67]. Over half of patients with bilateral tumors will also have multifocal disease [68]. Bilateral, multifocal (BMF) patients, whether hereditary or sporadic, pose challenges to the treating surgeon, as these patients are often at increased risk of requiring multiple interventions over a lifetime in order to definitively treat their condition. The traditional management of bilateral, multifocal RCC was bilateral nephrectomy and initiation of dialysis. Those individuals who did not demonstrate disease recurrence could be candidates for future renal transplantation [69–71]. Due to the significant cardiovascular morbidity associated with dialysis, partial nephrectomy in these patients has been considered imperative rather than elective. Various studies have demonstrated the safety of partial nephrectomy even in the setting of over a dozen renal tumors [72, 73]. This may involve simultaneous or staged bilateral renal interventions or may require repeat ipsilateral renal intervention. For example, in some syndromes, there is a high rate of ipsilateral tumor recurrence over time due to the presence of incipient microscopic tumors throughout the renal parenchyma and subsequent development of de novo tumors [19, 74]. Even in predominantly sporadic RCC series, multifocality by itself increases the likelihood of ipsilateral tumors [75]. Repeat renal surgeries pose the risk of increased complications and perioperative morbidity and blood loss [76–81].

The resection of multiple lesions requires specific surgical considerations over ischemia and margin status. Removing multiple lesions can lead to prolonged ischemia, placing the remaining normal parenchyma at risk. Therefore, when feasible, tumor removal without ischemia should be considered. While this leads to increased blood loss, tumor removal is performed in a coordinated, stepwise fashion, from the easiest to the most challenging tumor. This approach maximizes the number of lesions removed and allows the anesthesiologist to maintain hemodynamic stability. After each resection, hemostatic agents and pressure to the defect can control much of the venous bleeding. After several minutes, arterial and persistent venous bleeding can be oversewn.

Enucleation

Tumor enucleation is routinely performed in patients with VHL, HPRC, and BHD. Performing a wide margin on multiple lesions would lead to significant loss of adjacent parenchyma. When enucleation is employed in appropriate cases, most lesions can be enucleated without renal hilar clamping. First, the renal capsule is incised circumferentially around the tumor, and the renal parenchyma is gently separated bluntly. Once identified, the tumor capsule is followed typically with blunt dissection. The closed scissors in combination with gentle fenestrated bipolar are used to bluntly peel the tumor from the surrounding parenchyma. The assistant is critical during this portion to ensure visualization of the junction between the tumor capsule and the normal renal parenchyma. Placement of the suction catheter against the normal parenchyma with intermittent suction, with gentle retraction away from the tumor, while the surgeon gently retracts against the tumor creates an operating space in which the surgeon can identify the plane of dissection. While blunt dissection is usually sufficient to separate the tumor from the surrounding compressed renal parenchyma, perforating vessels are sometimes encountered. These can be controlled with bipolar cautery, point monopolar cautery, and small clips or can be cut sharply and later oversewn.

If the true enucleation plane is identified, then the surrounding parenchyma that is peeled away tends to have been compressed by the tumor growth. As such, it does not bleed as briskly as cutting into normal, non-compressed renal parenchyma. Once the tumor is completely removed from its defect, the base is inspected. If the true enucleation plane is followed throughout the dissection, the likelihood of entry into the collecting system and significant renal vasculature is minimal. Consequently, complex renorrhaphy involving the collecting system and major vasculature repair is often unnecessary. Generally, defects with arterial bleeding can be controlled using a running suture along the base. The defect is then filled with a hemostatic agent and Surgicel. Given the numerous tumors throughout the kidney, defects are not closed immediately because closed renal defects are difficult to image with ultrasound after the capsule is re-approximated. In addition, the ultrasound probe can be placed into the defect once hemostasis is achieved, which may allow for better imaging of and access to deeper lesions adjacent to the renal sinus fat and collecting system. Periodic intraoperative ultrasound is performed throughout the partial nephrectomy to ensure maximum removal of all clinically significant tumors. Repeated use of the ultrasound is critical because multi-tumor partial nephrectomy results in substantial distortion of the kidney, which may make finding target tumors more difficult. Serial use of the ultrasound allows the surgeon to keep real-time spatial relationships among tumors and intrarenal landmarks thereby facilitating complete excision of all targeted and clinically relevant lesions.

Wide Excision

For HLRCC and SDH renal tumors, our approach has been a wide surgical excision as we have observed an infiltrating pattern outside the pseudocapsule. Our institutional practice is to avoid robotic surgery in known HLRCC cases, as tumor spillage due to lack of haptic feedback can occur. Because normal parenchyma is transected, bleeding is more substantial than in enucleation, and it may be better suited to an approach that incorporates clamping the renal artery.

The role of enucleation surgery in the remaining hereditary cancer syndromes is unclear; however, as this approach has been proven safe with sporadic tumors, it likely is safe in these syndromes [82].

Systemic Therapy for Patients with Hereditary RCC

Systemic targeted therapy with bevacizumab and erlotinib has demonstrated particular efficacy in patients with HLRCC [83]. In patients with HLRCC, tumorigenesis is driven by genetic alterations to glucose metabolism. The combination of bevacizumab and erlotinib (inhibitors of vascular endothelial growth factor [VEGF] and epidermal growth factor receptor [EGFR], respectively) is hypothesized to inhibit effective glucose delivery to tumor cells, presenting a logical therapeutic approach to this disease. While this regimen is not FDA-approved for use in this patient population, its inclusion is supported by clinical trial data showing improved patient outcomes. In a phase II study investigating erlotinib/bevacizumab treatment in patients with HLRCC or sporadic papillary RCC, erlotinib/bevacizumab treatment led to a 64% ORR and a median PFS of 21.1 months in patients with HLRCC-associated RCC [83].

Patients with VHL disease often develop RCC and tumors and cysts in other organs including adrenal glands, CNS, retinal hemangioblastomas, and pancreas, and commonly undergo several surgical resections in their lifetime. Belzutifan specifically inhibits hypoxia-inducible factor-2alpha (HIF-2 alpha), a key protein regulated by the VHL pathway. Belzutifan was FDA-approved 2021 for VHL-associated RCC, CNS hemangioblastomas, or pancreatic neuroendocrine tumors (pNET), not requiring immediate surgery [84]. An open-label phase II trial enrolled 61 patients with VHL-associated RCC, 97% with previous tumor reduction procedures. The objective response rate (ORR) was 49% (95%CI 36–62) after a median follow-up of 21.8 months with 30 patients achieving a partial response. An additional 30 patients (49%) had stable disease (SD) as best response. Median time to response was 8.2 months and the median duration of response was not reached. Grade $\geq$ 3 treatment-related toxicities included anemia and hypertension, fatigue, as well as dyspnea and myalgias [84].

TSC is associated with mutations that result in activation of the mTOR pathway. Given this molecular understanding of TSC-associated AML, mTOR inhibitors have been explored as systemic therapeutic agents for managing this disease in TSC patients. Everolimus has been assessed in a phase III study among TSC- and LAM-associated AML [85]. The study showed a response rate of 42% (at least 50% reduction in volume), with 80% achieving at least a 30% reduction in size. Furthermore, no patient who had a tumor response suffered progression during follow-up, however, these tumors demonstrated growth after stopping treatment. Everolimus was FDA-approved in 2012 for therapy of asymptomatic, growing angiomyolipomas (AML) measuring >3 cm in diameter based on the EXIST-2 trial in TSC patients [85].

Conclusions

Patients with bilateral, multifocal, and early-onset kidney cancer frequently have hereditary kidney cancer syndrome. Genetic testing in those suspected of these syndromes is recommended. If a known syndrome is identified, family members should be tested in order to begin appropriate screening protocols. The management of several of the kidney cancer syndromes has been refined over the past few decades to prevent cancer dissemination, maximize kidney function, and minimize surgical morbidity. The molecular characterization of these syndromes may lead to exploitation of these aberrant pathways with a systemic therapy approach.

References

1. Moch H, Cubilla AL, Humphrey PA, Reuter VE, Ulbright TM. The 2016 WHO classification of tumours of the urinary system and male genital organs-part a: renal, penile, and testicular tumours. Eur Urol. 2016;70(1):93–105.
2. Linehan WM. Genetic basis of kidney cancer: role of genomics for the development of disease-based therapeutics. Genome Res. 2012;22(11):2089–100.
3. Siegel RL, Miller KD, Jemal A. Cancer statistics, 2019. CA Cancer J Clin. 2019;69(1):7–34.
4. Kletscher BA, Qian J, Bostwick DG, Andrews PE, Zincke H. Prospective analysis of multifocality in renal cell carcinoma: influence of histological pattern, grade, number, size, volume and deoxyribonucleic acid ploidy. J Urol. 1995;153(3 Pt 2):904–6.
5. Whang M, O'Toole K, Bixon R, Brunetti J, Ikeguchi E, Olsson CA, et al. The incidence of multifocal renal cell carcinoma in patients who are candidates for partial nephrectomy. J Urol. 1995;154(3):968–70. discussion 70–1
6. Gudbjartsson T, Jonasdottir TJ, Thoroddsen A, Einarsson GV, Jonsdottir GM, Kristjansson K, et al. A population-based familial aggregation analysis indicates genetic contribution in a majority of renal cell carcinomas. Int J Cancer. 2002;100(4):476–9.
7. Shuch B, Singer EA, Bratslavsky G. The surgical approach to multifocal renal cancers: hereditary syndromes, ipsilateral multifocality, and bilateral tumors. Urol Clin N Am. 2012;39:133–48.
8. Ball MW, Singer EA, Srinivasan R. Renal cell carcinoma: molecular characterization and evolving treatment paradigms. Curr Opin Oncol. 2017;29(3):201–9.
9. Nielsen SM, Rhodes L, Blanco I, Chung WK, Eng C, Maher ER, et al. Von Hippel-Lindau disease: genetics and role of genetic counseling in a multiple neoplasia syndrome. J Clin Oncol. 2016;34(18):2172–81.
10. Latif F, Tory K, Gnarra JR, Yao M, Duh FM, Orcutt ML, et al. Identification of the von Hippel-Lindau disease tumor suppressor gene. Science. 1993;260(5112):1317–20.
11. Tory K, Brauch H, Linehan WM, Barba D, Oldfield E, Filling-Katz M, et al. Specific genetic change in tumors associated with von Hippel-Lindau disease. J Natl Cancer Inst. 1989;81:1097–101.
12. Mandriota SJ, Turner KJ, Davies DR, Murray PG, Morgan NV, Sowter HM, et al. HIF activation identifies early lesions in VHL kidneys: evidence for site-specific tumor suppressor function in the nephron. Cancer Cell. 2002;1(5):459–68.
13. Beroud C, Joly D, Gallou C, Staroz F, Orfanelli MT, Junien C. Software and database for the analysis of mutations in the VHL gene. Nucleic Acids Res. 1998;26(1):256–8.
14. Nordstrom-O'Brien M, van der Luijt RB, van Rooijen E, van den Ouweland AM, Majoor-Krakauer DF, Lolkema MP, et al. Genetic analysis of von Hippel-Lindau disease. Hum Mutat. 2010;31(5):521–37.
15. Lonser RR, Glenn GM, Walther M, Chew EY, Libutti SK, Linehan WM, et al. von Hippel-Lindau disease. Lancet. 2003;361(9374):2059–67.
16. Poston CD, Jaffe GS, Lubensky IA, Solomon D, Zbar B, Linehan WM, et al. Characterization of the renal pathology of a familial form of renal cell carcinoma associated with von Hippel-Lindau disease: clinical and molecular genetic implications. J Urol. 1995;153(1):22–6.
17. Choyke PL, Filling-Katz MR, Shawker TH, Gorin MB, Travis WD, Chang R, et al. von Hippel-Lindau disease: radiologic screening for visceral manifestations. Radiology. 1990;174(3 Pt 1):815–20.
18. Duffey BG, Choyke PL, Glenn G, Grubb RL, Venzon D, Linehan WM, et al. The relationship between renal tumor size and metastases in patients with von Hippel-Lindau disease. J Urol. 2004;172(1):63–5.
19. Singer EA, Vourganti S, Lin KY, Gupta GN, Pinto PA, Rastinehad AR, et al. Outcomes of patients with surgically treated bilateral renal masses and a minimum of 10 years of follow-up. J Urol. 2012;188(6):2084–8.
20. Zbar B, Tory K, Merino MJ, Schmidt LS, Glenn GM, Choyke P, et al. Hereditary papillary renal cell carcinoma. J Urol. 1994;151(3):561–6.
21. Schmidt LS, Duh FM, Chen F, Kishida T, Glenn GM, Choyke P, et al. Germline and somatic mutations in the tyrosine kinase domain of the MET proto-oncogene in papillary renal carcinomas. Nat Genet. 1997;16(1):68–73.
22. Schmidt LS, Junker K, Weirich G, Glenn G, Choyke P, Lubensky I, et al. Two North American families with hereditary papillary renal carcinoma and identical novel mutations in the MET proto-oncogene. Cancer Res. 1998;58(8):1719–22.
23. Schmidt LS, Junker K, Nakaigawa N, Kinjerski T, Weirich G, Miller M, et al. Novel mutations of the MET proto-oncogene in papillary renal carcinomas. Oncogene. 1999;18(14):2343–50.
24. Lubensky IA, Schmidt LS, Zhuang Z, Weirich G, Pack S, Zambrano N, et al. Hereditary and sporadic papillary renal carcinomas with c-met mutations share a distinct morphological phenotype. Am J Pathol. 1999;155(2):517–26.
25. Ornstein DK, Lubensky IA, Venzon D, Zbar B, Linehan WM, Walther MM. Prevalence of microscopic tumors in normal appearing renal parenchyma of patients with hereditary papillary renal cancer. J Urol. 2000;163(2):431–3.

26. Zbar B, Glenn GM, Lubensky IA, Choyke P, Magnusson G, Bergerheim U, et al. Hereditary papillary renal cell carcinoma: clinical studies in 10 families. J Urol. 1995;153(3, Supplement 1):907–12.
27. Schmidt LS, Nickerson ML, Angeloni D, Glenn GM, Walther MM, Albert PS, et al. Early onset hereditary papillary renal carcinoma: germline missense mutations in the tyrosine kinase domain of the met protooncogene. J Urol. 2004;172(4, Part 1 Of 2):1256–61.
28. Birt AR, Hogg GR, Dube WJ. Hereditary multiple fibrofolliculomas with trichodiscomas and acrochordons. Arch Dermatol. 1977;113(12):1674–7.
29. Zbar B, Alvord WG, Glenn GM, Turner M, Pavlovich CP, Schmidt LS, et al. Risk of renal and colonic neoplasms and spontaneous pneumothorax in the Birt-Hogg-Dube syndrome. Cancer Epidemiol Biomarkers Prev. 2002;11(4):393–400.
30. Schmidt LS, Nickerson ML, Warren MB, Glenn GM, Toro JR, Merino MJ, et al. Germline BHD-mutation spectrum and phenotype analysis of a large cohort of families with Birt-Hogg-Dub, syndrome. Am J Hum Genet. 2005;76(6):1023–33.
31. Toro JR, Wei MH, Glenn GM, Weinreich M, Toure O, Vocke CD, et al. BHD mutations, clinical and molecular genetic investigations of Birt-Hogg-Dube syndrome: a new series of 50 families and a review of published reports. J Med Genet. 2008;45(6):321–31.
32. Schmidt LS, Linehan WM. Molecular genetics and clinical features of Birt-Hogg-Dube syndrome. Nat Rev Urol. 2015;12(10):558–69.
33. Pavlovich CP, Walther MM, Eyler RA, Hewitt SM, Zbar B, Linehan WM, et al. Renal tumors in the Birt-Hogg-Dub, syndrome. Am J Surg Pathol. 2002;26(12):1542–52.
34. Leung C, Pan S, Shuch B. Management of renal cell carcinoma in young patients and patients with hereditary syndromes. Curr Opin Urol. 2016;26(5):396–404.
35. Launonen V, Vierimaa O, Kiuru M, Isola J, Roth S, Pukkala E, et al. Inherited susceptibility to uterine leiomyomas and renal cell cancer. Proc Natl Acad Sci USA. 2001;98(6):3387–2.
36. Merino MJ, Torres-Cabala C, Pinto PA, Linehan WM. The morphologic spectrum of kidney tumors in hereditary leiomyomatosis and renal cell carcinoma (HLRCC) syndrome. Am J Surg Pathol. 2007;31(10):1578–85.
37. Grubb RL III, Franks ME, Toro J, Middelton L, Choyke L, Fowler S, et al. Hereditary leiomyomatosis and renal cell cancer: a syndrome associated with an aggressive form of inherited renal cancer. J Urol. 2007;177(6):2074–80.
38. Schmidt LS, Linehan WM. Hereditary leiomyomatosis and renal cell carcinoma. Int J Nephrol Renovasc Dis. 2014;7:253–60.
39. Toro JR, Nickerson ML, Wei MH, Warren MB, Glenn GM, Turner ML, et al. Mutations in the fumarate hydratase gene cause hereditary leiomyomatosis and renal cell cancer in families in North America. Am J Hum Genet. 2003;73(1):95–106.
40. Wei MH, Toure O, Glenn GM, Pithukpakorn M, Neckers L, Stolle C, et al. Novel mutations in FH and expansion of the spectrum of phenotypes expressed in families with hereditary leiomyomatosis and renal cell cancer. J Med Genet. 2006;43(1):18–27.
41. Tomlinson IP, Alam NA, Rowan AJ, Barclay E, Jaeger EE, Kelsell D, et al. Germline mutations in FH predispose to dominantly inherited uterine fibroids, skin leiomyomata and papillary renal cell cancer. Nat Genet. 2002;30(4):406–10.
42. Shuch B, Singer EA, Bratslavsky G. The surgical approach to multifocal renal cancers: hereditary syndromes, ipsilateral multifocality, and bilateral tumors. Urol Clin North Am. 2012;39(2):133–48. v.
43. Ricketts CJ, Shuch B, Vocke CD, Metwalli AR, Bratslavsky G, Middelton L, et al. Succinate dehydrogenase kidney cancer: an aggressive example of the Warburg effect in cancer. J Urol. 2012; https://doi.org/10.1016/j.juro.2012.08.030.
44. Gill AJ, Hes O, Papathomas T, Sedivcova M, Tan PH, Agaimy A, et al. Succinate dehydrogenase (SDH)-deficient renal carcinoma: a morphologically distinct entity: a clinicopathologic series of 36 tumors from 27 patients. Am J Surg Pathol. 2014;38(12):1588–602.
45. Rai K, Pilarski R, Cebulla CM, Abdel-Rahman MH. Comprehensive review of BAP1 tumor predisposition syndrome with report of two new cases. Clin Genet. 2016;89(3):285–94.
46. Farley MN, Schmidt LS, Mester JL, Pena-Llopis S, Pavia-Jimenez A, Christie A, et al. Germline BAP1 mutation predisposes to familial clear-cell renal cell carcinoma. Mol Cancer Res. 2013;11:1061.
47. Popova T, Hebert L, Jacquemin V, Gad S, Caux-Moncoutier V, Dubois-d'Enghien C, et al. Germline BAP1 mutations predispose to renal cell carcinomas. Am J Hum Genet. 2013;92(6):974–80.
48. Mir MC, Derweesh I, Porpiglia F, Zargar H, Mottrie A, Autorino R. Partial nephrectomy versus radical nephrectomy for clinical T1b and T2 renal tumors: a systematic review and meta-analysis of comparative studies. Eur Urol. 2016;71(4):606–17.
49. Kauffman EC, Ricketts CJ, Rais-Bahrami S, Yang Y, Merino MJ, Bottaro DP, et al. Molecular genetics and cellular features of TFE3 and TFEB fusion kidney cancers. Nat Rev Urol. 2014;11(8):465–75.
50. Argani P. MiT family translocation renal cell carcinoma. Semin Diagn Pathol. 2015;32(2):103–13.
51. Bertolotto C, Lesueur F, Giuliano S, Strub T, de Lichy M, Bille K, et al. A SUMOylation-defective MITF germline mutation predisposes to melanoma and renal carcinoma. Nature. 2011;480(7375):94–8.
52. Gorin MA, Ball MW, Pierorazio PM, Argani P, Allaf ME. Partial nephrectomy for the treatment of translocation renal cell carcinoma. Clin Genitourin Cancer. 2015;13(3):e199–201.
53. Crino PB, Nathanson KL, Henske EP. The tuberous sclerosis complex. N Engl J Med. 2006;355(13):1345–56.

54. Bjornsson J, Short MP, Kwiatkowski DJ, Henske EP. Tuberous sclerosis-associated renal cell carcinoma. Clinical, pathological, and genetic features. Am J Pathol. 1996;149(4):1–8.
55. Kothary N, Soulen MC, Clark TW, Wein AJ, Shlansky-Goldberg RD, Crino PB, et al. Renal angiomyolipoma: long-term results after arterial embolization. J Vasc Interv Radiol. 2005;16(1):45–50.
56. Cristescu M, Abel EJ, Wells S, Ziemlewicz TJ, Hedican SP, Lubner MG, et al. Percutaneous microwave ablation of renal angiomyolipomas. Cardiovasc Intervent Radiol. 2016;39(3):433–40.
57. Bissler JJ, McCormack FX, Young LR, Elwing JM, Chuck G, Leonard JM, et al. Sirolimus for angiomyolipoma in tuberous sclerosis complex or lymphangioleiomyomatosis. N Engl J Med. 2008;358(2):140–51.
58. Cohen AJ, Li FP, Berg S, Marchetto DJ, Tsai S, Jacobs SC, et al. Hereditary renal-cell carcinoma associated with a chromosomal translocation. N Engl J Med. 1979;301:592–5.
59. van Kessel AG, Wijnhoven H, Bodmer D, Eleveld M, Kiemeney L, Mulders P, et al. Renal cell cancer: chromosome 3 translocations as risk factors. J Natl Cancer Inst. 1999;91(13):1159–60.
60. Rodriguez-Perales S, Melendez B, Gribble SM, Valle L, Carter NP, Santamaria I, et al. Cloning of a new familial t(3;8) translocation associated with conventional renal cell carcinoma reveals a 5 kb microdeletion and no gene involved in the rearrangement. Hum Mol Genet. 2004;13(9):983–90.
61. Schmidt LS, Li F, Brown RS, Berg S, Chen F, Wei MH, et al. Mechanism of tumorigenesis of renal carcinomas associated with the constitutional chromosome 3;8 translocation. Cancer J Sci Am. 1995;1(3):191–5.
62. Steinbach F, Novick AC, Zincke H, Miller DP, Williams RD, Lund G, et al. Treatment of renal cell carcinoma in von Hippel-Lindau disease: a multicenter study. J Urol. 1995;153(6):1812–6.
63. Walther MM, Choyke PL, Glenn G, Lyne JC, Rayford W, Venzon D, et al. Renal cancer in families with hereditary renal cancer: prospective analysis of a tumor size threshold for renal parenchymal sparing surgery. J Urol. 1999;161(5):1475–9.
64. Pavlovich CP, Grubb RL 3rd, Hurley K, Glenn GM, Toro J, Schmidt LS, et al. Evaluation and management of renal tumors in the Birt-Hogg-Dube syndrome. J Urol. 2005;173(5):1482–6.
65. Al-Saleem T, Wessner LL, Scheithauer BW, Patterson K, Roach ES, Dreyer SJ, et al. Malignant tumors of the kidney, brain, and soft tissues in children and young adults with the tuberous sclerosis complex. Cancer. 1998;83(10):2208–16.
66. Bjornsson J, Short MP, Kwiatkowski DJ, Henske EP. Tuberous sclerosis-associated renal cell carcinoma. Clinical, pathological, and genetic features. Am J Pathol. 1996;149(4):1201–8.
67. Wunderlich H, Schlichter A, Zermann D, Reichelt O, Kosmehl H, Schubert J. Multifocality in renal cell carcinoma: a bilateral event? Urol Int. 1999;63(3):160–3.
68. Klatte T, Wunderlich H, Patard JJ, Kleid MD, Lam JS, Junker K, et al. Clinicopathological features and prognosis of synchronous bilateral renal cell carcinoma: an international multicentre experience. BJU Int. 2007;100(1):21–5.
69. Calne RY. Treatment of bilateral hypernephromas by nephrectomy, excision of tumour, and autotransplantation. Report of three cases. Lancet. 1973;2(7839):1164–7.
70. Clark JE. Transplantation for bilateral renal tumors. JAMA. 1970;211(8):1379.
71. Jochimsen PR, Braunstein PM, Najarian JS. Renal allotransplantation for bilateral renal tumors. JAMA. 1969;210(9):1721–4.
72. Fadahunsi AT, Sanford T, Linehan WM, Pinto PA, Bratslavsky G. Feasibility and outcomes of partial nephrectomy for resection of at least 20 tumors in a single renal unit. J Urol. 2011;185(1):49–53.
73. Walther MM, Choyke PL, Weiss G, Manolatos C, Long J, Reiter R, et al. Parenchymal sparing surgery in patients with hereditary renal cell carcinoma. J Urol. 1995;153(3 Pt 2):913–6.
74. Walther MM, Lubensky IA, Venzon D, Zbar B, Linehan WM. Prevalence of microscopic lesions in grossly normal renal parenchyma from patients with von Hippel-Lindau disease, sporadic renal cell carcinoma and no renal disease: clinical implications. J Urol. 1995;154(6):2010–4. discussion 4–5.
75. Zargar-Shoshtari K, Kim T, Simon R, Lin HY, Yue B, Sharma P, et al. Surveillance following nephron-sparing surgery: an assessment of recurrence patterns and surveillance costs. Urology. 2015;86(2):321–6.
76. Bratslavsky G, Liu JJ, Johnson AD, Sudarshan S, Choyke PL, Linehan WM, et al. Salvage partial nephrectomy for hereditary renal cancer: feasibility and outcomes. J Urol. 2008;179(1):67–70.
77. Johnson A, Sudarshan S, Liu J, Linehan WM, Pinto PA, Bratslavsky G. Feasibility and outcomes of repeat partial nephrectomy. J Urol. 2008;180(1):89–93. discussion
78. Liu NW, Khurana K, Sudarshan S, Pinto PA, Linehan WM, Bratslavsky G. Repeat partial nephrectomy on the solitary kidney: surgical, functional and oncological outcomes. J Urol. 2010;183(5):1719–24.
79. Maurice MJ, Ramirez D, Nelson R, Caputo P, Kara O, Malkoc E, et al. Multiple tumor excisions in ipsilateral kidney increase complications after partial nephrectomy. J Endourol. 2016;30:1200.
80. Minervini A, Serni S, Giubilei G, Lanzi F, Vittori G, Lapini A, et al. Multiple ipsilateral renal tumors: retrospective analysis of surgical and oncological results of tumor enucleation vs radical nephrectomy. Eur J Surg Oncol. 2009;35(5):521–6.

81. Shuch B, Linehan WM, Bratslavsky G. Repeat partial nephrectomy: surgical, functional and oncological outcomes. Curr Opin Urol. 2011;21(5):368–75.
82. Carini M, Minervini A, Masieri L, Lapini A, Serni S. Simple enucleation for the treatment of PT1a renal cell carcinoma: our 20-year experience. Eur Urol. 2006;50(6):1263–8. discussion 9–71
83. Srinivasan R, Gurram S, Al Harthy M, et al. Results from a phase II study of bevacizumab and erlotinib in subjects with advanced hereditary leiomyomatosis and renal cell cancer (HLRCC) or sporadic papillary renal cell cancer. J Clin Oncol. 2020;38:5004.
84. Jonasch E, Donskov F, Iliopoulos O, Rathmell WK, Narayan VK, Maughan BL, Oudard S, Else T, Maranchie JK, Welsh SJ, Thamake S, Park EK, Perini RF, Linehan WM, Srinivasan R, MK-6482-004 Investigators. Belzutifan for renal cell carcinoma in von Hippel-Lindau disease. N Engl J Med. 2021;385(22):2036–46.
85. Bissler JJ, Kingswood JC, Radzikowska E, Zonnenberg BA, Frost M, Belousova E, Sauter M, Nonomura N, Brakemeier S, de Vries PJ, et al. Everolimus for angiomyolipoma associated with tuberous sclerosis complex or sporadic lymphangioleiomyomatosis (EXIST-2): a multicentre, randomised, double-blind, placebo-controlled trial. Lancet. 2013;381(9869):817–24.

Pathology of Renal Cell Carcinoma

4

Ming Zhou

Introduction

Arising from the renal tubular epithelial cells, renal cell carcinomas (RCCs) account for more than 90% of the primary kidney tumors in adults. They are heterogeneous regarding clinical, pathological, and molecular characteristics as well as prognosis and therapeutic options and responses.

Pathological classification and many histological parameters obtained from biopsy and resection specimens provide invaluable information for management and prognostic prediction. In the current World Health Organization (WHO) classification published in 2022 [1–3], the major histological subtypes include clear cell, papillary, and chromophobe RCCs and oncocytomas and account for over 90% of the renal cell neoplasms. The molecular attributes are gradually integrated into the principally morphology-based classification. A new category, "molecularly defined renal carcinomas," was created in the WHO 2022 classification. The integration of clinical, pathological, and genetic features will ultimately enable prediction of individual tumor behavior more accurately, to tailor treatment for patients, and to pave the way for truly individualized and precision management.

M. Zhou (✉)
Department of Pathology, Molecular and Cell-based Medicine, Icahn School of Medicine at Mount Sinai, New York, NY, USA
e-mail: Ming.zhou@mountsinai.org

In this chapter, we review the pathological and molecular characteristics of major histological subtypes of RCC recognized in the 2022 WHO classification [1] along with several newly described subtypes, and those associated with inherited cancer syndromes. The management and prognostic implications of various histological parameters are also discussed. For detailed discussion of the molecular genetics of RCC, please refer to "Molecular Genetics of Renal Cell Carcinoma" of this book.

Pathological Classification of Renal Cell Neoplasms

The pathological classification of renal tumors is codified in the WHO classification [1], which was developed based on earlier classification schema, including Mainz [4], Heidelberg [5], and Rochester classifications [6]. All these classification systems attempted to separate a remarkably heterogeneous group of renal tumors into subgroups with similar pathological and molecular features, clinical outcomes, and therapeutic options. The classification was based initially on morphology and more recently on genetics. WHO classification is updated periodically using the best available evidence on clinical, morphological, and genetic features. It emphasizes the heterogeneity of renal tumors and defines distinct types with unique morphologic and genetic characteristics.

J. A. Libertino, J. R. Gee (eds.), *Renal Cancer*, https://doi.org/10.1007/978-3-031-97599-8_4

The current WHO classification was published in 2022. The major histologic RCC subtypes, namely, clear cell, papillary, and chromophobe RCC, account for 90–95% of renal carcinoma (Table 4.1). Other less common types include multilocular cystic renal neoplasm of low malignant potential, collecting duct carcinoma, mucinous tubular spindle cell RCC, tubulocystic RCC, acquired cystic disease-associated RCC, eosinophilic solid and cystic RCC, and clear cell papillary renal cell tumor. A new category, "molecularly defined renal cell carcinomas," was created to include those tumors with distinct molecular changes, such as *TFE3*-rearranged RCC, *TFEB*-rearranged RCC, fumarate hydratase (FH)-deficient RCC, succinate dehydrogenase-deficient RCC, SMARCB1-deficient renal medullary carcinoma, and *ALK*-rearranged RCC. Unclassified type, or "RCC, not otherwise specified," is assigned when a tumor cannot be classified as, yet clearly different from, any of the recognized subtypes. These 20 subtypes represent most renal tumors encountered clinically, but are obviously not all encompassing, as renal tumors with clinical, pathological, and genetic features distinct from these 20 tumors have been reported. It is certain that additional new subtypes will emerge when the molecular mechanisms of renal tumors become further elucidated. Molecular classification supplements and may eventually supplant the morphological classification.

Table 4.1 2022 WHO classification of renal cell tumors [1]

Clear cell renal cell carcinoma
Multilocular cystic renal neoplasm of low malignant potential
Papillary adenoma Papillary renal cell carcinoma
Oncocytoma Chromophobe renal cell carcinoma Other oncocytic tumors of the kidney
Collecting ducts carcinoma
Clear cell papillary renal cell tumor Mucinous tubular and spindle cell carcinoma Tubulocystic renal cell carcinoma Acquired cystic disease-associated renal cell carcinoma Eosinophilic solid cystic carcinoma Renal cell carcinoma, NOS TFE3-rearranged renal cell carcinoma TFEB-rearranged renal cell carcinoma
ELOC (formerly TCEB1)-mutated renal cell carcinoma Fumarate hydratase-deficient renal cell carcinoma
Succinate dehydrogenase (SDH)-deficient renal carcinoma
ALK-rearranged renal cell carcinoma MARCB1-deficient renal medullary carcinoma

Pathologic and Molecular Characteristics of RCC Subtypes

Renal Cell Carcinoma: Clear Cell Type (CCRCC)

Clinical Features

CCRCC is the most common histological subtype and accounts for 60–70% of all renal cell neoplasms. Reported in all age groups, it most commonly affects patients in their sixth to seventh decades of life with a male to female ratio of approximately 2:1 [1]. Most CCRCC arises sporadically; however, 2–4% of cases present as part of an inherited cancer syndrome, which includes von Hippel-Lindau syndrome, Cowden syndrome and constitutional chromosomal 3 translocation syndrome [7, 8]. As a general rule, familial CCRCC presents at a younger age and is more likely to be multifocal and bilateral.

Pathology

Grossly, CCRCC usually presents as a unilateral and unicentric, round and well-demarcated mass with a fibrous capsule. The mean diameter is 6.2 cm; however, smaller lesions are increasingly detected due to the wide use of imaging studies. The cut surface has a characteristic golden yellow color with a variable degree of hemorrhage, necrosis, cystic degeneration, and calcification (Fig. 4.1a). Bilaterality and/or multicentricity occur in <5% of sporadic cases but are more common in inherited cancer syndromes.

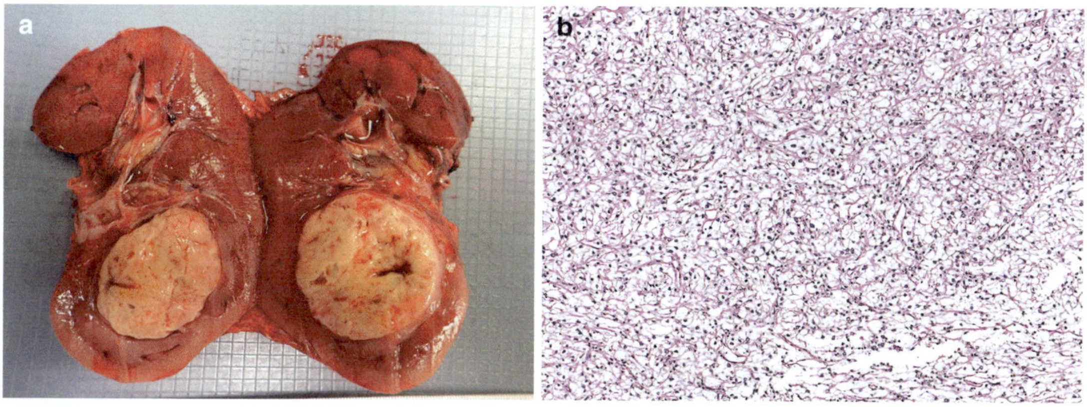

Fig. 4.1 Clear cell renal cell carcinoma is grossly a well-circumscribed solid mass with bright golden yellow color (**a**), composed of compact nests of tumor cells with clear cytoplasm separated by delicate arborizing vasculature (**b**)

Microscopically, the tumor cells are arranged in compact nests, sheets, or alveolar or acinar structures separated by thin-walled blood vessels. Tumor cells have clear cytoplasm (Fig. 4.1b) due to rich cytoplasmic lipid and glycogen content that is lost during tissue processing and slide preparation, imparting an empty or clear appearance. In high-grade and poorly differentiated tumors, cells no longer show cytoplasmic clearing but instead acquire a granular eosinophilic cytoplasm. In high-grade areas, loss of typical alveolar or acinar growth pattern is quite common. Solid and sometimes rhabdoid, papillary, or sarcomatoid morphology may be seen. Sarcomatoid and rhabdoid differentiation occurs in about 5% of cases and is regarded as a high-grade tumor with ominous prognosis.

Molecular Genetics

Nearly 90% of sporadic CCRCCs harbor chromosome 3p alterations that include deletion, mutation, or promoter methylation of several genes, including *von Hippel-Lindau* (*VHL*) gene on chromosome 3p25–26. 3p also contains other tumor suppressor genes that are lost or mutated in 15–40% of sporadic CCRCCs [9, 10]. These genes, including *PBRM1*, *SETD2*, and *BAP1*, are mostly involved in the chromatin remodeling complex [11]. *PBRM1* and *SETD2* are frequently mutated together, while *PBRM1* and *BAP1* tend to be mutually exclusive and render distinct morphologies. Additional driver mutations involve other histone-modifying genes (*KDM5C*, *KDM6A*), mTOR pathway genes, and chromosomes 14q, 4p, and 9p [12]. Clear cell RCC with *VHL* alterations is usually indolent. *PBRM1* mutations are usually an early event. Tumors with *BAP1* or multiple driver mutations tend to be high grade with an aggressive clinical course, early metastasis, and poor outcomes [13].

Somatic mutations in the *VHL* gene have been found in 18–82% of sporadic CCRCC cases. Loss of heterozygosity (LOH) at the *VHL* locus has been reported in up to 98% of cases [9]. Hypermethylation of the *VHL* gene promoter resulting in gene inactivation has been detected in 5–20% of patients without gene alteration. The vast majority of CCRCC showing somatic *VHL* mutations also exhibit allelic loss or loss of heterozygosity (LOH) at the second *VHL* locus, consistent with Knudson's two-hit model of tumorigenesis.

VHL protein plays a critical role in the cellular response to hypoxia [14] and regulates the cellular level of hypoxia-inducible factor (HIF). Under normoxic conditions, wild-type VHL binds to and targets hydroxylated HIF for ubiquitin-mediated degradation in proteasomes, thus keeping HIF levels low within normal cells under normoxic conditions. Under hypoxic conditions, however, HIF is not hydroxylated and cannot be recognized by VHL and therefore accumulates and activates many downstream hypoxia-driven genes, including genes that promote angiogenesis (vascular endothelial growth factor [*VEGF*] and platelet-derived growth factor β, *PDGF-β*), cell growth or survival (transforming growth factor α, *TGF-α*), anaerobic metabolism (*Glut-1*), acid-base balance (*CA IX*), and red cell production (*erythropoietin*). Along the way, numerous intracellular signal transduction pathways are activated, including PI3 kinase-Akt-mTOR pathway and Ras/Raf/ERK/MEK pathway, which are involved in various cellular processes, including the cell proliferation, survival, and differentiation. These signal transduction pathways serve a beneficial role by stimulating angiogenesis and compensatory metabolic changes in normal cells coping with hypoxia. When the *VHL* gene is inactivated by mutation or promoter hypermethylation, no functional VHL is produced. The result is activation of the aforementioned cellular processes that are no longer controlled by normal physiological mechanisms and therefore contribute to tumorigenesis and many of the clinical manifestations of CCRCC. The elucidation of these mechanisms has allowed the development of targeted therapies that specifically act within these pathways, including VEGF [15], VEGFR, and PDGFR using small molecule inhibitors of tyrosine kinase (TKI), EGFR, and mTOR [16]. More recently, an immune checkpoint inhibitor (ICI) and combination of ICI and TKIs have been approved as first-line therapy in advanced CCRCC [17].

Metastatic CCRCC shows unique molecular subsets with distinct drug responses [18, 19]. Tumors with a strong angiogenic gene expression signature are enriched for *PBRM1* loss and have a favorable response to anti-angiogenic therapies. CCRCCs with an inflamed microenvironment have a higher rate of *BAP1* mutations, more commonly harbor sarcomatoid change, have the highest expression of PD-L1, and show preferential response to immune checkpoint inhibitors [20].

Prognosis

In CCRCC, about 50% are stages I and II, 45% are stage III, and less than 5% are stage IV. Stage, nuclear grade, sarcomatoid and rhabdoid differentiation, and necrosis are significant predictors of clinical outcomes.

Renal Cell Carcinoma: Papillary Type (Papillary RCC, PRCC)

Clinical Features

PRCC is the second most common RCC subtype and accounts for ~15% of renal tumors. While the gender and age distribution are similar to CCRCC, the prognosis is quite different. Papillary RCC has a better prognosis with a 5-year survival approaching 90% [21]. Most tumors occur sporadically, but some develop in hereditary papillary renal carcinoma syndrome (HPRCC) [22]. Multifocal and bilateral tumors should raise the suspicion for a familial cancer syndrome but can occasionally be seen in a sporadic setting, as PRCC is more likely to be bilateral and multifocal than other types of RCC.

Pathology

Grossly, PRCC typically presents as a well-circumscribed mass enclosed within a pseudocapsule. Some tumors appear entirely necrotic and friable (Fig. 4.2a).

Microscopically, PRCC is composed of varying proportions of papillae, tubulopapillary and tubules (Fig. 4.2b). The papillae characteristically contain delicate fibrovascular cores infiltrated by foamy histiocytes. Necrosis, hemorrhage, acute and chronic inflammation, hemosiderin deposition, and psammoma bodies are common.

In earlier WHO classifications, PRCC was subclassified into two morphological patterns based on the morphology of tumor cells [23]. So-called "type 1" tumors contain papillae that are delicate and short and are lined with single layers of tumor cells with scant cytoplasm and low-grade nuclei (Fig. 4.2b). In contrast, papillae in "type 2" PRCC are large and lined with cells having abundant eosinophilic cytoplasm and large pseudostratified nuclei with prominent nucleoli (Fig. 4.2c). However, "type 2" tumors are a heterogeneous group. Some contain specific

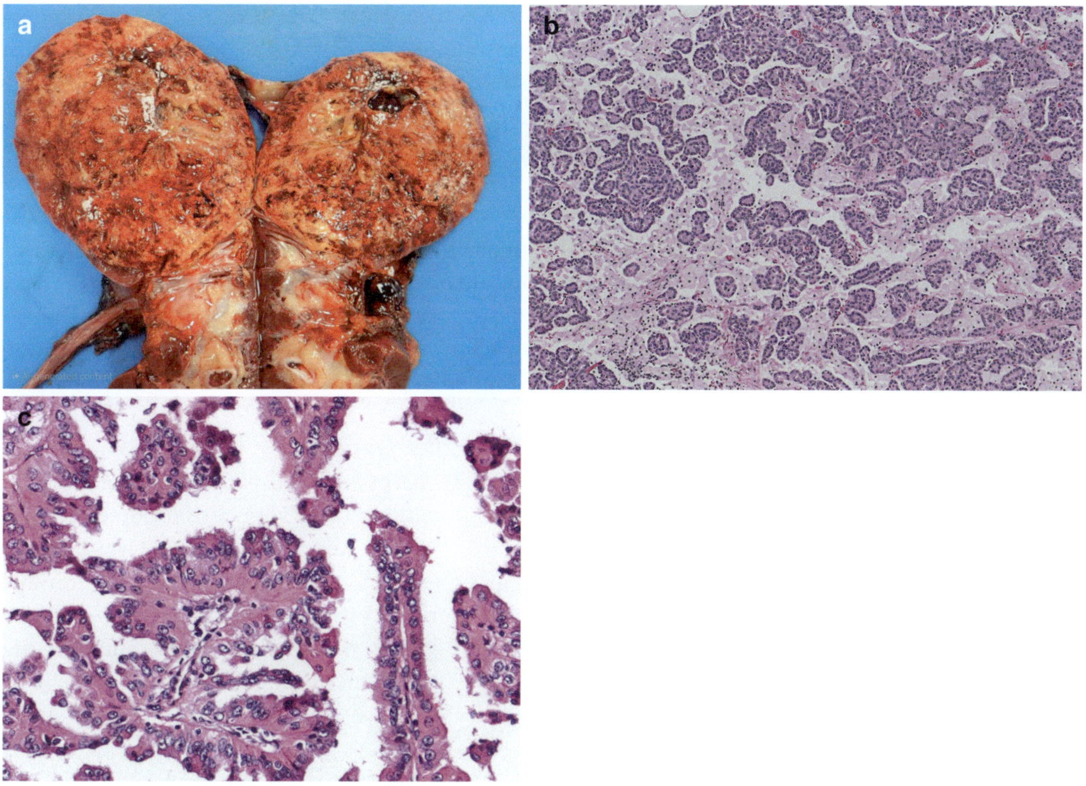

Fig. 4.2 Papillary renal cell carcinoma grossly has a thick fibrous capsule and is extensively necrotic (**a**). Low-grade PRCC is composed of papillae covered by a single layer of tumor cells with scant cytoplasm and low-grade nuclei. Abundant histiocytes are also present (**b**), while high-grade tumor cells have abundant eosinophilic cytoplasm and large pseudostratified nuclei with prominent nucleoli (**c**)

genetic changes, such as *TFE3* or *TFEB* translocation, mutations in TSC/mTOR pathway genes, and fumarate hydratase-deficiency. Those tumors are now excluded from the papillary RCC diagnosis and classified as specific molecularly defined entities. Therefore, the 2022 WHO classification no longer recommends the subtyping of PRCC.

Molecular Genetics

Trisomy or tetrasomy 7, trisomy 17, and loss of the Y chromosome (in men) are the most common cytogenetic changes in PRCC [24]. Additional gains of chromosomes 3, 12, 16, 20, and other chromosomes are often associated with tumor progression. Low-grade PRCC is characterized by alterations in cell signaling involving the *MET* gene with mutations or other alterations that affect its activity identified in 81% of the tumors. In contrast, high-grade PRCC was found to be more genetically heterogeneous [25] and is characterized by *CDKN2A* silencing, *SETD2* mutation, and increased expression of the NRF2-antioxidant response element pathway. A CpG island methylation phenotype (CIMP) was found in a distinct subgroup that was associated with the least favorable outcome. Across all high-grade PRCCs, 25% demonstrated decreased expression of *CDKN2A*, a tumor suppressor gene that regulates the cell cycle. Loss of *CDKN2A* expression was also associated with a less favorable outcome.

Prognosis

Papillary RCC has an overall low risk of recurrence and cancer death after nephrectomy. Predictors of outcome relate to stage and nuclear grade.

Renal Cell Carcinoma: Chromophobe Type (Chromophobe RCC, ChRCC)

Clinical Features

ChRCC accounts for approximately 5% of RCCs and is believed to arise from the intercalated cells of the collecting ducts [26]. ChRCC has a wide age range. Males and females are affected almost equally. The prognosis is significantly better than CCRCC with a disease recurrence in <5% of patients. Most cases arise sporadically, while some cases are associated with Birt-Hogg-Dube syndrome [27].

Pathology

ChRCC is typically a solitary, well-circumscribed and non-encapsulated mass with homogenous light brown solid cut surface. Hemorrhage and/or necrosis are uncommon. A central stellate scar can be seen in large tumors (Fig. 4.3a).

Microscopically, the tumor cells are arranged in solid sheets with tubulocystic architecture in some cases. The classic tumor consists of large and polygonal cells with finely reticulated cytoplasm due to numerous cytoplasmic microvesicles and prominent "plant cell-like" cell membrane. The nuclei are typically irregular, hyperchromatic, and wrinkled with perinuclear halos (Fig. 4.3b). Not infrequently, a tumor consists predominantly of cells with intensely eosinophilic cytoplasm, termed eosinophilic pattern (Fig. 4.3c) [1, 28].

Molecular Genetics

ChRCC harbors extensive chromosomal loss, most commonly involving chromosomes Y, 1, 2, 6, 10, 13, 17, and 21 [29, 30]. Occasionally, ChRCC occurs in Birt-Hogg-Dube syndrome, characterized by mutations in *Birt-Hogg-Dube (BHD)* gene on 17p11.2, which encodes the

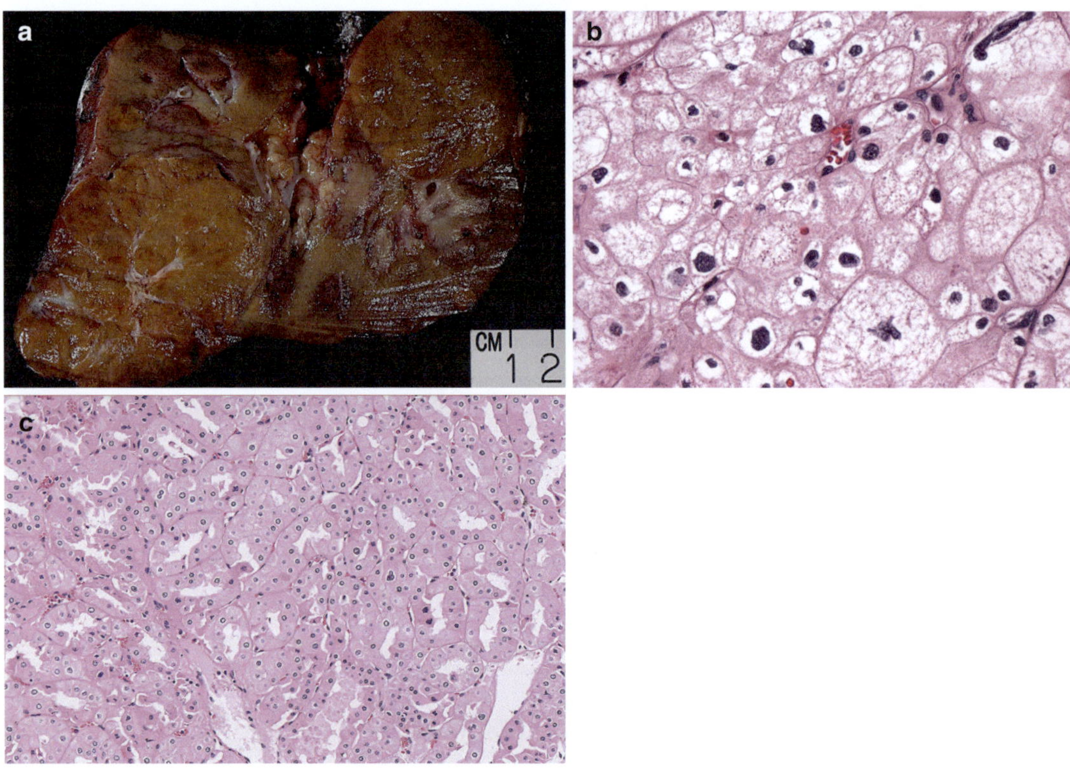

Fig. 4.3 Chromophobe renal cell carcinoma is a circumscribed, non-encapsulated mass with a homogenous yellow to light brown cut surface (**a**) and composed of large and polygonal tumor cells have finely reticulated cytoplasm, prominent cell border, and irregular nuclei with perinuclear clearing (**b**). Tumors of eosinophilic pattern are comprised predominantly of cells with intensely eosinophilic cytoplasm (**c**)

protein folliculin [31]. However, *BHD* mutations are rarely found in sporadic ChRCC. It has been suggested that ChRCC may evolve from an oncocytoma after acquiring additional cytogenetic abnormality. There are also multiple somatic mutations involving mitochondrial DNA and in *TP53* and *PTEN* genes, and rearrangements of the *TERT* promoter region in a significant subset of cases.

Prognosis

The prognosis is generally favorable except in a small subset that can show aggressive behavior with local recurrence, metastasis, and/or death due to disease. The adverse outcome with death of disease ranges from 0% to 15%. On multivariate analysis, sarcomatoid transformation, microscopic tumor necrosis, and higher pT stage were identified as independent predictors of aggressive biological behavior [32]. Tumors of "eosinophilic pattern" have an excellent prognosis with only rare instances of recurrence and metastasis after surgery [33]. However, the definition of "eosinophilic pattern" is not established in the WHO classification [1].

Other Uncommon Subtypes of Renal Cell Carcinoma

Other subtypes are uncommon and collectively account for less than 5% of RCC cases in the kidney and are summarized in Table 4.2. A newly created category, "molecularly defined renal cell carcinomas," refers to those tumors with characteristic genetic alterations (Table 4.3). Several other tumors have not been sufficiently characterized with regards to their clinicopathologic and genetic features and yet are deemed distinct from other RCC subtypes and are therefore included in the WHO classification as "emerging renal tumors" (Table 4.4).

Renal Cell Tumors with Somatic Mutations in TSC/mTOR Pathway Genes

Renal tumors reported in tuberous sclerosis complex (TSC) patients have a wide morphological range, but most of them exhibit eosinophilic differentiation (see Renal Cell Carcinomas in Inherited Cancer Syndromes). Tumors of the same morphologies and immunostaining patterns have also been reported in patients without TSC [34]. However, these tumors do harbor somatic mutations in *TSC1*, *TSC2*, or other genes of the TSC/mTOR pathway, such as *MTOR* and *RPTOR*, and therefore represent sporadic counterparts of the TSC tumors. The latter are far more common than those linked to TSC. They typically display an indolent course, though data is still evolving.

Eosinophilic solid and cystic RCC (ESC RCC) often affects young or middle-aged adult patients and is slightly more common in females [2]. They are generally indolent with minimal metastatic risk reported thus far. Surgical resection is curative, though long-term data remain scarce. Rare cases with lymph nodes or hematogenous metastasis have been reported and those patients may respond to mTOR pathway inhibitors. Grossly, these tumors are well-circumscribed and have solid and cystic areas with fibrous septa. Microscopically they are polygonal cells with abundant granular cytoplasm forming solid nests intermixed with cystic compartments. Coarse basophilic cytoplasmic granules, or basophilic stippling, are characteristic. Biallelic somatic inactivation of *TSC1/2* genes is reported in most of these tumors [35].

Low-grade oncocytic tumor (LOT) affects older patients with a mean age of 64.7 years [2, 33, 36]. They are more common in female patients and have benign clinical outcomes with no reports of recurrence or metastasis. The tumors are typically small, morphologically resembling oncocytomas and eosinophilic ChRCCs but have a distinct immunohistochemical pattern (CK7 diffusely positive and CD117 negative). Most of these tumors harbor somatic mutations in TSC/mTOR pathway genes.

Eosinophilic vacuolated tumors (EVTs) typically affect patients with a wide age range and are more common in female patients [37–39]. They have indolent clinical outcomes. Tumors present as small renal masses with large polygonal cells with frequent large cytoplasmic clear vacuoles and prominent nucleoli. The majority of these

Table 4.2 Clinical, pathological, and genetic features of uncommon RCC subtypes included in the 2022 WHO classification [1–3]

RCC subtype	Clinical Features	Pathology		Genetics	Prognosis
		Gross	Microscopic		
Multilocular cystic neoplasm of low malignant potential	<1% of renal tumors; mean age 55 years (range 18–84); male/female = 1.8:1	Related and morphologically similar to CCRCC; solitary, well-circumscribed, entirely cystic mass; no grossly visible nodules or necrosis	Variably sized cysts lined with one or several layers of flat or plump clear cells; no expansile cellular nodules exceeding 1 mm; low-grade nuclei (grade 1 or 2)	3p deletion as observed in CCRCC in 77% tumors	Excellent; No local or distant metastasis after complete surgical removal
Collecting duct carcinoma (Fig. 4.4a)	<1% of all renal tumors; arising in the collecting ducts of Bellini; often seen in fourth to seventh decade with mean age 55 years; male/female = 2:1	Poorly circumscribed; usually centrally located; cut surface grey, white, and firm	High-grade infiltrative tumor cells form complex tubulocystic structures; prominent desmoplastic stroma	Complex chromosomal aberrations, including allelic loss on chromosomes 1q, 6p, 8p,9p, 13q, 19q32, and 21q; *CDKN2A* loss; *NF2* and *SETD2* mutations	Poor; 1/3 presenting with metastasis; 2/3 patients dead of disease within 2 years of diagnosis
Mucinous tubular spindle cell carcinoma (Fig. 4.4b)	Mean age 53 years (range 13–82); Male/female = 1:4; incidental finding in many cases	Sharply circumscribed; grey-white with myxoid appearance; many have minimal hemorrhage and/or necrosis	Elongated compressed tubules and bland spindle cells with low-grade nuclei embedded in a myxoid stroma	Multiple chromosomal losses, most frequently involving chromosomes 1, 4, 6, 8, 9, 13, 14, 15, and 22; biallelic dysregulation of the Hippo pathway; *VSTM2A* overexpression	Favorable; majority of patients remain disease-free after surgical resection; high-grade transformation associated with metastasis and death
Tubulocystic carcinoma (Fig. 4.4d)	Occurs in fifth and sixth decade (range 30–94 years); male/female = 7:1	Usually solitary; circumscribed and unencapsulated; spongy cut surface resembling “bubble wrap”	Circumscribed collection of tubules and cysts with varied sizes; separated by fibrous stroma; no desmoplastic reaction; lining cells usually exhibit high-grade nuclei and eosinophilic cytoplasm; some cases with poorly differentiated foci and prominent nucleoli represent FH-deficient RCC	Gain in chromosome 17 and loss of 9 and Y; *KMT2C* and *KDM5C* mutations in some cases; frequent mutations in *ABL1* and *PDGFRA*	Majority cases have indolent clinical course; recurrence or metastasis in a few cases

Clear cell papillary renal cell tumor (Fig. 4.4e)	Vast majority incidental; mean age 60 years; male/female =1:1	Small tumor with mean size of 2.4 cm; cystic mass having prominent fibrous capsule or stroma	Branching tubules, acini, and/or clear cell ribbons with low-grade nuclei; positive for CK7 and CAIX, and negative for CD10	No known specific genetic abnormalities	Indolent; as the result, the name was changed from "carcinoma" to "tumor"
Acquired cystic kidney disease (ACD)-associated RCC (Fig. 4.4f)	Exclusively in patients with ACD after long-term dialysis; accounts for >1/3 of RCCs in patients with ESRD / ACD (2–7% RCC incidence in ACD patients; clear cell papillary RCC and PRCC are other common subtypes)	Frequently multicentric and bilateral; generally well circumscribed	Various architectures including papillary and solid; prominent intra- or inter-cytoplasmic lumina imparting sieve-like, cribriform appearance; frequent intratumoral calcium oxalate crystals	Recurrent mutations in *KMT2C* (in tumors with "sieve-like" morphology) and *TSC2* (in tumors with PRCC morphology)	Mostly indolent behavior with rare metastasis, usually in cases with dedifferentiated pathology

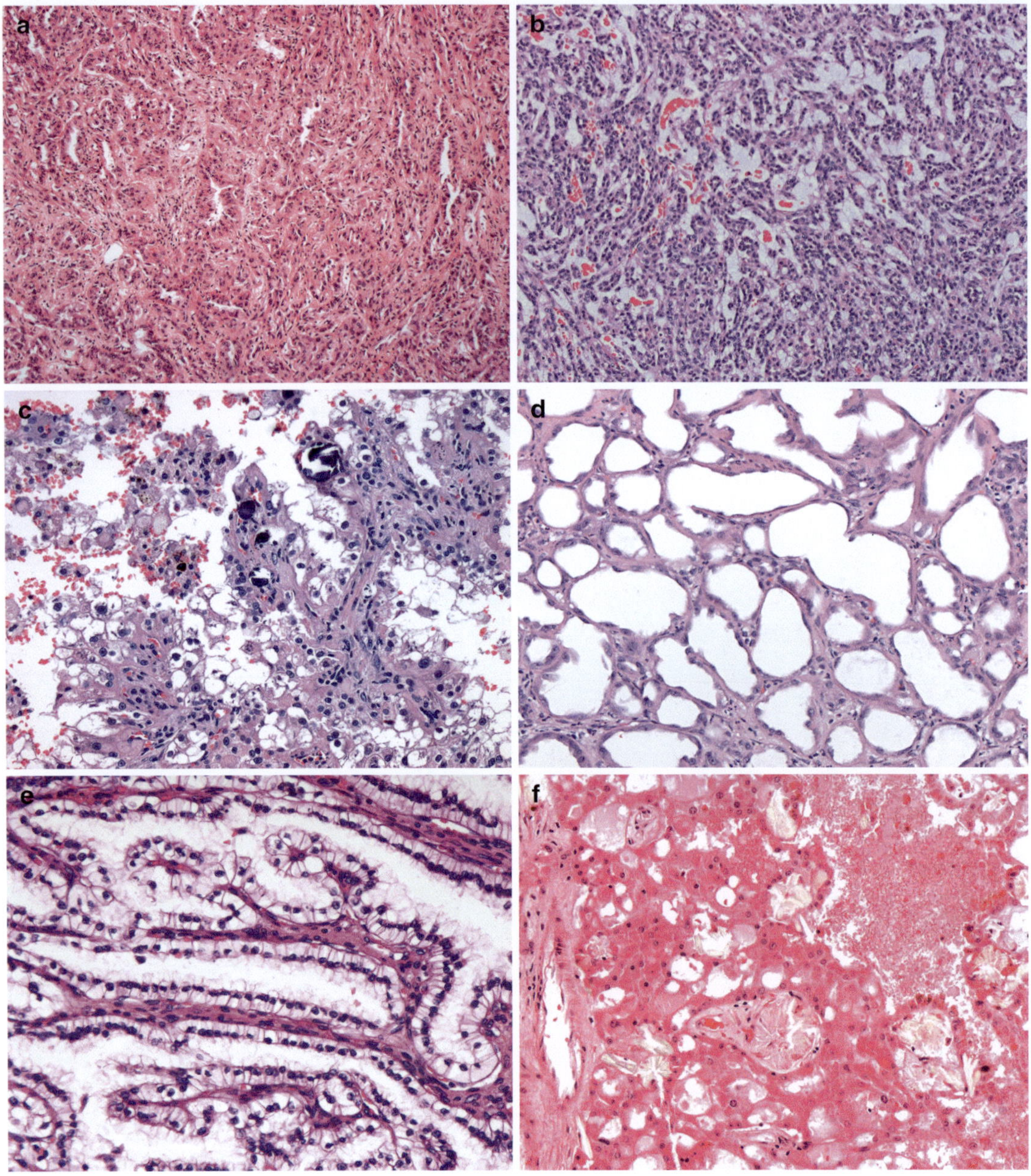

Fig. 4.4 Uncommon renal cell carcinoma subtypes. Collecting duct carcinoma consists of high-grade tumor cells forming complex tubules or tubulopapillary structures embedded in a remarkably desmoplastic stroma (**a**). Mucinous tubular and spindle cell carcinoma is composed of elongated cords and collapsed tubules with slit-like spaces embedded in a lightly basophilic myxoid background. The tumor cells have low-grade nuclear features (**b**). *TFE3*-rearranged renal cell carcinoma with characteristic papillary structure lined with tumor cells with abundant partly clear, partly eosinophilic cytoplasm and high-grade nuclei. Psammomatous calcification is also present (**c**). Tubulocystic renal cell carcinoma is composed of closely packed tubules and cysts separated by thin, fibrous septae (**d**). Clear cell papillary renal cell tumor comprises tubules and stubby papillae lined with cells with clear cytoplasm and low-grade nuclei, the latter characteristically aligned towards luminal surface (**e**). Acquired cystic disease-associated renal cell carcinoma is composed of cribriform nests of cells with abundant eosinophilic cytoplasm. Calcium oxalate crystals with "sun-burst" appearance are often found in the tumor (**f**)

Table 4.3 Clinical, pathological, and genetic features of "molecularly defined renal cell carcinomas" included in the 2022 WHO classification [1–3]

RCC subtype	Clinical Features	Pathology		Genetics	Prognosis
		Gross	Microscopic		
TFE3-rearranged RCC	40% of pediatric RCCs and 1.6–4% of adult RCCs	No characteristic gross appearance	Papillae lined with epithelioid clear cells with abundant psammomatous calcification; other uncommon patterns reminiscent of MLCNLMP, oncocytoma and epithelioid AML; under-expressing epithelial markers	Fusions of *TFE3* with one of many partner genes	Similar to CCRCC but worse than PRCC; distant metastasis and older age at presentation predict death; pediatric patients have better prognosis
TFEB-altered RCC	Rare; mean age 31 years; older patients with *TFEB*-amplified RCCs; clinical presentations not specific	Not specific	Overlap with *TFE3*-RCCs; biphasic pattern with nests of larger epithelioid cells and smaller cells clustered around basement membrane material is characteristic; *TFEB*-amplified RCC often show high-grade, poorly differentiated RCC with frequent oncocytic and papillary features	*TFEB*-rearranged RCC: fusion between *TFEB* and various partner genes, mainly *MALAT1*; *TFEB*-amplified RCC: amplification of 6p21, resulting in amplification of *TFEB* and other genes (*VEGFA*, *CCND3* etc.)	*TFEB*-rearranged RCC more indolent than *TFE3*-RCCs *TFEB*-amplified RCC more aggressive
ELOC-mutated RCC	Rare; median age 60 years; majority in male patients	Small (pT1) and well-circumscribed tumors	Clear cells forming nodules with thick fibromuscular capsule and stroma	Mutations involve VHL protein binding site in *ELOC* gene, leading to HIF1α overexpression	Indolent with rare reports of metastasis from tumors with high nuclear grade
FH-deficient RCC (Fig. 4.5)	Prevalence unknown; male/female = 1.9:1; young patients with early onset uterine leiomyoma and skin leiomyomas; frequently with flank pain and hematuria;	Solitary; solid or solid and cystic	Multiple admixed morphological patterns, including papillary, solid, tubulocystic, cribriform and cystic; eosinophilic macronucleoli common although nonspecific; negative IHC for FH and strong staining for 2SC	Germline, and in a subset somatic, mutations in fumarate hydratase (*FH*) gene	Aggressive; a subset with a favorable prognosis

(continued)

Table 4.3 (continued)

RCC subtype	Clinical Features	Pathology		Genetics	Prognosis
		Gross	Microscopic		
SDH-deficient RCC (Fig. 4.6)	Rare, <0.05–0.2% of all RCCs; young adults (median age: 35 years), slight male predominance	Usually circumscribed with a tan-brown cut surface; mostly solid	Sheets or compact nests of bland eosinophilic cells with pale, bubbly cytoplasm due to inclusion containing lightly eosinophilic or basophilic material; occasionally high-grade transformation with denser cytoplasm, increased nuclear atypia, necrosis and sarcomatoid changes; loss of SDHB expression on IHC	Inactivation of any one of the *SDH* genes, most commonly *SDHB*, usually due to germline mutations	Favorable prognosis in tumors with low-grade morphology; tumors with high-grade transformation have risk of metastasis as high as 70%
ALK-rearranged RCC	Rare; occurs in both children and adults; both sexes affected equally; pediatric patients with sickle cell trait	Usually solitary; small and confined to the kidney; solid or solid-cystic	Variable mixed patterns, often mucinous or myxoid stroma; medullary carcinoma-like in children; ALK+	*ALK* rearrangement with various fusion partners	Limited; metastasis and death in ¼ cases
SMARCB1-deficient medullary RCC	Wide age range; male/female-2:1; most cases in patients of African ancestry with sickle cell trait or hemoglobinopathy	Large, poorly circumscribed; centered in the renal medulla	High-grade infiltrative growth; marked myxoid desmoplastic reaction with inflammatory cell infiltrate; sickled red blood cells present; loss of SMARCB1 protein; OCT3/4 + in 50% cases	Biallelic loss of SMARCB1 in vast majority of cases	Extremely poor prognosis

Table 4.4 Emerging renal cell tumors (2022 WHO classification) [1–3]

RCC subtype	Clinical features	Pathology		Genetics	Prognosis
		Gross	Microscopic		
Thyroid-like follicular carcinoma	Very rare; mean age 45 years	Wide size range; tan to brown; well-circumscribed	Prominent pseudocapsule; micro- and macro-follicles lined with low-grade cells; colloid-like material present in >50% of follicles; thyroid IHC markers negative	Limited data; no distinctive IHC or molecular marker	Mostly indolent, with rare cases reporting distant metastases
Biphasic hyalinizing psammomatous renal cell carcinoma	Older adults; more common in men	Not specific	Solid and papillary growth; biphasic cell population: larger cells and smaller cells clustered around basement membrane material ("glomeruloid pattern"); hyalinized stroma with psammoma bodies	Somatic mutations in *NF2* gene	Very limited; generally indolent with a favorable prognosis; occasional reports of recurrence or metastasis
Papillary neoplasm with reverse polarity	Middle-aged or old patients; no sex predilection; incidental finding	Small, well-circumscribed with tan and yellow cut surface	Papillary structures lined by a single layer of cells with abundant eosinophilic cytoplasm; nuclei oriented away from the basement membrane (reverse polarity); lack significant nuclear atypia; psammoma bodies common	Recurrent KRAS mutations	Indolent
RCC with fibromyomatous stroma	Variable	Variable	Nests and nodules of clear cells arranged in tubulopapillary pattern; prominent smooth muscle and vascular stroma	Negative for 3p deletions and trisomy 7, 17; association with *TSC* gene mutations; rarely with *ELOC* gene mutation	Mostly favorable prognosis

tumors harbor somatic mutations in TSC/mTOR pathway genes.

RCCs with fibromyxomatous stroma contain nests or nodules of tumor cells with abundant clear or slightly eosinophilic cytoplasm embedded in a dense fibrous and smooth muscle stroma [34, 40]. These tumors may overlap considerably in morphology with clear cell RCCs and clear cell papillary tumours. They frequently contain mutations in *TSC1*, *TSC2*, and *MTOR* genes. Although morphology and immunophenotype are often suggestive, a definitive diagnosis can only be made after sequencing of these genes. Of note, RCCs of similar morphology are reported to harbor mutations in *ELOC* gene [41].

Renal Cell Carcinoma: Unclassified Type

RCC, unclassified type, is a term for RCC that does not fit into any of the accepted RCC diagnoses in WHO classification [42]. It is important to understand that this is a diagnostic category rather than a true biological entity. These tumors represent a heterogeneous group with poorly defined clinical, morphological, or genetic features and therefore cannot be classified using the current criteria. Most but not all unclassified tumors are poorly differentiated and are associated with a poor prognosis. However, with increasing molecular diagnostics, some "unclassified" tumors can be classified if they show hallmark genetic events (e.g., *ALK* rearrangements, *ELOC* mutations). As our understanding of RCC improves, this category is destined to diminish and perhaps eventually disappear.

Renal Cell Carcinomas in Inherited Cancer Syndromes

Less than 5% of RCC occur in the setting of inherited cancer syndromes, including von Hippel-Lindau disease (VHLD), hereditary papillary renal cell carcinoma (HPRCC), hereditary leiomyomatosis and renal cell carcinoma (HLRCC), Birt-Hogg-Dube (BHD) syndrome, and others such as familial pheochromocytoma paraganglioma syndrome and tuberous sclerosis complex [43–45]. Each inherited cancer syndrome is featured with distinct subtypes of RCC which often affect patients at a younger age and are more likely to be bilateral and multifocal than sporadic cases.

von Hippel-Lindau Disease (VHLD)

VHLD is an autosomal-dominant hereditary condition with stigmata including CCRCCs, central nervous system hemangioblastomas, pheochromocytomas, pancreatic cysts, and endolymphatic sac tumors of the inner ear [25533676]. Germline mutations in the *VHL* gene are causative. VHLD patients are born with a germline defect in one of the alleles, and the second allele is inactivated by somatic alterations. Renal lesions in VHLD are always CCRCC and tend to be bilateral and multifocal. Dozens or even hundreds of microscopic tumor foci can be identified in resected kidney specimens. RCC develops early with a mean age of onset of 37 years as compared with 61 years for sporadic CCRCC. Although metastasis typically only occurs when tumors are greater than 3 cm, RCC is nevertheless the leading cause of death in this syndrome. However, VHLD patients with renal involvement fare better in 10-year survival than their sporadic counterparts [46, 47]. New surveillance protocols suggest biannual imaging and early intervention with ablative therapies to preserve renal function and delay surgical nephrectomy. Hypoxia-inducible factors (HIF-1α and HIF-2α) play a critical role in tumor progression, leading to the development of HIF-2α inhibitors such as belzutifan as a systemic therapy for advanced VHLD RCC.

Hereditary Papillary Renal Cell Carcinoma (HPRCC)

HPRCC is characterized by a predisposition to bilateral multiple papillary renal tumors. To date, the kidney is the only organ affected in these patients [48]. HPRCC is associated with a germline mutation in the tyrosine kinase domain of the *c-met* proto-oncogene on chromosome 7q31 which encodes a cell surface receptor protein for hepatocyte growth factor (HGF) and has tyrosine kinase activity [49]. Gain-of-function mutations result in activated cellular processes that contribute to carcinogenesis, including angiogenesis, cell motility, proliferation, and morphogenic differentiation. MET inhibitors, such as tepotinib and capmatinib, have shown promise in treatment of metastatic HPRCC. *MET* amplification renders resistance to targeted therapies, suggesting combination strategies for treatment.

Hereditary Leiomyomatosis and Renal Cell Carcinoma (HLRCC)

HLRCC is an autosomal dominant characterized by cutaneous leiomyomas and early-onset uterine leiomyomas, occasional uterine leiomyosarcoma, and RCCs [3, 50, 51]. RCC develops in ~15% of patients, and it usually behaves in an aggressive fashion with frequent metastasis to regional lymph nodes, adrenal gland, liver, or

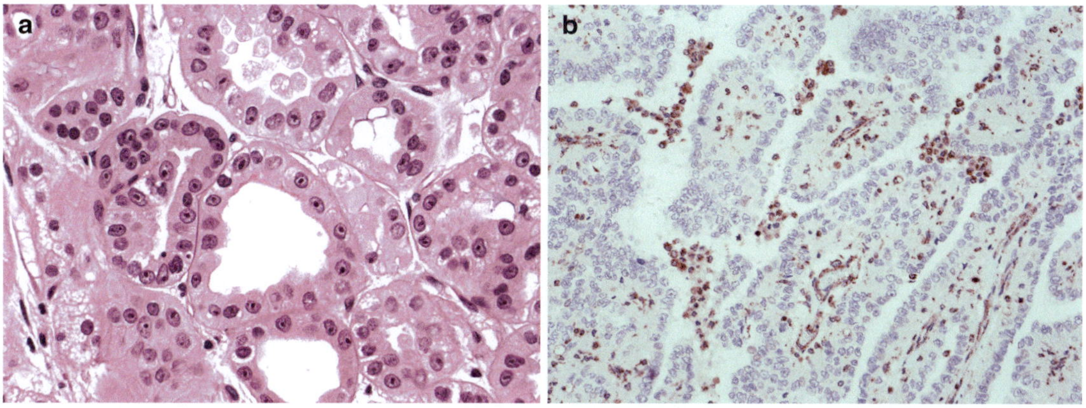

Fig. 4.5 Fumarate hydratase-deficient renal cell carcinoma in hereditary leiomyomatosis/renal cell carcinoma syndrome. Tumor cells have large nuclei with prominent eosinophilic nucleoli surrounded by clear halos (**a**). Immunohistochemically, tumor cells show loss of FH protein expression in contrast to positive expression in stromal cells (**b**)

lung, even when the tumor is small. Grossly, the renal tumor is usually solitary and unilateral, unlike other renal tumors in inherited cancer syndromes. Histologically, the tumor characteristically shows mixed architectural patterns with papillary, tubular, tubulopapillary, solid, and cystic configurations. Sometimes, collecting duct carcinoma-like or tubulocystic carcinoma-like patterns can also be observed. The most characteristic feature is large nuclei with prominent eosinophilic nucleoli surrounded by clear halos (cytomegaloviral inclusion-like) (Fig. 4.5a), which may also be observed in uterine leiomyomas. Immunohistochemically, HLRCC tumors show loss or marked reduced expression of fumarate hydratase protein (Fig. 4.5b). Genetically, somatic mutation of the fumarate hydratase (*FH*) gene or loss of heterozygosity is observed in addition to *FH* germline mutation on chromosome 1 (1q42.3–43) in most cases. FH is required to convert fumarate to malate in the Krebs cycle and inactivation of *FH* impairs it, thereby activating anaerobic metabolism and upregulation of HIF and hypoxia-inducible genes. The term "FH-deficient" RCC is used when tumors show the typical histomorphology and immunohistochemical profile described above but lack or have uncertain information regarding clinical or family history and genetic status. Suspected cases should be confirmed by *FH* gene sequencing. Radical nephrectomy, including adrenal gland resection and regional lymphadenectomy, is the choice of therapy. Advances in molecular studies highlight fumarate-mediated epigenetic reprogramming as a potential therapeutic target. Clinical trials involving FH inhibitors and immune checkpoint inhibitors are ongoing.

Renal Cell Carcinomas in Hereditary Pheochromocytoma Paraganglioma Syndrome

Hereditary pheochromocytoma paraganglioma syndrome is an autosomal dominant syndrome with incomplete penetrance, caused by germline mutations in succinate dehydrogenase (SDH) genes (*SDHA, B, C, D*, and *SDHAF2*), and epimutation in *SDHC*, leading to disruption of the mitochondrial complex 2 on the inner membrane of mitochondria [52], which plays a critical role in the Krebs cycle, and subsequent accumulation of oncometabolites that contribute to carcinogenesis. Patients are predisposed to develop pheochromocytoma, paraganglioma, or gastrointestinal stromal tumor and RCC. SDHB is mutated in the vast majority of cases. SDH-deficient RCC tends to affect young adults. The tumor is grossly well-circumscribed, and the cut surface demonstrates tan to brown color.

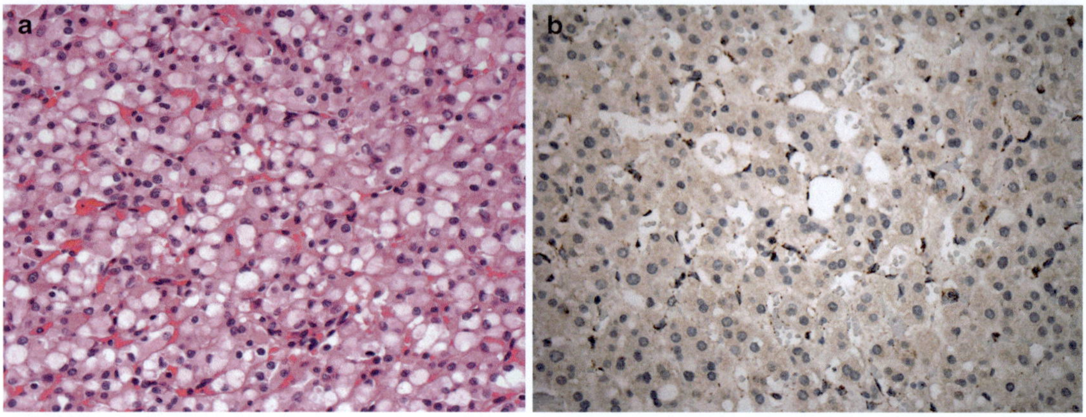

Fig. 4.6 Succinate dehydrogenase-deficient renal cell carcinoma is composed of cuboidal to oval cells with eosinophilic cytoplasm and "bubbly" appearance due to presence of intracytoplasmic vacuoles (**a**). Tumor cells are negative for SDHB staining immunohistochemically with vascular endothelial cells as positive control with brown chunky granular staining (**b**)

Histologically, the tumor is composed of round to oval cells with eosinophilic cytoplasm and "bubbly" appearance due to the presence of intracytoplasmic vacuoles (Fig. 4.6a), which by ultrastructural studies have shown to be giant mitochondria [3, 52]. Nuclei are generally of low grade, but high grade including sarcomatoid change may occur. Immunohistochemically, tumor cells are negative for SDHB staining (Fig. 4.6b). Because mutations in any of the SDH subunits destabilize the mitochondrial complex 2 and lead to loss of SDHB proteins, SDHB IHC is a very effective way to screen for SDH mutations. Surgical resection is the choice of treatment. Tumors behave in an indolent fashion, but those with high-grade component or coagulative necrosis are likely to behave aggressively [3, 52].

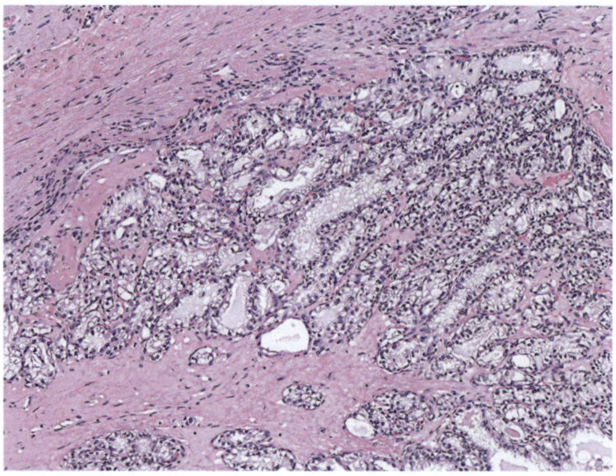

Fig. 4.7 Renal cell carcinoma with fibromyomatous stroma in tuberous sclerosis complex contains nests or nodules of tumor cells with abundant clear or slightly eosinophilic cytoplasm embedded in a dense fibrous and smooth muscle stroma

Renal Tumors in Tuberous Sclerosis Complex (TSC)

Tuberous sclerosis complex (TSC), an autosomal dominant syndrome with inactivating mutations in tumor suppressor genes *TSC1* and *TSC2*, affects the central nervous system and other organs [53]. In the kidney, TSC is most associated with the development of angiomyolipomas (in ~80% of cases). RCC occurs in 2–4% of patients [54–56] and presents at a young age with a female predominance and multiple lesions in half of the patients. A wide array of tumors has been reported, including clear cell RCC, papillary RCC, chromophobe RCC, unclassified RCC, and renal oncocytoma, as well as newly described entities like RCC with fibromyxomatous stroma (Fig. 4.7), eosinophilic-solid cystic RCC, low-grade oncocytic tumor (LOT) and eosinophilic vacuolated tumor (EVT). Concurrent renal angiomyolipoma is frequent (also see discussion in "angiomyolipoma" below). For treatment, surgical resection has been performed for most patients. These tumors generally pursue an indolent clinical course, but nodal metastases have been reported.

Birt-Hogg-Dube Syndrome (BHD)

RCC is also part of the Birt-Hogg-Dube syndrome, an autosomal dominant disorder characterized by benign skin tumors (fibrofolliculomas, trichodiscomas of hair follicles, and skin tag), renal epithelial neoplasms, lung cysts, and spontaneous pneumothorax [27, 57, 58]. Renal neoplasms are almost always multifocal and bilateral, the most common being hybrid oncocytic tumors (50%) with features of both ChRCC and oncocytoma but diagnostic of neither [59]. Intermixed oncocytic and clear cells with "checkerboard" mosaic pattern is characteristic [60] (Fig. 4.8). *BHD*, the gene implicated in the syndrome, on 17p11.2, is a potential tumor suppressor gene and encodes the protein folliculin. The oncocytic tumors in BHD generally have favorable prognosis.

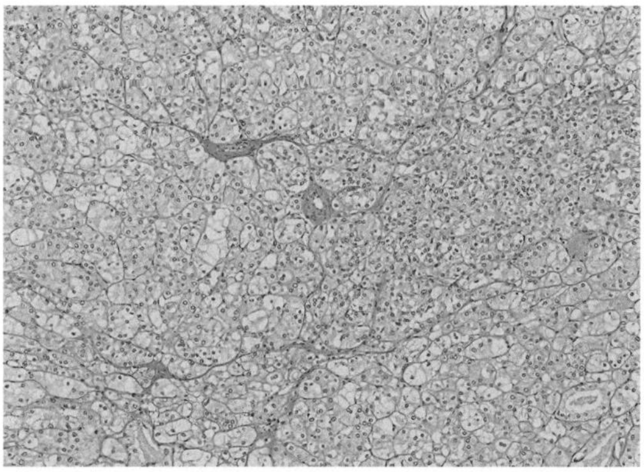

Fig. 4.8 Hybrid oncocytic tumor in Birt-Hogg-Dube syndrome shows intermixed oncocytic and clear cells in a checkerboard pattern

Common Benign Renal Tumors

Papillary Adenoma

Papillary adenomas are unencapsulated epithelial neoplasms up to 15 mm in size with papillary and/or tubular architecture, composed of tumor cells with low-grade nuclei [1].

Clinical Features

Papillary adenoma is the most common renal cell neoplasm, frequently seen as incidental findings in nephrectomy specimens or at autopsy. In one autopsy study, papillary adenomas were found in up to 40% of patients older than 70 years of age. Its incidence increases with age and in patients who are on long-term dialysis.

Pathology

Papillary adenomas appear as small (<15 mm by definition), well-circumscribed, yellow or white nodules in the renal cortex. They have papillary, tubular, or tubulopapillary architecture like papillary RCC but are usually unencapsulated. The tumor cells have uniform small nuclei and inconspicuous nucleoli equivalent to WHO/ISUP grade 1 or 2 nuclei.

Molecular Genetics

KMT2C mutations are probably an important early event during the development of papillary adenomas. They share many genetic alterations with PRCC, including combined gains of chromosomes 7 and 17 and loss of the Y chromosome in men. PRCCs acquire additional genetic alterations, including trisomy 12, 16, or 20. The cytogenetic findings support the hypothesis that papillary adenoma is a precursor of PRCC [1].

Renal Oncocytoma

Clinical Features

Renal oncocytoma accounts for 5% of surgically resected renal neoplasms. Patients vary in age with a peak incidence in the seventh decade of life. The male to female ratio is 2: 1. Most cases are sporadic, although familial cases have been reported in association with Birt-Hogg-Dube syndrome and familial renal oncocytoma syndrome. They are benign.

Pathology

Oncocytoma is typically solitary and well-circumscribed and has varying degrees of encapsulation. The cut surface exhibits a characteristic homogeneous mahogany-brown color (Fig. 4.9a). A central stellate scar can be seen in 1/3 of the cases, more common in larger tumors. More than 10% of cases are multifocal or bilateral.

Microscopically, oncocytoma is characterized by bright eosinophilic cells, termed oncocytes, arranged in nested, acinar, or microcystic pattern associated with a loose hypocellular and hyalinized stroma (Fig. 4.9b). Extension of oncocytoma into the perinephric fat, or rarely into vascular space, can be found sometimes and does not adversely affect the benign prognosis of the lesion.

Molecular Genetics

Many oncocytomas have a normal karyotype [61]. Some tumors show recurrent chromosomal losses involving 1, 14, 21, X, and Y [62]. A subset shows CCND1 rearrangements at the 11q13 locus [63]. Mutations of mitochondrial genes have also been reported in oncocytoma [63]. Oncocytoma can be a manifestation of Birt-Hogg-Dube syndrome.

Whether oncocytoma and ChRCC are related is still controversial. They not only have overlapping morphological features but also share some cytogenetic changes, such as the loss of heterozygosity at chromosome 1. However, monosomy of chromosomes 2, 10, 13, 17, and 21 occurred exclusively in ChRCC [64].

Angiomyolipoma

Clinical Features

Angiomyolipoma (AML) is a renal mesenchymal tumor comprising variable proportions of adipose tissue, smooth muscle bundles, and blood vessels. The prevalence in autopsies is 0.3% and 0.1% in ultrasound-screened patients. It accounts for 0.3–3% of all renal tumors in surgically resected renal neoplasms. AMLs are usually sporadic but in a minority of cases associated with TSC [65], in which most individuals have multiple AMLs affecting both kidneys. Patients with TSC develop AML earlier (mean age at diagnosis at 25–35 years with TSC versus 40–45 years without TSC). The male–to-female ratio in surgical series is 1: 4. AMLs, particularly those associ-

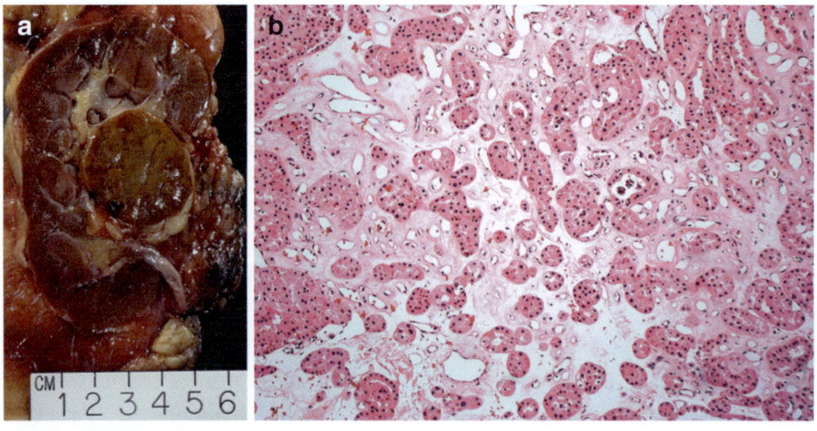

Fig. 4.9 Renal oncocytoma is a solitary, well-circumscribed, non-encapsulated mass with homogeneous dark-brown cut surface (**a**), and consists of bright eosinophilic cells nested in a loose stroma. The tumor cells are uniform, round to polygonal with granular eosinophilic cytoplasm, and regular round nuclei (**b**)

ated with TSC, are usually asymptomatic and detected by imaging studies. Intra-abdominal bleeding owing to rupture may be an uncommon presentation initially or during follow-up. Fat-poor AML is challenging to diagnose radiologically and may be mistaken for an RCC. Classic AMLs are benign.

Pathology

AML is typically well-circumscribed, non-capsulated mass with or without lobulation and sometimes with subtle infiltrative edges. The cut surface depends on the relative amount of three tissue components.

As its name implies, AML consists of thick-walled blood vessels, spindle cells with smooth muscle features, and mature adipose tissue in variable proportions (Fig. 4.10). Blood vessels typically have an eccentrically thickened wall with spindle cells spun off the wall. Spindle cells range from mature-appearing smooth muscle cells to immature spindle cells, epithelioid cells, and even bizarre cells with atypical nuclear features. Mature adipose tissue may have cytological atypia. Melanocytic markers, including Melan-A and HBM-45, are positive in AMLs and are often used to confirm the diagnosis. Other markers such as Cathepsin K, smooth muscle markers, and CD68 may be positive. Classical AMLs are benign. However, ¼ to 1/3 of epithelioid AML are malignant with local and distant metastasis. Pathological features that correlate with adverse outcomes include large size, tumor necrosis, atypical mitosis, and diffuse atypical nuclei.

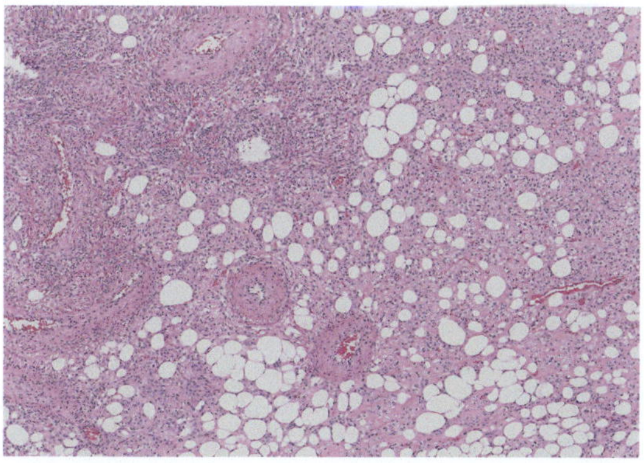

Fig. 4.10 Angiomyolipoma consists of thick-walled blood vessels, spindle cells with smooth muscle features, and mature adipose tissue in variable proportions

Molecular Genetics

AML belongs to the so-called perivascular epithelioid tumor (PEComa). AMLs in TSC show evidence of bi-allelic inactivation of the *TSC1* or *TSC2* gene, corresponding to the germline mutation present in such individuals. With loss of heterozygosity for the *TSC2* region, *TSC2* inactivation by mutation is likely a necessary genetic event in the pathogenesis of most sporadic AMLs [66, 67].

Pathological Prognosis Parameters for Renal Cell Carcinoma

Stage

The AJCC (8th Edition) staging system for RCC (Table 4.5), published in 2017 [68], remains critical for assessing prognosis, guiding treatment, and stratifying patients for clinical trials.

No major staging revisions have been made to the AJCC seventh edition, but clarifications have reinforced the importance of renal sinus invasion (T3a) as an adverse prognostic factor. Invasion into perinephric fat and renal sinus fat is both staged as pT3a. Recent studies suggest that invasion of renal sinus is more ominous prognostically [69, 70]. While organ-confined renal tumors that are >7 cm in size are staged as pT2, these are uncommon. Studies have shown large kidney tumors very frequently show extrarenal invasion, usually in the renal sinus, when subjected to careful gross sampling [71, 72].

This staging method applies to RCCs. There should be histological confirmation of the tumor. The regional lymph nodes are the hilar, abdominal para-aortic and paracaval nodes. Metastasis to lymph nodes other than regional is considered distant metastasis. pM1 denotes distant metastasis confirmed microscopically. pM0 and pMx are not valid categories.

Table 4.5 Pathology stage of primary renal cell carcinoma (AJCC 2017) [68]

Primary tumor (T)	
TX	Primary tumor cannot be assessed
T0	No evidence of primary tumor
T1	Tumor 7 cm or less in greatest dimension, limited to the kidney
T1a	Tumor 4 cm or less in greatest dimension, limited to the kidney
T1b	Tumor more than 4 cm but not more than 7 cm in greatest admission, limited to the kidney
T2	Tumor more than 7 cm in greatest dimension, limited to the kidney
T2a	Tumor more than 7 cm but less than or equal to 10 cm in greatest dimension, limited to the kidney
T2 b	Tumor more than 10 cm, limited to the kidney
T3	Tumor extends into major veins or perinephric tissues but not into the ipsilateral adrenal gland and not beyond Gerota's fascia
T3a	Tumor extends into the renal vein or its segmental branches, or tumor invades the pelvicalyceal system or tumor invades perirenal and/or renal sinus fat but not beyond Gerota's fascia
T3b	Tumor extends into the vena cava below the diaphragm
T3c	Tumor extends into the vena cava above the diaphragm or invades the wall of the vena cava
T4	Tumor invades beyond Gerota's fascia including contiguous extension into the ipsilateral adrenal gland
Regional lymph nodes (N)	
Nx	Regional lymph nodes cannot be assessed
N0	No regional lymph node metastasis
N1	Metastasis in regional lymph node(s)
Distant metastasis (M)	
M1	Distant metastases

Grading of Renal Cell Carcinomas

The WHO/International Society of Urological Pathology (WHO/ISUP) grading of renal cell carcinomas employs a 4-tier system (Table 4.6) [73, 74]. Grades 1–3 are defined by the degree of nucleolar prominence, and grade 4 is defined by the nuclear pleomorphism, tumor giant cells, and sarcomatoid and rhabdoid differentiation. This grading system is recommended for CCRCC and PRCC with adequate validated data for clinical use [1]. The nuclear grading is clearly not applicable for chromophobe RCC [75] and *TFE3*-rearranged RCC. It is potentially useful for SDH-deficient RCC, mucinous tubular and spindle cell carcinoma, *ELOC*-mutated RCC, *TFEB*-altered RCC, FH-deficient RCC and RCC-NOS; however, more studies are needed to validate the use in these tumors. Some renal cell carcinomas are inherently aggressive regardless of the nuclear grading, including collecting duct carcinoma and *SMARCB1*-deficient medullary carcinoma. For tumors such as tubulocystic RCC, acquired cystic disease-associated RCC, eosinophilic and cystic RCC and EVT, nuclear grading is potentially misleading because these tumors often have high-grade nuclei despite their overall indolent clinical behavior. There is no or limited data on the predictive value of grading for such tumors as *ALK*-rearranged RCC and other oncocytic tumors.

Table 4.6 WHO/ISUP grading system for renal cell carcinoma [24025520] [1]

Grade	Nucleolar features
1	Nucleoli absent or inconspicuous and basophilic at 400× magnification
2	Nucleoli conspicuous and eosinophilic at 400× magnification, visible but not prominent at 100× magnification
3	Nucleoli conspicuous and eosinophilic at 100× magnification
4	Marked nuclear pleomorphism and/or multinucleate giant cells and/or rhabdoid and/or sarcomatoid differentiation

Sarcomatoid and Rhabdoid Differentiation

Sarcomatoid differentiation is present in about 5% of RCCs and is found in any RCC subtype [76]. Therefore, sarcomatoid RCC is not considered a distinct subtype of RCC; rather, it is thought to represent a high-grade and poorly differentiated component. It is associated with poor clinical outcomes, including high metastatic potential and median survival <1 year in advanced disease. Any RCC with sarcomatoid differentiation is assigned a WHO/ISUP grade 4.

RCC with sarcomatoid differentiation typically has other adverse pathological features, including large tumor size, extension into perinephric fat and vessels, and presence of hemorrhage and necrosis [77]. Sarcomatoid components usually appear as white to grey, firm and fibrous cut surfaces. Histologically, the sarcomatoid component ranges from malignant spindle cells to occasionally those resembling leiomyosarcoma, fibrosarcoma, angiosarcoma, rhabdomyosarcoma, and other sarcomas. The co-existing RCC component, including clear cell, papillary, and chromophobe RCC, can often be identified and is used to subtype the RCC with sarcomatoid differentiation. Rarely, the sarcomatoid component overruns RCC epithelial components and renders subtyping impossible in such cases.

Molecular features of the sarcomatoid RCCs include high genomic instability with frequent alterations in *TP53*, *CDKN2A*, and *RB1* tumor suppressor genes [78]. There is strong association with *VHL* mutations and dysregulation of the PI3K/AKT/mTOR pathway, particularly in clear cell RCC. Expression of immune checkpoints like PD-L1 is enriched, indicating potential for immune evasion.

Therapeutically, sarcomatoid RCC has limited response to conventional therapies, including VEGF-targeted agents [79]. Immune checkpoint inhibitors (e.g., nivolumab + ipilimumab) have shown promise, leveraging PD-L1 expression for improved survival in advanced cases.

Rhabdoid differentiation can be identified in approximately 5% of RCCs with tumor cells having large eccentric nuclei, macronucleoli, and prominent acidophilic globular cytoplasm [24025520]. The presence of rhabdoid component is also associated with high grade and high stage with frequent extrarenal extension. It is a marker of high risk for metastasis and poor prognosis even when the rhabdoid component is limited. It is assigned a WHO/ISUP grade 4. Rhabdoid differentiation arises through clonal evolution although less is known of specific genomic alterations in rhabdoid cells. Therapeutically, tumors show poor response to conventional therapies such as VEGF inhibitors in CCRCC. Immune checkpoint inhibitors show emerging promise, especially in tumors with high PD-L1 expression [80, 81].

Tumor Necrosis

Tumor necrosis is linked to hypoxia and ischemia within the tumor microenvironment [82]. It is frequently associated with mutations or alterations in genes regulating angiogenesis and hypoxia responses, such as VHL and HIF pathways, especially in clear cell RCC. TP53 mutations and immune evasion markers (e.g., PD-L1 expression) are more prevalent in necrotic tumors, suggesting a link to aggressive tumor biology [83]. Tumor necrosis correlates with high expression of pro-inflammatory cytokines and pathways associated with epithelial-to-mesenchymal transition (EMT) [84].

Tumor necrosis is a recognized independent marker of poor prognosis in RCC, and is associated with higher tumor grade and stage, increased metastatic potential and recurrence risk and reduced overall survival and progression-free survival [85]. Tumor necrosis is incorporated into some prognostic scoring systems, including the SSIGN score, used for risk stratification in clear cell RCC [86].

Tumors with extensive necrosis often show resistance to anti-angiogenic therapies due to a hypoxic microenvironment fostering angiogenesis [87]. High necrotic burden may correlate with increased PD-L1 expression, supporting the use of immune checkpoint inhibitors [83]. Tumor necrosis may serve as a biomarker for aggressive treatment strategies, including multimodal approaches combining targeted therapy and immunotherapy.

Microvascular Invasion

Microvascular invasion (MVI) defined as neoplastic cells invading the vessel wall or neoplastic emboli within vascular spaces (small veins or lymphatics) adjacent to or within the primary tumor is present in 13.6–44.6% of RCC [88]. It is more common in RCC of high stage and grade and large size. Unlike macrovascular invasion, presence of MVI does not change the pathologic stage of RCCs. It is associated with advanced primary tumor stage, high pathological grades, high tumor size, high clinical symptoms and lymph node invasion, worse cancer specific survival [88, 89]. However, it does not seem to be an independent predictor of cancer survival mortality. Its prognostic value is therefore uncertain and requires further studies to better define its prognostic significance.

Histological Subtyping in Localized and Metastatic RCC

Reflecting biological behavior and metastatic potential, histological subtyping significantly influences prognosis [21, 90]. In the era of partial nephrectomies for RCC, histological subtyping remains a significant predictor of survival, regardless of type of surgical resection or tumor stage. CCRCC has worse outcomes than other subtypes for equivalent stages, with higher metastatic potential and more aggressive clinical courses. PRCC often has indolent clinical courses and favorable prognosis, although high-grade PRCC has poorer outcomes, higher aggressiveness and metastatic risk. Chromophobe RCC has a generally favorable prognosis and low metastatic potential. It rarely progresses, but late recurrences can occur. FH-deficient carcinoma is highly aggressive with early metastasis and has an extremely poor clinical outcome. For unclassified RCC, its prognosis is variable and depends on the grade and is often worse for poorly differentiated ones.

Similarly, histologic subtyping has prognostic and therapeutic potential in metastatic RCC as well. Intermediate and high-risk metastatic non-clear cell RCCs appear to have an inferior prognosis as compared to clear cell RCC; however, such a difference vanishes in favorable risk tumors [91].

Treatment for metastatic RCC has transformed from cytokine-based regimens to tyrosine kinase inhibitors (TKIs) such as targeted agent therapy against vascular endothelial growth factor (VEGF) and platelet-derived growth factor (PDGF), and most recently to immune checkpoint inhibitor (ICI) and combination of ICI and TKIs. The subtyping of metastatic RCC also significantly impacts treatment decisions, as different subtypes respond differently to targeted therapies [17]. ICI-based combinations primarily benefit CCRCC. MET inhibitors in combination with ICIs have been proven effective in treating metastatic papillary RCC. RCC with sarcomatoid differentiation has demonstrated preferential responsiveness to ICIs.

Summary

Renal cell carcinomas include many tumors with diverse clinical, pathological, and molecular characteristics as well as distinct prognosis and therapeutic responses. These tumors are classified based primarily on morphology, but genetic features of renal tumors have been increasingly incorporated into the classification scheme. The classification is codified in the WHO classification system, which is updated periodically based on the available data. Many histological parameters obtained from pathological examination of renal tumors provide invaluable prognostic value and treatment guidance. The clinical, pathological, and genetic features in combination will eventually enable urologists to predict individual tumor behavior and stratify patients into more sophisticated risk groups, ultimately rendering individualized management and treatment options.

References

1. WHO Classification of Tumours Editorial Board. Urinary and male genital Tumours, vol. 8. 5th ed. Lyon, France: International Agency for Research on Cancer; 2022. (WHO Classification of Tumours Series). https://publications.iarc.fr/610
2. Trpkov K, Williamson SR, Gill AJ, Adeniran AJ, Agaimy A, Alaghehbandan R, et al. Novel, emerging and provisional renal entities: the genitourinary pathology society (GUPS) update on renal neoplasia. Mod Pathol. 2021;34(6):1167–84.
3. Trpkov K, Hes O, Williamson SR, Adeniran AJ, Agaimy A, Alaghehbandan R, et al. New developments in existing WHO entities and evolving molecular concepts: the Genitourinary Pathology Society (GUPS) update on renal neoplasia. Mod Pathol. 2021;34(7):1392–424.
4. Thoenes W, Störkel S, Rumpelt HJ. Histopathology and classification of renal cell tumors (adenomas, oncocytomas and carcinomas). The basic cytological and histopathological elements and their use for diagnostics. Pathol Res Pract. 1986;181(2):125–43.
5. Kovacs G, Akhtar M, Beckwith BJ, Bugert P, Cooper CS, Delahunt B, et al. The Heidelberg classification of renal cell tumours. J Pathol. 1997;183(2):131–3.
6. Störkel S, Eble JN, Adlakha K, Amin M, Blute ML, Bostwick DG, et al. Classification of renal cell carcinoma: Workgroup No. 1. Union Internationale Contre le Cancer (UICC) and the American Joint Committee on Cancer (AJCC). Cancer. 1997;80(5):987–9.
7. Al-Obaidy KI, Alruwaii ZI, Williamson SR, Cheng L. The pathological and molecular genetic landscape of the hereditary renal cancer predisposition syndromes. Histopathology. 2022;81(1):15–31.
8. Yanus GA, Kuligina ES, Imyanitov EN. Hereditary renal cancer syndromes. Med Sci (Basel). 2024;12(1):12.
9. Cotta BH, Choueiri TK, Cieslik M, Ghatalia P, Mehra R, Morgan TM, et al. Current landscape of genomic biomarkers in clear cell renal cell carcinoma. Eur Urol. 2023;84(2):166–75.
10. Pezzicoli G, Ciciriello F, Musci V, Salonne F, Ragno A, Rizzo M, et al. Genomic profiling and molecular characterization of clear cell renal cell carcinoma. Curr Oncol. 2023;30(10):9276–90.
11. Cancer Genome Atlas Research Network. Comprehensive molecular characterization of clear cell renal cell carcinoma. Nature. 2013;499(7456):43–9. https://doi.org/10.1038/nature12222. Epub 2013 Jun 23
12. Klatte T, Rao PN, de Martino M, LaRochelle J, Shuch B, Zomorodian NS, et al. Cytogenetic profile predicts prognosis of patients with clear cell renal cell carcinoma. J Clin Oncol. 2009;27(5):746–53.
13. Peña-Llopis S, Vega-Rubín-de-Celis S, Liao A, Leng N, Pavía-Jiménez A, Wang S, et al. BAP1 loss defines a new class of renal cell carcinoma. Nat Genet. 2012;44(7):751–9.
14. Liao C, Hu L, Zhang Q. Von Hippel-Lindau protein signalling in clear cell renal cell carcinoma. Nat Rev Urol. 2024;21(11):662–75.
15. Garcia J, Hurwitz HI, Sandler AB, Miles D, Coleman RL, Deurloo R, et al. Bevacizumab (Avastin®) in cancer treatment: a review of 15 years of clinical experience and future outlook. Cancer Treat Rev. 2020;86:102017.
16. Choueiri TK, Kaelin WG Jr. Targeting the HIF2-VEGF axis in renal cell carcinoma. Nat Med. 2020;26(10):1519–30. https://doi.org/10.1038/s41591-020-1093-z. Epub 2020 Oct 5. Erratum in: Nat Med. 2024 ;30(10):3027
17. Tenold M, Ravi P, Kumar M, Bowman A, Hammers H, Choueiri TK, et al. Current approaches to the treatment of advanced or metastatic renal cell carcinoma. Am Soc Clin Oncol Educ Book. 2020;40:1–10.
18. Brugarolas J, Rajaram S, Christie A, Kapur P. The evolution of angiogenic and inflamed tumors: the renal cancer paradigm. Cancer Cell. 2020;38(6):771–3.
19. Motzer RJ, Banchereau R, Hamidi H, Powles T, McDermott D, Atkins MB, et al. Molecular subsets in renal cancer determine outcome to checkpoint and angiogenesis blockade. Cancer Cell. 2020;38(6):803–17.
20. Joseph RW, Millis SZ, Carballido EM, Bryant D, Gatalica Z, Reddy S, et al. PD-1 and PD-L1 expression in renal cell carcinoma with sarcomatoid differentiation. Cancer Immunol Res. 2015;3(12):1303–7.
21. Cheville JC, Lohse CM, Zincke H, Weaver AL, Blute ML. Comparisons of outcome and prognostic features among histologic subtypes of renal cell carcinoma. Am J Surg Pathol. 2003;27(5):612–24.
22. Adeniran AJ, Shuch B, Humphrey PA. Hereditary renal cell carcinoma syndromes: clinical, pathologic, and genetic features. Am J Surg Pathol. 2015;39(12):e1–e18.
23. Delahunt B, Eble JN, McCredie MR, Bethwaite PB, Stewart JH, Bilous AM. Morphologic typing of papillary renal cell carcinoma: comparison of growth kinetics and patient survival in 66 cases. Hum Pathol. 2001;32(6):590–5.
24. Pitra T, Pivovarcikova K, Alaghehbandan R, Hes O. Chromosomal numerical aberration pattern in papillary renal cell carcinoma: review article. Ann Diagn Pathol. 2019;40:189–99.
25. Cancer Genome Atlas Research Network. Comprehensive molecular characterization of

papillary renal-cell carcinoma. N Engl J Med. 2016;374(2):135–45.
26. Garje R, Elhag D, Yasin HA, Acharya L, Vaena D, Dahmoush L. Comprehensive review of chromophobe renal cell carcinoma. Crit Rev Oncol Hematol. 2021;160:103287.
27. Wu J, Lu J, Wu CL, Lu M. Birt-Hogg-Dubé syndrome in an overall view: focus on the clinicopathological prospects in renal tumors. Semin Diagn Pathol. 2024;41(3):119–24.
28. Moch H, Ohashi R. Chromophobe renal cell carcinoma: current and controversial issues. Pathology. 2021;53(1):101–8.
29. Davis CF, Ricketts CJ, Wang M, Yang L, Cherniack AD, Shen H, et al. The somatic genomic landscape of chromophobe renal cell carcinoma. Cancer Cell. 2014;26(3):319–30.
30. Ricketts CJ, De Cubas AA, Fan H, Smith CC, Lang M, Reznik E, et al. The cancer genome atlas comprehensive molecular characterization of renal cell carcinoma. Cell Rep. 2018;23(12):3698. https://doi.org/10.1016/j.celrep.2018.06.032. Erratum for: Cell Rep. 2018 Apr 3;23(1):313-326.e5
31. Schmidt LS, Linehan WM. FLCN: the causative gene for Birt-Hogg-Dubé syndrome. Gene. 2018;640:28–42.
32. Finley DS, Shuch B, Said JW, Galliano G, Jeffries RA, Afifi AA, Castor B, Magyar C, Sadaat A, Kabbinavar FF, Belldegrun AS, Pantuck AJ. The chromophobe tumor grading system is the preferred grading scheme for chromophobe renal cell carcinoma. J Urol. 2011;186(6):2168–74.
33. Alghamdi M, Chen JF, Jungbluth A, Koutzaki S, Palmer MB, Al-Ahmadie HA, et al. L1 cell adhesion molecule (L1CAM) expression and molecular alterations distinguish low-grade oncocytic tumor from eosinophilic chromophobe renal cell carcinoma. Mod Pathol. 2024;37(5):100467.
34. Shah RB, Mehra R. Renal cell carcinoma associated with TSC/MTOR genomic alterations: an update on its expanding Spectrum and an approach to clinicopathologic work-up. Adv Anat Pathol. 2024;31(2):105–17.
35. Munari E, Settanni G, Caliò A, Segala D, Lonardi S, Sandrini S, et al. TSC loss is a clonal event in eosinophilic solid and cystic renal cell carcinoma: a multiregional tumor sampling study. Mod Pathol. 2022;35(3):376–85.
36. Kapur P, Gao M, Zhong H, Chintalapati S, Mitui M, Barnes SD, et al. Germline and sporadic mTOR pathway mutations in low-grade oncocytic tumor of the kidney. Mod Pathol. 2022;35(3):333–43.
37. Farcaş M, Gatalica Z, Trpkov K, Swensen J, Zhou M, Alaghehbandan R, et al. Eosinophilic vacuolated tumor (EVT) of kidney demonstrates sporadic TSC/MTOR mutations: next-generation sequencing multi-institutional study of 19 cases. Mod Pathol. 2022;35(3):344–51.
38. He H, Trpkov K, Martinek P, Isikci OT, Maggi-Galuzzi C, Alaghehbandan R, et al. "High-grade oncocytic renal tumor": morphologic, immunohistochemical, and molecular genetic study of 14 cases. Virchows Arch. 2018;473(6):725–38.
39. Chen YB, Mirsadraei L, Jayakumaran G, Al-Ahmadie HA, Fine SW, Gopalan A. Somatic mutations of TSC2 or MTOR characterize a morphologically distinct subset of sporadic renal cell carcinoma with eosinophilic and vacuolated cytoplasm. Am J Surg Pathol. 2019;43(1):121–31.
40. Tjota MY, Sharma A, Wanjari P, Fitzpatrick C, Segal J, Antic T. TSC/MTOR mutated renal cell carcinoma with leiomyomatous stroma is a distinct entity: a comprehensive study of 12 cases. Hum Pathol. 2023;134:124–33.
41. Hakimi AA, Tickoo SK, Jacobsen A, Sarungbam J, Sfakianos JP, Sato Y, et al. TCEB1-mutated renal cell carcinoma: a distinct genomic and morphological subtype. Mod Pathol. 2015;28(6):845–53.
42. Sirohi D, Smith SC, Agarwal N, Maughan BL. Unclassified renal cell carcinoma: diagnostic difficulties and treatment modalities. Res Rep Urol. 2018;10:205–17.
43. Carlo MI. Hereditary renal cell carcinoma syndromes. Hematol Oncol Clin North Am. 2023;37(5):841–8.
44. Wu CL. Pathology of hereditary renal cell carcinoma syndromes. Semin Diagn Pathol. 2024;41(3):118.
45. Maher ER. Hereditary renal cell carcinoma syndromes: diagnosis, surveillance and management. World J Urol. 2018;36(12):1891–8.
46. Li Z, Zhang J, Zhang L, Yao L, Zhang C, He Z, et al. Natural history and growth kinetics of clear cell renal cell carcinoma in sporadic and von Hippel-Lindau disease. Transl Androl Urol. 2021;10(3):1064–70.
47. Capitanio U, Rosiello G, Erdem S, Rowe I, Kara O, Roussel E, et al. Kidney Cancer Working Group of the Young Academic Urologists (YAU) Working Party of the European Association of Urology (EAU). Clinical, surgical, pathological and follow-up features of kidney cancer patients with Von Hippel-Lindau syndrome: novel insights from a large consortium. World J Urol. 2021;39(8):2969–75.
48. Jacoba IM, Lu Z. Hereditary papillary renal cell carcinoma. Semin Diagn Pathol. 2024;41(1):28–31.
49. Lindor NM, Dechet CB, Greene MH, Jenkins RB, Zincke MT, Weaver AL, Wilson M, Zincke H, Liu W. Papillary renal cell carcinoma: analysis of germline mutations in the MET proto-oncogene in a clinic-based population. Genet Test. 2001;5(2):101–6.
50. Merino MJ, Torres-Cabala C, Pinto P, Linehan WM. The morphologic spectrum of kidney tumors in hereditary leiomyomatosis and renal cell carcinoma (HLRCC) syndrome. Am J Surg Pathol. 2007;31(10):1578–85.
51. Grubb RL 3rd, Franks ME, Toro J, Middelton L, Choyke L, Fowler S, Torres-Cabala C, Glenn GM, Choyke P, Merino MJ, Zbar B, Pinto PA, Srinivasan R, Coleman JA, Linehan WM. Hereditary leiomyomatosis and renal cell cancer: a syndrome associated with an aggressive form of inherited renal cancer. J Urol. 2007;177(6):2074–9. discussion 2079-80

52. Rogala J, Zhou M. Hereditary succinate dehydrogenase-deficient renal cell carcinoma. Semin Diagn Pathol. 2024;41(1):32–41.
53. Peron A, Au KS, Northrup H. Genetics, genomics, and genotype-phenotype correlations of TSC: insights for clinical practice. Am J Med Genet C Semin Med Genet. 2018;178(3):281–90.
54. Machacek ME, Wu CL, Cornejo KM. Pathology of hereditary renal cell carcinoma syndromes: tuberous sclerosis complex (TSC). Semin Diagn Pathol. 2024;41(1):8–19.
55. Argani P, Mehra R. Renal cell carcinoma associated with tuberous sclerosis complex (TSC)/mammalian target of rapamycin (MTOR) genetic alterations. Mod Pathol. 2022;35(3):296–7.
56. Henske EP, Cornejo KM, Wu CL. Renal cell carcinoma in tuberous sclerosis complex. Genes (Basel). 2021;12(10):1585.
57. Gupta N, Sunwoo BY, Kotloff RM. Birt-Hogg-Dubé Syndrome. Clin Chest Med. 2016;37(3):475–86.
58. Menko FH, van Steensel MA, Giraud S, Friis-Hansen L, Richard S, Ungari S, Nordenskjöld M, Hansen TV, Solly J, Maher ER, European BHD Consortium. Birt-Hogg-Dubé syndrome: diagnosis and management. Lancet Oncol. 2009;10(12):1199–206.
59. Furuya M, Hasumi H, Yao M, Nagashima Y. Birt-Hogg-Dubé syndrome-associated renal cell carcinoma: histopathological features and diagnostic conundrum. Cancer Sci. 2020;111(1):15–22.
60. Wang XM, Mannan R, Zhang Y, Chinnaiyan A, Rangaswamy R, Chugh S, et al. Hybrid oncocytic tumors (HOTs) in Birt-Hogg-Dubé syndrome patients-a tale of two cities: sequencing analysis reveals dual lineage markers capturing the 2 cellular populations of HOT. Am J Surg Pathol. 2024;48(2):163–73.
61. Füzesi L, Frank D, Nguyen C, Ringert RH, Bartels H, Gunawan B. Losses of 1p and chromosome 14 in renal oncocytomas. Cancer Genet Cytogenet. 2005;160(2):120–5.
62. Liu YJ, Ussakli C, Antic T, Liu Y, Wu Y, True L, Tretiakova MS. Sporadic oncocytic tumors with features intermediate between oncocytoma and chromophobe renal cell carcinoma: comprehensive clinicopathological and genomic profiling. Hum Pathol. 2020;104:18–29.
63. Joshi S, Tolkunov D, Aviv H, Hakimi AA, Yao M, Hsieh JJ, Ganesan S, Chan CS, White E. The genomic landscape of renal oncocytoma identifies a metabolic barrier to tumorigenesis. Cell Rep. 2015;13(9):1895–908.
64. Yusenko MV, Kuiper RP, Boethe T, Ljungberg B, van Kessel AG, Kovacs G. High-resolution DNA copy number and gene expression analyses distinguish chromophobe renal cell carcinomas and renal oncocytomas. BMC Cancer. 2009;9:152.
65. Nair N, Chakraborty R, Mahajan Z, Sharma A, Sethi SK, Raina R. Renal manifestations of tuberous sclerosis complex. J Kidney Cancer VHL. 2020;7(3):5–19.
66. Giannikou K, Malinowska IA, Pugh TJ, Yan R, Tseng YY, Oh C, et al. Whole exome sequencing identifies TSC1/TSC2 biallelic loss as the primary and sufficient driver event for renal angiomyolipoma development. PLoS Genet. 2016;12(8):e1006242.
67. Qin W, Bajaj V, Malinowska I, Lu X, MacConaill L, Wu CL, et al. Angiomyolipoma have common mutations in TSC2 but no other common genetic events. PLoS One. 2011;6(9):e24919.
68. Amin MB, Edge SB, Greene FL, et al., editors. AJCC cancer staging manual. 8th ed. Springer; 2017.
69. Rezaee ME, Pallauf M, Fletcher SA, Pavlovich CP, Baraban E, Ged Y, Singla N. Prognostic significance of pT3a staging subclassifications in renal cell carcinoma: not all pT3a are equal. Urol Oncol. 2024;42(4):119.e23–9.
70. Brookman-May SD, May M, Wolff I, Zigeuner R, Hutterer GC, Cindolo L, et al. Evaluation of the prognostic significance of perirenal fat invasion and tumor size in patients with pT1-pT3a localized renal cell carcinoma in a comprehensive multicenter study of the CORONA project. Can we improve prognostic discrimination for patients with stage pT3a tumors? Eur Urol. 2015;67(5):943–51.
71. Bonsib SM. T2 clear cell renal cell carcinoma is a rare entity: a study of 120 clear cell renal cell carcinomas. J Urol. 2005;174(4 Pt 1):1199–202. discussion 1202
72. Thompson RH, Blute ML, Krambeck AE, Lohse CM, Magera JS, Leibovich BC, Kwon ED, Frank I, Cheville JC. Patients with pT1 renal cell carcinoma who die from disease after nephrectomy may have unrecognized renal sinus fat invasion. Am J Surg Pathol. 2007;31(7):1089–93.
73. Delahunt B, Cheville JC, Martignoni G, Humphrey PA, Magi-Galluzzi C, McKenney J, Egevad L, Algaba F, Moch H, Grignon DJ, Montironi R, Srigley JR, Members of the ISUP Renal Tumor Panel. The International Society of Urological Pathology (ISUP) grading system for renal cell carcinoma and other prognostic parameters. Am J Surg Pathol. 2013;37(10):1490–504.
74. Delahunt B, Eble JN, Egevad L, Samaratunga H. Grading of renal cell carcinoma. Histopathology. 2019;74(1):4–17.
75. Avulova S, Cheville JC, Lohse CM, Gupta S, Potretzke TA, Tsivian M, et al. Grading chromophobe renal cell carcinoma: evidence for a four-tiered classification incorporating coagulative tumor necrosis. Eur Urol. 2021;79(2):225–31.
76. Cheville JC, Lohse CM, Zincke H, Weaver AL, Leibovich BC, Frank I, Blute ML. Sarcomatoid renal cell carcinoma: an examination of underlying histologic subtype and an analysis of associations with patient outcome. Am J Surg Pathol. 2004;28(4):435–41.
77. Adeniran AJ, Shuch B, Humphrey PA. Sarcomatoid and Rhabdoid renal cell carcinoma: clinical, pathologic, and molecular genetic features. Am J Surg Pathol. 2024;48(7):e65–88.
78. Bakouny Z, Braun DA, Shukla SA, Pan W, Gao X, Hou Y, et al. Integrative molecular characterization of

sarcomatoid and rhabdoid renal cell carcinoma. Nat Commun. 2021;12(1):808.
79. Blum KA, Gupta S, Tickoo SK, Chan TA, Russo P, Motzer RJ, Karam JA, Hakimi AA. Sarcomatoid renal cell carcinoma: biology, natural history and management. Nat Rev Urol. 2020;17(12):659–78.
80. Hahn AW, Surasi DS, Viscuse PV, Bathala TK, Wiele AJ, Campbell MT, et al. Treatment outcomes in patients with metastatic renal cell carcinoma with Sarcomatoid and/or Rhabdoid dedifferentiation after progression on immune checkpoint therapy. Oncologist. 2024;29(5):392–9.
81. Kiyozawa D, Takamatsu D, Kohashi K, Kinoshita F, Ishihara S, Toda Y, et al. Programmed death ligand 1/indoleamine 2,3-dioxygenase 1 expression and tumor-infiltrating lymphocyte status in renal cell carcinoma with sarcomatoid changes and rhabdoid features. Hum Pathol. 2020;101:31–9.
82. Emami Nejad A, Najafgholian S, Rostami A, Sistani A, Shojaeifar S, Esparvarinha M, et al. The role of hypoxia in the tumor microenvironment and development of cancer stem cell: a novel approach to developing treatment. Cancer Cell Int. 2021;21(1):62.
83. Reiniger L, Téglási V, Pipek O, Rojkó L, Glasz T, Vágvölgyi A, et al. Tumor necrosis correlates with PD-L1 and PD-1 expression in lung adenocarcinoma. Acta Oncol. 2019;58(8):1087–94.
84. van Loo G, Bertrand MJM. Death by TNF: a road to inflammation. Nat Rev Immunol. 2023;23(5):289–303. https://doi.org/10.1038/s41577-022-00792-3.
85. Zhang L, Zha Z, Qu W, Zhao H, Yuan J, Feng Y, Wu B. Tumor necrosis as a prognostic variable for the clinical outcome in patients with renal cell carcinoma: a systematic review and meta-analysis. BMC Cancer. 2018;18(1):870.
86. Parker WP, Cheville JC, Frank I, Zaid HB, Lohse CM, Boorjian SA, Thompson RH, et al. Application of the stage, size, grade, and necrosis (SSIGN) score for clear cell renal cell carcinoma in contemporary patients. Eur Urol. 2017;71(4):665–73.
87. Haibe Y, Kreidieh M, El Hajj H, Khalifeh I, Mukherji D, Temraz S, et al. Resistance mechanisms to anti-angiogenic therapies in cancer. Front Oncol. 2020;10:221.
88. Bedke J, Heide J, Ribback S, Rausch S, de Martino M, Scharpf M, et al. Microvascular and lymphovascular tumour invasion are associated with poor prognosis and metastatic spread in renal cell carcinoma: a validation study in clinical practice. BJU Int. 2018;121(1):84–92.
89. Xu J, Tan Y, Gao S, Lee W, Ye Y, Deng G, et al. Microvascular invasion is associated with poor prognosis in renal cell carcinoma: a retrospective cohort study and meta-analysis. Front Oncol. 2024;14:1417630.
90. Nguyen DP, Vertosick EA, Corradi RB, Vilaseca A, Benfante NE, Touijer KA, et al. Histological subtype of renal cell carcinoma significantly affects survival in the era of partial nephrectomy. Urol Oncol. 2016;34(6):259.e1-8.
91. de Velasco G, McKay RR, Lin X, Moreira RB, Simantov R, Choueiri TK. Comprehensive analysis of survival outcomes in non-clear cell renal cell carcinoma patients treated in clinical trials. Clin Genitourin Cancer. 2017;15(6):652–60.e1

Imaging of Renal Cancer

5

Jalil Afnan, Rose-Anna Voog, and Christoph Wald

Renal Imaging

The most recent data for adult renal cancer estimate around 82,000 new cases of renal cancer annually within the United States in 2024, with a 2:1 male-to-female predominance and over 14,000 associated annual deaths [1]. The predominant subtype of renal cell carcinoma (RCC), is associated with multifactorial etiologies [2, 3], and incidence continues to rise at least in part due to increasing overall image utilization in the United States and elsewhere, which has been observed in the inpatient as well as outpatient setting [4, 5]. Consensus guidelines for further evaluation of incidentally identified renal lesions, typically on a non-contrast CT study, continue to recommend the use of multiphasic CT or MRI for further characterization [6]. Despite earlier reports of approximately 50% mortality at 5 years, the larger number of cancers detected at an earlier stage and often organ-confined disease is leading to a more favorable overall prognosis [7] most likely associated with a lead time bias, permitting earlier and possibly definitive treatment.

J. Afnan (✉) · R.-A. Voog · C. Wald
Department of Radiology, Lahey Hospital & Medical Center, Burlington, MA, USA
e-mail: jalil.afnan@lahey.org; Rose-Anna.Voog@lahey.org; Christoph.Wald@lahey.org

Renal cancer is detected either during the evaluation of genitourinary tract-related symptoms, such as flank pain and hematuria, or during workup of unrelated medical issues for a variety of abdomino-pelvic conditions or, for instance, during colon cancer screening with CT colonography. It should be noted that many computed tomography (CT) examinations of the chest may include at least a portion of the kidneys. Therefore, future potential risk population screening for lung cancer may lead to a further increase in incidental renal cancer discovery. Certain groups of patients, such as those with Von Hippel Lindau (VHL) and other hereditary renal cancer syndromes, may undergo active surveillance [8].

A variety of imaging techniques and modalities are at the clinician's disposal, to appropriately characterize and stage a renal tumor and subsequently use in disease surveillance. These range from basic grayscale ultrasound to advanced cross-sectional imaging, including CT and magnetic resonance tomography imaging (MRI). The various modalities will be considered, together with the refinements necessary to maximize their respective strengths. Imaging may also play a central role in the treatment of renal cancer, such as high-intensity-focused ultrasound ablation (HIFU) [9, 10], and image-guided percutaneous ablation [11, 12]. These techniques and the functional radionuclide analysis will be reviewed separately.

J. A. Libertino, J. R. Gee (eds.), *Renal Cancer*, https://doi.org/10.1007/978-3-031-97599-8_5

Intravenous Pyelogram (IVP)

Intravenous pyelography, or excretory urography, is a noninvasive, sequential fluoroscopic evaluation of the kidneys, ureters, and urinary bladder before and after administration of iodinated contrast. An initial X-ray may identify an area of increased density, a density (mass) with irregular margins, or calcifications, which is intrinsic to the kidneys or resulting in local mass effect (Fig. 5.1).

However, soft tissue contrast resolution of plain radiography and fluoroscopy are limited and the resulting images are a two-dimensional representation of a three-dimensional object inherently subject to superimposition of anatomical structures interfering with detection and precise localization of structures of interest. Following administration of an intravenous contrast agent, usually an iodine-based dye, additional serial X-rays are used to evaluate the same structures during excretory phase imaging (Fig. 5.2).

Sometimes, conventional tomography is employed to focus the examination on intrinsic abnormalities of the collecting system or portions of the bladder. As a result of these limitations, IVP is of limited value in the context of renal cancer detection (especially of early-stage, treatable disease), which is reflected in the low reported sensitivity and specificity of 60% and 48%, respectively [13]. As such, in current practice, an IVP alone cannot be considered sufficient for renal mass evaluation and will likely be complemented by an ultrasound or dedicated cross-sectional imaging. Even in terms of evaluating

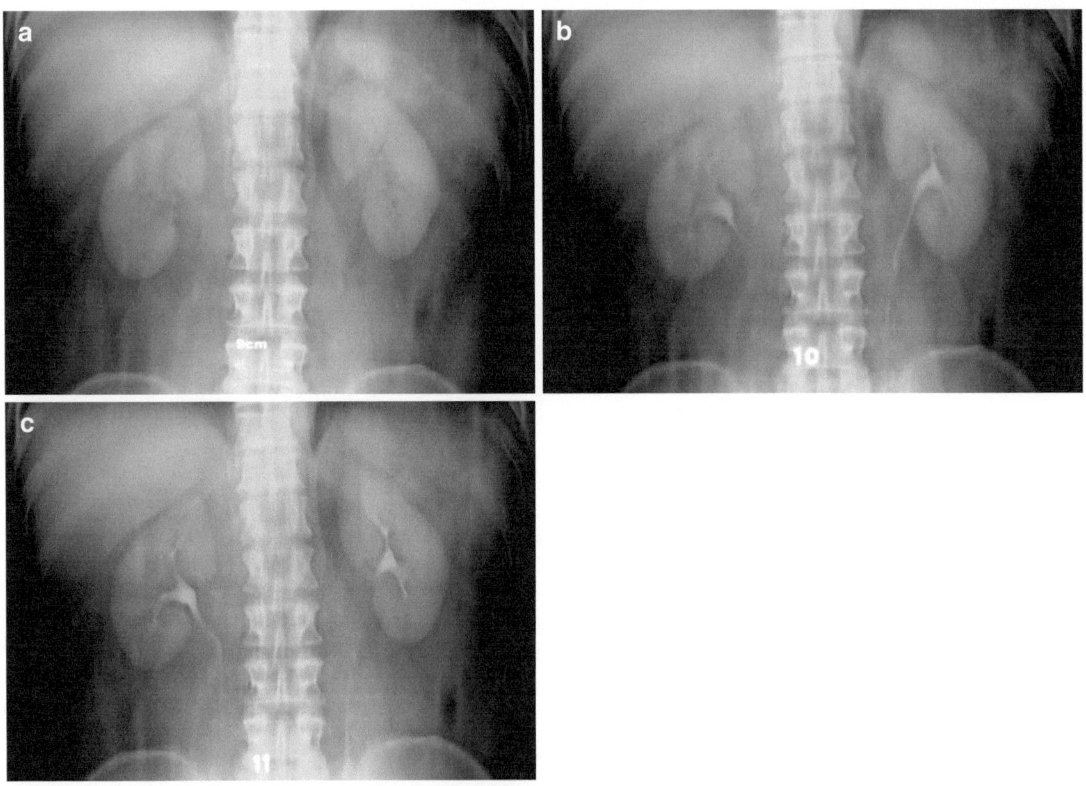

Fig. 5.1 Sequential frontal abdominal radiographs from an intravenous pyelogram (IVP), performed for hematuria, with no apparent abnormalities. Blurring of adjacent intra-abdominal structures while keeping the collecting system in focus is deliberately achieved with controlled tube-table translation during image acquisition. Distinct phases of contrast excretion typically evaluated are renal cortical phase (**a**) and calyceal opacification with early (**b**) and excretory phase (**c**)

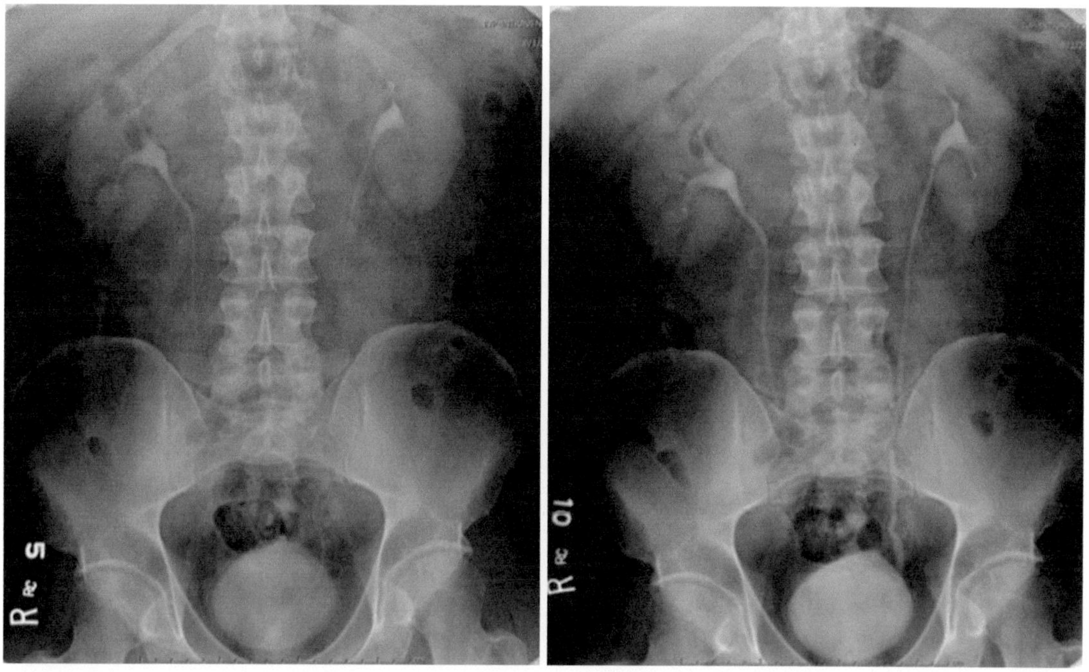

Fig. 5.2 KUB images in the late excretory phase, to further delineate the ureters and bladder. Prone imaging may be helpful to show ureters to advantage. Post-micturition images are subsequently acquired

renal function and further characterizing the renal tract, CT or MR urography, or radionuclide-based tests are now more commonly performed in most practices. Finally, the use of ionizing radiation, albeit at a low dose, and the use of an intravenous contrast agent are additional considerations when utilizing this test.

Ultrasound (US)

Since its introduction into the medical arena in the 1950s, ultrasound has distinguished itself as a readily available, cost-effective imaging modality relying on the differential penetrance and reflectivity of sound waves and notably being performed without the use of ionizing radiation. Ultrasonic waves are generated by mechanical oscillation of certain crystals and ceramics, typically generating frequencies in the range of 2–15 MHz. The ultrasound beam is focused either mechanically or electronically. The ultrasound wave is subjected to attenuation, reflection, scattering, refraction, and diffraction within human tissues due to the inherent differences in the acoustic impedance of the tissue components. Analysis of the reflected wave generates a predictable 2D or 3D grayscale image with information about the constituent elements of a lesion, its distance from the transducer, and degree of vascularity if Doppler is utilized (Fig. 5.3).

Certain processing techniques, such as harmonic imaging, may be employed to reduce background echoes, which can be helpful, for instance, when attempting to clarify borderline echogenic signals within a suspected (simple) cyst.

Ultrasound readily differentiates cystic from solid lesions, often the first step in assessing whether a renal lesion is likely benign or malignant. A typical benign renal cystic lesion is a well-circumscribed and anechoic structure with posterior acoustic enhancement on the United States. The back wall of the lesion should appear sharp and smooth, and positive "through transmission" or un-attenuated ultrasound waves should be observed beyond the lesion, from

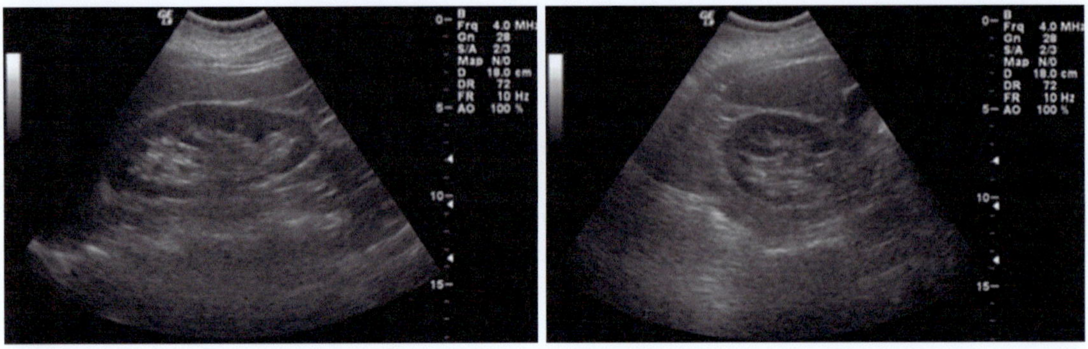

Fig. 5.3 Normal ultrasound images of the kidney, in sagittal and transverse planes. Grayscale ultrasound images were acquired with a 4.0 MHz curvilinear probe and demonstrate typical central echogenic structures of the renal sinus, and overlying hypoechoic cortex

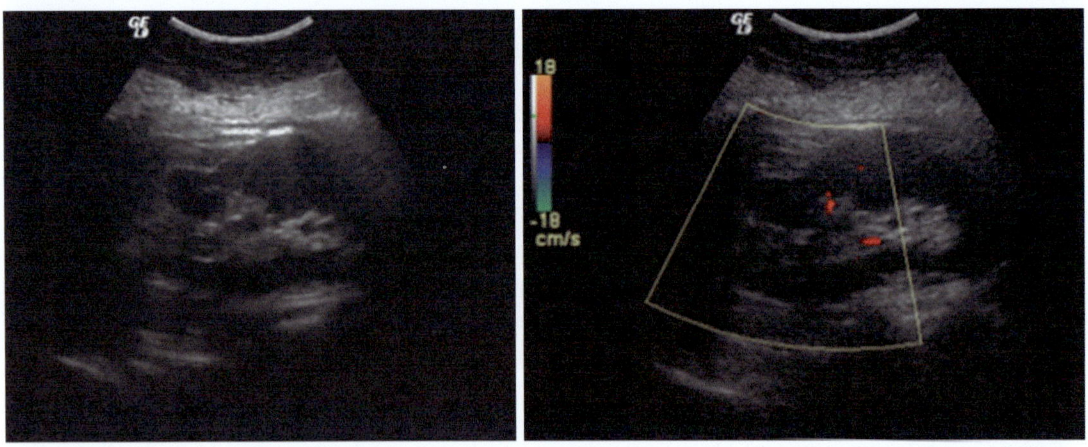

Fig. 5.4 Ultrasound images of the kidney, in sagittal plane. On the left, a grayscale ultrasound image demonstrates a well-circumscribed, partially exophytic, anechoic, thin-walled cortical cyst with posterior acoustic enhancement. On the right, a color Doppler evaluation (inside yellow-framed region of interest) confirms absence of abnormal blood flow in the cyst; findings are typical for a simple renal cyst

which the simple nature of the fluid within the lesion is inferred (Fig. 5.4).

Complex features include debris indicative of proteinaceous content or prior hemorrhage and necrosis, thickened irregular septations, soft tissue mural nodularity, and the presence of calcifications (Fig. 5.5).

Renal cell carcinoma (RCC) may exhibit a variety of characteristics on grayscale ultrasound, usually hyperechoic or isoechoic to the surrounding renal cortex with a hypoechoic rim or pseudocapsule. It is typically hypervascular around the periphery of the mass, although papillary-type RCC is hypovascular and less locally invasive. Color Doppler may also evaluate renal vein and IVC patency, or the presence of tumor thrombus. Larger lesions often exhibit hypoechoic areas of central necrosis on ultrasound. Although renal cell carcinoma may be fat-containing, a typical solid, fat-containing renal mass is most likely a benign angiomyolipoma. Occasionally, renal carcinomas can exhibit predominantly cystic features [14] (Fig. 5.6).

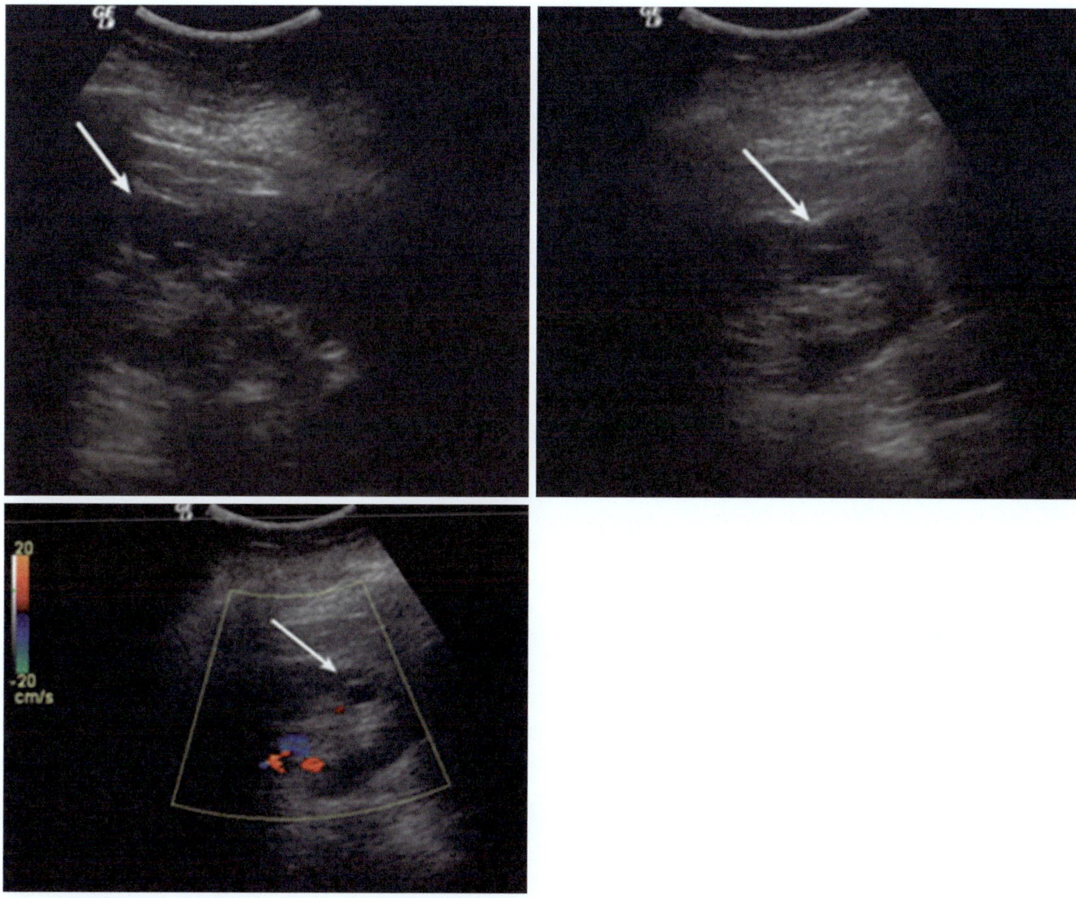

Fig. 5.5 Grayscale ultrasound images demonstrate a predominantly hypoechoic renal cortical lesion, containing a well-defined linear echogenic septation (solid white arrow). There is no evidence of vascular flow within the septation, and no associated soft tissue mass or mural nodule. Findings are consistent with a minimally complex, septated cyst

A possible mimic to RCC are oncocytomas, a benign renal mass appearing as a well circumscribed mass, isoechoic to the surrounding renal cortex with a central stellate scar.

Studies have matched ultrasound against CT and MRI in the evaluation of renal masses prior to surgical resection and found it to be equivalent in determining tumor size [15]. A recent study determined that contrast-enhanced ultrasound performed as well as, or better than contrast-enhanced CT or MRI in the diagnosis of renal masses. It is possible to distinguish between clear cell carcinoma and non-clear cell renal tumors, based on grayscale heterogeneity, lesion washout, grade of contrast enhancement, and quantitative measure of peak intensity [16]. The utility of contrast-enhanced ultrasound (CEUS), employing injected intravascular microbubbles, may be an accurate diagnostic test for patients with chronic renal impairment in whom intravenous contrast is contraindicated [17]. In addition to sonographic evaluation of the lesion, CEUS permits vascular architectural analysis and multiphasic analysis of contrast enhancement and washout. A sensitivity of 96% and specificity of 50% have been demonstrated for malignancy in patients with normal renal function. The sensitivity, although slightly reduced in patients with chronic renal impairment, remains high at 90%, with a similar specificity of 55% [18].

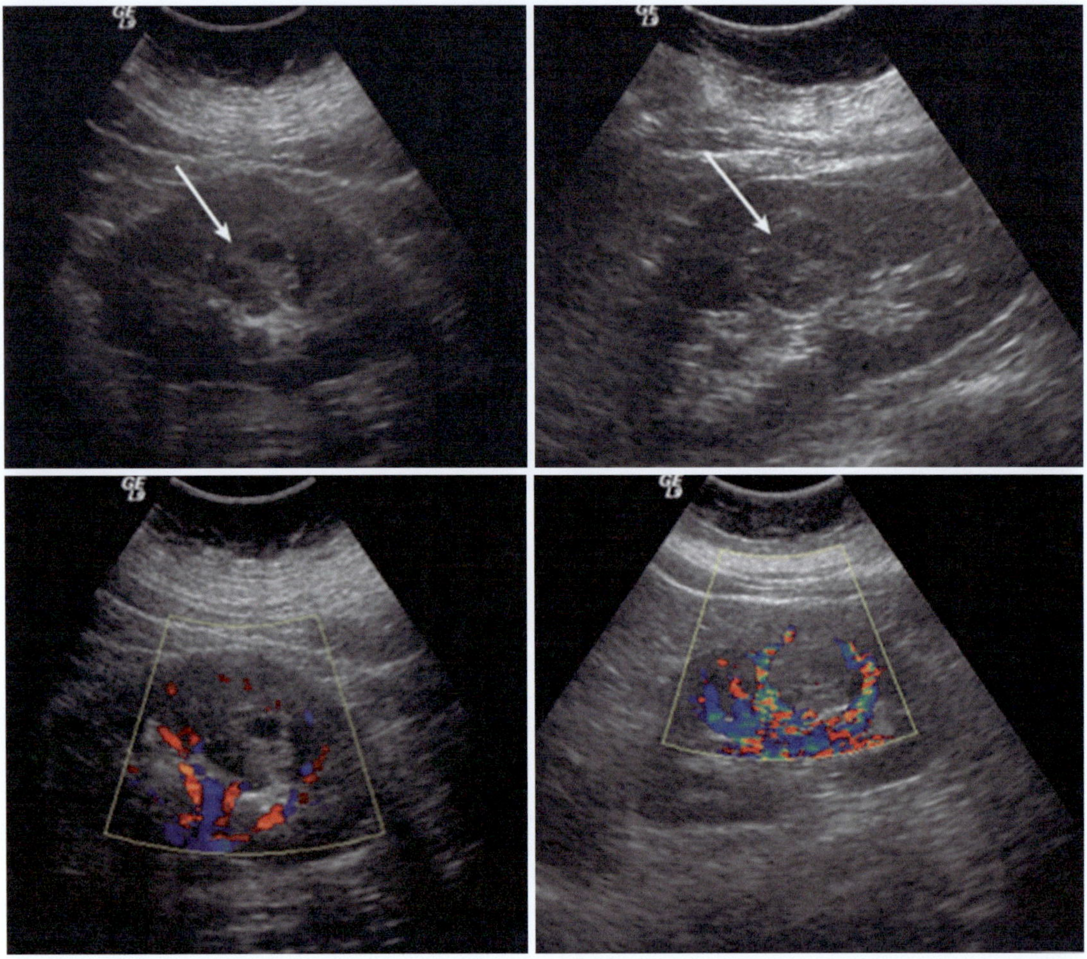

Fig. 5.6 Well-circumscribed mass of heterogeneous echogenicity is centered in the renal cortex. Trace vascular flow is seen on color Doppler images. Findings are consistent with a complex renal mass; multiphasic cross-sectional imaging would typically be recommended for further evaluation

Small renal masses which are defined as less than 4 cm in size are usually managed conservatively, following an active surveillance monitoring paradigm [19]. The majority are statistically likely to be benign [20]. Although locally aggressive features and metastases may be seen in renal cell carcinomas of all sizes, a large prospectively collected population-based registry identified that small RCCs (less than 4 cm) are likely to be an organ-confined disease with a limited malignant potential around 5% [21].

Although ultrasound may identify a variety of specific morphologic characteristics to aid diagnosis, it is incapable of categorizing tumor biology that may ultimately play a more significant role in predicting disease progression.

Ultrasound is also utilized to guide local thermal coagulation and cryoablation of renal lesions, both techniques requiring percutaneous puncture and direct placement of probes within the target tumor. A separate role for high-intensity focused ultrasound (HIFU) is well-described, whereby energy absorbed by biologic tissue in the path of a wave of ultrasound energy, focused on a specific location, results in temperatures exceeding the threshold level of protein denaturation, effecting coagulative necrosis [22]. The intraoperative use of ultrasound to assist with the guidance of nephron-sparing partial nephrectomy has become

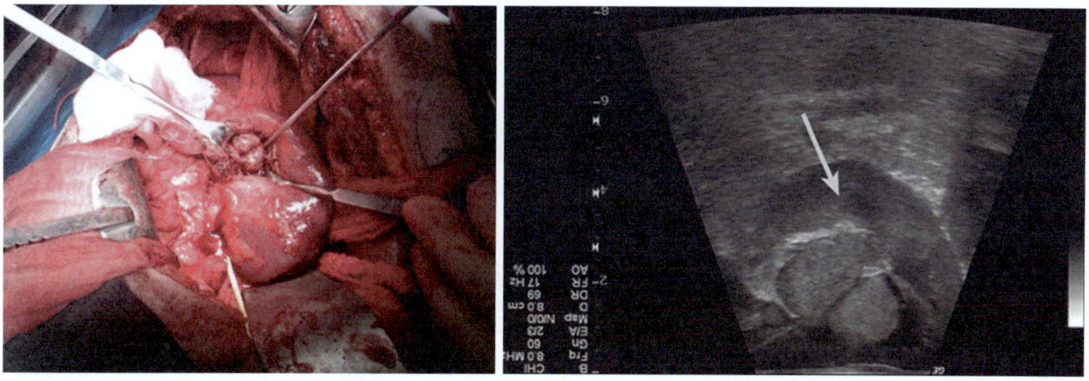

Fig. 5.7 Intraoperative photograph on the left, demonstrating open, partial nephrectomy for renal mass within the upper pole of the kidney. Intraoperative real-time ultrasound image on the right is used routinely to identify tumor and evaluate extent of local invasion during nephron-sparing surgery

standard of care at Lahey Hospital and Medical Center and many other institutions (Fig. 5.7).

Ultrasound is, therefore, most commonly utilized as a screening tool for RCC, to document stability of known lesions over time and may be considered for ongoing surveillance following tumor resection. If a lesion is identified, initial further characterization and staging of disease by contrast-enhanced multiphasic cross-sectional imaging with either CT or MRI is recommended.

Computed Tomography (CT)

It is a common finding on abdominal imaging studies, to identify at least one renal lesion, unrelated to the patient's presenting illness or the known medical history. Studies estimate 40% of patients will have at least one renal cyst [23, 24]. Since CT has become a widely utilized means of urgent assessment of abdominal and pelvic conditions, as well as a screening tool for colon cancer and lately lung cancer, many renal tumors will, therefore, come to light as an incidental finding during the evaluation of a separate clinical issue. Such incidental findings invariably present a diagnostic dilemma, not least because the findings are rarely found on studies with protocols optimized for evaluation of a renal mass. Furthermore, the clinical relevance of any asymptomatic, incidental small renal mass must be critically considered in the global clinical context for a given patient to temper any potential downstream diagnostic or therapeutic activity. Increasing evidence that many incidentally identified renal masses, whether cystic or solid, are benign resulted in the practice guidelines provided by the American College of Radiology (ACR) Incidental Findings committee recommendations [25].

An optimized renal CT study is a multiphasic examination of the abdomen and pelvis, utilizing a precontrast and at least one postcontrast phase, often during the excretory or nephrogenic phase (80–100 s post-injection). An arterial phase (between 20 and 30 s) may be considered, although this is usually not necessary to make a diagnosis of a renal mass, but rather aids depiction of the renal vasculature (Fig. 5.8a, b).

Thin section axial imaging sufficient to discriminate between lesions less than 3 mm in size should be employed on a multidetector CT, equipped to modulate patient dose and better, yet, capable of acquiring low-dose images of quality comparable to full-dose images through use of newer iterative image reconstruction techniques. Low KV imaging should also be considered in follow-up CT studies when a lesion has already been characterized. Studies have demonstrated that 1 mm thick axial images in multiphase acquisition have the capability of diagnosing stage I renal cell cancer with 96% sensitivity and 93% specificity in detection of perirenal fat infiltra-

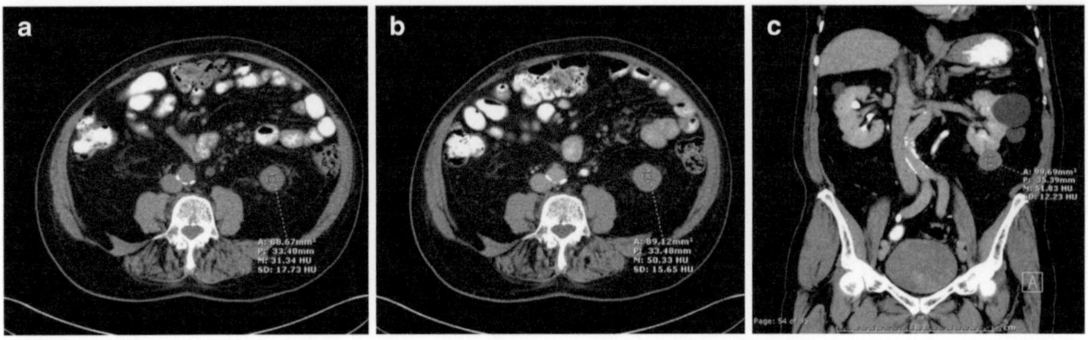

Fig. 5.8 Multiphasic CT study demonstrates precontrast (**a**), and nephrogenic phase (**b**) axial images, and excretory phase (**c**) coronal reformat of an enhancing left renal lower pole lesion. Enhancement is quantified in Hounsfield units (HU), evaluated by manually placing a region of interest (ROI) on the target. Mean HU increased from 31 to 50, suspicious for neoplasm. Incidental note of several benign appearing, non-enhancing upper pole renal cortical cysts

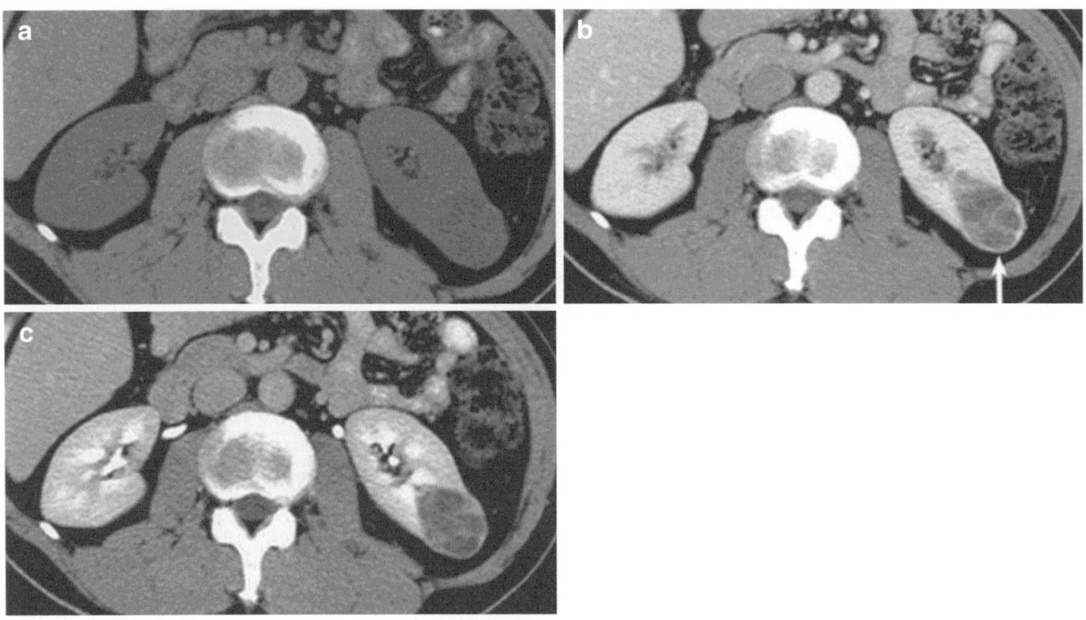

Fig. 5.9 Multiphasic CT study demonstrates precontrast (**a**), arterial phase (**b**) and nephrogenic phase (**c**) axial images of a well-circumscribed, exophytic renal cortical mass in the posterior left kidney. Septations seen on pre-contrast imaging demonstrate enhancement, a suspicious feature. The mass corresponded to a clear cell type renal cell carcinoma

tion, with 100% positive predictive value [26] (Figs. 5.9, 5.10a, b, and 5.11).

However, the benefit of multiphasic imaging data (requiring multiple imaging acquisitions) should be weighed against the associated increase in radiation dose. Post-processing technology should be available to construct dedicated 3D models of the kidneys, identify tumor foci, and further characterize the renal hilar vasculature. Although not essential to diagnosis, additional

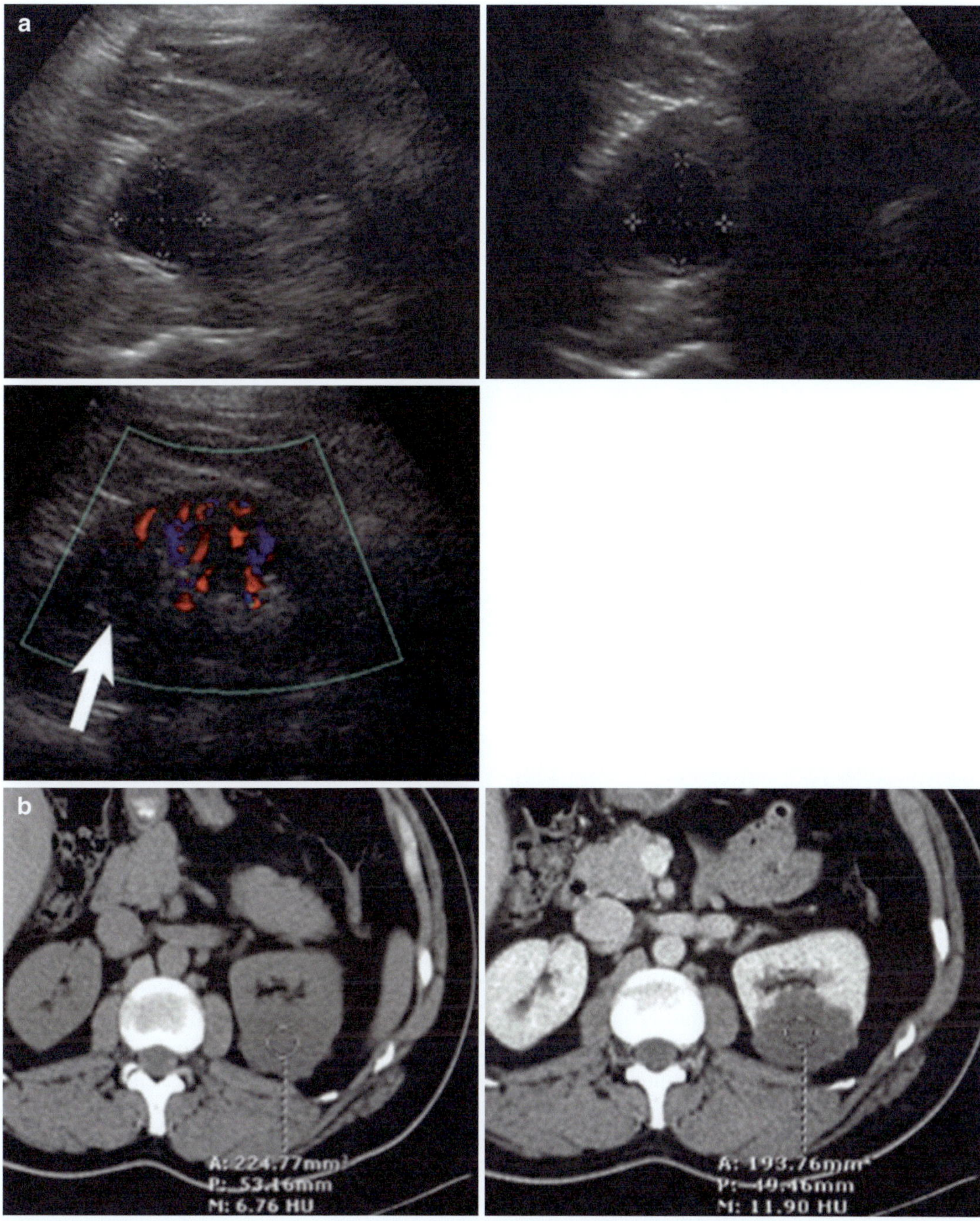

Fig. 5.10 (**a**) Grayscale ultrasound images in sagittal and transverse planes, of the left kidney, demonstrate a well-circumscribed, hypoechoic cortical lesion, without apparent vascularity. (**b**) Precontrast and late arterial phase axial CT image demonstrates a lobulated, hypodense lesion in the left posterior interpolar region, without significant enhancement (6 HU to 12 HU). The lesion was resected due to associated hematuria and pain; pathology demonstrated a renal cell carcinoma, clear cell type. Imaging features are atypical

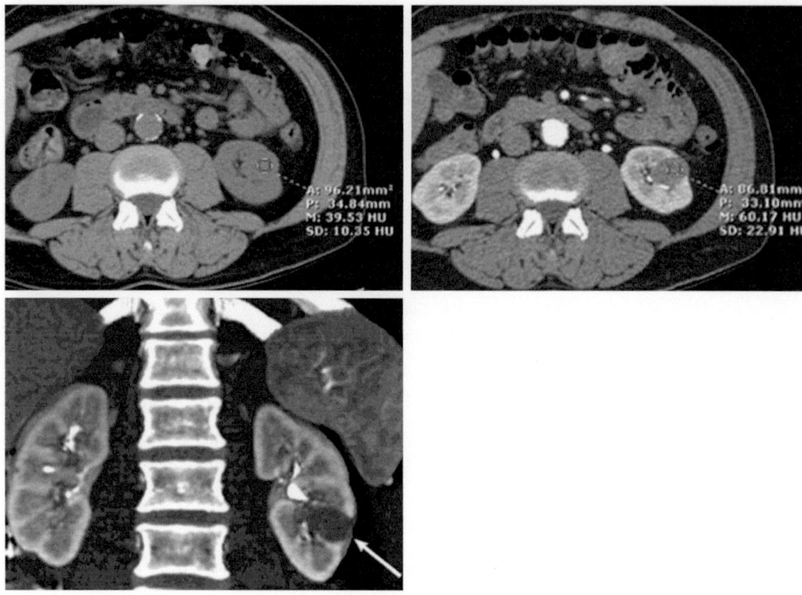

Fig. 5.11 Precontrast (left), nephrogenic phase (middle) and coronal reformat (right) demonstrate a hypodense, enhancing cortical lesion, abutting the collecting system. Significant differential enhancement of 21 HU is noted; pathology confirmed renal cell carcinoma, papillary type

information is provided for treatment planning, including operative approach. To complete disease staging, a CT scan of the chest and contrast-enhanced MRI of the brain may each be considered (Figs. 5.12, 5.13 and 5.14).

Staging for renal cell cancer was first introduced in 1958 [27] and revised in 1963 [28]. Following the introduction of the TNM system in 1978 and its subsequent iterations, the most recent American Joint Committee on Cancer (AJCC) guidelines on renal cancer staging from 2010 incorporate recent advances in survival characteristics between different groups. The framework allows for standardization of treatment, appropriate inclusion into research trials, and utilization of experimental therapies and provides more accurate prognostic indicators, all of which depend upon imaging.

The relative radiodensity of a region of interest on a CT image is defined according to the Hounsfield reference scale that measures the linear attenuation coefficient against that of water. Fluid and solid tissue are, therefore, given a relative positive numerical designation; fat and air are defined with relative negative values. The majority of adult renal cancers appear as a solid, enhancing, cortically based mass. An increase of at least 15 Hounsfield units (HU) measured within a representative region of interest (ROI) represents significant enhancement on a CT scan [29]. Enhancement of less than 10 HU strongly suggests a benign process, well-established criteria [30].

On pre-contrast imaging, and also on ultrasound, a simple cystic renal lesion, which is almost certainly benign, will demonstrate simple fluid density, Hounsfield units between 0 and 20, the upper end of this spectrum indicating proteinaceous or possibly hemorrhagic content. Cystic lesions are well-characterized by the eponymous Bosniak classification system, which has evolved particularly in the categorization of complex lesions, in large part due to outcomes since its initial introduction in 1986 [31, 32]. A recent systematic review demonstrated the Bosniak classification system to retain a high level of accuracy and efficacy for grading complex lesions (Bosniak classes II, IIF, and IV), while proposing some refinements of image characterization [33] (Table 5.1).

Although definitive subtyping of renal cell cancer is not consistently achievable by CT, certain characteristic features may be exhibited. Clear cell type tends to enhance, avidly and het-

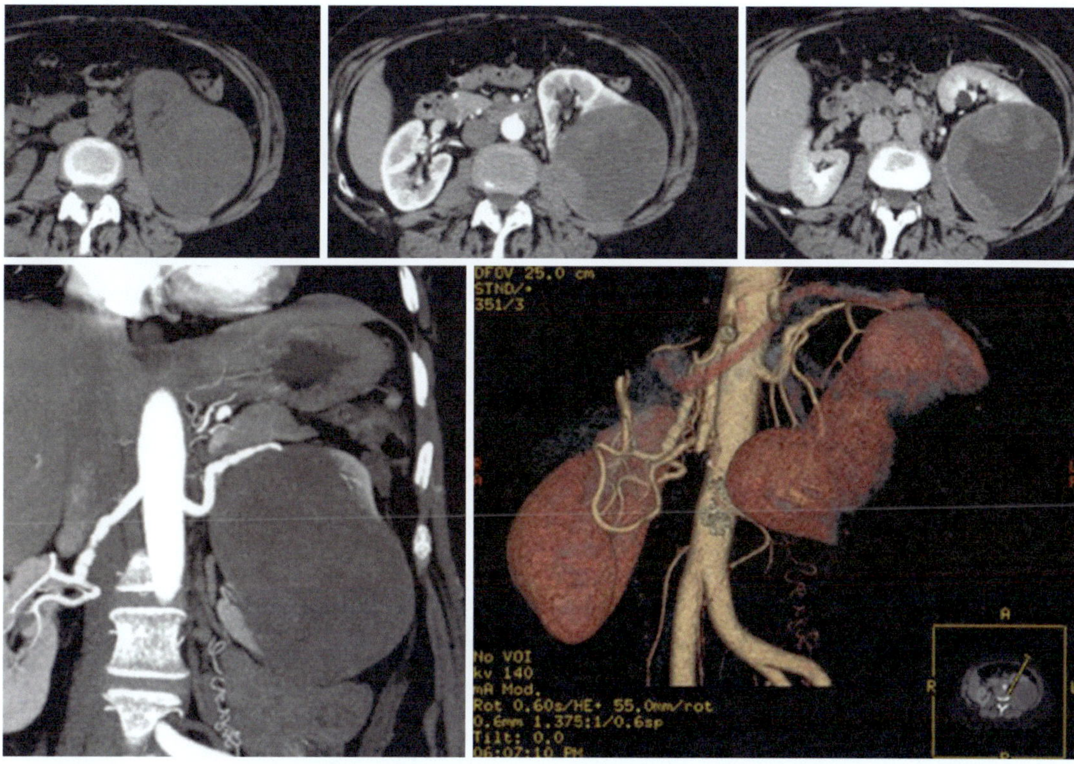

Fig. 5.12 Multiphasic axial CT images in precontrast (upper left), arterial (upper middle), and nephrogenic phases (upper right), demonstrate a large, heterogeneous mass arising from the left kidney, centrally cystic and peripherally nodular in appearance. Coronal reformat (lower left), and volume-rendered subtracted image (lower right) provide further information about the blood supply

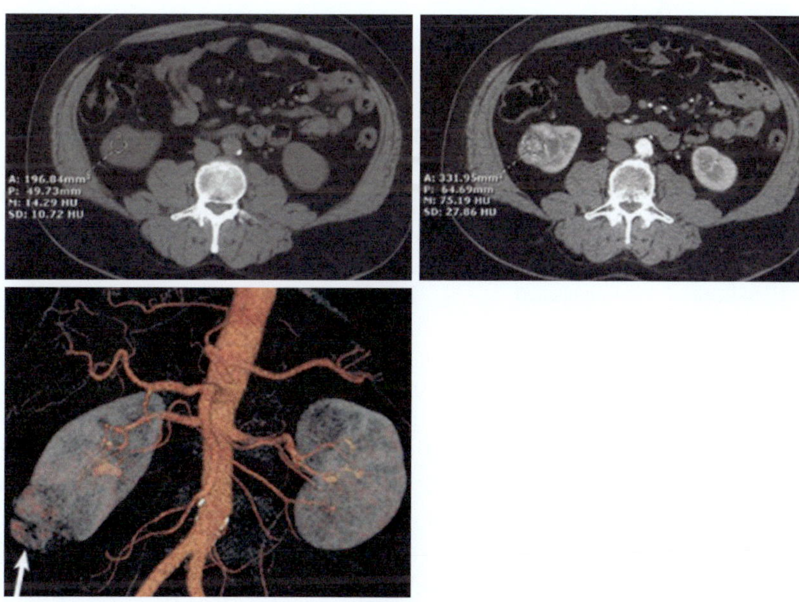

Fig. 5.13 Precontrast (left) and arterial phase (middle) CT images demonstrate a heterogeneous, right lower pole cortical tumor with avid enhancement of 61 HU. The tumor and vascular supply are well-demonstrated on the volume-rendered subtracted image (right), useful for operative planning

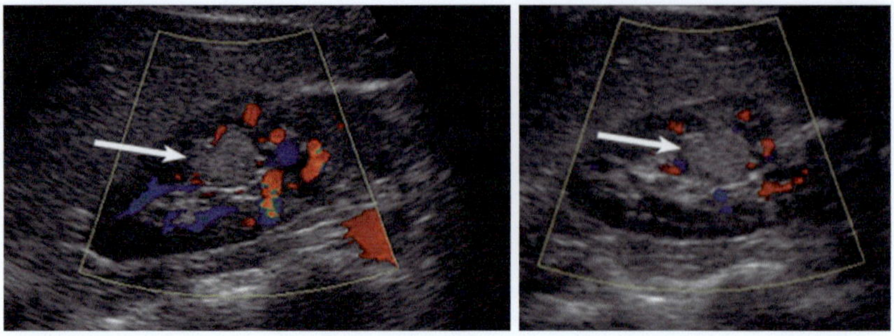

Fig. 5.14 Sagittal and transverse ultrasound images of the right kidney, with superimposed Doppler, demonstrate a well-circumscribed, heterogeneous, slightly hyperechoic lesion. There is no significant vascularity

Table 5.1 The Bosniak renal cyst classification. A classification system used worldwide, to evaluate and categorize cystic renal masses into one of five groups. It is not a pathological classification system, rather an imaging and clinical management system

Category	Criteria and management
I	A benign simple cyst with a hairline-thin wall that does not contain septa, calcifications, or solid components; it has water attenuation and does not enhance; no intervention is needed
II	A benign cystic lesion that may contain a few hairline-thin septa in which perceived (not measurable) enhancement may be appreciated; fine calcification or a short segment of slightly thickened calcification may be present in the wall or septa; uniformly high-attenuating lesions (<3 cm) that are sharply marginated and do not enhance are included in this group; no intervention is needed[a]
IIF[b]	Cysts may contain multiple hairline-thin septa; perceived (not measurable) enhancement of a hairline-thin smooth septum or wall can be identified; there may be minimal thickening of wall or septa, which may contain calcification that may be thick and nodular, but no measurable contrast enhancement is present; there are no enhancing soft-tissue components; totally intrarenal nonenhancing high-attenuating renal lesions (>3 cm) are also included in this category; these lesions are generally well marginated; they are thought to be benign but need follow-up to prove their benignity by showing stability[a]
III	Cystic masses with thickened irregular or smooth walls or septa in which measurable enhancement is present; these masses need surgical intervention in most cases, as neoplasm cannot be excluded; this category includes complicated hemorrhagic or infected cysts, multilocular cystic nephroma, and cystic neoplasms; these lesions need histologic diagnosis, as even gross observation by the urologist at surgery or the pathologist at gross pathologic evaluation is frequently indeterminate
IV	Clearly malignant cystic masses that can have all of the criteria of category III but also contain distinct enhancing soft-tissue components independent of the wall or septa; these masses are clearly malignant and need to be removed

Adapted from [33]

[a] Perceived enhancement refers to enhancement of hairline-thin or minimally thickened walls or septa that can be visually appreciated when comparing unenhanced and contrast-enhanced CT images side-by-side and on subtracted MR imaging datasets. This "enhancement" occurs in hairline-thin or smooth minimally thickened septa/walls and, therefore, cannot be measured or quantified. The authors believe tiny capillaries supply blood (and contrast material) to these septa/walls, which are appreciated because of higher doses of intravenous contrast material and thinner CT and MR imaging sections

[b] "F" indicates follow-up needed

erogeneously, typically an increase of more than 80 HU on postcontrast imaging, differentiating this from non-clear cell type renal cell cancer, with a sensitivity of 74% and specificity of 100% [34]. Homogeneous enhancement and lower tumor to parenchyma enhancement ratio is noted in non-papillary type renal cell carcinoma, particularly in smaller tumors [35].

Additional features include a peripheral enhancement pattern and decreased vascularity that have been noted in chromophobe tumors, although these characteristics are not always seen. Medullary renal cell cancer is usually central in location and exhibits a variable enhancement pattern, but is seen in young patients with concomitant sickle cell disease. Oncocytomas, although benign, cannot be readily differentiated from chromophobe renal cell cancer, or necrotic clear cell tumors, the latter subtype mimicking the central scar sometimes associated with oncocytomas. Thus, frequently subjected to biopsy and surgical resection (Fig. 5.15).

A greater awareness of radiation dose associated with CT is reflected in the principles of ALARA enshrined in the American College of Radiology Appropriateness Criteria ensure minimum standards are established at all accredited imaging centers. Technical and hardware advances drive lower CT radiation dose, including dose modulation, lower tube current, and individualization of the kilovoltage to patient body habitus, all of which afford significantly lower doses of radiation administered with CT studies and the possibility of more focused examinations of the upper abdomen with decreased dose in follow-up studies. Furthermore, evolving hybrid (HIR) and model-based iterative reconstruction (MIR) algorithms have been established, in contrast to earlier adaptive statistical iterative reconstruction (ASIR) algorithms that permit lower radiation doses without sacrificing image quality. Finally, recent developments in dual-energy CT, which utilize different methodologies to generate low- and high-energy spectra, have demonstrated the potential to improve renal lesion and calcification characterization [36]. CT

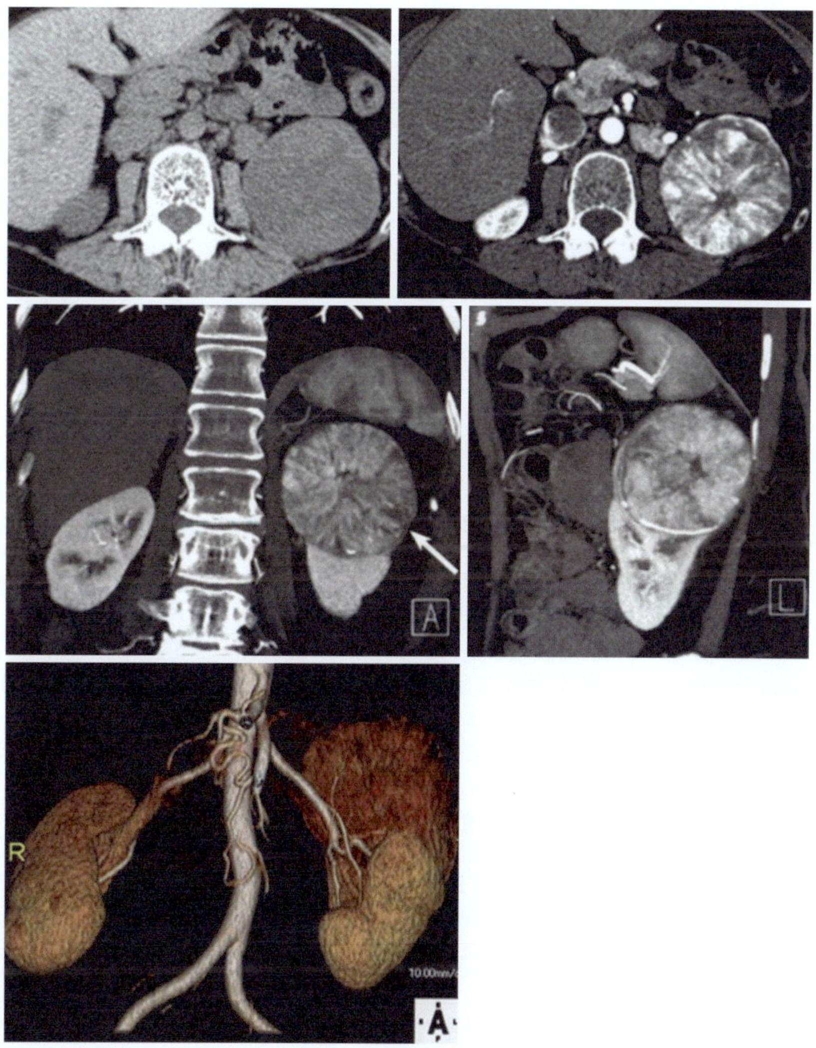

Fig. 5.15 Multiphasic axial CT images, including precontrast (upper left), arterial phase (upper right), coronal and sagittal reformatted images (middle row), demonstrate a large, heterogeneously enhancing mass in the upper pole of the left kidney. There is a “spoke wheel” pattern noted on axial imaging. Imaging findings are typical for oncocytoma, a benign solid renal tumor, confirmed by pathology. However, this diagnosis is often rendered at time of surgery due to the common close resemblance of oncocytoma and renal carcinoma

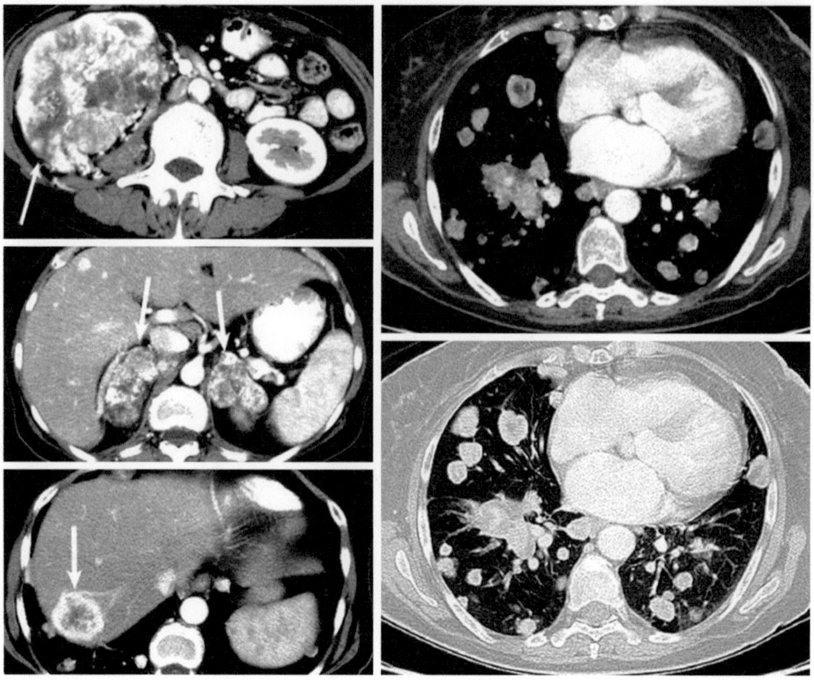

Fig. 5.16 Multiple contrast-enhanced axial CT images demonstrate evidence of numerous metastatic lesions from a renal cell carcinoma primary. The large, heterogeneous enhancing mass in the right kidney (upper left) was the primary tumor. Metastases to both adrenal glands are evident (middle left), and a hypervascular metastasis to the liver (lower left). Numerous large, hypervascular metastases are noted within the lungs

remains a mainstay of imaging in both the elective and emergent settings, generating images of high quality that guide diagnosis, therapy, and surveillance.

Posttreatment imaging remains an integral component of surveillance due to the risk of local or metastatic recurrent disease. The highest recurrence rate occurs in those with an initial tumor greater than 5 cm in size, a higher Fuhrman grade, and stage at presentation. T1 tumors recur between 38 and 45 months, while T3 tumors recur between 17 and 28 months following initial nephrectomy [37]. Metastatic recurrence correlates directly with tumor stage and has been reported as 7.1% in stage T1 disease, 26.5% in stage T2 disease, and 39.4% in stage T3 disease [38]. Although the recurrence rate is close to 85% within the first three postoperative years, recurrence continues to occur up to and beyond 10 years posttreatment [39]. Although some variability in surveillance guidelines for metastatic disease exists [40], imaging is suggested at 6-month intervals for the first 3 years, followed by annual surveillance [41]. Recurrent renal cell carcinoma is typically seen as hypervascular lesions within the lung, liver, bone, and brain and is more commonly multifocal [42]. Surveillance strategies following surgery are considered in more detail in another chapter (Fig. 5.16).

Thermal ablation with either radiofrequency ablation (RFA) or cryoablation is an alternative treatment to partial nephrectomy in a patient population with comorbid conditions that preclude surgery or in those who elect to undergo a minimally invasive procedure [42]. It is of paramount importance to correctly interpret the images of a renal tumor that has been subjected to thermal ablation and recognize its variable appearance. Immediately following thermal ablation, and up to 2 months later, an ablation cavity larger than the original tumor forms, particularly if the mass was less than 3 cm^3 in volume [43]. Between 12 and 24 months after thermal ablation, the ablation cavity reduces to less than half the original volume. The ablation cavity is typically of higher density than surrounding normal parenchyma, likely residual blood products. Postcontrast images demonstrate lower attenuation cavities due to lack of viable tissue. Perinephric stranding may persist indefinitely associated with the intense heat during RFA, resulting in a localized inflammatory response. The stranding is partially replaced by a halo of fibrous tissue within 1–2 months. Finally, later fat invagination, particularly with exophytic lesions, is seen [44] (Fig. 5.17a, b).

In cases where contrast-enhanced CT (or MR) imaging raises the suspicion for recurrent tumor but fails to unequivocally demonstrate its presence, examination with 18F FDG PET/CT or even a combination thereof with a blood flow agent such as Rubidium PET/CT may provide clues to the diagnosis.

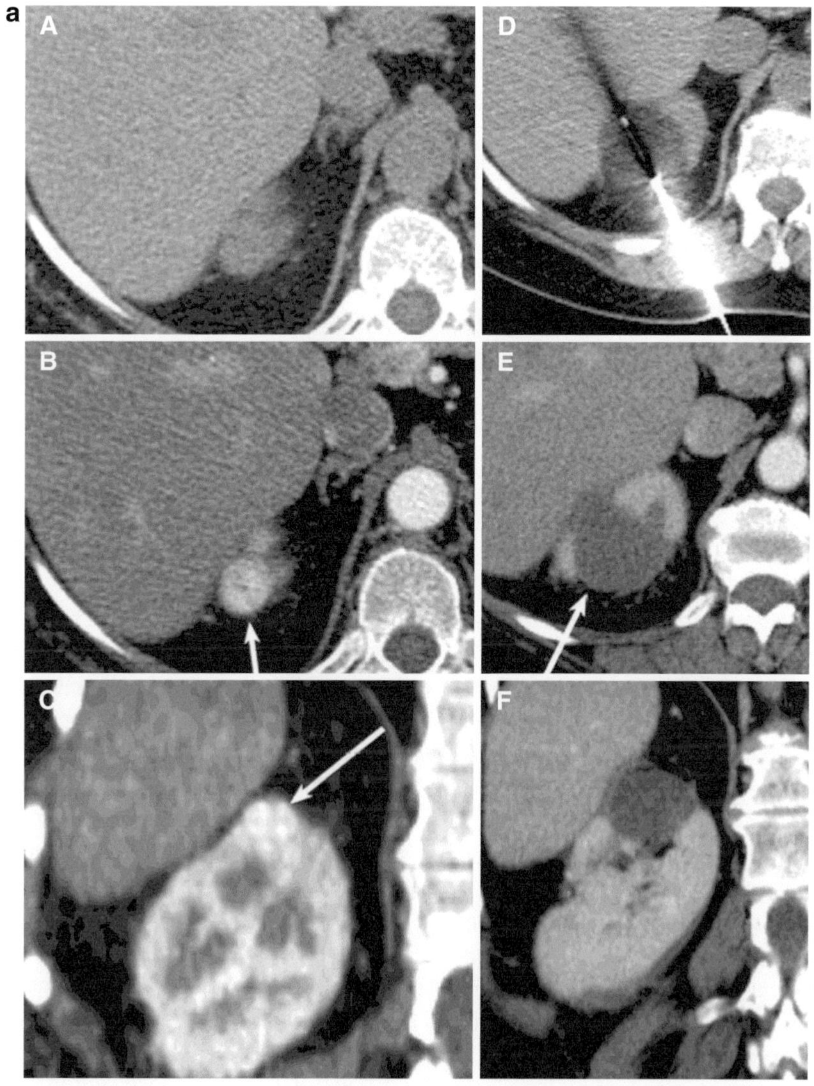

Fig. 5.17 (**a**) Axial precontrast (A) and postcontrast (B) CT images demonstrate a hypervascular upper pole lesion, better seen on coronal reformat (C). This was proven renal cell cancer by biopsy and treated with cryoablation (D). Post-ablation contrast-enhanced CT images in the axial (E) and coronal (F) plane demonstrate infarcted tissue, no definite evidence of recurrence. (**b**) Dynamic phase T1-weighted, subtracted precontrast (left) and postcontrast (middle and right) MR images demonstrate no evidence of recurrent disease

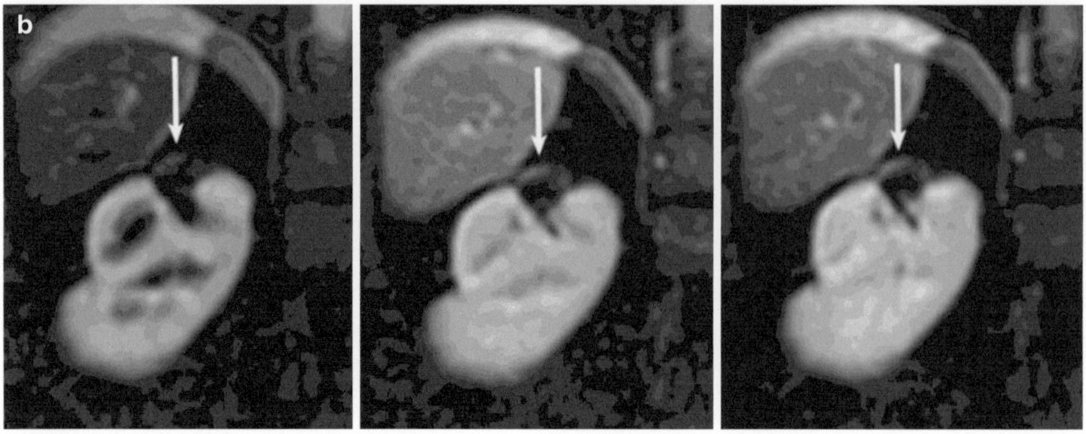

Fig. 5.17 (continued)

Magnetic Resonance Imaging (MRI)

MRI represents a powerful tool alongside ultrasonography and CT in the detection, characterization, and staging of renal masses. The intrinsic properties of MRI allow multiplanar soft tissue characterization, without ionizing radiation, and the available variety of imaging sequences is continually evolving to address specific questions.

A complete abdominal MR examination consists of many individual short component exams, often termed sequences which are named after the radiofrequency pulse schemas which drive each interrogation of the target tissue. Each sequence is designed to produce images which are optimized for the characterization of one or several tissue types of interest. MRI has a much higher intrinsic soft tissue contrast resolution, which means it is better suited to visualize subtle differences between tissue types. Furthermore, some MR sequences are exquisitely sensitive to the detection and degree of acuity of blood products or other fluid. Typical sequences used in renal imaging include T1, T2, in- and opposed-phase imaging, diffusion-weighted images (DWI), and post contrast T1 sequences employing breath hold technique. The T2-weighted sequence may be used to evaluate renal cysts; simple cysts are T2 bright with thin walls, while proteinaceous or hemorrhagic cysts will appear heterogeneous to low signal intensity. Septae and mural nodules are quickly identified against the fluid background. Precontrast images of proteinaceous or hemorrhagic cysts are intrinsically T1 bright. Chemical shift imaging is utilized to identify tumoral fat content and incidental findings such as hepatic steatosis and fat-containing adrenal lesions such as adenoma. Postcontrast imaging, typically following intravenous administration of an extracellular contrast agent such as gadopentetate dimeglumine, is acquired dynamically in corticomedullary, nephrographic, and excretory phases. Subtraction imaging may assist with identification of small lesions (Figs. 5.18 and 5.19).

The most common renal cell cancer subtype is clear cell, comprising up to 80% of all RCC, and associated with a poorer prognosis than papillary or chromophobe [45, 46]. Typical MR characteristics of clear cells include T1 isointense and T2 hyperintense with surrounding parenchyma, and signal drop on opposed phase imaging consistent with cytoplasmic fat is seen in 60% of clear cell tumors. Central necrosis and intratumoral hemorrhage are common and may appear different on T1- and T2-weighted images, depending on the age of the hemorrhage. Subacute hemorrhage is T1 and T2 hyperintense, while chronic hemorrhage is T1 and T2 hypointense from hemosiderin. Postcontrast images demonstrate a hypervascular tumor. A surrounding T1 and T2 pseudocapsule is often identified and, if interrupted, may indicate capsular extension.

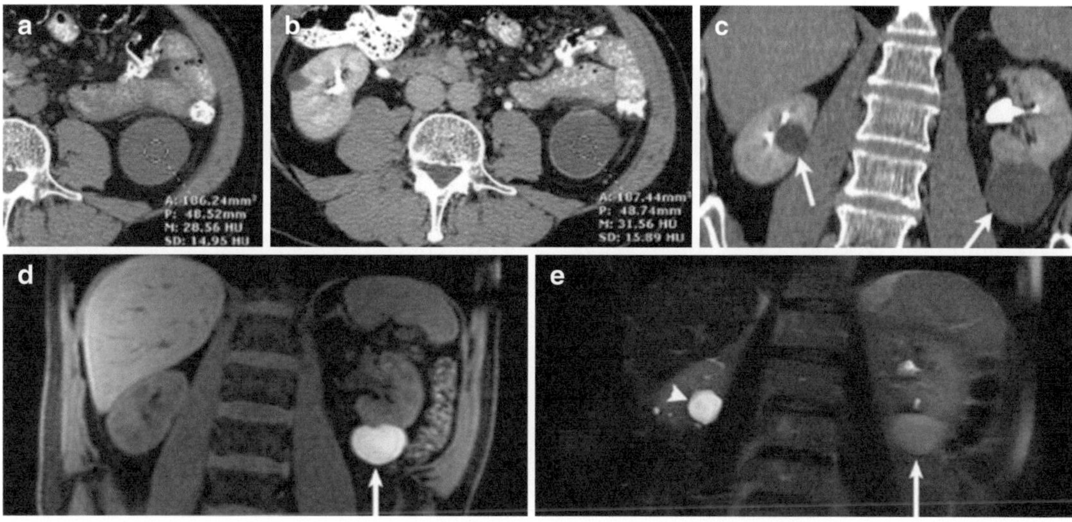

Fig. 5.18 Prominent exophytic left lower pole hypodense lesion seen on precontrast CT (**a**). Lesion is measured at 28 HU, more than would be expected for simple fluid. There is no significant enhancement on nephrogenic phase axial (**b**) or coronal (**c**) images. T1-weighted, fat-suppressed coronal MRI (**d**) confirms bright signal, likely proteinaceous rather than hemorrhagic content, given the CT appearance. Fluid-sensitive T2-weighted sequence (**e**) demonstrates isointense left lower pole lesion, and more typical simple fluid-density cyst in the right kidney (arrowhead). Interpretation of images from different modalities by an expert radiologist often yields the most specific lesion characterization

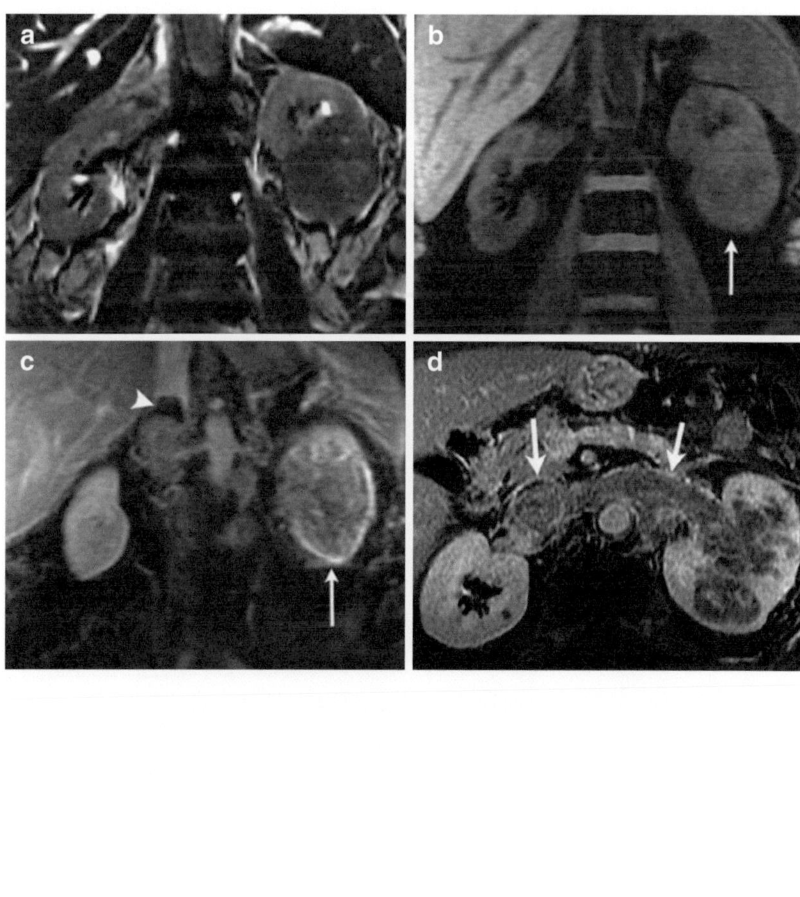

Fig. 5.19 Coronal T2-weighted sequence (**a**) demonstrates hypointense lesion in the left lower pole. This appears to be heterogeneously enhanced on T1-weighted, fat-suppressed precontrast (**b**) and postcontrast (**c**) coronal images. Note is made of a filling defect within the suprarenal IVC (arrowhead), better seen on the postcontrast, T1-weighted fat-suppressed axial image (**d**), with enlargement and apparent occlusion of the left renal vein, through to the IVC

The second group of RCC is papillary type, comprising up to 15% of all RCC, and may appear necrotic and hemorrhagic (type 1) or more heterogeneous (type 2). Enhancing papillary projections at the periphery of a cystic, hemorrhagic mass is noted, together with a fibrous capsule.

The third main type of RCC is chromophobe, which appears as a solid mass with central cystic areas. Certain macroscopic features may be similar to clear cell RCC, although it carries a more favorable prognosis. In addition, chromophobe-type RCC may appear very similar to an oncocytoma, as mentioned in the description of CT imaging (Fig. 5.20).

Benign entities within the kidneys include angiomyolipoma (AML) and oncocytoma. AML is the most common benign renal lesion and is a

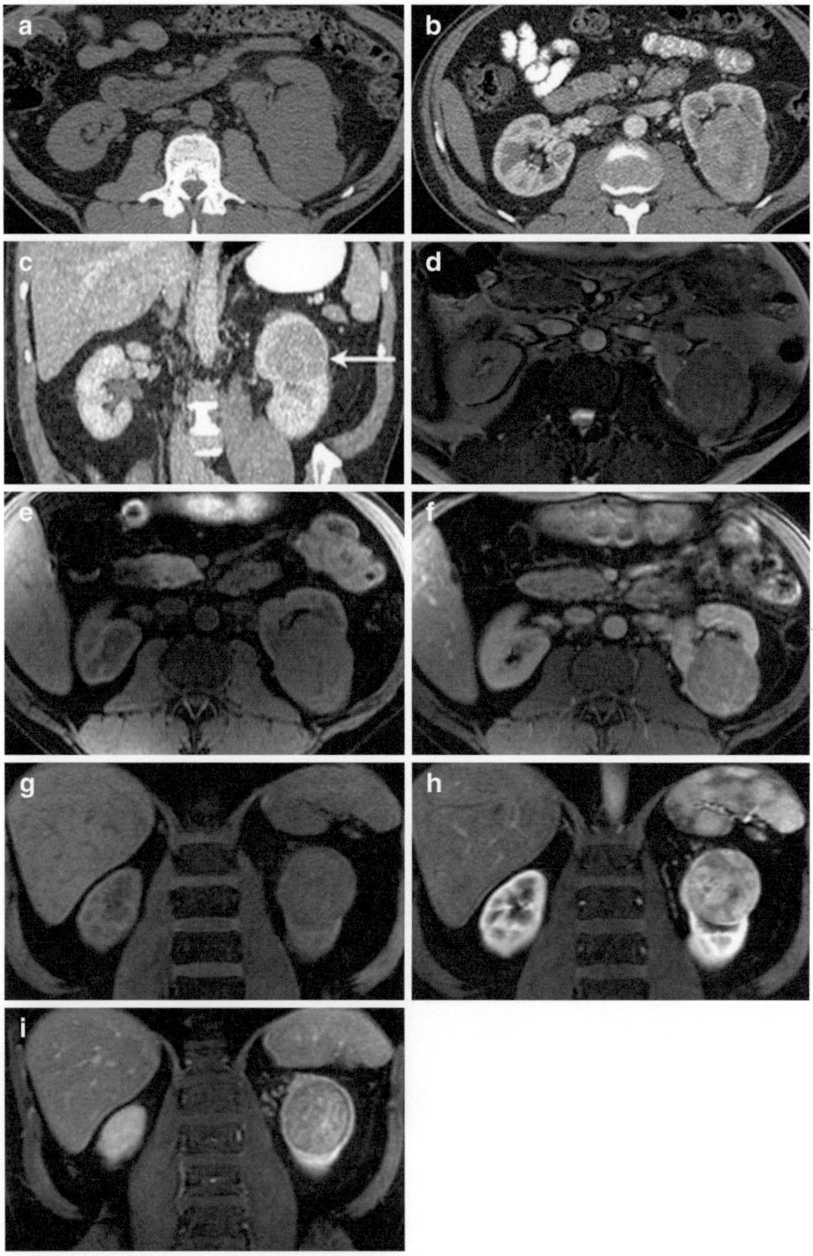

Fig. 5.20 Multiphasic CT images, including axial precontrast (**a**), nephrogenic phase (**b**), and coronal postcontrast (**c**), demonstrating a lobular, hypointense mass with heterogeneous enhancement. Axial T2-weighted (**d**), T1-weighted precontrast (**e**) and postcontrast (**f**) images confirm the left interpolar mass with heterogeneous enhancement. Coronal precontrast T1-weighted (**g**), early (**h**) and late (**i**) T1-weighted postcontrast images demonstrate heterogeneous enhancement with delayed washout. Imaging findings are similar to those of an oncocytoma, pathologically proven chromophobe type, renal cell carcinoma

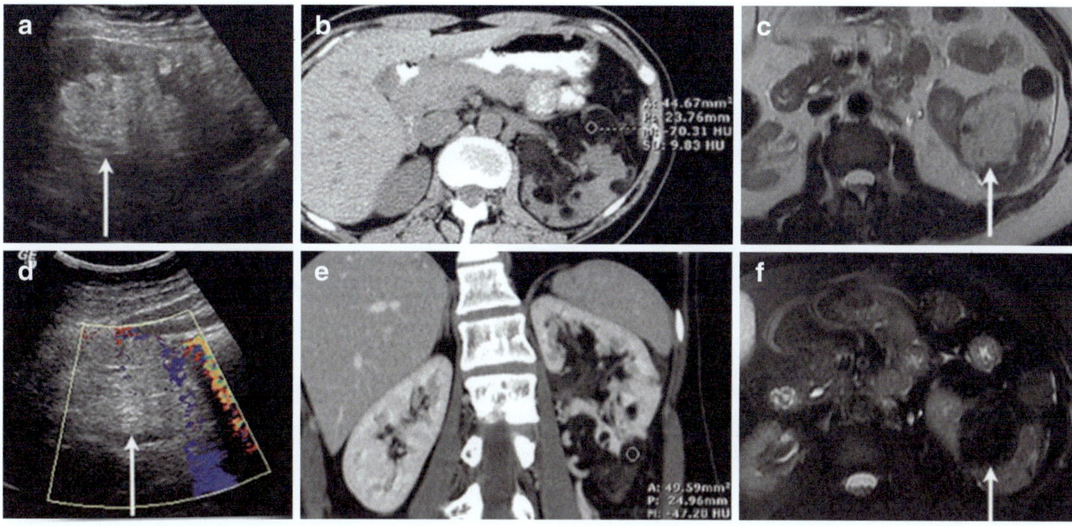

Fig. 5.21 Grayscale (**a**) and Doppler (**d**) images demonstrate an echogenic renal mass without vascular flow. Axial (**b**) and coronal (**e**) CT images demonstrate multiple fat-density lesions (between −40 and −70 HU) within the left kidney. T1-weighted axial MR image (**c**) demonstrates T1 hyperintense left renal mass, which loses signal on fat-suppressed image (**f**), consistent with angiomyolipoma

hamartomatous mass that can be associated with life-threatening hemorrhage if greater than 4 cm in size. Fat suppression pulse sequences are based on a technique which nulls signal arising from tissue areas composed of macroscopic fat, and opposed phase imaging demonstrates classic "India-ink" artifact surrounding the kidney, indicating a fat–water interface. Since RCC may rarely be fat-containing [47], the presence of macroscopic fat is not entirely pathognomonic for AML. It is suggested that central necrosis is a feature of RCC and not AML [48] (Figs. 5.21 and 5.22).

Renal oncocytoma is the second most common benign renal neoplasm, after angiomyolipoma, and is found in up to 7% of solid renal masses; morphologically appearing spherical and well-defined, often peripheral in location, with mildly decreased signal on T1-weighted sequences, slightly T2 hyperintense in comparison with surrounding parenchyma. Homogeneously enhanced with a hypointense central stellate scar. These lesions may be heterogeneous, although less likely to contain cysts, subacute hemorrhage, hemosiderin, and microscopic fat. There is often a stellate, central scar that enhances on delayed post contrast imaging. These various imaging features are shared with chromophobe type renal cell cancer, the third most common subtype; both lesions sharing a common origin renal progenitor cell. Another distinctive feature of an oncocytoma is termed "segmental enhancement inversion" in reference to areas of hyalinized stroma, resulting in relative hypovascularity in comparison with the renal cortex at the start of each phase of imaging. This may also be seen in chromophobe RCC. Although a capsule is seen in up to 50% of oncocytomas, it is also seen in an equivalent number of renal cell cancers [49].

Diffusion-weighted imaging (DWI) is an increasingly utilized sequence in abdominal imaging to evaluate inflammatory and neoplastic processes. Malignant tumors often cause relative impedance to unrestricted diffusion and transit of water molecules, normally seen as a function of Brownian motion. Apparent diffusion coefficient (ADC) values are derived as a measure of diffusion, and ranges can be established that may be used to evaluate for benign versus malignant mass. ADC values typically range from 1.0 to 4.0×10^{-3} mm^2/s; lower values are indicative of higher-grade tumors [50]. The ADC value should be independent of MR scanner field strength, but

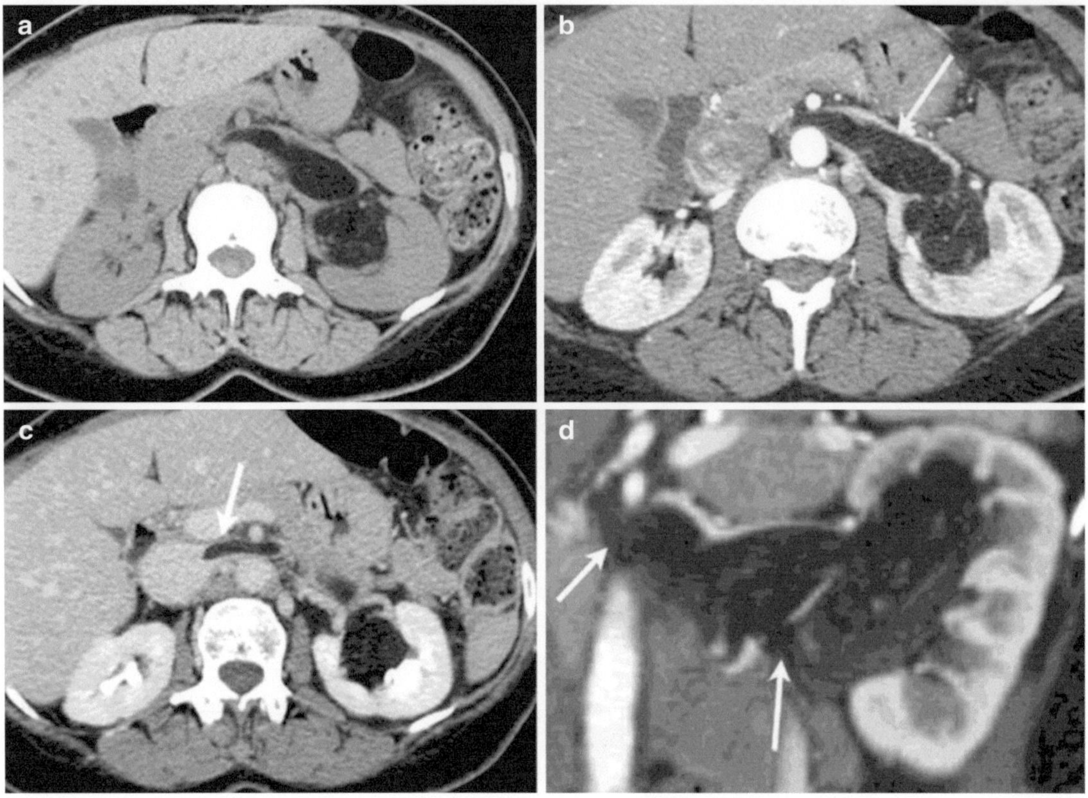

Fig. 5.22 Multiphasic axial CT images, precontrast (**a**), arterial phase (**b**), and nephrogenic phase (**c**) demonstrate a homogeneous, non-enhancing, fat-density mass within the left kidney with extension to the IVC, consistent with a large renal AML An Ultrasound image of the same lesion, shows an echogenic mass (**d**)

may be affected by field inhomogeneities, such that a lower ADC value will be recorded in a 3 Tesla MRI scanner, as compared with a 1.5 Tesla scanner. DWI sequences provide additional functional information, conferring improved diagnostic accuracy and detection of neoplastic processes without requiring intravenous contrast administration [51] (Figs. 5.23 and 5.24).

Differentiation between solid and cystic renal masses has been demonstrated based on ADC values. Mean ADC values of 2.18×10^{-3} mm^2/s were obtained for normal renal parenchyma. Solid renal tumors demonstrate significantly lower ADC values, with a median of 1.16×10^{-3} mm^2/s, compared with a median of 2.73×10^{-3} mm^2/s for cystic tumors. Bosniak category I simple cysts had a mean ADC value of 3.09×10^{-3} mm^2/s. Furthermore, different histologic subtypes exhibited significantly different ADC values; chromophobe cell carcinoma 1.41×10^{-3} mm^2/s, clear cell carcinoma 1.23×10^{-3} mm^2/s, and papillary cell carcinoma 0.90×10^{-3} mm^2/s [50].

In a different study, analysis of a variety of renal masses prior to surgical resection with subsequent pathologic histological correlation noted that, in clear cell type RCC, ADC values greater than 2.12×10^{-3} mm^2/s indicated low-grade tumor, and less than 1.50×10^{-3} mm^2/s indicating high-grade cancer. An ADC value of 1.87×10^{-3} mm^2/s or less corresponded to high-grade, clear cell type renal cell cancer, with a sensitivity and specificity of 90% and 71%, respectively [52]. These findings have been cor-

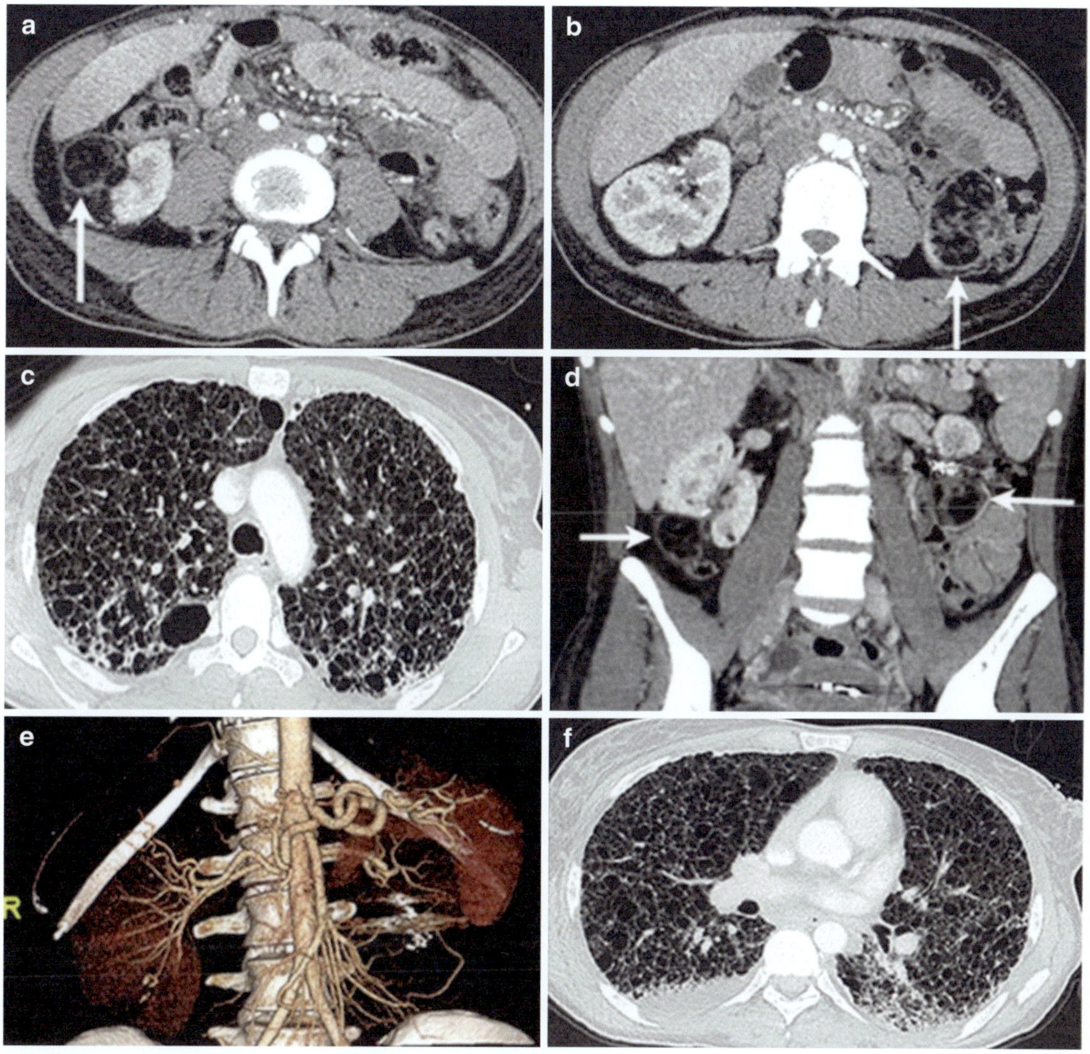

Fig. 5.23 Axial (**a**, **b**) and coronal (**d**) postcontrast images demonstrate multiple fat-density lesions within both kidneys. Corresponding lucent masses are seen on the volume-rendered image (**e**). Evaluation of the lung parenchyma (**c**, **f**) demonstrates innumerable thin-walled cysts and small pleural effusions. The unifying diagnosis is tuberous sclerosis, associated with multiple renal angiomyolipomas (AML) and lymphangioleiomyomatosis (LAM)

roborated in more recent retrospective analyses, including a potential diagnostic role for DWI in distinguishing high- from low-grade clear cell renal cell carcinoma, which may assist with a treatment plan [53].

Further refinement and standardization in the acquisition of DWI sequences and generation of ADC maps may provide information on the histologic subtype and degree of differentiation of a renal tumor with increased accuracy.

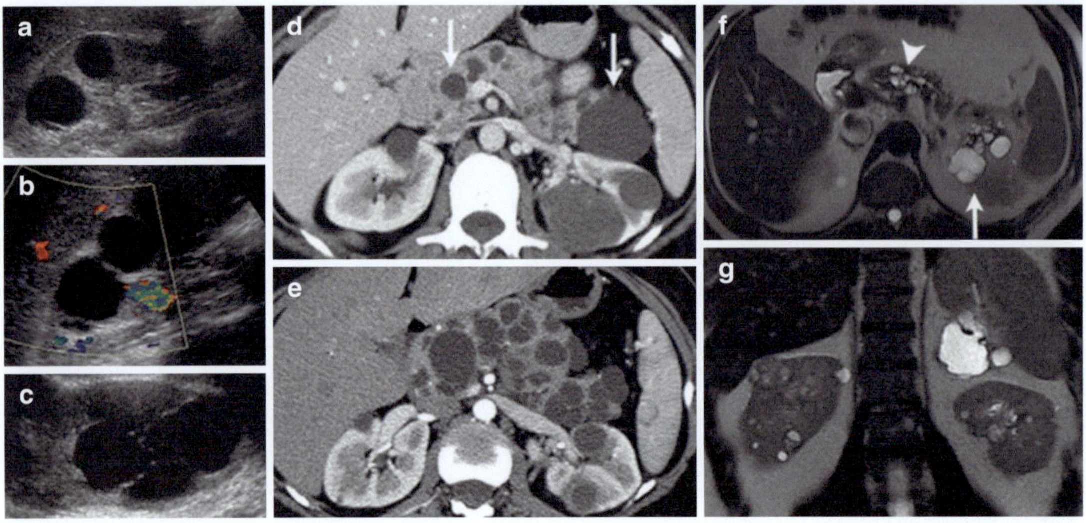

Fig. 5.24 Multiple well-circumscribed, anechoic, avascular cysts are seen within both kidneys on grayscale and Doppler ultrasound (**a**–**c**). Axial CT images in the arterial phase demonstrate multiple non-enhancing, thin-walled renal and pancreatic cysts of varying sizes (**d**, **e**). These findings are also seen on T2-weighted axial and coronal images (**f**, **g**). The underlying condition is Von-Hippel-Lindau disease

Future Directions

The future of renal cancer imaging features a variety of novel techniques, including DECT, functional or molecular imaging, radiomics, and artificial intelligence.

Dual energy CT (DECT). DECT allows for the acquisition of dual-energy images simultaneously, typically at 80 and 140 kVp, without an increase in radiation dose [54]. This technique is used to estimate elemental composition of an object. Additionally, DECT can generate synthetic, virtually unenhanced images by removing the iodine signal from contrast-enhanced images, resulting in a reduction in radiation dose for CT renal mass examinations by approximately 10%–36% [55].

Functional or molecular imaging remains an exciting frontier of imaging, targeting a physiologic pathway or mechanism. Novel pharmaceutical agents used in conjunction with positron emission tomography (PET), combine the highly sensitive and specific antigen-antibody reaction (that may be further tailored by altering the Fc binding domain) with the high resolution of PET imaging. As an example, Tc-99m Sestamibi SPECT/CT, primarily used in cardiac and parathyroid imaging, may aid in differentiating RCC from oncocytoma and hybrid oncocytic/chromophobe tumors. The use of Sestamibi in imaging solid tumors is due to its affinity for accumulating in mitochondria-rich tissues, including tumors. Most RCCs contain very little or no mitochondria, in contrast to oncocytomas, which are rich in mitochondria. This results in avid uptake of the Tc-99m Sestamibi radiotracer by oncocytomas, compared to very low uptake by RCCs. A 2022 meta-analysis showed a sensitivity and specificity of 92% and 88%, respectively, for Tc-99m Sestamibi SPECT/CT in differentiating renal oncocytomas from other renal lesions [56, 57]. Additionally, prostate-specific membrane antigen (PSMA) is known to be overexpressed in the endothelial cells of tumoral neovasculature. A correlation between ^{68}Gallium-PSMA PET/CT and pathologic T stage, grade, and adverse pathologic features has been shown [58], however, additional research investigation is needed.

Active targeting of renal cancer with nanoparticles for the purpose of diagnosis or treatment, including antibody and antibody fragment-based imaging, remains an area of interest, resulting from passive or active tumoral uptake [59]. Monoclonal antibody recognition of a determinant on carbonic anhydrase IX (CA-IX), which has near ubiquitous overexpression in clear cell-type renal cell carcinomas and is not expressed in benign tumors, has been proven successful in animal models. This may provide future direction as a form of radio immunetherapy combined with tyrosine kinase, for the treatment of both primary and metastatic renal cell carcinoma. A benefit has been demonstrated in risk stratification of renal masses, in particular when anatomic imaging provides limited information [60].

Artificial intelligence (AI), machine learning (ML), and the subset of ML termed deep learning (DL) with multi-layered computational models designed to learn representations of data and simulate complex, abstract thought processes will disrupt this and many other fields. Allied with radiomics (extracting quantitative metrics from imaging studies), and in combination with demographic, histologic, genomic, or proteomic data, greater prospective diagnostic and prognostic accuracy may be achieved. It is anticipated that healthcare will be directed toward more personalized medicine and the potential for individualized treatment of renal cancer [61]. Experimental models have created synthetic contrast-enhanced CT images from non-contrast CT studies, and used a deep learning neural network to identify the renal cancer with a high concordance rate compared with real contrast-enhanced CT images [62]. Others have demonstrated successful differentiation of benign renal oncocytoma from chromophobe-type renal cell carcinoma on a limited CT dataset [63]. Despite the potential of these technologies to support renal cancer diagnosis and surveillance imaging, significant ongoing research efforts will be needed, to assure consistent performance and applicability across novel data sets, without error, or bias.

References

1. NIH National Cancer Institute, Surveillance, Epidemiology and End Results (SEER) Program; 2024.
2. Bukavina L, Bensalah K, Bray F, et al. Epidemiology of renal cell carcinoma: 2022 update. Eur Urol. 2022;82(5):529–42.
3. Padala S, Barsouk A, Thandra K, et al. Epidemiology of renal cell carcinoma. World J Oncol. 2020;11(3):79–87.
4. Sun M, Thuret R, Abdollah F, et al. Age-adjusted incidence, mortality, and survival rates of stage-specific renal cell carcinoma in North America: a trend analysis. Eur Urol. 2011;59(1):135–41.
5. Agarwal R, Bergey M, Sonnad S, et al. Inpatient CT and MRI utilization: trends in the academic hospital setting. J Am Coll Radiol. 2010;7(12):949–55.
6. Herts B, Silverman S, Hindman N, et al. Management of the incidental renal mass on CT: a white paper of the ACR incidental findings committee. J Am Coll Radiol. 2018;15(2):264–73.
7. Young M, Jackson-Spence F, Beltran L, et al. Renal cell carcinoma. Lancet. 2024;404(10451):476–91.
8. McIntosh AG, Ristau BT, Ruth K, et al. Active surveillance for localized renal masses: tumor growth, delayed intervention rates, and >5-yr clinical outcomes. Eur Urol. 2018;74(2):157–64.
9. Klatte T, Marberger M. High-intensity focused ultrasound for the treatment of renal masses: current status and future potential. Curr Opin Urol. 2009;19(2):188–91.
10. Ljungberg B, Bensalah K, Canfield S, et al. EAU guidelines on renal cell carcinoma: 2014 update. Eur Urol. 2015;67(5):913–24.
11. Ginzburg S, Tomaszewski J, Kutikov A, et al. Focal ablation therapy for renal cancer in the era of active surveillance and minimally invasive partial nephrectomy. Nat Rev Urol. 2017;14(11):669–82.
12. Long CJ, Kutikov A, Canter DJ, et al. Percutaneous vs surgical cryoablation of the small renal mass: is efficacy compromised? BJU Int. 2011;107(9):1376–80.
13. O'Connor OJ, McSweeney SE, Maher MM. Imaging of hematuria. Radiol Clin North Am. 2008;46(1):113–32, vii.
14. Bai X, Wu CL. Renal cell carcinoma and mimics: pathologic primer for radiologists. Am J Roentgenol. 2012;198(6):1289–93.
15. Mucksavage P, Ramchandani P, Malkowicz SB, Guzzo TJ. Is ultrasound imaging inferior to computed tomography or magnetic resonance imaging in evaluating renal mass size? Urology. 2012;79(1):28–31.
16. Furrer M, Spycher S, Büttiker S. Comparison of the diagnostic performance of contrast-enhanced ultrasound with that of contrast-enhanced computed tomography and contrast-enhanced magnetic resonance imaging in the evaluation of renal masses: a systematic review and meta-analysis. Eur Urol Oncol. 2020;3(4):464–73.

17. Dietrich CF, Averkiou M, Nielsen MB, et al. How to perform contrast-enhanced ultrasound (CEUS). Ultrasound Int Open. 2018;4(1):E2–E15.
18. Chang EH, Chong WK, Kasoji SK, et al. Diagnostic accuracy of contrast-enhanced ultrasound for characterization of kidney lesions in patients with and without chronic kidney disease. BMC Nephrol. 2017;18:266.
19. Finelli A, Ismaila N, Bro B, et al. Management of small renal masses: American Society of Clinical Oncology clinical practice guideline. J Clin Oncol. 2017;35(6):668–680s.
20. Pahernik S, Ziegler S, Roos F, et al. Small renal tumors: correlation of clinical and pathological features with tumor size. J Urol. 2007;178(2):414–7; discussion 416–7.
21. Guðmundsson E, Hellborg H, Lundstam S, et al. Swedish Kidney Cancer Quality Register Group. Metastatic potential in renal cell carcinomas ≤7 cm: Swedish Kidney Cancer Quality Register data. Eur Urol. 2011;60(5):975–82.
22. Marberger M, Schatzl G, Cranston D, Kennedy JE. Extracorporeal ablation of renal tumours with high-intensity focused ultrasound. BJU Int. 2005;95(Suppl 2):52–5.
23. Bradley A, Lim Y, Singh F. Imaging features, follow-up, and management of incidentally detected renal lesions. Clin Radiol. 2011;66(12):1129–39.
24. Israel GM, Silverman SG. The incidental renal mass. Radiol Clin North Am. 2011;49(2):369–83.
25. Herts B, Silverman S, Hindman N, et al. Management of the incidental renal mass on CT: a white paper of the ACR Incidental Findings Committee. J Am Coll Radiol. 2018;15(2):264–73.
26. Catalano C, Fraioli F, Laghi A, et al. High-resolution multidetector CT in the preoperative evaluation of patients with renal cell carcinoma. Am J Roentgenol. 2003;180(5):1271–7.
27. Flocks RH, Kadesky MC. Malignant neoplasms of the kidney; an analysis of 353 patients followed five years or more. J Urol. 1958;79(2):196–201.
28. Robson CJ. Radical nephrectomy for renal cell carcinoma. J Urol. 1963;89:37–42.
29. Hartman DS, Choyke PL, Hartman MS. From the RSNA refresher courses: a practical approach to the cystic renal mass. Radiographics. 2004;24(Suppl 1):S101–15.
30. Bosniak MA. The small (less than or equal to 3.0 cm) renal parenchymal tumor: detection, diagnosis, and controversies. Radiology. 1991;179(2):307–17.
31. Bosniak MA. The current radiological approach to renal cysts. Radiology. 1986;158(1):1–10.
32. Bosniak MA. The Bosniak renal cyst classification: 25 years later. Radiology. 2012;262(3):781–5.
33. Silverman S, Pedrosa I, Ellis J, et al. Bosniak classification of cystic renal masses, version 2019: an update proposal and needs assessment. Radiology. 2019;292:475–88.
34. Kim JK, Kim TK, Ahn HJ, et al. Differentiation of subtypes of renal cell carcinoma on helical CT scans. Am J Roentgenol. 2002;178(6):1499–506.
35. Herts BR, Coll DM, Novick AC, et al. Enhancement characteristics of papillary renal neoplasms revealed on triphasic helical CT of the kidneys. Am J Roentgenol. 2002;178(2):367–72.
36. Pourvaziri A, Mojtahed A, Hahn P, et al. Renal lesion characterization: clinical utility of single-phase dual-energy CT compared to MRI and dual-phase single-energy CT. Eur Radiol. 2023;33:1318–28.
37. Lam JS, Leppert JT, Figlin RA, Belldegrun AS. Surveillance following radical or partial nephrectomy for renal cell carcinoma. Curr Urol Rep. 2005;6(1):7–18. Review.
38. Levy DA, Slaton JW, Swanson DA, Dinney CP. Stage specific guidelines for surveillance after radical nephrectomy for local renal cell carcinoma. J Urol. 1998;159(4):1163–7.
39. Motzer RJ, Bander NH, Nanus DM. Renal-cell carcinoma. N Engl J Med. 1996;335(12):865–75. Review.
40. Scatarige JC, Sheth S, Corl FM, Fishman EK. Patterns of recurrence in renal cell carcinoma: manifestations on helical CT. Am J Roentgenol. 2001;177(3):653–8.
41. Williamson TJ, Pearson JR, Ischia J, et al. Guideline of guidelines: follow-up after nephrectomy for renal cell carcinoma. BJU Int. 2016;117(4):555–62.
42. Lam JS, Shvarts O, Pantuck AJ. Changing concepts in the surgical management of renal cell carcinoma. Eur Urol. 2004;45(6):692–705. Review.
43. Kawamoto S, Permpongkosol S, Bluemke DA, et al. Sequential changes after radiofrequency ablation and cryoablation of renal neoplasms: role of CT and MR imaging. Radiographics. 2007;27(2):343–55.
44. Davenport MS, Caoili EM, Cohan RH, et al. MRI and CT characteristics of successfully ablated renal masses: imaging surveillance after radiofrequency ablation. Am J Roentgenol. 2009;192(6):1571–8.
45. Bostwick DG, Murphy GP. Diagnosis and prognosis of renal cell carcinoma: highlights from an international consensus workshop. Semin Urol Oncol. 1998;16(1):46–52. Review.
46. Beck SD, Patel MI, Snyder ME, et al. Effect of papillary and chromophobe cell type on disease-free survival after nephrectomy for renal cell carcinoma. Ann Surg Oncol. 2004;11(1):71–7.
47. Schuster TG, Ferguson MR, Baker DE, et al. AJR papillary renal cell carcinoma containing fat without calcification mimicking angiomyolipoma on CT. Am J Roentgenol. 2004;183(5):1402–4.
48. Pedrosa I, Sun MR, Spencer M, et al. MR imaging of renal masses: correlation with findings at surgery and pathologic analysis. Radiographics. 2008;28(4):985–1003.
49. Rosenkrantz AB, Hindman N, Fitzgerald EF, et al. MRI features of renal oncocytoma and chromophobe renal cell carcinoma. Am J Roentgenol. 2010;195(6):W421–7.

50. Inci E, Hocaoglu E, Aydin S, Cimilli T. Diffusion-weighted magnetic resonance imaging in evaluation of primary solid and cystic renal masses using the Bosniak classification. Eur J Radiol. 2012;81(5):815–20.
51. Sasaguri K, Takahashi N. CT and MR imaging for solid renal mass characterization. Eur J Radiol. 2018;99:40–54.
52. Sandrasegaran K, Sundaram CP, Ramaswamy R, et al. Usefulness of diffusion-weighted imaging in the evaluation of renal masses. Am J Roentgenol. 2010;194(2):438–45.
53. Woo S, Suh CH, Kim SY, Cho JY, Kim SH. Diagnostic performance of DWI for differentiating high- from low-grade clear cell renal cell carcinoma: a systematic review and meta-analysis. Am J Roentgenol. 2017;209(6):W374–81.
54. Schawkat K, Krajewski K. Insights into Renal Cell Carcinoma with Novel Imaging Approaches. Hematol Oncol Clin North Am. 2023;37(5):863–75.
55. Xiao J, Hippe D, Zecevic M, et al. Virtual unenhanced dual-energy CT images obtained with a multi material decomposition algorithm: diagnostic value for renal mass and urinary stone evaluation. Radiology. 2021;298(3):611–9.
56. Campbell S, Tzortzakis A, Javadi M, et al. 99mTc-sestamibi SPECT/CT for the characterization of renal masses: a pictorial guide. Br J Radiol. 2018;91(1084):20170526.
57. Wilson M, Katlariwala P, Murad M, et al. Diagnostic accuracy of 99mTc-sestamibi SPECT/CT for detecting renal oncocytomas and other benign renal lesions: a systematic review and meta-analysis. Abdom Radiol (NY). 2020;45(8):2532–41.
58. Aggarwal P, Singh H, Das CK, et al. Potential role of 68Ga-PSMA PET/CT in metastatic renal cell cancer: a prospective study. Eur J Radiol. 2024;170:111218.
59. Paluszkiewicz P, Martuszewski A, Zaręba N, et al. The application of nanoparticles in diagnosis and treatment of kidney diseases. Int J Mol Sci. 2021;23(1):131.
60. Rowe S, Islam Z, Viglianti B, et al. Molecular imaging for non-invasive risk stratification of renal masses. Diagn Interv Imaging. 2024;105(9):305–10.
61. Raman A, Fisher D, Yap F, et al. Radiomics and artificial intelligence: renal cell carcinoma. Urol Clin North Am. 2024;51(1):35–45.
62. Sassa N, Kameya Y, Takahashi T, et al. Creation of synthetic contrast-enhanced computed tomography images using deep neural networks to screen for renal cell carcinoma. Nagoya J Med Sci. 2023;85(4):713–24.
63. Baghdadi A, Aldhaam N, Elsayed A, et al. Automated differentiation of benign renal oncocytoma and chromophobe renal cell carcinoma on computed tomography using deep learning. BJU Int. 2020;125:553–60.

6 Molecular Imaging for Renal Cell Carcinoma

Brandon Koo, Yamin Dou, and Eric Dietsche

Introduction

Molecular imaging has gained widespread use in recent years as an important adjunct in oncologic imaging due to its ability to highlight not only key anatomic but also physiologic aspects of malignancy. The advent of positron emission tomography (PET) and PET/CT, with utilization of different radiotracers, such as fluorodeoxyglucose (FDG) and prostate-specific membrane antigen (PSMA), has allowed for more accurate and reliable staging of malignancy for the purposes of treatment planning and assessment of therapeutic response. As immunotherapy and targeted therapies have become part of the standard of practice for many malignancies, molecular imaging is likely to play an even greater role in future treatment selection and in monitoring treatment response. Special attention has been devoted to the development of new tracers for better evaluation of both tumor burden and immunotherapy/targeted therapy response. In this chapter, we will outline the clinical utility of PET/CT and provide a brief discussion of new radiotracers for the imaging of renal cell carcinoma (RCC).

B. Koo · E. Dietsche (✉)
Department of Radiology, Rhode Island Hospital, Warren Alpert Medical School of Brown University, Providence, RI, USA
e-mail: bkoo@brownhealth.org; eric.dietsche@brownhealth.org

Y. Dou
Nuclear Medicine, Department of Radiology, Veterans Affairs Boston Healthcare System, West Roxbury, MA, USA
e-mail: yamin.dou@va.gov

Renal cell carcinoma (RCC) accounts for approximately 4% of all adult cancers and 85% of all primary renal tumors, with 70% of those having a clear cell histology [1]. RCC is the seventh most common cancer in men and the ninth most common in women. Known factors that increase the risk of RCC are smoking, obesity, chronic kidney disease, and hypertension [2]. The incidence of RCC has risen over time, which is partially attributable to the increased utilization of cross-sectional imaging. Choudhary and colleagues estimated 50–60% of RCCs are found incidentally on imaging for an unrelated indication [1]. Small incidental renal masses can then be further characterized through invasive tissue biopsy, which carries known procedural complications, potential sampling errors, and the possibility of metastasis seeding along the biopsy tract. Non-invasive molecular imaging modalities such as PET/CT and ^{99m}Tc-Sestamibi SPECT/CT may serve as useful adjuncts in the initial diagnosis of RCC, as well as differentiation of RCC from benign incidental renal tumors.

To date, the role of FDG PET in the initial detection and diagnosis of RCC is still limited and controversial and is not currently recommended under the 2024 NCCN guidelines. However, FDG PET has shown promise in the detection of distant metastases and local recurrence, as well as prediction of RCC tumor

J. A. Libertino, J. R. Gee (eds.), *Renal Cancer*, https://doi.org/10.1007/978-3-031-97599-8_6

differentiation and prognosis. FDG PET has also shown utility in limited data assessing response to immunotherapy, which stymies standard criteria for response assessment due to delayed response and initial pseudoprogression occurring in some patients. Alternative targeted therapies for metastatic RCC (mRCC), such as tyrosine kinase inhibitors (TKIs), are aimed at specific biologic molecules or processes to modify response or signal transduction. These drugs are primarily cytostatic rather than cytotoxic, and inhibit growth rather than induce tumor regression. Conventional imaging techniques such as CT and MRI that rely on size-based criteria for treatment response may be suboptimal in the evaluation of early posttreatment change. Molecular imaging has become more important in evaluating response in the setting of these cytostatic agents, with changes in FDG uptake on PET scans before and after therapy serving as a strong indicator of biological response to TKIs.

In this chapter, we will examine the current application of molecular imaging techniques including PET/CT, Tc99m-sestamibi, and novel tracers for the detection of primary RCC, as well as locoregional and distant metastases to the liver, lung, and bone. We will also discuss the prognostic value of PET/CT and the utility of PET/CT for monitoring therapeutic response for mRCC.

Primary Renal Cell Carcinoma Diagnosis

Although RCC was once considered to be a single disease entity, it is now known that there are numerous histologic patterns of RCC with variable clinical courses and different responses to therapy [3]. The Heidelberg classification identifies five distinct malignant subtypes: clear cell, papillary, chromophobe, collecting duct, and RCC unclassified. Benign renal tumors have been subclassified into metanephric adenoma and adenofibroma, papillary renal cell adenoma, and renal oncocytoma [4]. Approximately 54% of overall renal masses and 70% of RCCs are the clear cell carcinoma subtype [3].

The initial diagnosis of a renal mass is usually made with ultrasound, CT, or MRI. Most cases are discovered incidentally during studies performed for other indications [5]. CT is currently the imaging modality of choice to stage and detect metastasis in patients with RCC, which is essential for both prognostic evaluation and surgical planning. Surgical resection by either partial or radical nephrectomy remains the standard of care for localized disease, with percutaneous ablation available for higher-risk, non-surgical candidates.

Among molecular imaging techniques, FDG PET has gained increasing acceptance for the diagnosis of cancer, although its application in the detection of RCC remains limited. Early studies using FDG PET reported a broad range of accuracy for detecting primary RCC. Ramdave et al. [6] studied 17 patients with known or suspected primary tumors and found true positives in 15, 1 true negative, and 1 false negative. The accuracy of FDG PET and CT was identical (94%). Similar results were also reported by Goldberg et al. [7]. Two other studies [8, 9] with larger samples of 53 and 66 patients showed different results. Aide et al. [8] reported a sensitivity, specificity, and accuracy of 47%, 80%, and 51%, respectively. Kang et al. [9] reported a sensitivity of 60% and a specificity of 100% for PET versus 91.7% sensitivity and 100% specificity for CT. Kang and colleagues concluded that the role of FDG PET in the detection of primary RCC is limited by low sensitivity. However, the superior specificity of the PET may have a complementary role in equivocal cases on conventional imaging [9]. Several factors may explain the large ranges of variation of sensitivity. First, due to the heterogeneity of RCC, some have low FDG uptake due to low glucose transporter-1 expression [10]. In a study with 44 primary clear cell RCC, SUVmax (maximum standardized uptake value) ranges from 2.5 to 18.4, with an average SUVmax of 6.8 [11]. Second, the kidneys and collecting system are the route for radiotracer FDG excretion; this makes the diagnosis of small parenchymal masses difficult, even with hydration and diuretics [12]. Third, due to the limited resolution and the lack of anatomic (CT) correlation of old-generation non-hybrid PET-only scanners, small lesions are very difficult to detect. The main disadvantage of FDG PET for RCC is the relatively high false-negative results. Another drawback of FDG PET is the lower spatial resolution of PET-only images when compared to conventional CT. There is known false-positive uptake in infection and inflammation for PET as well. It is worth noting that most articles published regarding RCC were based on PET-only scanners, which may lower the sensitivity and specificity by about 5–10%. The newer generation of hybrid PET/CT scanners with improved resolution has markedly improved the localization of lesions and diagnostic accuracy compared to either CT or PET stand-alone applications. A more recent study with FDG PET/CT by Kayani et al. detected 41/43 of primary RCC, with the smallest tumor measuring less than 2.5 cm [11].

There is limited data regarding the ability to predict the histological diagnosis based on anatomic imaging findings [13]. Clear cell RCC is the most common type of renal malignancy. It can have a variable appearance on pre-contrast CT, and may be hypodense, isodense, or hyperdense relative to normal parenchyma. Clear cell RCC has notable post-contrast enhancement and can appear heterogeneous due to regions of non-enhancing necrosis [14]. Most clear cell RCC tumors demonstrate increased FDG uptake above the background renal parenchyma activity (Fig. 6.1). SUVmax (maximum standardized uptake value) has been reported ranging from 2.5 to 18.4 with an average of 6.5 [11].

Oncocytomas are benign solid renal tumors originating from collecting tubule cells. Oncocytomas can be difficult to differentiate from RCC on CT; they usually appear as well-demarcated masses that are isodense or hypodense to renal parenchyma on noncontrast CT, with heterogeneous post-contrast enhancement. Oncocytomas may demonstrate a central scar in a third of cases, although this imaging feature overlaps with RCC. In contrast to RCC however, oncocytomas typically do not demonstrate increased FDG avidity on PET/CT [15], although individual cases of FDG avid oncocytomas have been reported [16], as have RCCs with uptake similar to background renal parenchyma. Overall, imaging features on CT and FDG PET have a significant amount of overlap, making differentiation between RCC and oncocytoma on these modalities extremely challenging. Historically, enhancing renal masses seen on CT or MRI are treated as an RCC until proven otherwise. A typical appearance of oncocytoma is shown in Fig. 6.2.

More recently, there have been attempts to further differentiate benign oncocytomas from RCC through the use of ^{99m}Tc-sestamibi SPECT/CT. Sestamibi is a lipophilic radiotracer that localizes to mitochondria-rich cells, which are commonly found in benign renal tumors such as oncocytic neoplasms (Fig. 6.3); in contrast, aggressive RCCs often express multidrug-resistant pumps, which actively efflux the tracer (Fig. 6.4). This difference in sestamibi uptake has been used to distinguish between oncocytoma and RCC, although its efficacy has yet to be fully explored in the literature. Parihar et al. reported a sensitivity and specificity of 66.7% and 86.7% compared to 10% and 75% for ^{99m}Tc-sestamibi SPECT/CT and contrast-enhanced CT, respectively, in the detection of non-concerning renal lesions in a cohort of 42 patients [17]. In another

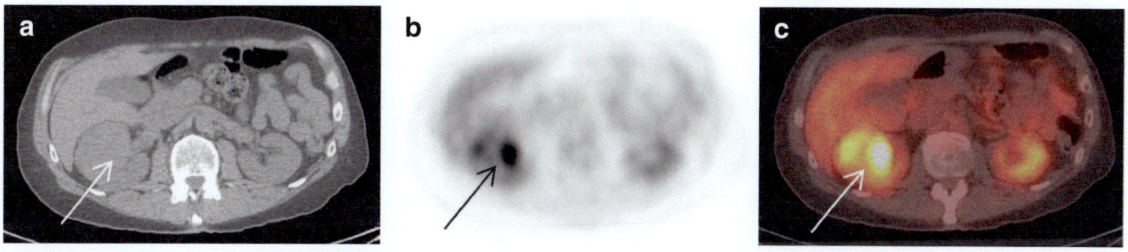

Fig. 6.1 Clear cell renal carcinoma. (**a**) Noncontrast CT shows a 5-cm right renal mass. (**b**) FDG PET demonstrates heterogeneous increased uptake in right renal mass. SUVmax 5.7. (**c**) Fused PET/CT image

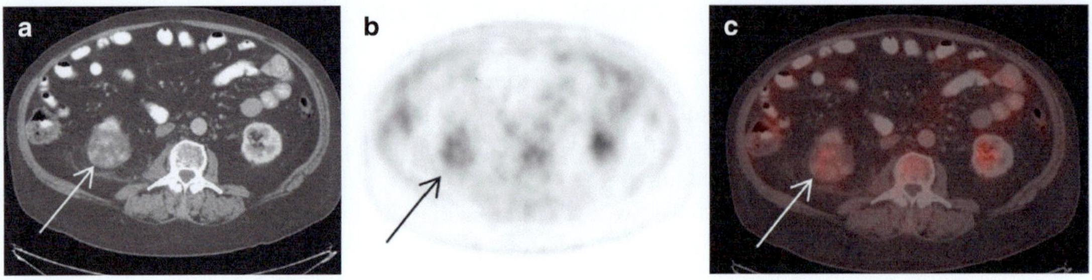

Fig. 6.2 Oncocytoma. (**a**) CT with IV contrast shows a well-defined 5-cm mass with mild heterogeneous enhancement. (**b**) FDG PET shows mild increased uptake. SUVmax 2.9. (**c**) Fused PET/CT image

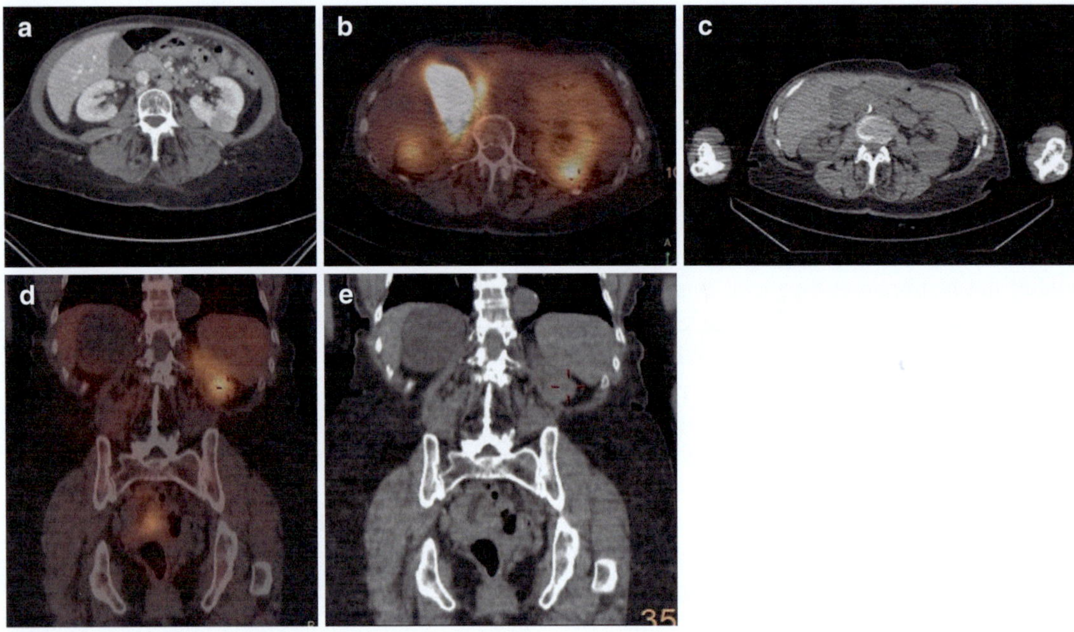

Fig. 6.3 Oncocytoma. (**a**) CT with IV contrast shows a well-defined enhancing mass in the left kidney. (**b**) Fused axial Tc-99m sestamibi SPECT/CT demonstrates uptake greater than background parenchyma in the lesion, which is localized on low dose noncontrast CT (**c**). (**d**, **e**) Coronal fused sestamibi SPECT/CT and low dose noncontrast CT images, respectively. (Images courtesy of Yana Studentsova, MD)

prospective study by Gorin et al., the use of ^{99m}Tc-sestamibi SPECT/CT in detecting oncocytomas was assessed in 50 presurgical patients with T1 renal masses, and results were compared to final surgical pathologies [18]. The authors found a sensitivity of 87.5% and a specificity of 95.2% in differentiating oncocytomas from hybrid oncocytic/chromophobe tumors.

Angiomyolipoma (AML) is the most common benign tumor of the kidney. These lesions characteristically contain variable amounts of abnormal blood vessels, adipose tissue, and smooth muscle elements. The majority of angiomyolipomas can be accurately diagnosed on unenhanced CT as the lesions contain macroscopic fat (Fig. 6.5). There is limited literature on the role of FDG PET in the diagnosis of angiomyolipoma. Kochhar et al. [15] showed a renal angiomyolipoma without significant FDG uptake similar to our case in Fig. 6.5.

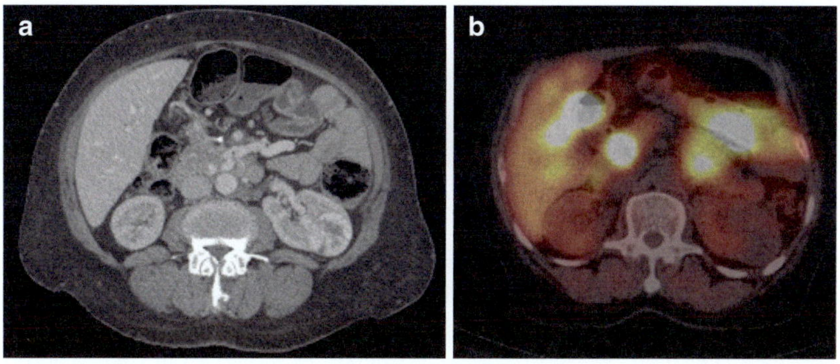

Fig. 6.4 Mixed clear cell and papillary RCC. (**a**) CT with IV contrast shows a well-defined heterogeneously enhancing mass in the left kidney with possible central scar. (**b**) Fused axial Tc-99m sestamibi SPECT/CT demonstrates uptake less than background renal parenchyma in the lesion, compatible with biopsy proven RCC. (Images courtesy of Merissa Zeman, MD)

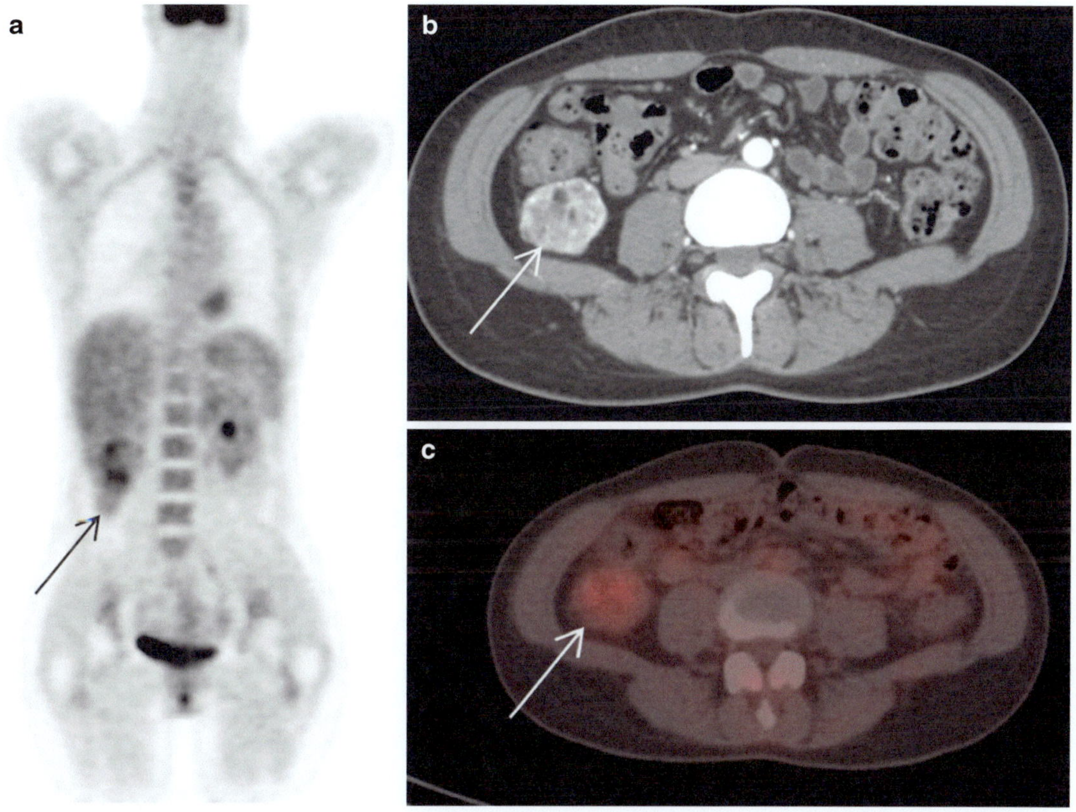

Fig. 6.5 Angiomyolipoma of the kidney. (**a**) FDG PET shows mild uptake equal to or less than background renal parenchymal activity, SUVmax 1.9. (**b**) A right renal lesion with areas of macroscopic fat attenuation seen on CT scan (arrow), highly suggestive of angiomyolipoma. (**c**) Fused PET/CT image

Locoregional Metastasis

Approximately 18% of patients with RCC have metastases at the time of diagnosis [19]. CT and MRI are currently the studies of choice to evaluate tumor extension, vascular invasion, and regional metastasis. MRI in particular has a special role in assessing RCC tumor thrombus extent, which has clinical significance in both prognosis and management, with different surgical approaches and surgical mortality rates depending on the extent of vascular invasion. Metastatic lymphadenopathy remains a major challenge for cross-sectional imaging due to considerable overlap between the appearance of nodal metastatic disease and reactive adenopathy. FDG PET provides an alternative to size- and appearance-based criteria in contrast-enhanced CT by demonstrating the metabolic activity of suspected nodal disease, although data regarding detection rates between CT and PET remain limited [20].

FDG PET plays a vital role in the detection of small metastatic nodes that would fall below size threshold on standard cross-sectional imaging (Fig. 6.6). Kang et al. [9] reported 75% sensitivity and 100% specificity for retroperitoneal lymph node metastases and/or local recurrence by PET, while abdominal CT demonstrated 92.6% sensitivity and 98.1% specificity. Aide et al. [8] reported two cases of RCC with local nodal metastasis. FDG PET was able to detect one of these cases, while contrast-enhanced CT was able to detect both.

Kocher et al. [21] compared the results of FDG PET with histology in patients with suspected RCC. They found true regional lymph node metastasis in three patients and true negative in seven. Ramdave et al. [6] reported two cases of locoregional lymph node metastasis detected on FDG PET but not on CT.

Although some publications have suggested that only tumor and infected thrombi show increased FDG uptake, a few reports showed that bland thrombus may have this appearance as well, a finding consistent with the acute inflammatory phase of aseptic deep venous thrombosis, with uptake attributed to normal macrophage activity [22]. It seems that FDG PET is not useful in recognizing the cause of the thrombus because FDG uptake relies on the degree of reactive inflammation, which is variable and does not correlate with bland or tumor thrombus. However, there is generally accepted consensus that tumor thrombi have higher uptake than bland thrombus. A case with tumor thrombosis is shown in Fig. 6.6.

The incidence of local recurrence ranges from 1.8% to 27% after nephrectomy [23]. CT interpretation of the renal bed is difficult because of migration of the adjacent normal organs into the renal fossa, postoperative scarring, and artifacts from surgical clips. In addition, patients may develop renal failure after nephrectomy which makes IV contrast injection relatively contraindicated. The metabolic activity of the tumor is not altered by these factors, which increases the utility of FDG PET for evaluation of renal bed recurrence of RCC (Fig. 6.7). Ramdave et al. [6] showed that in the eight patients referred for this condition, PET was able to clearly differentiate tumor recurrence from fibrosis or necrosis. The diagnostic accuracy of FDG PET was calculated to be 100%. In comparison, the diagnostic accuracy of CT was 88%.

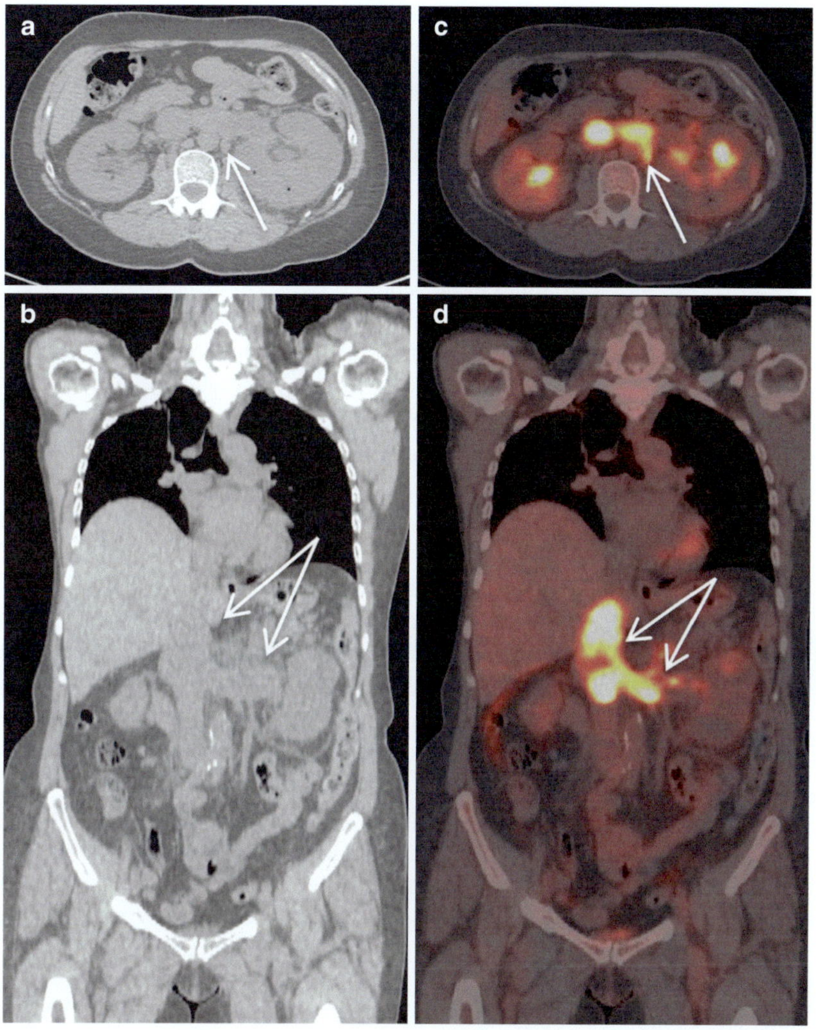

Fig. 6.6 Papillary renal cell carcinoma with local small nodal metastasis and tumor invading renal vein and IVC. (**a**) Staging FDG PET/CT demonstrates a large left renal mass and a 10-mm left para-aortic node (arrow) on noncontrast CT. (**b**) There is a markedly dilated left renal vein and IVC (arrows). (**c**) Fused FDG PET/CT images demonstrate heterogeneous uptake in the left renal mass, SUVmax 11, and corresponding uptake in a 10-mm left para-aortic lymph node (arrow), suggesting metastatic disease. (**d**) There is intense FDG uptake in the left renal vein and IVC (arrows), consistent with intravascular tumor extension

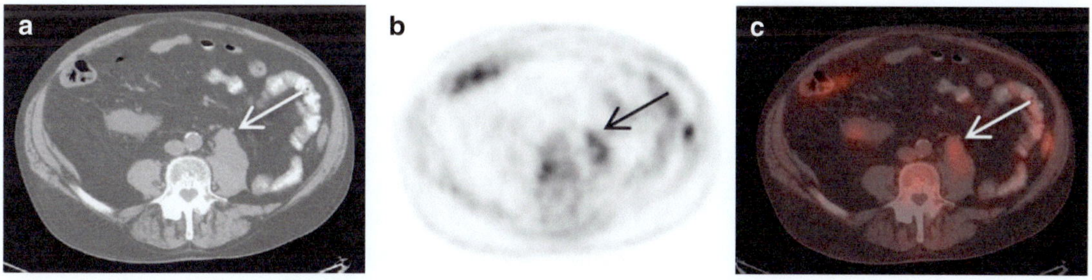

Fig. 6.7 Chromophobe renal cell cancer with FDG avid local recurrence. (**a**) Re-staging FDG PET/CT demonstrates a left retroperitoneal soft-tissue mass on noncontrast CT with differential, including postsurgical change versus local recurrence. Axial FDG PET (**b**) and fused FDG PET/CT (**c**) demonstrates uptake associated with the soft tissue, SUVmax 2.5, consistent with recurrent disease

Distant Metastasis

FDG PET/CT is very useful in evaluating distant metastases, partially attributable to the field of view (routine skull base to mid-thigh) of the scan. It has shown promising results with RCC, with sensitivity ranging from 60% to 100% and the specificity close to 100% for the majority of cases [8, 20, 24–28]. Majhail et al. reported two cases of unsuspected distant metastasis detected by FDG PET not seen by CT in 17 patients evaluated for primary RCC [24]. In another study [29], FDG PET detected 77/112 of the metastatic lesions. Of those, 32 lesions had not been detected by any form of purely anatomic imaging. The results of CT and FDG PET for detecting distant metastases from RCC were comparable, with sensitivities of 70% and 69%, respectively. Safaei et al. [30] reported a study of 20 patients with 25 lesions biopsied. FDG PET accurately identified 21/25 metastases and demonstrated a sensitivity of 87% and a specificity of 100%. Park et al. [20] evaluated FDG PET/CT for the postoperative surveillance of advanced RCC and found that it has 89.5% sensitivity, 83.3% specificity, 77.3% PPV, 92.6% NPV, and 85.7% accuracy in detecting local recurrent and distant metastasis. A study by Aide et al. [8] showed no metastases detected by CT that were missed by FDG PET. In fact, FDG PET was able to detect additional metastatic sites, leading to better accuracy compared with CT.

Lung Metastasis

Lung is the most common site of mRCC and accounts for 50–60% of metastasis [31, 32]. Patients with lung-only metastases have a better survival rate than patients with other sites of metastases [33]. Pulmonary metastases usually appear as well-circumscribed round or ovoid nodules on both chest radiography and CT. They can be solitary though are often multiple and typically range in size from 0.5 to 2 cm in diameter. They are one of the well-known causes of "cannonball" metastases [34]. CT with IV contrast is the current study of choice to evaluate lung metastases with high sensitivity. However, CT evaluation alone is limited due to lower specificity in differentiating benign from malignant nodules. FDG PET assesses the metabolic activity of the lesions and is useful in evaluating malignant potential. A large study of 585 patients by Bryant and colleagues showed the greater the SUV, the greater the likelihood of malignancy [35]. Fortes et al. [36] evaluated 83 patients with metastatic pulmonary nodules from different primaries and found that FDG PET is positive in only 67.5% of them. Nodule size and grade affect the sensitivity of FDG PET. For nodules ranging from 1 to 5 mm, the sensitivity of FDG PET was 23.5% (4/17); however, for nodules greater than 25 mm in diameter, the sensitivity of FDG PET was 88.5% (23/26). The evaluation of smaller nodules is limited by the spatial resolution of PET, which is widely recognized as about 8 mm.

With FDG PET, Majhail et al. [24] reported a sensitivity of 63.2% and 100% PPV in detecting pulmonary metastasis from RCC. The mean size of lung metastases in patients with true-positive FDG PET was 2.0 cm (95% CI, 1.3–2.7 cm) compared with 0.8 cm (95% CI, 0.5–1.2 cm) in patients with false-negative FDG PET.

Hybrid PET/CT scanning, which is the standard of care at this time, takes advantage of the high sensitivity from CT and the greater specificity of FDG PET which results in increasing accuracy as compared to either modality alone. Small pulmonary metastasis from RCC even without significant metabolic activity can be seen by CT (Fig. 6.8). A pulmonary nodule with corresponding FDG uptake is highly suspicious for metastasis in a patient with a history of RCC (Fig. 6.9). Due to overlapping FDG uptake between inflammatory cells and cancer cells, false-positive metastasis is not uncommonly seen on FDG PET/CT (Fig. 6.10).

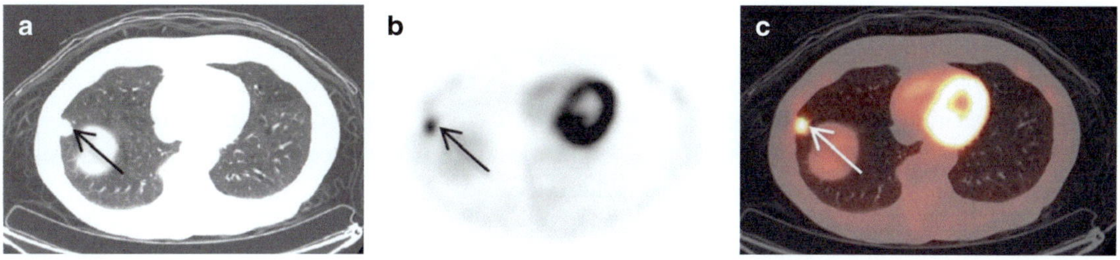

Fig. 6.8 Clear cell renal cancer with FDG avid lung metastasis. (**a**) Noncontrast CT component of FDG PET/CT scan shows a 2.0 cm solitary right lower lobe pulmonary nodule. (**b**) FDG PET demonstrates intense uptake, SUVmax 6.4, which corresponds to the pulmonary nodule, as seen on fused FDG PET/CT images (**c**)

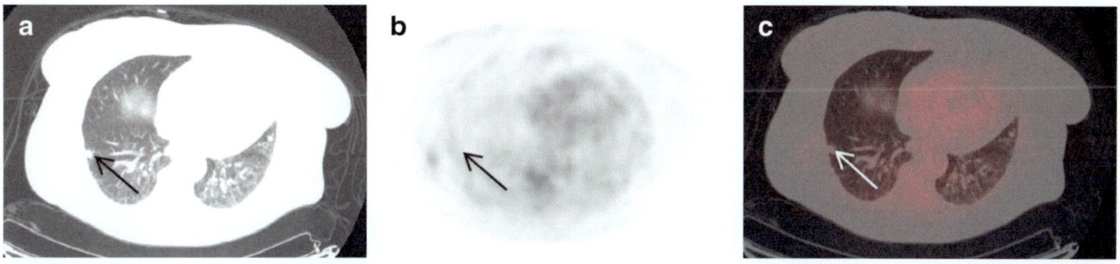

Fig. 6.9 Lung metastases from clear cell renal cancer without discernible FDG uptake. FDG PET/CT in a 63-year-old female with clear cell renal cancer and biopsy-proven pulmonary metastases. (**a**) Multiple pulmonary nodules are present, largest measuring 10 mm (arrow) on axial noncontrast CT. (**b**) No significant FDG uptake corresponding to these small nodules on PET or fused PET/CT (**c**) images

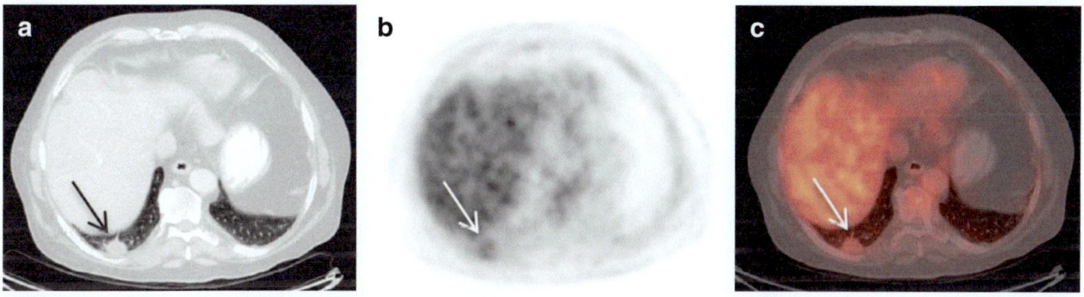

Fig. 6.10 FDG avid pulmonary nodule in a patient with clear cell renal carcinoma, biopsy proven necrotic inflammatory tissue without malignancy detected. (**a**) Axial noncontrast CT shows a 2.7 × 1.7 cm pulmonary nodule (arrow), which has FDG uptake (SUVmax 2.7) on PET (**b**) and fused PET/CT (**c**) images

Bone Metastasis

Osseous metastasis accounts for 30–40% of distant metastasis in RCC [37]. Bone metastases classically appear as large expansile lytic lesions on plain radiography and noncontrast CT, most commonly in the axial skeleton [34]. Contrast-enhanced CT shows bone destruction with or without the presence of an enhancing soft-tissue mass. Bone scans are not routinely performed for RCC patients due to the predominantly lytic nature of the osseous metastatic lesions. The general consensus is to order a bone scan only for patients with symptomatic bone pain and elevated serum alkaline phosphatase [30, 38].

FDG PET has been reported to be very accurate to stage bone metastases in breast and lung cancers [39, 40]. FDG PET is expected to offer improved specificity over bone scintigraphy in the detection of RCC bone metastases (Fig. 6.11). Another advantage of PET over bone scans is the evaluation of both bone and soft tissue in a single study. Solitary bone metastasis from RCC is not uncommon, and a subtle bone lesion is not easily seen on a CT scan (Fig. 6.12). Wu et al. [41] showed that for detecting bone metastasis, FDG PET had both sensitivity and accuracy of 100% compared with 77.5% and 59.6%, respectively, for bone scintigraphy. Kang et al. [9] showed that positive predictive value and negative predictive value for bone metastases were 99% and 93.2%, respectively, and indicated that FDG PET is the most sensitive test for imaging bone metastasis of RCC.

As expected, NaF-18 PET has been shown to be more accurate than ^{99m}Tc-diphosphonate SPECT for identifying both malignant and benign lesions of the skeleton [42]. Combining the NaF-18 PET with CT using a PET/CT scanner can improve the specificity and overall accuracy of detecting skeletal metastasis.

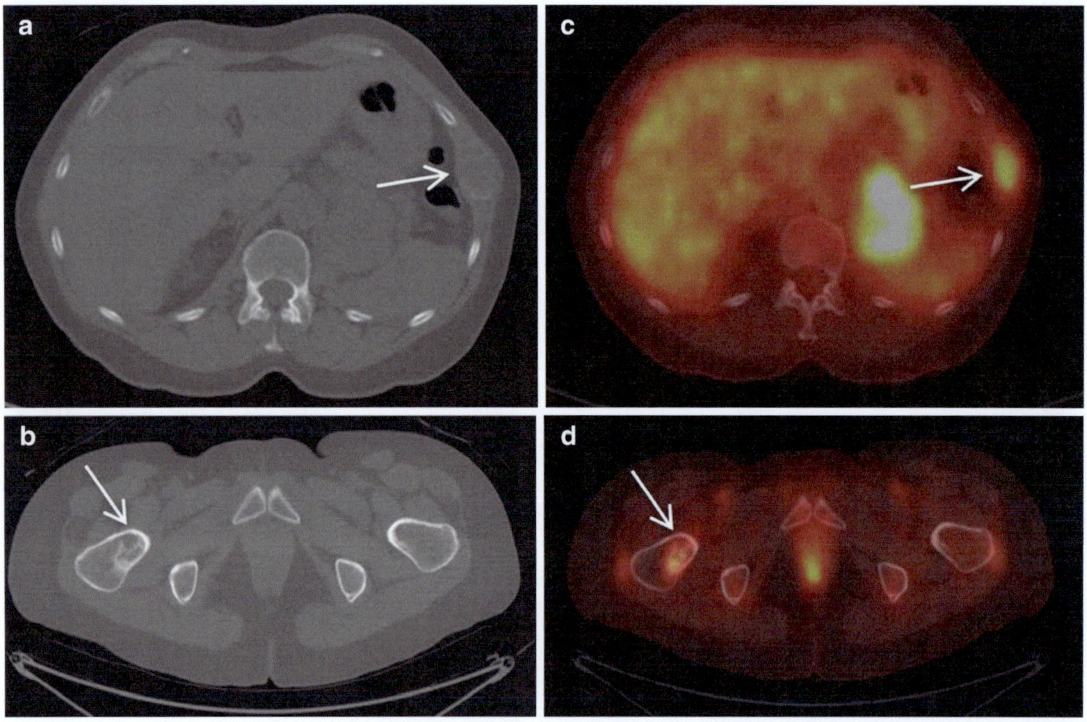

Fig. 6.11 Multiple bone metastases from clear cell renal carcinoma. (**a**, **b**) Re-staging scan demonstrates an expansile destructive lesion in a left anterior rib and a mixed lytic and sclerotic lesion in the right proximal femur on CT (arrows). (**c**, **d**) Fused axial PET/CT images demonstrate moderate FDG uptake corresponding to the known osseous lesions, compatible with metastases

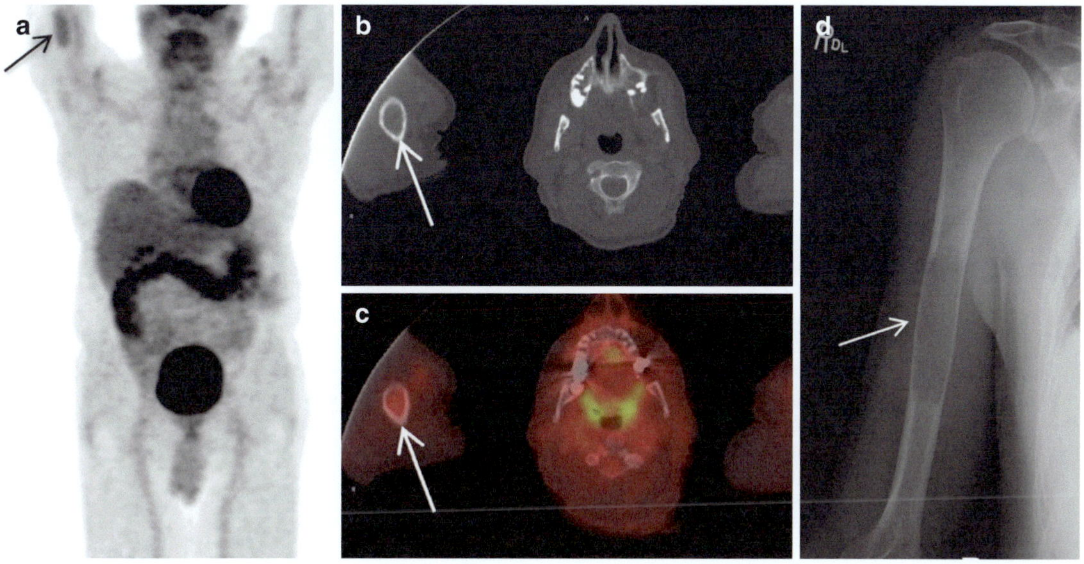

Fig. 6.12 Solitary FDG avid bone metastasis from clear cell renal carcinoma. (**a**) Re-staging FDG PET/CT in a 63-year-old male with clear cell renal carcinoma. PET demonstrates focal moderate FDG uptake in the right humerus. (**b**) On the corresponding CT, there is a subtle lesion with cortical thinning. (**c**) Fused PET/CT image clearly demonstrates abnormal uptake in the marrow with likely extension to the cortex. (**d**) Subsequently performed plain film of the right humerus more obviously shows the lytic osseous metastasis

Liver Metastasis

The liver is the third most common site of metastasis for RCC after lung and bone, and accounts for 15–20% of metastasis in RCC [31, 32]. Liver metastasis is associated with poor prognosis [33]. CT is the mainstay of imaging in the detection of intra-abdominal metastases. On CT, liver metastases can appear as ill-defined low-attenuation lesions that may show peripheral enhancement or appear as hypervascular masses with or without central necrosis [34]. On a noncontrast FDG PET/CT scan, lesions on the CT component are most often subtle. In general, there is a high target-to-background ratio of uptake seen on FDG PET, which makes metastatic lesions easier to detect (Fig. 6.13). Kang et al. [9] showed FDG PET has a sensitivity of 61.5% and a specificity of 100% for liver metastases. In contrast, CT has a sensitivity of 76.9% and a specificity of 94.1%. FDG PET detected 2/13 metastases that were negative on CT. In a study conducted by Park et al. [20], FDG PET/CT was shown to have a sensitivity of 100% for liver metastasis.

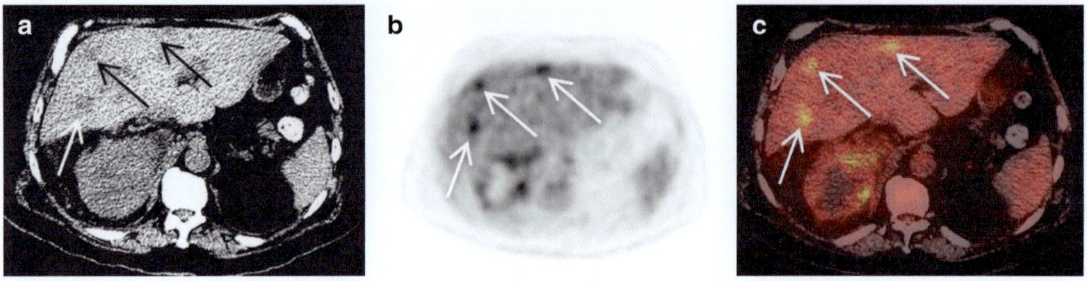

Fig. 6.13 Clear cell renal cancer with liver metastases. (**a**) Noncontrast axial CT shows a large right renal mass and subtle hypoattenuating liver lesions (arrows). (**b**) Axial FDG PET and (**c**) fused axial FDG PET/CT images show intense heterogeneous uptake in the right renal mass with central photopenia suggestive of necrosis and multiple foci of uptake within the liver corresponding to the hypoattenuating lesions seen on CT, compatible with hepatic metastases (arrows)

Surveillance

The mean time of tumor recurrence post resection of RCC is 17 months, with 83% of recurrence occurring within 2 years of surgery [32]. Most guidelines currently recommend anatomical and conventional imaging to monitor relapse and recurrence of RCC. FDG PET has been shown to identify relapse and/or recurrence more readily than conventional imaging with higher sensitivity and specificity [20]. One advantage of FDG PET/CT imaging is that IV contrast is not essential to perform the study, thus avoiding potential renal injury, which is of particular importance in RCC patients who may have impaired renal function at baseline. Nakatani et al. [43] reviewed 28 scans in 23 patients who had undergone FDG PET scans after surgery. They correlated the FDG PET findings with other imaging and histology or by clinical follow-up for at least 6 months and reported overall sensitivity, specificity, and diagnostic accuracy of 81%, 71%, and 79%, respectively. FDG PET correctly detected local recurrence and metastases in all cases in the peritoneum, bone, muscle, and adrenal glands. Their experience suggested FDG PET would be useful for postoperative surveillance in patients with RCC.

Prognostic Values of FDG PET for RCC

A prognostic model has been developed by Motzer et al. [44]. Patients were categorized into favorable, intermediate, or poor prognostic groups based on five risk factors: Karnofsky performance status, elevated lactate dehydrogenase (>1.5 times the upper limit of normal), low hemoglobin (less than normal), high corrected calcium, and absence of prior nephrectomy. Patients with no risk factors (favorable risk) had a median survival of 20 months; with one to two risk factors (intermediate risk), 10 months; and with three or more risk factors (poor risk), 4 months. Furthermore, Motzer et al. [45] performed a retrospective study to identify prognostic factors for survival in previously treated patients with advanced RCC. They found risk factors for shorter survival were low Karnofsky performance status, low hemoglobin level, and high-corrected serum calcium. The median time to death in patients with zero risk factors was 22 months. The median survival in patients with one of these prognostic factors was 11.9 months. Patients with two or three risk factors had a median survival of 5.4 months.

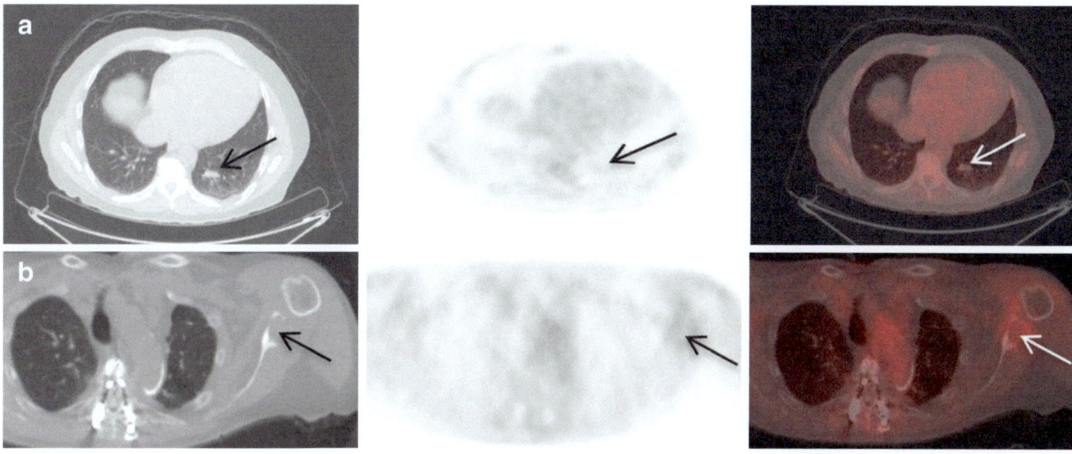

Fig. 6.14 Low FDG uptake in metastatic mRCC lesions demonstrates long-term survival. This 75-year-old male was diagnosed with clear cell renal carcinoma in 2001 and developed a left lower lobe pulmonary nodule (**a**). FDG PET/CT showed minimal uptake. He underwent wedge resection of this nodule which was later confirmed as metastatic renal cell carcinoma. Subsequently, the patient developed multiple new mildly FDG avid metastases. He survived more than 10 years after the initial diagnosis of mRCC. The most recent FDG PET/CT showed a new mildly FDG avid lytic bone lesion in the left scapula (**b**), compatible with a new osseous metastasis

Studies have shown the metabolic tumor burden (MTB) and/or metabolic tumor volume (MTV) on FDG PET/CT is an independent prognostic factor in lung, head, and neck, and esophageal cancers [46–48]. Other studies showed that FDG SUVmax predicts prognosis in various cancers [49–51]. The role of FDG uptake such as SUVmax or MTB as a prognostic factor has not been fully established in RCC, but it is generally accepted that a more aggressive tumor has a higher SUV since it will be more metabolically active and take up more FDG. One study showed that RCC patients with SUVmax equal to or above 8.8 demonstrated poor prognosis [52]. Kayani et al. [11] showed a SUVmax of 7.1 was the most significant level to predict overall survival. In another study, Revheim et al. [53] found that patients with relatively low FDG uptake before treatment (defined as an SUVmax <5) had significantly longer progression-free survival than those with relatively high initial 18F-FDG uptake (SUVmax >5). Patients with low FDG uptake in their metastatic lesions are favorable for longer survival (Fig. 6.14). These findings suggest that SUVmax should be considered as a criterion to incorporate in future prognostic models.

Monitoring Therapeutic Response

Immunotherapy has become a cornerstone treatment for mRCC. Based on the CheckMate-214 trial [54], the European Association of Urology has recommended the combination of two immune checkpoint inhibitors, ipilimumab and nivolumab, as the first-line therapy for mRCC [55]. The NCCN recommends multiple possible therapeutic regimens for relapsed or stage IV disease, many of which are combined therapies including tyrosine kinase inhibitors such as axitinib and PD-1/PDL-1 inhibitors, such as pembrolizumab. Conventional standard criteria for response assessment are not suitable to immunotherapy based on the fact that early pseudoprogression of existing lesions and small new lesions

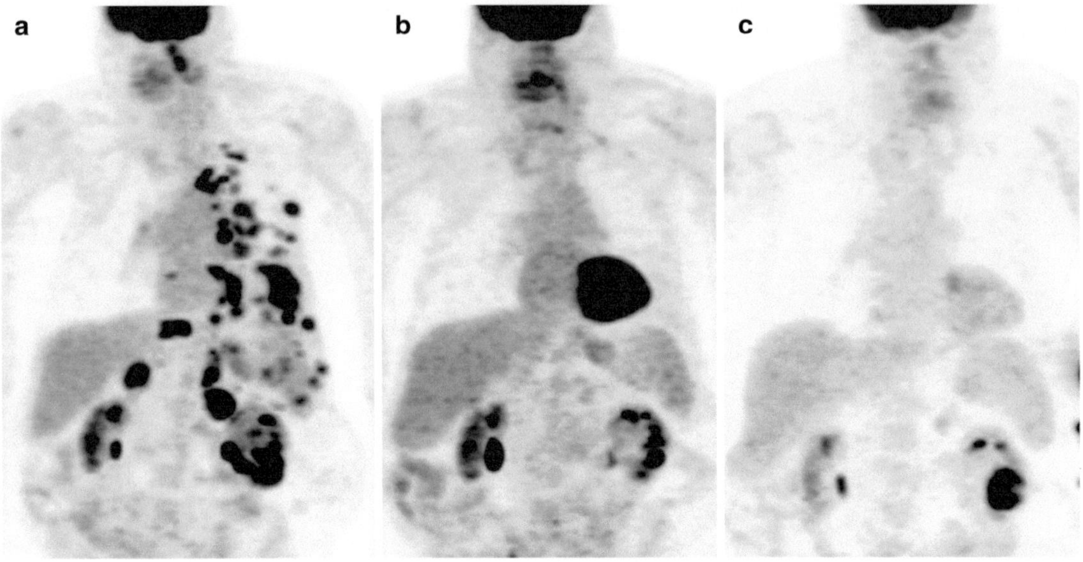

Fig. 6.15 Monitoring of immunotherapy response by FDG PET/CT. A 75-year-old male presented with a large left renal clear cell carcinoma with extensive metastasis to bilateral adrenals, right lung, right pleura, and bone with negative PD-1 expression (**a**). He was treated with combined checkpoint inhibitors (Nivo + Ipi). After four cycles of therapy, restaging FDG PET/CT showed dramatic response to therapy (**b**). Follow-up scan demonstrated continued treatment response of metastatic disease. Worsening of uptake in the primary left renal lesion may represent pseudoprogression (**c**)

can occur in these late responders [56]. Therefore, immune-related response criteria were proposed by Wolchok et al. [56]. It is hypothesized that the initial pseudoprogression in some patients treated with immunotherapy is due to inflammatory cell infiltrates. Given that both cancer and immune infiltrates can be FDG avid, it is a challenge for FDG PET/CT to differentiate cancer progression with pseudoprogression. Several studies have been conducted to explore the role of non-FDG radiotracers, the "immuno-PET" for the evaluation of immunotherapy [57, 58]. Nevertheless, a negative FDG PET/CT after immunotherapy indicates good response to therapy (Fig. 6.15).

Alternative therapies are also used for the treatment of mRCC. These include TKIs such as sorafenib and sunitinib, inhibitors of mammalian target of rapamycin (mTOR) such as temsirolimus and everolimus, and other biologic agents, such as bevacizumab. Currently, TKIs are still agents of choice for favorable-risk patients with mRCC [55]. These agents block cell signaling through various mechanisms and demonstrate better outcomes in patients with advanced clear cell RCC compared with standard therapies [22, 59].

Most and nearly all of these new agents can induce stabilization of RCC. A decrease in primary tumor diameter >30% while on targeted therapy is rare [60]. Since these therapies induce tumor necrosis with little tumor shrinkage, an unchanged residual mass does not necessarily imply poor therapeutic responses. This makes anatomic imaging less suitable for monitoring treatment response for mRCC. In addition, differentiation between vital tumors and fibrosis or necrosis is difficult using anatomic imaging. Thus, molecular imaging such as FDG PET can

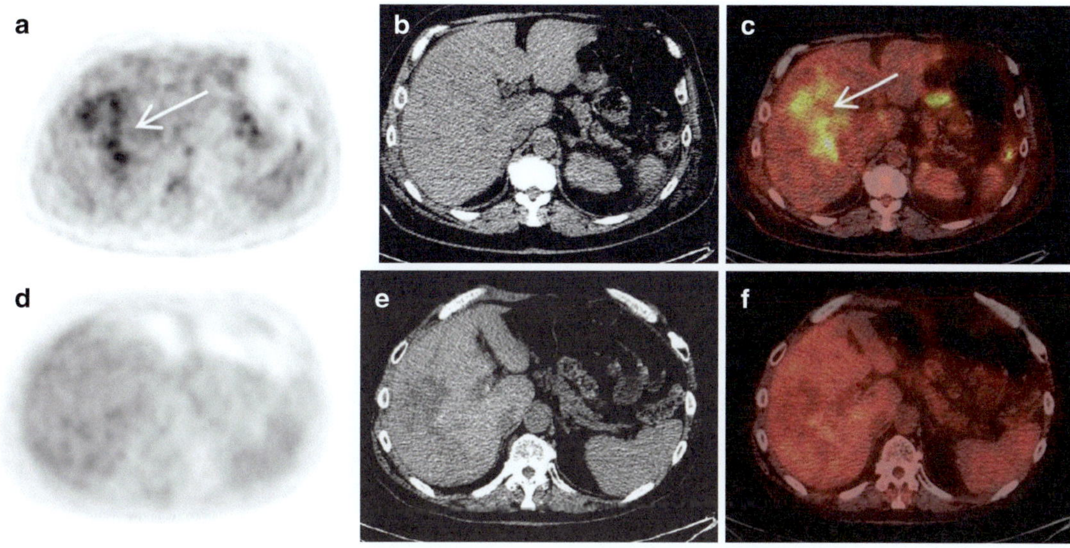

Fig. 6.16 Good response to therapy. FDG PET/CT in a 61-year-old male with bilateral renal cell cancer and liver metastasis. Top row: (**a**) pre-therapy staging scan shows large heterogeneous conglomerate of abnormal uptake in the right hepatic lobe (arrow), SUVmax 6.5, which corresponds to a subtle hypodense lesion on noncontrast CT (**b**). (**c**) Fused PET/CT image. Bottom row: (**d**) 6 months after sorafenib treatment, there is marked improvement of uptake in liver metastasis. (**e**) Large lesions in the liver are now easily seen on CT without contrast. (**f**) Fused PET/CT image. Patient's disease has been stable with sorafenib treatment 4 years after initial diagnosis

be an attractive alternative to morphological imaging for this purpose. RECIST 1.1 allows for the use of functional imaging in the response assessment [61, 62]. Data is now available on the monitoring of the therapeutic response of mRCC using FDG PET and FDG PET/CT [63–65]. A recent study [53] demonstrated that in patients with metastatic RCC, a high baseline FDG uptake indicates aggressive disease, and patients with a partial metabolic response or stable metabolic disease after two courses of sunitinib had improved prognosis as compared with those with progressive metabolic disease. They concluded that the inclusion of the PET results seems to improve the clinical counseling of patients with advanced disease.

Early metabolic response monitoring is possible with molecular imaging since the signal change at the cellular level takes quite some time to translate into size change (Fig. 6.16). Interestingly, in a multicenter phase II study, Kayani et al. [11] found that after 4 weeks of sunitinib, metabolic response occurred in 24/42 (57%) patients, but this did not correlate with progression-free survival (PFS) or overall survival (OS). After 16 weeks of treatment, disease progression on FDG PET/CT occurred in 28% of patients which correlated with a decreased OS and PFS.

FDG PET might be useful to identify nonresponding patients early in the treatment phase of TKIs (Fig. 6.17). This can guide a personalized treatment plan and avoid unnecessary therapy; the potential benefits to patients, the medical community, and the economy could be enormous.

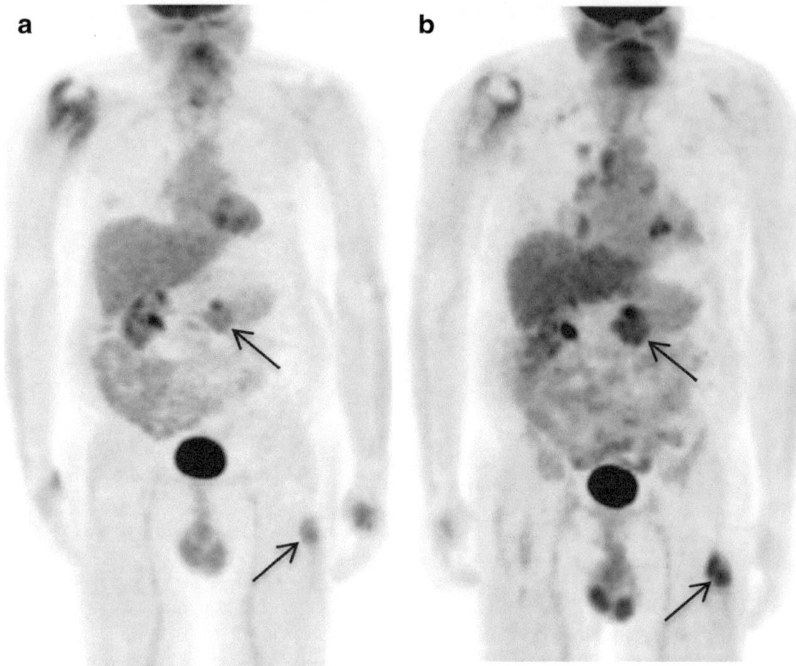

Fig. 6.17 Progression of metastatic disease. FDG PET/CT scans in a 70-year-old male with metastatic clear cell renal cancer. (**a**) Pre-therapy FDG PET/CT scan shows disease in left paraspinal soft tissue and left thigh (arrows). There is postsurgical/radiation uptake in right humeral metastasis. (**b**) Post-therapy with sunitinib, FDG PET/CT scan shows interval increased in size and intensity of FDG uptake in left paraspinal mass and left thigh soft-tissue mass (arrows). There are multiple new pulmonary and mediastinal metastases, compatible with progression of disease

Influence on Management

Studies demonstrate that FDG PET commonly alters the management of patients with mRCC. In one study [6], FDG PET was completed in 25 patients with known or suspected primary RCC and/or metastasis, and the results were compared to those that received conventional imaging techniques. Normally all patients would go to surgery post-conventional imaging, but PET scan altered the treatment plan for 6 (35%); 3 could be treated with partial nephrectomy rather than radical surgery, and 3 avoided surgery owing to confirmation of benign pathology or detection of unsuspected metastasis leading to systemic therapy. Similar results were reported by others as well [8, 9, 30, 38].

The National Oncologic PET Registry (NOPR) conducted a large study to evaluate the impact of FDG PET on Medicare cancer patients. The results of the NOPR were published in several high impact journals through a peer review process [66–68]. The first paper was published in the *Journal of Clinical Oncology* in May 2008 with over 22,000 studies analyzed [66]. This large, prospective, nationally representative registry of elderly cancer patients found that physicians often change their intended management on the basis of PET scan results across the full spectrum of its potential uses. In this article, there were 1600 cases of kidney and other urinary tract cancer patients, which account for 7% of total cases. Overall, physicians changed their intended management in 36.5% (95% CI, 35.9–37.2) of cases after FDG PET scan.

Another article was published in the *Journal of Nuclear Medicine* by the same group at the end of 2008 with similar findings and more details [68]:

including 895 cases for initial staging of RCC, with a 41.1% change in management; 979 cases for RCC restaging, with a 34.4% change in management; and 1003 cases for monitoring response, with a 32.4% change in management. Given the evidence-based large population study results, FDG PET was approved by CMS for virtually all cancer types as the initial treatment strategy in mid-2009.

Novel Tracers and Future

18F-DCFPyl

18F-DCFPyl is a tracer that has been recently FDA approved in the initial staging and evaluation of biochemical recurrence of prostate cancer. This tracer binds to prostate specific membrane antigen, or PSMA, which is a type II transmembrane glycoprotein that is typically highly expressed in prostate cancer cells; however, despite its name, it has also been demonstrated to be overexpressed within endothelial cells constituting solid tumor neovasculature, including RCC [69]. PSMA expression varies among RCC histologic subtypes; however, it has been shown to be most strongly expressed in ccRCC. In a small series of 5 patients with known metastatic RCC, there was a higher sensitivity for 18F-DCFPyl compared to conventional imaging in the detection of metastatic RCC (94.7% vs. 78.9%) [70]. In a meta-analysis of 9 studies with a pool of 152 patients with RCC (133 of which were ccRCC), Sadaghiani et al. reported a 0.74 and 0.87 detection rate of primary and metastatic RCC respectively using PSMA PET/CT, highlighting its potential as a promising alternative modality in the assessment of metastatic/recurrent ccRCC [71].

Carbonic Anhydrase IX

Carbonic anhydrase IX (CA IX) is a membrane protein that is overexpressed in ccRCC and is found in 94% of ccRCCs. Decreased CA IX levels are independently associated with poor survival in advanced RCC [72]. G250 is a monoclonal antibody to CA IX that has high affinity binding to ccRCC with tumor uptake approaching 0.5% of the injected dose per gram of tumor tissue [73]. This antibody was initially tagged to 131I, then to 124I and 89Zr [74–77]. Multiple studies had previously been performed with 124I-cG250 with the goal of determining the subtype of RCC prior to the initiation of therapy in a non-invasive manner, as a renal tumor with a positive scan had a likelihood of being a ccRCC approaching 100%, while a negative scan was suggestive of a non-clear cell subtype of RCC (90% accuracy) [76] (Figs. 6.18 and 6.19). Metastatic lesions could also be diagnosed on this type of scan with a high level of confidence. However, research into this tracer has since moved away from 124I and more toward other tracers using 68Ga and 89Zr, as discussed below.

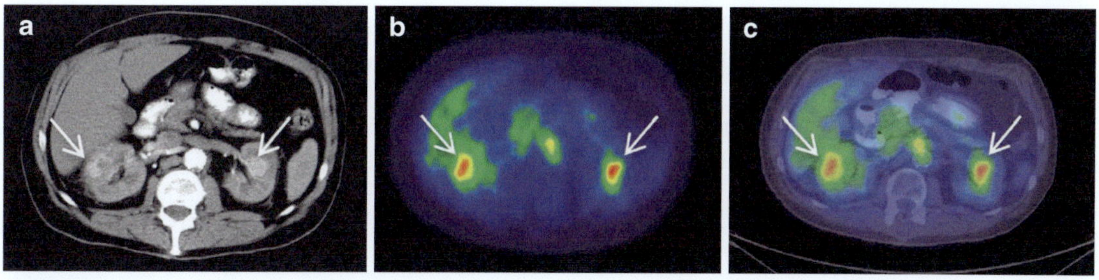

Fig. 6.18 Bilateral clear cell renal carcinoma. 124I-cG250 PET/CT in a 65-year-old male with bilateral renal masses. (**a**) Triphasic CT shows a 5-cm enhancing lesion in the right kidney and a 2-cm enhancing lesion in the left kidney (arrows). (**b**) 124I-cG250 PET and (**c**) fused PET/CT image shows intense uptake in both renal lesions, compatible with clear cell renal carcinoma

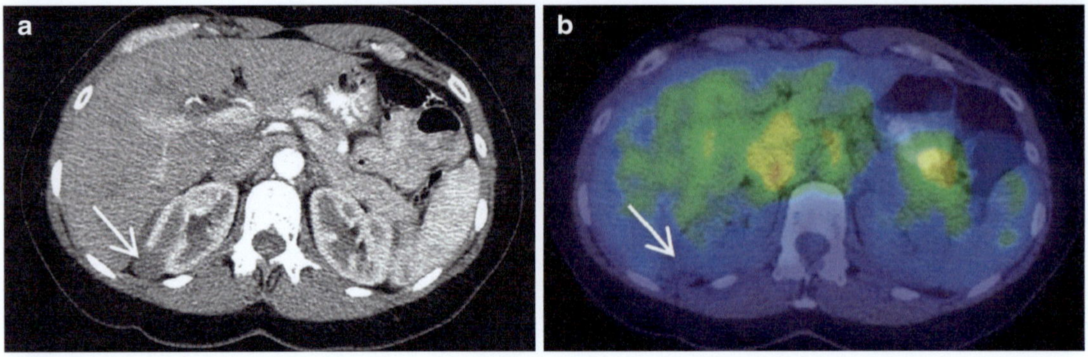

Fig. 6.19 Papillary renal cell carcinoma. 124I-cG250 PET/CT scan in a 49-year-old female with a right kidney mass. (**a**) A triphasic CT scan demonstrates a non-enhancing indeterminate lesion in the right kidney (arrow), HU 41. (**b**) On fused PET/CT images, there is no significant 124I-cG250 uptake corresponding to this renal mass, suggesting non-clear cell renal tumor

68Ga-DPI-4452 is a radiolabeled peptide which also binds to CA IX. In an open-label, nonrandomized, multicenter phase ½ study (NCT05706129) aiming to assess the safety, tolerability, and imaging characteristics of the tracer (part A) and the safety, efficacy, and therapeutic potential of 177Lu-DPI-4452 (parts B and C) in patients with unresectable locally advanced or metastatic solid tumors, 68Ga-DPI-4452 showed exceptional tumor uptake in patients with ccRCC, with very high tumor-to-background ratios and no significant adverse events [78]. This tracer shows early promise in diagnostic and therapeutic applications.

89Zr-DFO-girentuximab is a monoclonal antibody that also targets CA IX. Results from the ZIRCON phase 3 study demonstrated sensitivity and specificity at 86% and 87%, respectively, for coprimary endpoints and 85% and 90% for key secondary endpoints. Positive and negative predictive values were ≥91.7% and ≥73.7%, respectively [79, 80]. This compound has also been bound to I-124 for the detection of ccRCC by Divgi et al in the form of 124I-girentuximab, with imaging taking place 2 to 6 days after administration of the radiotracer. Sensitivity and specificity were 86.2% and 85.9%, respectively [90].

Other Novel Tracers

The previously discussed novel tracers are meant to target processes that are unique to RCC or some of its subtypes. Other tracers are less specific for RCC but target common disease pathways/control points, such as metabolism, proliferation, hypoxia, angiogenesis, and apoptosis. FDG has been extensively discussed as it relates to metabolism. The below discussed tracers evaluate some of these other key points in disease pathways.

18F-labeled thymidine (FLT), an analog of the nucleic acid thymidine, is a tracer that evaluates cellular proliferation. In one study, 18F-FLT was used to characterize and quantify changes in RCC tumor proliferation during sunitinib exposure and temporary withdrawal [77]. Data regarding the clinical use of 18F-FLT in RCC is still limited and has not progressed since the last edition of this book.

Hypoxia is another phenomenon commonly studied with novel PET tracers and PET imaging. 18F-FMISO appears to be the most commonly used tracer for imaging hypoxia. In a study, 18F-FMISO was performed in 17 patients with presumed RCC and showed only minimal increased uptake in RCC compared to normal renal tissue [81]. The mean SUV for RCC was 1.3, while that in the normal contralateral kidney was 1.1. A more recent study [82] with 53 patients evaluated the relationship between initial hypoxia-induced metastasis and after 1 month of sunitinib treatment using FMISO-PET scans. They concluded that sunitinib reduced hypoxia in hypoxic metastases but did not induce significant hypoxia in non-hypoxic lesions. This research has also not progressed since the last edition of this book.

18F-labeled choline has been used for PET imaging of other tumors [83–86] such as lung and prostate. Middendorp and colleagues [87] published their initial experience with 18F-fluoroethylcholine PET/CT in staging and monitoring therapy response of advanced renal cell carcinoma. 18F-fluoroethylcholine PET/CT detected 56% of mRCC lesions on the baseline scan. Further study, ideally in comparison with FDG PET, should be investigated, but has not been published in the last several years.

Acetate is another compound of interest. 11C-acetate has shown increased uptake in primary RCC and metastasis [88] as well, though this was not verified in other settings, as an additional study showed decreased uptake [89]. 11C-acetate has been used for early prediction of sunitinib response in metastatic RCC with some success [88]. The use of this agent is limited due to the short half-life of 11C (20 min) requiring the need for an on-site cyclotron or one very near to the imaging facility to produce. Recently available 18F-labeled acetate makes the delivery and commercialization of this tracer possible. Research into this tracer as it pertains to RCC also appears stalled, however.

Conclusion

Although PET/CT is widely used in oncologic imaging, its current role in the detection of RCC is limited. FDG PET/CT is currently not a first-line modality in the initial diagnosis of primary RCC; however, it plays a complementary role to anatomic imaging in the detection of locoregional and metastatic disease, with a higher sensitivity in detecting small nodal metastases, locoregional recurrence post-nephrectomy, as well as osseous metastases. In addition, PSMA PET/CT has shown promise in limited studies in the detection of metastatic clear cell RCC. Overall, despite these possible new radiotracers and therapies, 18F FDG remains the radiotracer of choice in the molecular imaging evaluation of RCC.

Monitoring immunotherapy response of metastatic RCC by FDG PET/CT requires further validation; however, it has shown promise in the evaluation of response to targeted cytostatic therapies. The information provided by molecular imaging, such as maximum standardized uptake value (SUVmax) has been shown to be an independent prognostic factor for RCC, and its role in future prognostic models warrants further investigation.

Finally, some new theranostic agents, such as 177Lu-DPI-4452, are in later clinical trials and may soon be available for the treatment of patients with RCC that are not surgical candidates.

References

1. Choudhary S, Sudarshan S, Choyke PL, Prasad SR. Renal cell carcinoma: recent advances in genetics and imaging. Semin Ultrasound CT MR. 2009;30(4):315–25.
2. Motzer RJ, et al. NCCN guidelines® insights: kidney cancer, version 2.2024. J Natl Compr Cancer Netw. 2024;22(1):4–16. https://doi.org/10.6004/jnccn.2024.0008.
3. Linehan WM, Walther MM, Zbar B. The genetic basis of cancer of the kidney. J Urol. 2003;170(6 Pt 1):2163–72.
4. Kovacs G, Akhtar M, Beckwith BJ, Burgert P, Cooper CS, Delahunt B, Eble JN, Fleming S, Ljungberg B, Medeiros J, et al. The Heidelberg classification of renal cell tumours. J Pathol. 1997;183:131–3.
5. Vasudevan A, Davies RJ, Shannon BA, Cohen RJ. Incidental renal tumours: the frequency of benign lesions and the role of preoperative core biopsy. BJU Int. 2006;97(5):946–9.
6. Ramdave S, Thomas GW, Berlangieri SU, Bolton DM, Davis I, Danguy HT, et al. Clinical role of F-18 fluorodeoxyglucose positron emission tomography for detection and management of renal cell carcinoma. J Urol. 2001;166(3):825–30.
7. Goldberg MA, Mayo-Smith WW, Papanicolaou N, Fischman AJ, Lee MJ. FDG PET characterization of renal masses: preliminary experience. Clin Radiol. 1997;52(7):510–5.
8. Aide N, Cappele O, Bottet P, Bensadoun H, Regeasse A, Comoz F, et al. Efficiency of [(18)F]FDG PET in characterising renal cancer and detecting distant metastases: a comparison with CT. Eur J Nucl Med Mol Imaging. 2003;30(9):1236–45.
9. Kang DE, White RL Jr, Zuger JH, Sasser HC, Teigland CM. Clinical use of fluorodeoxyglucose F 18 positron emission tomography for detection of renal cell carcinoma. J Urol. 2004;171(5):1806–9.

10. Lidgren A, Bergh A, Grankvist K, Rasmuson T, Ljungberg B. Glucose transporter-1 expression in renal cell carcinoma and its correlation with hypoxia inducible factor-1 alpha. BJU Int. 2008;101(4):480–4.
11. Kayani I, Avril N, Bomanji J, Chowdhury S, Rockall A, Sahdev A, Nathan P, Wilson P, Shamash J, Sharpe K, Lim L, Dickson J, Ell P, Reynolds A, Powles T. Sequential FDG-PET/CT as a biomarker of response to Sunitinib in metastatic clear cell renal cancer. Clin Cancer Res. 2011;17(18):6021–8. Epub 2011 Jul 8.
12. Bouchelouche K, Oehr P. Recent developments in urologic oncology: positron emission tomography molecular imaging. Curr Opin Oncol. 2008;20(3):321–6.
13. Krajewski KM, Giardino AA, Zukotynski K, Van den Abbeele AD, Pedrosa I. Imaging in renal cell carcinoma. Hematol Oncol Clin North Am. 2011;25(4):687–715.
14. Zhang J, Lefkowitz RA, Ishill NM, Wang L, Moskowitz CS, Russo P, Eisenberg H, Hricak H. Solid renal cortical tumors: differentiation with CT. Radiology. 2007;244(2):494–504.
15. Kochhar R, Brown RK, Wong CO, Dunnick NR, Frey KA, Manoharan P. Role of FDG PET/CT in imaging of renal lesions. J Med Imaging Radiat Oncol. 2010;54(4):347–57.
16. Blake MA, McKernan M, Setty B, Fischman AJ, Mueller PR. Renal oncocytoma displaying intense activity on 18F-FDG PET. Am J Roentgenol. 2006;186(1):269–70.
17. Parihar AS, et al. Diagnostic accuracy of ^{99m}Tc-sestamibi SPECT/CT for characterization of solid renal masses. J Nucl Med. 2023;64(1):90–5. https://doi.org/10.2967/jnumed.122.264329.
18. Gorin MA, et al. Prospective evaluation of (99m) Tc-sestamibi SPECT/CT for the diagnosis of renal oncocytomas and hybrid oncocytic/chromophobe tumors. Eur Urol. 2016;69(3):413–6. https://doi.org/10.1016/j.eururo.2015.08.056.
19. Siegel R, Naishadham D, Jemal A. Cancer statistics, 2012. CA Cancer J Clin. 2012;62(1):10–29.
20. Park JW, Jo MK, Lee HM. Significance of 18F-fluorodeoxyglucose positron-emission tomography/computed tomography for the postoperative surveillance of advanced renal cell carcinoma. BJU Int. 2009;103(5):615–9.
21. Kocher F, Grimmel S, Hautmann R, et al. Preoperative lymph node staging in patients with kidney and urinary bladder neoplasm. J Nucl Med Suppl. 1994;35:223.
22. Khosa F, Otero HJ, Prevedello LM, Rybicki FJ, Di Salvo DN. Imaging presentation of venous thrombosis in patients with cancer. Am J Roentgenol. 2010;194(4):1099–108. Review.
23. Itano NB, Blute ML, Spotts B, Zincke H. Outcome of isolated renal cell carcinoma fossa recurrence after nephrectomy. J Urol. 2000;164:322–5.
24. Majhail NS, Urbain JL, Albani JM, Kanvinde MH, Rice TW, Novick AC, et al. F-18 fluorodeoxyglucose positron emission tomography in the evaluation of distant metastases from renal cell carcinoma. J Clin Oncol. 2003;21(21):3995–4000.
25. Schroder H, Larson SM. Positron emission tomography for prostate, bladder, and renal cancer. Semin Nucl Med. 2004;34(4):274–92.
26. Mueller-Lisse UG, Mueller-Lisse UL, Meindl T, Coppenrath E, Degenhart C, Graser A, et al. Staging of renal cell carcinoma. Eur Radiol. 2007;17(9):2268–77.
27. Hyodo T, Sugawara Y, Tsuda T, Yanagihara Y, Aoki K, Tanji N, et al. Widespread metastases from sarcomatoid renal cell carcinoma detected by (18)F-FDG positron emission tomography/computed tomography. Jpn J Radiol. 2009;27(2):111–4.
28. Kumar R, Shamim SA, Shandal V, Sharma P, Gadodia A, Malhotra A. FDG PET/CT in detection of adrenal metastasis in patients with renal cell carcinoma. Clin Nucl Med. 2011;36(7):513–7.
29. Brouwers AH, Dorr U, Lang O, et al. 131I-cG250 monoclonal antibody immunoscintigraphy versus [18F] FDG-PET imaging in patients with metastatic renal cell carcinoma: a comparative study. Nucl Med Commun. 2002;23:229–36.
30. Safaei A, Figlin R, Hoh CK, Silverman DH, Seltzer M, Phelps ME, et al. The usefulness of F-18 deoxyglucose whole-body positron emission tomography (PET) for re-staging of renal cell cancer. Clin Nephrol. 2002;57(1):56–62.
31. Eggener SE, Yossepowitch O, Pettus JA, Snyder ME, Motzer RJ, Russo P. Renal cell carcinoma recurrence after nephrectomy for localized disease: predicting survival from time of recurrence. J Clin Oncol. 2006;24:3101–6.
32. Chae EJ, Kim JK, Kim SH, Bae SJ, Cho KS. Renal cell carcinoma: analysis of postoperative recurrence patterns. Radiology. 2005;234:189–96.
33. Flanigan RC, Salmon SE, Blumenstein BA, et al. Nephrectomy followed by interferon alfa-2b compared with interferon alfa-2b alone for metastatic renal-cell cancer. N Engl J Med. 2001;345:1655–9.
34. Griffin N, Gore ME, Sohaib SA. Imaging in metastatic renal cell carcinoma. Am J Roentgenol. 2007;189(2):360–70.
35. Bryant AS, Cerfolio RJ. The maximum standardized uptake values on integrated FDG-PET/CT is useful in differentiating benign from malignant pulmonary nodules. Ann Thorac Surg. 2006;82(3):1016–20.
36. Fortes DL, Allen MS, Lowe VJ, Shen KH, Wigle DA, Cassivi SD, et al. The sensitivity of 18F-fluorodeoxyglucose positron emission tomography in the evaluation of metastatic pulmonary nodules. Eur J Cardiothorac Surg. 2008;34(6):1223–7.
37. Kollender Y, Bickels J, Price WM, et al. Metastatic renal cell carcinoma of bone: indications and technique of surgical intervention. J Urol. 2000;164:1505–8.
38. Dilhuydy MS, Durieux A, Pariente A, de Clermont H, Pasticier G, Monteil J, et al. PET scans for decision-making in metastatic renal cell carcinoma: a single-institution evaluation. Oncology. 2006;70(5):339–44.

39. Cook GJ, Houston S, Rubens R, Maisey MN, Fogelman I. Detection of bone metastases in breast cancer by 18FDG PET: differing metabolic activity in osteoblastic and osteolytic lesions. J Clin Oncol. 1998;16:3375–9.
40. Bury T, Barreto A, Daenen F, Barthelemy N, Ghaye B, Rigo P. Fluorine-18 deoxyglucose positron emission tomography for the detection of bone metastases in patients with non-small cell lung cancer. Eur J Nucl Med. 1998;25:1244–7.
41. Wu HC, Yen RF, Shen YY, Kao CH, Lin CC, Lee CC. Comparing whole-body 18F-2-deoxyglucose positron emission tomography and technetium-99m methylene diphosphate bone scan to detect bone metastases in patients with renal cell carcinomas: a preliminary report. J Cancer Res Clin Oncol. 2002;128:503–6.
42. Grant FD, Fahey FH, Packard AB, Davis RT, Alavi A, Treves ST. Skeletal PET with 18F-fluoride: applying new technology to an old tracer. J Nucl Med. 2008;49(1):68–78.
43. Nakatani K, Nakamoto Y, Saga T, Higashi T, Togashi K. The potential clinical value of FDG-PET for recurrent renal cell carcinoma. Eur J Radiol. 2011;79(1):29–35.
44. Motzer RJ, Mazumdar M, Bacik J, Berg W, Amsterdam A, Ferrara J. Survival and prognostic stratification of 670 patients with advanced renal cell carcinoma. J Clin Oncol. 1999;17:2530–40.
45. Motzer RJ, Bacik J, Schwartz LH, Reuter V, Russo P, Marion S, et al. Prognostic factors for survival in previously treated patients with metastatic renal cell carcinoma. J Clin Oncol. 2004;22(3):454–63.
46. Zhu D, Ma T, Niu Z, Zheng J, Han A, Zhao S, et al. Prognostic significance of metabolic parameters measured by (18)F-fluorodeoxyglucose positron emission tomography/computed tomography in patients with small cell lung cancer. Lung Cancer. 2011;73:332–7.
47. Seol YM, Kwon BR, Song MK, Choi YJ, Shin HJ, Chung JS, et al. Measurement of tumor volume by PET to evaluate prognosis in patients with head and neck cancer treated by chemo-radiation therapy. Acta Oncol. 2010;49:201–8.
48. Hyun SH, Choi JY, Shim YM, Kim K, Lee SJ, Cho YS, et al. Prognostic value of metabolic tumor volume measured by 18F-fluorodeoxyglucose positron emission tomography in patients with esophageal carcinoma. Ann Surg Oncol. 2010;17:115–22.
49. Allal AS, Slosman DO, Kebdani T, Allaoua M, Lehmann W, Dulguerov P. Prediction of outcome in head-and-neck cancer patients using the standardized uptake value of 2-[18F]fluoro-2-deoxy-D-glucose. Int J Radiat Oncol Biol Phys. 2004;59:1295–3000.
50. Downey RJ, Akhurst T, Gonen M, Vincent A, Bains MS, Larson S, Rusch V. Preoperative F-18 fluorodeoxyglucose-positron emission tomography maximal standardized uptake value predicts survival after lung cancer resection. J Clin Oncol. 2004;22:3255–60.
51. Lee YY, Choi CH, Kim CJ, Kang H, Kim TJ, Lee JW, Lee JH, Bae DS, Kim BG. The prognostic significance of the SUVmax (maximum standardized uptake value for F-18 fluorodeoxyglucose) of the cervical tumor in PET imaging for early cervical cancer: preliminary results. Gynecol Oncol. 2009;115:65–8.
52. Namura K, Minamimoto R, Yao M, Makiyama K, Murakami T, Sano F, Hayashi N, Tateishi U, et al. Impact of maximum standardized uptake value (SUVmax) evaluated by 18-fluoro-2-deoxy-D--glucose positron emission tomography/computed tomography (18F-FDG-PET/CT) on survival for patients with advanced renal cell carcinoma: a preliminary report. BMC Cancer. 2010;10:667.
53. Revheim ME, Winge-Main AK, Hagen G, Fjeld JG, Fossa SD, Lilleby W. Combined positron emission tomography/computed tomography in sunitinib therapy assessment of patients with metastatic renal cell carcinoma. Clin Oncol (R Coll Radiol) 2011;23(5):339–43.
54. Escudier B, Tannir NM, McDermott DF, et al. CheckMate 214: efficacy 316 and safety of nivolumab plus ipilimumab vs sunitinib for treatment-naïve 317 advanced or metastatic renal cell carcinoma, including 318 IMDC risk and PD-L1 expression subgroups. Ann Oncol. 2017;28(Suppl 5):v605–49. LBA5, ESMO 319 2017.
55. Powles T, Albiges L, Staehler M, Bensalah K, Dabestani S, Giles RH, Hofmann F, Hora M, Kuczyk MA, Lam TB, Marconi L, Merseburger AS, Fernández-Pello S, Tahbaz R, Volpe A, Ljungberg B, Bex A. Updated European Association of Urology guidelines: recommendations for the treatment of first-line metastatic clear cell renal cancer. Eur Urol. 2018;73:311–5.
56. Wolchok JD, Hoos A, O'Day S, et al. Guidelines for the evaluation of immune therapy activity in solid tumors: immune-related response criteria. Clin Cancer Res. 2009;15:7412–20.
57. Higashikawa K, Yagi K, Watanabe K, Kamino S, Ueda M, Hiromura M, Enomoto S. 64Cu-DOTA-anti-CTLA-4 mAb enabled PET visualization of CTLA-4 on the T-cell infiltrating tumor tissues. PLoS One. 2014;9:e109866.
58. Maute RL, Gordon SR, Mayer AT, McCracken MN, Natarajan A, Ring NG, Kimura R, Tsai JM, Manglik A, Kruse AC, et al. Engineering high-affinity PD-1 variants for optimized immunotherapy and immuno-PET imaging. Proc Natl Acad Sci U S A. 2015;112:E6506–14.
59. Murdoch D, Sager J. Will targeted therapy hold its promise? An evidence-based review. Curr Opin Oncol. 2008;20(1):104–11.
60. Abel EJ, Culp SH, Tannir NM, Matin SF, Tamboli P, Jonasch E, et al. Primary tumor response to targeted agents in patients with metastatic renal cell carcinoma. Eur Urol. 2011;59(1):10–5.
61. Eisenhauer EA, Therasse P, Bogaerts J, Schwartz LH, Sargent D, Ford R, et al. New response evaluation

criteria in solid tumours: revised RECIST guideline (version 1.1). Eur J Cancer. 2009;45(2):228–47.
62. Schwartz LH, Bogaerts J, Ford R, Shankar L, Therasse P, Gwyther S, et al. Evaluation of lymph nodes with RECIST 1.1. Eur J Cancer. 2009;45(2):261–7.
63. Jennens RR, Rosenthal MA, Lindeman GJ, Michael M. Complete radiological and metabolic response of metastatic renal cell carcinoma to SU5416 (semaxanib) in a patient with probable von Hippel-Lindau syndrome. Urol Oncol. 2004;22(3):193–6.
64. Lyrdal D, Boijsen M, Suurkula M, Lundstam S, Stierner U. Evaluation of sorafenib treatment in metastatic renal cell carcinoma with 2-fluoro-2-deoxyglucose positron emission tomography and computed tomography. Nucl Med Commun. 2009;30(7):519–24.
65. Vercellino L, Bousquet G, Baillet G, Barre E, Mathieu O, Just PA, et al. 18F-FDG PET/CT imaging for an early assessment of response to sunitinib in metastatic renal carcinoma: preliminary study. Cancer Biother Radiopharm. 2009;24(1):137–44.
66. Hillner BE, Siegel BA, Liu D, Shields AF, Gareen IF, Hanna L, et al. Impact of positron emission tomography/computed tomography and positron emission tomography (PET) alone on expected management of patients with cancer: initial results from the National Oncologic PET registry. J Clin Oncol. 2008;26(13):2155–61.
67. Hillner BE, Siegel BA, Shields AF, Duan F, Gareen IF, Hanna L, et al. Impact of dedicated brain PET on intended patient management in participants of the National Oncologic PET registry. Mol Imaging Biol. 2011;13(1):161–5.
68. Hillner BE, Siegel BA, Shields AF, Liu D, Gareen IF, Hunt E, et al. Relationship between cancer type and impact of PET and PET/CT on intended management: findings of the National Oncologic PET registry. J Nucl Med. 2008;49(12):1928–35.
69. Baccala A, et al. Expression of prostate-specific membrane antigen in tumor-associated neovasculature of renal neoplasms. Urology. 2007;70(2):385–90. https://doi.org/10.1016/j.urology.2007.03.025.
70. Rowe SP, et al. Imaging of metastatic clear cell renal cell carcinoma with PSMA-targeted ^{18}F-DCFPyL PET/CT. Ann Nucl Med. 2015;29(10):877–82. https://doi.org/10.1007/s12149-015-1017-z.
71. Sadaghiani MS, et al. Utility of PSMA PET/CT in staging and restaging of renal cell carcinoma: a systematic review and metaanalysis. J Nucl Med. 2024;65(7):1007–12. https://doi.org/10.2967/jnumed.124.267417.
72. Bui MH, Seligson D, Han KR, et al. Carbonic anhydrase IX is an independent predictor of survival in advanced renal clear cell carcinoma: implications for prognosis and therapy. Clin Cancer Res. 2003;9:802–11.
73. Steffens MG, Boerman OC, Oosterwijk-Wakka JC, et al. Targeting of renal cell carcinoma with iodine-131-labeled chimeric monoclonal antibody G250. J Clin Oncol. 1997;15:1529–37.
74. Brouwers AH, Dorr U, Lang O, Boerman OC, Oyen WJ, Steffens MG, et al. 131 I-cG250 monoclonal antibody immunoscintigraphy versus [18 F]FDG-PET imaging in patients with metastatic renal cell carcinoma: a comparative study. Nucl Med Commun. 2002;23(3):229–36.
75. Brouwers A, Verel I, Van Eerd J, Visser G, Steffens M, Oosterwijk E, et al. PET radioimmuno scintigraphy of renal cell cancer using 89Zr-labeled cG250 monoclonal antibody in nude rats. Cancer Biother Radiopharm. 2004;19(2):155–63.
76. Divgi CR, Pandit-Taskar N, Jungbluth AA, Reuter VE, Gonen M, Ruan S, et al. Preoperative characterisation of clear-cell renal carcinoma using iodine-124-labelled antibody chimeric G250 (124I-cG250) and PET in patients with renal masses: a phase I trial. Lancet Oncol. 2007;8(4):304–10.
77. Liu G, Jeraj R, Vanderhoek M, Perlman S, Kolesar J, Harrison M, et al. Pharmacodynamic study using FLT PET/CT in patients with renal cell cancer and other solid malignancies treated with sunitinib malate. Clin Cancer Res. 2011;17(24):7634–44.
78. Hofman MS, et al. First-in-human safety, imaging, and dosimetry of a carbonic anhydrase IX-targeting peptide, [^{68}Ga]Ga-DPI-4452, in patients with clear cell renal cell carcinoma. J Nucl Med. 2024;65(5):740–3. https://doi.org/10.2967/jnumed.123.267175.
79. Shuch B, et al. [^{89}Zr]Zr-girentuximab for PET-CT imaging of clear-cell renal cell carcinoma: a prospective, open-label, multicentre, phase 3 trial. Lancet Oncol. 2024;25(10):1277–87. https://doi.org/10.1016/S1470-2045(24)00402-9.
80. Calais J, et al. 89Zr-DFO-girentuximab PET/CT imaging can accurately detect clear cell renal cell carcinoma primary and secondary lesions in patients with renal masses at conventional imaging, results from ZIRCON phase 3 study. J Nucl Med. 2023;64:P1113.
81. Lawrentschuk N, Poon AM, Foo SS, Putra LG, Murone C, Davis ID, et al. Assessing regional hypoxia in human renal tumours using 18F-fluoromisonidazole positron emission tomography. BJU Int. 2005;96(4):540–6.
82. Hugonnet F, Fournier L, Medioni J, Smadja C, Hindie E, Huchet V, et al. Metastatic renal cell carcinoma: relationship between initial metastasis hypoxia, change after 1 month's sunitinib, and therapeutic response: an 18F-fluoromisonidazole PET/CT study. J Nucl Med. 2011;52(7):1048–55.
83. Bansal A, Shuyan W, Hara T, Harris RA, Degrado TR. Biodisposition and metabolism of [(18)F] fluorocholine in 9L glioma cells and 9L glioma-bearing fisher rats. Eur J Nucl Med Mol Imaging. 2008;35(6):1192–203.
84. DeGrado TR, Coleman RE, Wang S, Baldwin SW, Orr MD, Robertson CN, et al. Synthesis and evaluation of 18F-labeled choline as an oncologic tracer for positron emission tomography: initial findings in prostate cancer. Cancer Res. 2001;61(1):110–7.
85. Pieterman RM, Que TH, Elsinga PH, Pruim J, van Putten JW, Willemsen AT, et al. Comparison of (11) C-choline and (18)F-FDG PET in primary diagnosis

and staging of patients with thoracic cancer. J Nucl Med. 2002;43(2):167–72.
86. Schillaci O, Calabria F, Tavolozza M, Ciccio C, Carlani M, Caracciolo CR, et al. 18F-choline PET/CT physiological distribution and pitfalls in image interpretation: experience in 80 patients with prostate cancer. Nucl Med Commun. 2010;31(1):39–45.
87. Middendorp M, Maute L, Sauter B, Vogl TJ, Grunwald F. Initial experience with 18F-fluoroethylcholine PET/CT in staging and monitoring therapy response of advanced renal cell carcinoma. Ann Nucl Med. 2010;24(6):441–6.
88. Maleddu A, Pantaleo MA, Castellucci P, Astorino M, Nanni C, Nannini M, et al. 11C-acetate PET for early prediction of sunitinib response in metastatic renal cell carcinoma. Tumori. 2009;95(3):382–4.
89. Kotzerke J, Linne C, Meinhardt M, Steinbach J, Wirth M, Baretton G, et al. [1-(11)C]acetate uptake is not increased in renal cell carcinoma. Eur J Nucl Med Mol Imaging. 2007;34(6):884–8.
90. Divgi CR, Uzzo RG, Gatsonis C, Bartz R, Treutner S, Yu JQ, Chen D, Carrasquillo JA, Larson S, Bevan P, Russo P. Positron emission tomography/computed tomography identification of clear cell renal cell carcinoma: results from the REDECT trial. J Clin Oncol. 2013;31(2):187–94.

Interventional Radiology and Angioinfarction Transcatheter Embolization of Renal Tumors

7

Sebastian Flacke

Indications for Renal Artery Embolization

The key indications for renal artery embolization include:

- Angioinfarction or tumor infarction prior to resection or ablation.
- Palliation of unresectable renal malignancies.
- Management of renal angiomyolipomas.
- Life-threatening or debilitating hematuria.
- Arteriovenous fistulas (spontaneous or iatrogenic).
- Vascular malformations.
- Renal artery aneurysm or pseudoaneurysm.
- End-stage renal disease [1, 2].
- Uncontrollable hypertension [3, 4].

Technical Details

The techniques and materials used for the embolization of the kidney vary depending on the level of occlusion within the renal vascular tree. The selection of the site and the material used to achieve vascular occlusion will determine the degree of complexity of the procedure and potential risks.

All endovascular procedures have in common the vascular access in the femoral, brachial, or radial artery with the insertion of a catheter sheath. In patients with very tortuous iliac arteries, a longer (35–45 cm) 5 or 6 French sheath can be positioned in the infrarenal aorta, facilitating access to the renal artery ostium. Embolization procedures are performed under strict aseptic conditions, and prophylactic administration of antibiotics is recommended for permanent embolization of larger areas of renal parenchyma. All endovascular procedures bear the risk associated with access to the arterial system. As imaging during the procedure relies on the injection of iodine contrast, poor renal function may further deteriorate [5]. It is, therefore, beneficial if the patient is sufficiently hydrated prior to the procedure.

In principle, four types of occlusion can be differentiated based on the level of occlusion within the arterial system.

Central Occlusion

A central occlusion is usually achieved by the deployment of larger platinum coils, a vascular occluder device, or a detachable balloon in the main renal artery through a 5 French or larger guiding catheter in hockey-stick or cobra configuration. The shape and size of the coils vary

S. Flacke (✉)
Department of Radiology at UMass Chan-Lahey, Lahey Hospital and Medical Center, Burlington, MA, USA
e-mail: Sebastian.Flacke@lahey.org

J. A. Libertino, J. R. Gee (eds.), *Renal Cancer*, https://doi.org/10.1007/978-3-031-97599-8_7

according to the size of the vessel to be occluded. Coils may contain small pieces of textile to enhance clot formation after deployment.

In the presence of a renal artery aneurysm, detachable microcoils, which can be introduced through a 3F or smaller microcatheter, are used to occlude the diseased area while preserving flow to the kidney. Coil deployment within an aneurysm may be facilitated with balloon or stent-assisted coiling (Fig. 7.1).

Multiple coils are usually needed to obtain complete stasis in the main renal artery. Complete stasis can be documented with the injection of iodine contrast through the guiding catheter. The catheter is placed sufficiently deep into the renal artery to avoid inadvertent dislodgement of a coil into the aorta. If main renal artery embolization is performed prior to surgery, the coils should be deployed at least about 2 cm distant from the branching point of the aorta to allow for surgical ligation without the risk of coil displacement into the aorta.

A vascular occluder (Amplatzer Vascular Plug AGA Medical Corporation, Plymouth, MN) consists of a nitinol cage filled with thrombogenic polyester filaments. The size of the occluder is chosen according to the size of the vessel to be occluded. A vascular occluder provides very rapid occlusion and is ideal for high-flow situations.

Detachable balloons have been largely replaced by coils and plugs despite the fact that

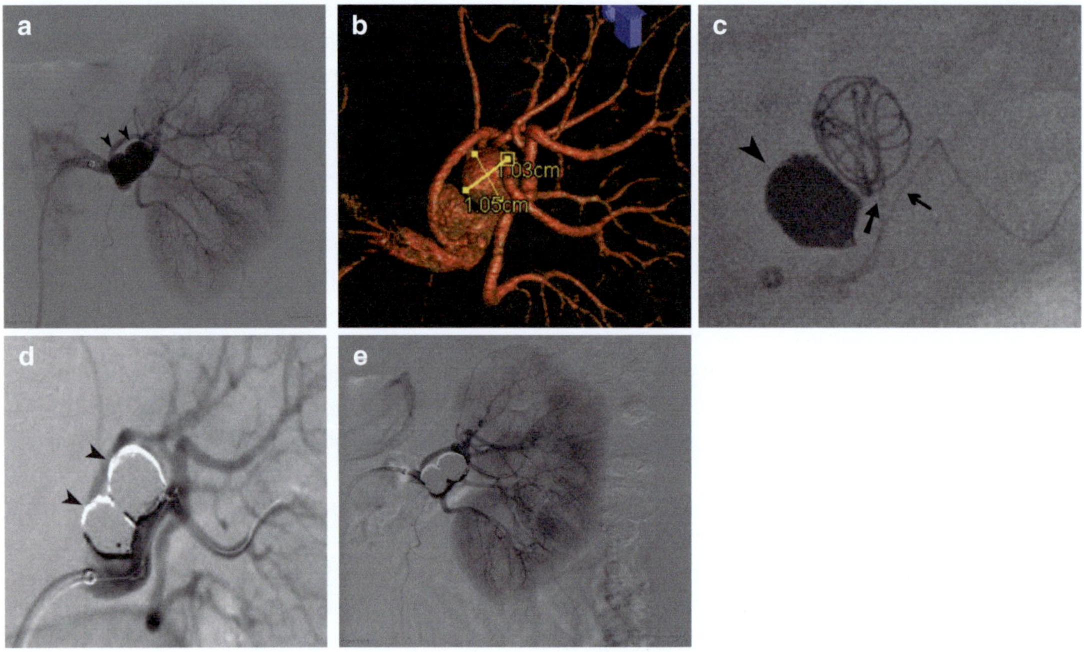

Fig. 7.1 Saccular aneurysm arising from the main renal artery in a 73-year-old patient with a planned contralateral partial nephrectomy for renal cancer. Both aneurysms were detected on cross-sectional imaging, and selective coil embolization was performed prior to surgery. Initially, a 6 French vascular sheath was positioned in the proximal portion of the main renal artery. This sheath secured safe access to the main renal artery during the entire procedure. Both aneurysms are seen as a saccular outpouching of the main renal artery (**a**, arrowheads). A rotational angiogram and three-dimensional surface-rendered reconstructions were obtained, which helped to determine the dimensions of the aneurysm and the best projection angle of the C-arm (**b**). Balloon-assisted coiling of both aneurysms was performed using detachable microcoils. After embolization of the first aneurysm (**c**, arrowhead) the microcatheter used for coil delivery is entered into the second aneurysm (**c**, arrow). A second microcatheter holding a balloon is inserted into the main renal artery (**c**, rounded arrow). The balloon is inflated if portions of the coils protrude into the main renal artery. An arteriogram of the main renal artery after dense packing of both aneurysms (**d**, arrowhead) shows patency of the main renal artery. These angiograms are obtained by injecting the guiding sheath. The parenchymal phase (**e**) shows patency of the entire vascular tree without embolic events

they provide large-volume occlusion with great precision. However, deployment is difficult, and the shape and persistence of the inflation of these balloons are variable and change over time.

Combined Central and Peripheral Occlusion

This type of embolization aims to occlude the renal artery and first- and second-order branches. A coaxial catheter system using a 3 French or smaller microcatheter and a guiding catheter positioned in the main renal artery to reach the second-order branches. The use of a coaxial catheter system provides additional safety as the inner catheter can be withdrawn at any time without losing access to the renal artery and the added option to inject iodine contrast through the guiding catheter. A variety of embolic materials can be used.

Micro- and macro coils can be deployed by either pushing the coil with a guidewire or flushing the coils into the artery with a small bolus of saline injected using a 1 mL syringe.

A multitude of prefabricated inert embolic particles are available, ranging from 40 to 1200 μm. Particles larger than 100 μm will not reach the capillary bed and may be used for this type of embolization. Different types of particles are available: polyvinyl alcohol (Ivalon, Unipoint Laboratories, High Point, NC), acrylic polymer microspheres (Embospheres Microspheres, Biosphere Medical, Rockland, MA), polymer-coated particles with a hydrogel core (Embozene Color-Advanced Microspheres, CeloNova Biosciences, Newnan, GA) and polyvinyl alcohol microspheres (Beadblock, Biocompatibles Inc., Oxford, CT). These particles can be dry or diluted in aqueous solution. They are usually mixed with iodine contrast prior to injection to facilitate visualization. Care must be taken to carefully assess for large arteriovenous shunting, which bears the danger of embolizing into the renal vein and from there into the lungs. With the reduction of forward flow during embolization, the risk of reflux increases. A control angiogram after embolization with particles should be performed with care (Fig. 7.2). A gentle injection may confirm stasis of blood flow, and a more forceful injection may wash out some of the injected particles, leading to inadvertent nontarget embolization.

Embolization with resorbable material is another inexpensive option for this type of embolization. Sterile synthetic gelatin sponge is a biodegradable material that is reabsorbed within 2 weeks to 3 months after the embolization.

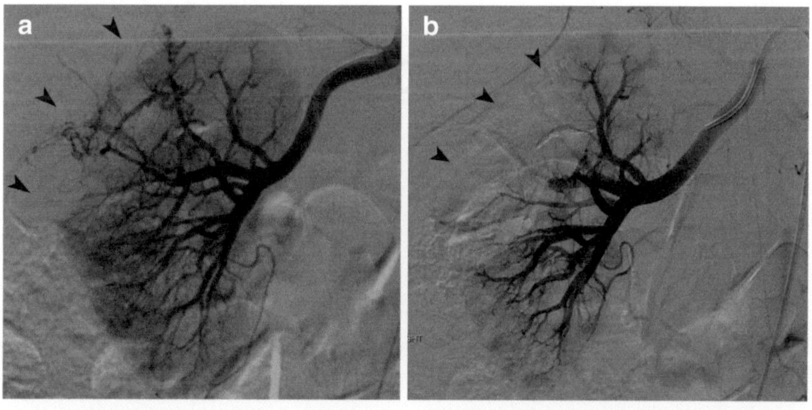

Fig. 7.2 Preventive embolization of a large angiomyolipoma in a 54-year-old female with recurrent hematuria. A selective angiogram of the left kidney shows a rounded, poorly defined mass of approximately 5 cm in diameter in the left upper pole of the kidney (**a**). Superselective embolization of three segmental branches using a 3 French microcatheter and 300–500 μm microspheres was performed to completely devascularized the mass (**b**, arrowheads). Final angiography shows the preserved portions of the kidney

Various commercial preparations are available: Gelfoam (Pharmacia & Upjohn Company, MI), Curaspon (CuraMedical BV, Amsterdam, The Netherlands), and Gelitaspon (Gelita Medical BV, Amsterdam, The Netherlands). The foam particles can be cut to the appropriate size by the operator. They are then mixed with saline and contrast and can be injected into the target area. Although immediate occlusion can be achieved relatively quickly, there is a chance of recanalization of the targeted vessel territory over time as the gelfoam particles may be reabsorbed.

Capillary Occlusion

Capillary occlusion aims to occlude the entire arterial compartment from the capillary bed to the main artery to create an infarct of a portion of the entire organ or total angioinfarction with permanent occlusion of all glomeruli.

Capillary occlusion can be achieved using small caliber inert embolic particles of about 40–100 μm. Small particles are the preferred agents for smaller parenchymal areas, such as a small tumor, due to the ease of administration.

Liquid embolic agents are an alternative and the preferred agents for the embolization of a larger vascular bed. *N*-butyl-2 cyanoacrylate biological glue (Histoacryl, B/Braun, Tutlingen Germany) can be injected through a microcatheter using a coaxial approach. Prior to the injection, cyanoacrylate is mixed with ethiodized oil (Ethiodol/Lipiodol, Guerbet, Bloomington, In), a poppy seed oil used as a radiopaque contrast agent and diluent of the tissue glue. The speed of embolization is influenced by the quantity of added Ethiodol. In a mixture containing 0.5 mL of tissue glue and 0.5 mL of Ethiodol, the polymerization of the tissue glue occurs within 0.5–1 s [6]. Mixtures of 1:1 to 1:3 ratios of biological glue and ethiodized oil are favored for capillary occlusion. The microcatheter is flushed with concentrated glucose or dextrose, which binds anions by osmosis prior to the injection of the biological glue to avoid polymerization within the microcatheter. If injected in small aliquots using a 1 mL syringe, adhesion of the microcatheter tip to the vessel wall can be avoided. However, it is recommended to withdraw the microcatheter into the guiding catheter after each injection, as a small portion of the tissue glue may stick to the tip and require an exchange of the catheter. The use of a coaxial catheter approach is warranted. The advantage of the use of tissue glue is the fact that it will create immediate vascular occlusion, even in the presence of impaired clotting. Complications related to inadvertent displacement of tissue glue are scarce and mostly related to an inappropriate technique, often due to not relying on a coaxial catheter set-up. Tissue glue can create a foreign body giant cell reaction within the first weeks of administration but does not lead to the development of secondary tumors.

Onyx (EV3 endovascular, Plymouth, MN), another liquid embolic agent, is comprised of ethylene vinyl alcohol (EVOH) copolymer dissolved in dimethyl sulfoxide (DMO) and suspended micronized tantalum powder to provide contrast for visualization under fluoroscopy. It can be injected as a liquid in a very controlled fashion and solidifies in contact with ionic solutions from the outside to the inside. It has potential application in vascular disease, but experience in the renal vasculature is still limited [7].

The most widely used liquid embolic agent to create a complete renal infarction is highly concentrated alcohol [8]. The injection of alcohol into the renal artery for complete infarction requires the use of an occlusion balloon, which is positioned in the proximal renal artery to avoid a spillover of the injected alcohol into the aorta and control the blood flow through the kidney. If a coaxial approach is chosen, a sheath can be positioned in the aorta close to the ostium of the renal artery, and the balloon catheter is inserted through the sheath. The coaxial approach has the benefit of allowing verification of the tightness of the inflated balloon with the injection of iodine contrast through the sheath (Fig. 7.3). If only a small region of the kidney is targeted, a coaxial approach using a microcatheter is sufficient. Alcohol can be injected in a single fast injection or in fractionated smaller doses. If a single fast injection is used, 10–15 mL of alcohol is injected through the tightly inflated

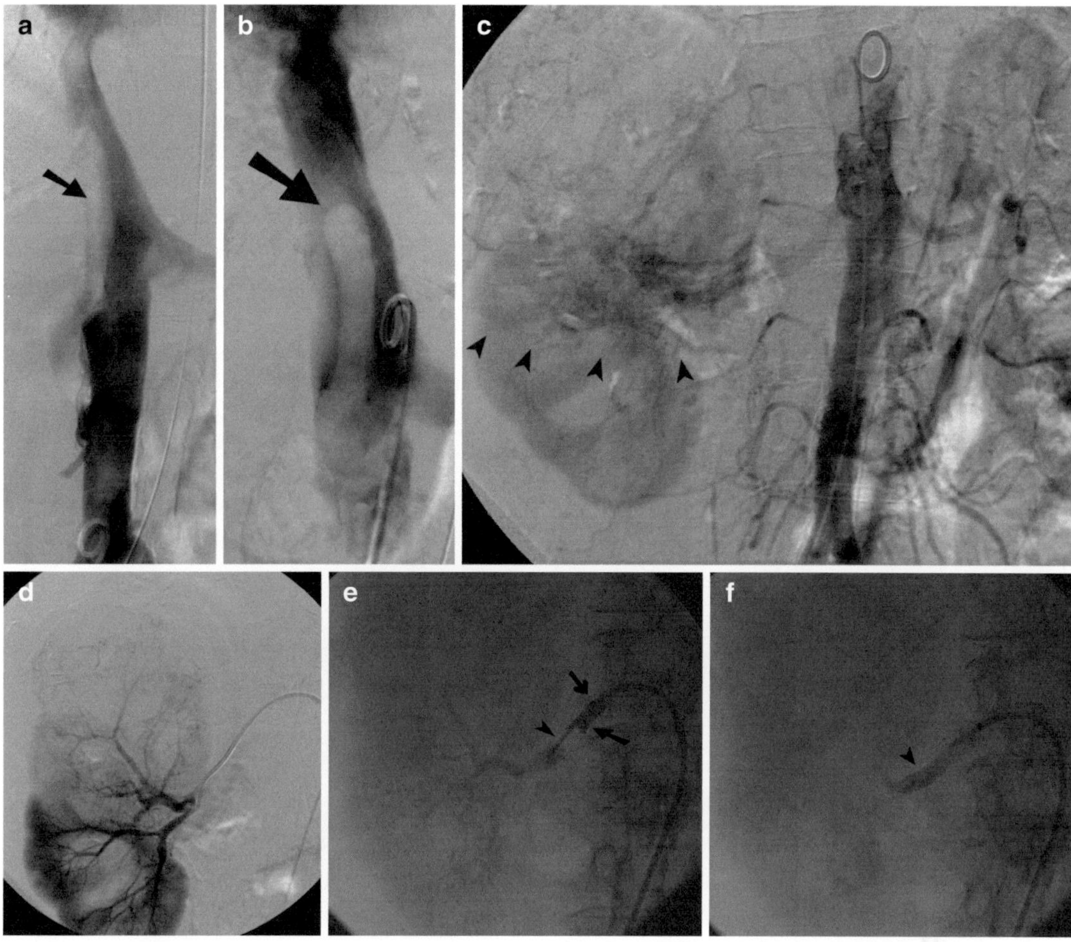

Fig. 7.3 Angioinfarction of a large left renal mass with extension into the inferior vena cava. An initial venogram of the inferior vena cava obtained after injection of a pigtail catheter placed at the level of the common iliac vein shows a filling defect in the IVC (**a**, arrow). A second injection with the pigtail catheter placed in the suprarenal IVC delineates the large tumor thrombus (**b**, arrow) extending into the intrahepatic segment of the IVC. An aortogram shows the extent of the large renal mass, which has replaced the upper 2/3 of the kidney (**c**, arrowheads). The uninvolved portion of the kidney fed by the lower pole segmental artery is better appreciated with a selective injection (**d**). Angioinfarction with high concentrated alcohol is performed through a balloon occlusion catheter (**e**, arrow head). The balloon occlusion catheter is introduced through a 6 French guiding sheath placed into the proximal main renal vein (**e**, rounded arrow). Once the balloon occlusion catheter is inflated, blood flow through the main renal artery into the kidney is completely blocked. A contrast injection into the guiding sheath allows for verifying the tightness of the occlusion. The injected contrast remains in the proximal stem of the main renal artery (**e**, arrow). After an injection of 15 mL of alcohol and an occlusion of 15 min, the balloon was deflated. The injected contrast filled the space occupied by the balloon (**f**, arrowhead), but secondary thrombosis of the renal vasculature had already occurred and prevented the contrast from flowing into the kidney

occlusion balloon. The balloon remains inflated for at least 10 min before iodine contrast is injected to document secondary thrombosis of the arterial system. If the degree of occlusion is not satisfactory, the procedure will be repeated. In the fractionated approach, 4–10 mL are injected over several minutes. The degree of thrombosis will be documented with the injection of iodine contrast after each alcohol injection until complete stasis is reached. Both techniques require the same amount of time and approximately 20 mL of alcohol; however, in a few cases, up to 50 mL can be used. A total dose of 0.5 mL/kg body weight of alcohol should not be exceeded. Many complications associated with the embolization of the kidney with alcohol have been reported in the early days of embolization. The complications were mostly related to the reflux of the embolic material into other vessel territories, resulting in necrosis of the colon, skin, and spinal cord [8–10]. The appropriate use of an occlusion balloon has drastically reduced complications.

Capillary occlusion of the kidney requires appropriate pain medication during and after the procedure. We usually use intravenous analgesics and opioids for 12 h after the embolization procedure. The anticipated degree of pain is inversely correlated to the degree of tumor infiltration of the renal capsule. Embolization of a large tumor that has replaced the kidney will be better tolerated than whole kidney embolization for small tumor burden. A more targeted approach to smaller tumors is often more appropriate (Fig. 7.4).

Moderate hematuria may be observed after embolization as a result of hemorrhagic infarction in the first days after embolization.

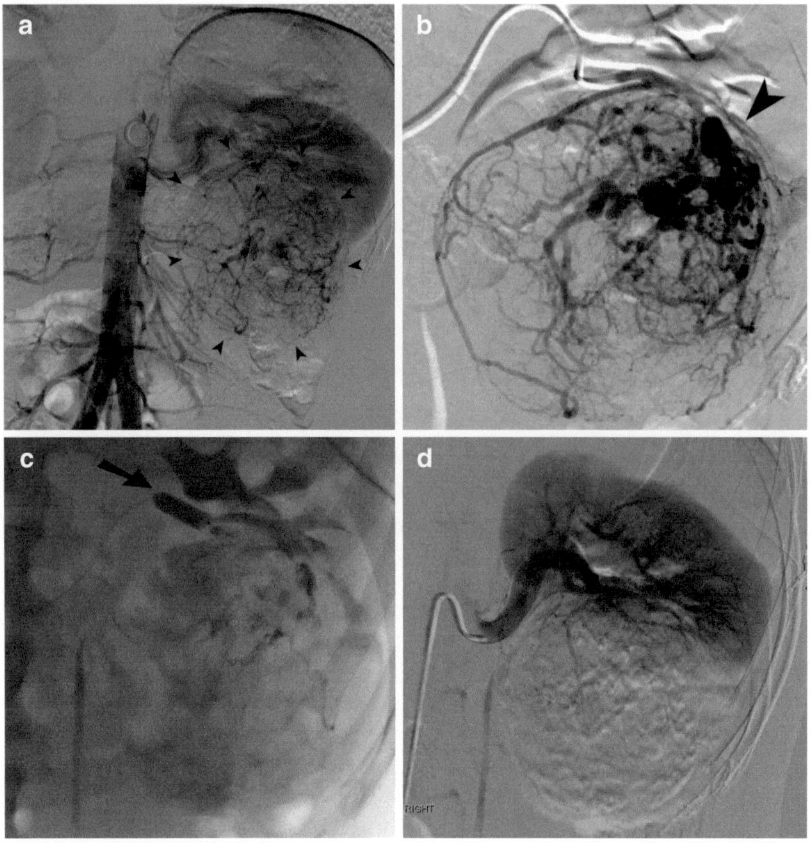

Fig. 7.4 Embolization of large angiomyolipoma in a 32-year-old female with recurrent retroperitoneal bleeding prior to intended partial nephrectomy. The initial aortogram shows a large, 7.6 cm in diameter, exophytic right lower pole renal mass (**a**, arrowheads) with pathological vessels. Aneurysmal dilatation of the intratumoral vessels (**b**, arrowhead) is better appreciated with a selective angiogram. A small percutaneous transluminal angioplasty (PTA) balloon was advanced into the tumor-feeding segmental artery. After the inflation of the balloon catheter, 12 mL of concentrated alcohol was injected (**c**). The PTA balloon remains inflated for 20 min. A final selective angiogram shows complete devascularization of the tumor with preserved perfusion of the uninvolved upper pole (**d**)

Post-embolization syndrome with flank pain, fever, paralytic ileus, nausea, vomiting, and headache can be observed in about 4% of patients after whole kidney embolization. Laboratory assessment shows an increased white blood cell count and increased level of plasmatic lactate dehydrogenase. The leading symptom is flank pain, which should be controlled with appropriate pain medication. Increased temperature may be present for hours or days but usually subsides shortly after the procedure. The syndrome generally resolves with symptomatic treatment in a few days.

Transient increases in arterial blood pressure is frequent during and immediately after the procedure, which could be associated with the increasing level of pain. Persistent arterial hypertension may indicate the presence of residual ischemic but not infarcted tissue [11].

During follow-up, small gas inclusion within the necrotic area can be found in cross-sectional imaging. These bubbles are not of a septic origin but represent normal aseptic necrosis and usually do not require treatment as an abscess [12, 13].

Superselective Embolization

Superselective embolization is performed through a microcatheter or a balloon occlusion microcatheter (Sniper, Embolx, Sunnyvale, CA), which is introduced in the coaxial technique through a 5-7F guiding catheter. The microcatheter is advanced as close to the target area as possible prior to the injection of the embolic material. Microcoils, particles, tissue glue, alcohol, or onyx may all be used in various circumstances. The choice of the embolic material is dependent on the blood flow and target. High blood flow with the chance of false embolization into the venous system usually requires the placement of microcoils, detachable balloons, or tissue glue. Microcoils are among the safest embolic materials in these situations (Fig. 7.5). The selective deployment of such coils in small branches up to the interlobular artery level allows for a very selective embolization, sparing the remaining parenchyma (Fig. 7.6). Care must be taken not to overestimate the embolic effect of a single coil, as vasospasm associated with the deployment may falsely create the impression of a complete occlusion. Superselective embolization is the method of choice for focal renal arterial bleeding associated with false aneurysm, A-V fistulas, trauma, angiodysplasia, or post-biopsy or resection (Fig. 7.7). Superselective embolization may also be considered to reduce tumor bleeding prior to or during focal resection or percutaneous ablation [14, 15] (Fig. 7.8).

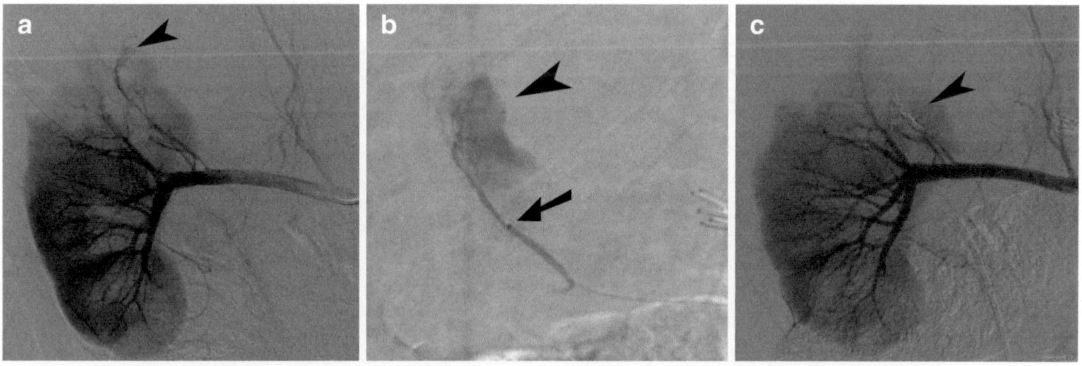

Fig. 7.5 Superselective embolization of a bleeding segmental artery after partial nephrectomy in a 67-year-old male. A selective angiogram of the left kidney shows a faint blush (**a**, arrowhead) next to an upper pole segmental artery after resection of a portion of the upper pole. A 2.3 French microcatheter (**b**, arrow) was placed close to the bleeding site. The superselective angiogram delineates the full extent of the bleeding (**b**, arrowheads). The placement of two microcoils into this artery (**c**, arrowhead) occluded the vessel and stopped the bleeding with minimal parenchymal damage

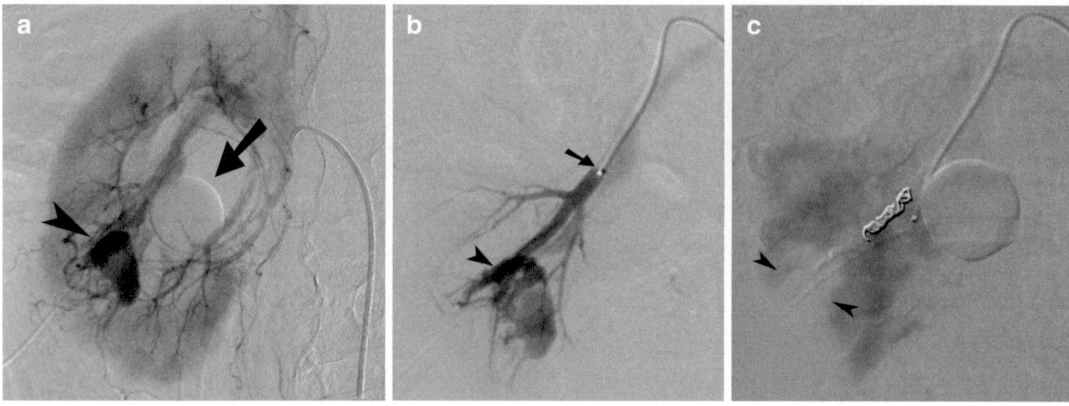

Fig. 7.6 Embolization of a false aneurysm after percutaneous nephrolithotomy. A selective angiogram of the left renal artery shows a false aneurysm (**a**, arrowhead) arising from the access site into the kidney. A Foley catheter (**a**, arrow) was placed initially to tamponade the bleeding. A 3 French microcatheter (arrow) was advanced into the bleeding segmental artery. A superselective angiogram using the microcatheter demonstrates the vascular injury to the artery (**b**, arrowhead). Coil embolization of the artery using three microcoils was performed, leading to a small cortical defect (**c**, arrowheads)

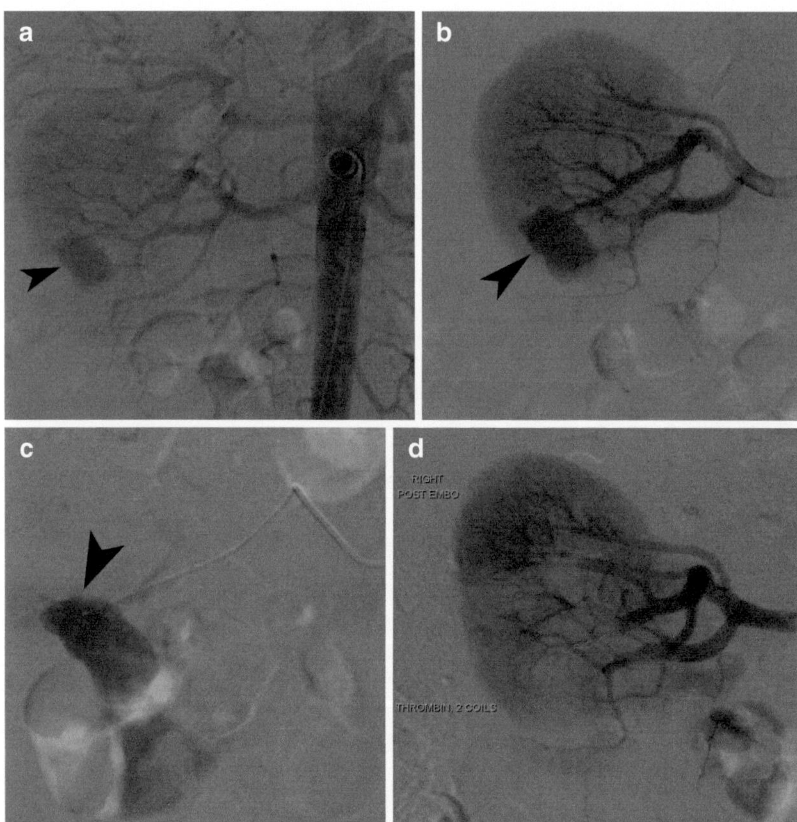

Fig. 7.7 Embolization of a false aneurysm in a 64-year-old male with massive hematuria after left lower pole partial nephrectomy. The initial aortogram shows a largely contained contrast extravasation (**a**, arrowhead) near the resection plane of the lower pole. The total extent of the false aneurysm is better appreciated with a selective angiogram (**b**, arrowhead). A microcatheter was advanced into the false aneurysm (**c**, arrowhead), and 1000 units of thrombin were injected before the withdrawal of the microcatheter from the false aneurysm and coiling of the feeding artery with two microcoils. The final selective angiogram shows complete exclusion of the aneurysm with no parenchymal defect (**d**)

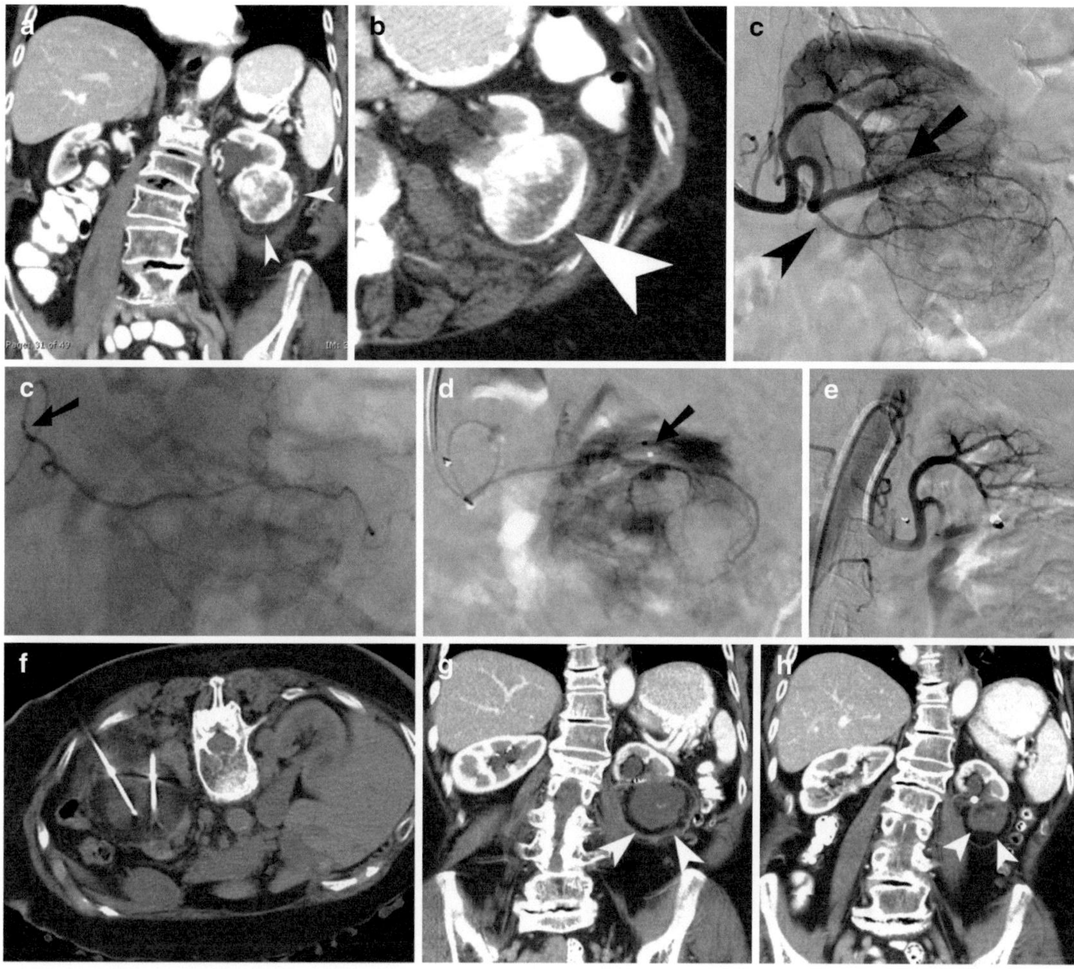

Fig. 7.8 Combined selective embolization and cryoablation of a large lower pole renal mass in a 91-year-old female with multiple comorbidities. A fast-growing 5.8 cm in diameter mass of the lower pole of the right kidney (**a**, **b**, arrowheads) was treated at the patient's request. Embolization was performed 24 h prior to cryoablation of the lesion. A selective angiogram demonstrated the blood supply to the tumor area. A capsular branch (**c**, arrowhead) arising from the adrenal artery and the lower pole artery (arrow) were identified as contributors. A 2.3 French microcatheter was advanced into the capsular artery (**d**, arrow), and a small amount of alcohol was injected with the catheter in a wedge position. A microcoil was then deployed before the withdrawal of the microcatheter. The lower pole artery and tumor were then embolized through a microcatheter (**e**, arrowheads) using concentrated alcohol, 300–500 microspheres, and proximal microcoils. The final selective angiogram showed complete devascularization of the tumor with preserved perfusion of the upper pole. Cryoablation (**f**) was performed using four cryoablation probes under monitored anesthesia care (MAC) anesthesia from a dorsal approach. Follow-up CT images in the coronal plane obtained at 3 (**g**) and 12 months (**h**) after the procedure showed good control of the tumor (arrowheads) without any residual enhancement and slow retraction over time. The upper kidney and collecting system were well preserved

Clinical Value of Transcatheter Tumor Embolization

To date, embolization is considered in two different situations: preoperative and palliative. The majority of published data on renal tumor embolization is centered around preoperative embolization, approximately 1/3 around palliative embolization.

Preoperative Embolization

Superselective, targeted embolization of small malignant renal tumors prior to minimal invasive nephron-sparing surgery or percutaneous ablation may be considered to reduce intraprocedural bleeding in patients with larger lesions or increased bleeding risks [14–17]. The effectiveness of the percutaneous ablation will be enhanced by creating larger ablation zones if performed shortly after the embolization. Published evidence regarding the combination of embolization and ablation is still small but promising.

Renal angioinfarction in locally advanced renal cell carcinoma is discussed controversially in the literature. Protagonists emphasize the benefit of embolization on intraoperative blood loss [18], edema in the resection planes creating a better cleavage plane [19] and earlier control of the renal pedicle due to decompression of vascular structures, thus facilitating radical nephrectomy [20–22]. It is also believed that embolization may improve control of large tumor thrombus within the vena cavae extending to the liver (grade III) or above the diaphragm (grade IV) by reducing the cephalad extension [23]. Survival benefit has been found in patient cohorts who underwent embolization prior to radical nephrectomy [24]. However, an extensive body of literature refutes the benefit of the embolization procedure, which may be associated with a longer hospital stay, questioning the need for this procedure even in advanced cases of renal cell carcinoma with vena cava involvement [21, 25–27]. Further discussion surrounds the optimal time interval between embolization and surgery. Twenty-four hours is favored by many authors, but a longer time interval may allow for tumor shrinkage and encapsulation of the necrotic kidney [23]. At our institution, embolization precedes surgery by more than 20 days (Fig. 7.9).

Despite the fact that more than several thousand cases of embolization have been published,

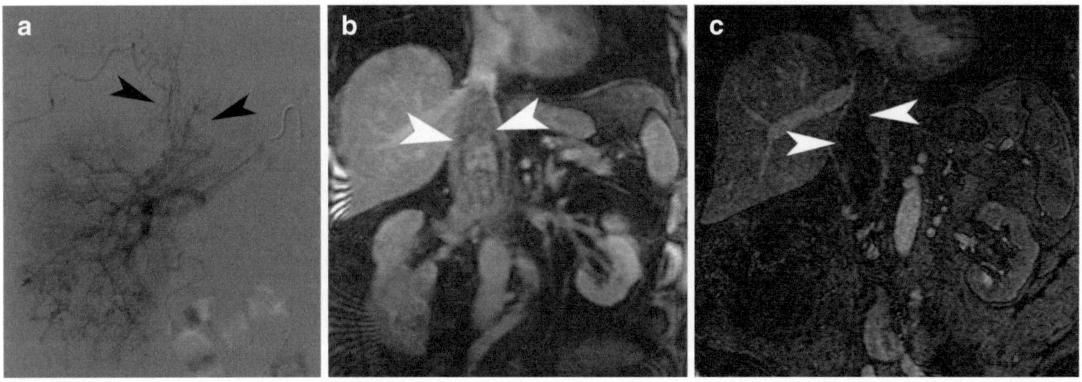

Fig. 7.9 Angiogram prior to angioinfarction of a large renal mass with inferior vena cava involvement in a 74-year-old man. The large mass has infiltrated and replaced the entire lower left kidney. Small arteries (**a**, arrowheads) are seen extending from the renal hilum into the large tumor thrombus within the inferior vena cava. MR images before and after the embolization are displayed in **b**, **c**. 3D-T1-weighted images show the avid enhancement of the tumor and the IVC tumor thrombus extending into the diaphragmatic portion of the IVC after administration of gadolinium-containing contrast. A follow-up MR imaging study obtained 4 weeks after angioinfarction shows complete devascularization of the renal mass and IVC thrombus (**c**, arrowhead). The thrombus has not significantly shrunken in cranio-caudal directions but appears less voluminous

we still do lack clear evidence of the benefits of renal angioinfarction. Randomized controlled trials should be undertaken to compare the treatment of locally advanced renal carcinoma with and without embolization. To date, routine angioinfarction of renal cell carcinoma prior to resection is based on weak evidence. However, for a complicated radical nephrectomy and inferior vena cava (IVC) thrombectomy, several nuances exist in the surgical approach, which may require presurgical embolization in selected cases.

Palliative Embolization

Renal Cell Carcinoma

Much less controversy exists regarding the value of embolization in a palliative setting [21, 28]. Palliation of unresectable renal cell carcinoma aims to stop hematuria, paraneoplastic syndromes, or tumor-associated pain. Survival is if at all a secondary target [29]. Success rates of permanent control of hematuria vary significantly in the literature, but this is related, to some extent, to the level of embolization and the material used. Liquid embolic agents usually provide prompt symptomatic improvement of hematuria. The extent of the embolization should be limited to what is necessary to control the symptoms. Angioinfarction of the entire kidney, which may result in a notable deterioration of kidney function, increase the risk of infection, and be associated with a post-embolization syndrome, is often not necessary.

Angiomyolipoma

Embolization of hypervascular angiomyolipoma is justified in the presence of bleeding, but it is also performed to prevent imminent bleeding. Hypervascular lesions may contain a multitude of vessels with impaired vessel wall function due to a lack of elastic fibers and are thus prone to aneurysm formation (Fig. 7.4). Rupture of these aneurysms creates perirenal bleeding or massive hematuria [30]. Hemorrhagic complications occur more frequently in tumors greater than 4 cm in diameter, in the order of one out of five per year [31, 32]. This is why prophylactic embolization of renal angiomyolipomas may be considered in hypervascular lesions exceeding 4 cm in diameter. The risk of overtreatment has to be balanced against the possible morbidity associated with the procedure [33]. The goal of the embolization procedure is to devascularized the tumor nodule while preserving as much healthy renal parenchyma as possible. This is especially important in the presence of multiple lesions [32]. Long-term control can be achieved with superselective capillary occlusion of the hypervascular tumor nodules [34–36]. Resorbable material and coil embolization bear a substantial risk of revascularization.

Embolization of the Primary Renal Mass in the Presence of Metastasis

Based on the observation that resection of the primary tumor in the kidney has beneficial effects on lung metastases, embolization of the primary renal mass has been advocated [29]. A survival benefit has been described, but these findings could not be confirmed independently [37].

Embolization of a Nonfunctioning Renal Graft

Embolization of a nonfunctioning renal graft could be considered in poor surgical candidates. This procedure is usually well tolerated if the relatively frequent post-embolization syndrome is appropriately managed [38].

References

1. Keller FS, Coyle M, Rosch J, Dotter CT. Percutaneous renal ablation in patients with end-stage renal disease: alternative to surgical nephrectomy. Radiology. 1986;159:447–51.
2. Olivero JJ, Frommer JP, Gonzalez JM. Medical nephrectomy: the last resort for intractable complications of the nephrotic syndrome. Am J Kidney Dis. 1993;21:260–3.
3. Teigen CL, Mitchell SE, Venbrux AC, Christenson MJ, McLean RH. Segmental renal artery embolization for treatment of pediatric renovascular hypertension. J Vasc Interv Radiol. 1992;3:111–7.

4. Kunzendorf U, Keller F, Schweitzer G, Sorensen R, Distler A. Control of renovascular hypertension by renal embolization. Am J Nephrol. 1990;10:339–43.
5. Lammer J, Justich E, Schreyer H, Pettek R. Complications of renal tumor embolization. Cardiovasc Intervent Radiol. 1985;8:31–5.
6. Cromwell LD, Kerber CW. Modification of cyanoacrylate for therapeutic embolization: preliminary experience. Am J Roentgenol. 1979;132:799–801.
7. Rennert J, Herold T, Schreyer AG, et al. [Evaluation of a liquid embolization agent (Onyx) for transcatheter embolization for renal vascular lesions]. Rofo. 2009;181:996–1001.
8. Ellman BA, Green CE, Eigenbrodt E, Garriott JC, Curry TS. Renal infarction with absolute ethanol. Investig Radiol. 1980;15:318–22.
9. Cox GG, Lee KR, Price HI, Gunter K, Noble MJ, Mebust WK. Colonic infarction following ethanol embolization of renal-cell carcinoma. Radiology. 1982;145:343–5.
10. Nurmi M, Satokari K, Puntala P. Renal artery embolization in the palliative treatment of renal adenocarcinoma. Scand J Urol Nephrol. 1987;21:93–6.
11. Probert CS, Osborn DE, Watkin EM. Malignant hypertension due to embolisation of a clear cell renal carcinoma. Br J Urol. 1992;70:95–6.
12. Jafri SZ, Ellwood RA, Amendola MA, Farah J. Therapeutic angio infarction of renal carcinoma: CT follow-up. J Comput Assist Tomogr. 1989;13:443–7.
13. Weckermann D, Schlotmann R, Tietze W, Hackel T. Gas formation after renal artery embolisation: genesis and clinical relevance. Urol Int. 1992;49:211–4.
14. Simone G, Papalia R, Guaglianone S, Forestiere E, Gallucci M. Preoperative superselective transarterial embolization in laparoscopic partial nephrectomy: technique, oncologic, and functional outcomes. J Endourol. 2009;23:1473–8.
15. Woodrum DA, Atwell TD, Farrell MA, Andrews JC, Charboneau JW, Callstrom MR. Role of intra arterial embolization before cryoablation of large renal tumors: a pilot study. J Vasc Interv Radiol. 2010;21:930–6.
16. Nakasone Y, Kawanaka K, Ikeda O, Tamura Y, Yamashita Y. Sequential combination treatment (arterial embolization and percutaneous radiofrequency ablation) of inoperable renal cell carcinoma: single-center pilot study. Acta Radiol. 2012;53:410.
17. Singh VK, Sarma D, Agarwal S, Bagchi PK, Phukan M, Das N, Barua SK. Preoperative superselective embolization vs "on-clamp" laparoscopic partial nephrectomy for T1 renal tumors—a prospective randomized study. J Kidney Cancer VHL. 2024;11(2):18–26.
18. Bakal CW, Cynamon J, Lakritz PS, Sprayregen S. Value of preoperative renal artery embolization in reducing blood transfusion requirements during nephrectomy for renal cell carcinoma. J Vasc Interv Radiol. 1993;4:727–31.
19. Kaisary AV, Williams G, Riddle PR. The role of preoperative embolization in renal cell carcinoma. J Urol. 1984;131:641–6.
20. Klimberg I, Hunter P, Hawkins IF, Drylie DM, Wajsman Z. Preoperative angio infarction of localized renal cell carcinoma using absolute ethanol. J Urol. 1985;133:21–4.
21. Lanigan D, Jurriaans E, Hammonds JC, Wells IP, Choa RG. The current status of embolization in renal cell carcinoma—a survey of local and national practice. Clin Radiol. 1992;46:176–8.
22. Schwartz MJ, Smith EB, Trost DW, Vaughan ED Jr. Renal artery embolization: clinical indications and experience from over 100 cases. BJU Int. 2007;99:881–6.
23. Craven WM, Redmond PL, Kumpe DA, Durham JD, Wettlaufer JN. Planned delayed nephrectomy after ethanol embolization of renal carcinoma. J Urol. 1991;146:704–8.
24. Zielinski H, Szmigielski S, Petrovich Z. Comparison of preoperative embolization followed by radical nephrectomy with radical nephrectomy alone for renal cell carcinoma. Am J Clin Oncol. 2000;23:6–12.
25. Bakke A, Goethlin J, Hoisaeter PA. Renal malignancies: outcome of patients in stage 4 with or without embolization procedure. Urology. 1985;26:541–3.
26. May M, Brookman-Amissah S, Pflanz S, Roigas J, Hoschke B, Kendel F. Pre-operative renal arterial embolisation does not provide survival benefit in patients with radical nephrectomy for renal cell carcinoma. Br J Radiol. 2009;82:724–31.
27. Subramanian VS, Stephenson AJ, Goldfarb DA, Fergany AF, Novick AC, Krishnamurthi V. Utility of preoperative renal artery embolization for management of renal tumors with inferior vena caval thrombi. Urology. 2009;74:154–9.
28. Kalman D, Varenhorst E. The role of arterial embolization in renal cell carcinoma. Scand J Urol Nephrol. 1999;33:162–70.
29. Kauffmann GW, Richter GM, Rohrbach R, Wenz W. Prolonged survival following palliative renal tumor embolization by capillary occlusion. Cardiovasc Intervent Radiol. 1989;12:22–8.
30. Steiner MS, Goldman SM, Fishman EK, Marshall FF. The natural history of renal angiomyolipoma. J Urol. 1993;150:1782–6.
31. Soulen MC, Faykus MH Jr, Shlansky-Goldberg RD, Wein AJ, Cope C. Elective embolization for prevention of hemorrhage from renal angiomyolipomas. J Vasc Interv Radiol. 1994;5:587–91.
32. Williams JM, Racadio JM, Johnson ND, Donnelly LF, Bissler JJ. Embolization of renal angiomyolipoma in patients with tuberous sclerosis complex. Am J Kidney Dis. 2006;47:95–102.
33. Ryan JW, Farelly C, Georgehegan T. What are the indications for prophylactic embolization of renal angiomyolipomas? A review of current evidence in the literature. Can Assoc Radiol J. 2018;69(3):236–9.

34. Davis C, Boyett T, Caridi J. Renal artery embolization: application and success in patients with renal cell carcinoma and angiomyolipoma. Semin Intervent Radiol. 2007;24:111–6.
35. Han YM, Kim JK, Roh BS, et al. Renal angiomyolipoma: selective arterial embolization—effectiveness and changes in angio myogenic components in long-term follow-up. Radiology. 1997;204:65–70.
36. Thulasidasan N, Sriskandakumar S, Ilyas S, Sabharwal T. Renal angiomyolipoma: mid to long term results following embolization with Onyx. Cardiovasc Intervent Radiol. 2016;39(12):1759–64.
37. Kim SH, Kim JK, Park B, Joo J, Joung JY, Seo HK, Lee KH, Chung J. Effects of renal embolization in patients with synchronous metastatic renal cell carcinoma: a retrospective comparison of cytoreductive nephrectomy and systemic medical therapy. Oncotarget. 2007;8(30):49615–24.
38. Takase HM, Contii MM, Bravin AM, Valiatti MF, El-Dib RP, Madeli de Andrade LG. Nephrectomy versus embolization on non-functioning renal graft: a systematic review with a proportional meta-analysis. Ann Transplant. 2018;23:207–17.
39. Dotter CT, Goldman ML, Rosch J. Instant selective arterial occlusion with isobutyl 2-cyanoacrylate. Radiology. 1975;114:227–30.
40. Loffroy R, Abualsaud B, Delgal A, et al. [Role of percutaneous arterial embolization in renal pathology]. Prog Urol. 2010;20:161–71.
41. Fechner G, Hauser S, Flacke S, Gerhard T, Muller SC. [The role of superselective transcatheter arterial embolisation in management of complications after kidney surgery]. Aktuelle Urol. 2008;39:229–33.

Natural History, Diagnostic Evaluation, and Active Surveillance of Small Renal Masses

8

Robert S. Wang, Andres F. Correa, Robert G. Uzzo, David Y. T. Chen, and Benjamin T. Ristau

Introduction

Renal masses less than 4 cm in size are referred to as small renal masses, or SRMs. When malignant, they are usually staged as T1a according to the American Joint Committee on Cancer (AJCC) Tumor/Node/Metastasis (TNM) staging system [1]. Increasing use of cross-sectional imaging over the past few decades has led to a phenomenon of "stage migration" where more renal cell carcinomas (RCCs) are being found incidentally, and at earlier stages. In the United States, the proportion of new RCC cases diagnosed at stage I increased from 43% in 1993, to 57% in 2004, and to 70% by 2015, with a concomitant drop in other stages [2, 3]. At the same time, the overall incidence of new RCC diagnoses has steadily grown while the mortality rate has decreased, suggesting that a majority of new RCC diagnosis involve small and/or indolent tumors [4].

These trends mirror those of prostate cancer detection and treatment early on in the era of PSA screening, where concerns for missed diagnoses and undertreatment transformed into concerns over cancer overdiagnosis and overtreatment, ultimately leading to the adoption of active surveillance (AS) as an initial management strategy for low-risk disease [5, 6]. While the overall prognosis for early-stage RCC following treatment is excellent, the natural history of SRMs is also very indolent, with slow rates of growth and very low rates of metastasis. As such, similar concerns have been raised regarding the necessity of intervention for every SRM, in particular in patients of advanced age and comorbidity.

In this chapter, we will review the natural history and behavior of SRMs—their risks of malignancy, histologies, and rates of growth and metastasis. Then, we will describe current diagnostic tools used to evaluate SRMs, evaluating their strengths and weaknesses. Finally, we will provide a comprehensive overview of active surveillance as a management strategy for small renal masses.

Natural History of Untreated Renal Masses

Historically, the natural history of untreated small renal masses was poorly understood as standard management was immediate surgical excision

R. S. Wang (✉)
Department of Urology, Massachusetts General Hospital – Mass General Brigham, Boston, MA, USA
e-mail: rswang@mgb.org

A. F. Correa · R. G. Uzzo · D. Y. T. Chen
Department of Urology, Fox Chase Cancer Center – Temple University Health System, Philadelphia, PA, USA

B. T. Ristau
Department of Surgery/Division of Urology, UConn Health, Farmington, CT, USA

J. A. Libertino, J. R. Gee (eds.), *Renal Cancer*, https://doi.org/10.1007/978-3-031-97599-8_8

shortly after diagnosis. Our current understanding comes from the last two decades of experience of centers applying surveillance in select elderly and comorbid patients with incidentally found SRMs, with or without delayed intervention, prior to the more recent adoption of formal active surveillance protocols. The majority of the initial data was from small, retrospective series of selected SRMs monitored with serial abdominal imaging at variable intervals prior to extirpation [7–10] and single institution series investigating outcomes in medically high-risk patients managed over the long term with AS alone [11–24]. However, as data from prospectively collected institutional cohorts have matured [25–27], a clearer picture has emerged regarding the natural history of incidentally detected SRMs, confirming their typically indolent behavior. Understanding how an incidentally detected SRM is expected to evolve over time can guide the choice between surveillance and treatment, distinguishing lesions that might be safely surveilled from those that may benefit from immediate definitive intervention.

Benign Versus Malignant SRMs

Approximately 80–85% of small renal masses are malignant; conversely, 15–20% prove benign upon resection [28–31]. Of malignant tumors, 70–80% are clear cell RCC (ccRCC), 15% are papillary RCC, and 5% are chromophobe RCC, with the remainder divided between rarer tumor subtypes [30, 32]. Among resected benign masses, approximately 70–75% are oncocytomas, 15–25% are angiomyolipomas (AMLs), and 5% are papillary adenomas [33]. At the demographic level, a 2016 meta-analysis of 20 studies including 12,149 patients found male sex to be an independent risk factor for malignancy (effect size 2.71, 95% CI 2.39–3.02), while age, BMI, and incidental detection were not [34]. While smoking has been identified as an independent risk factor for the development of renal carcinoma [35], it is unknown whether it is specifically a risk factor for malignancy in patients who are incidentally found to have a renal mass.

Though the overall risk of malignancy in SRMs is well-established, accurate prediction of *which* masses are benign versus malignant in the absence of a tissue biopsy remains the holy grail of management, as it would allow for the avoidance of unnecessary treatment in those with benign pathology. Currently, no single test or combination of tests has been shown to make this distinction with >95% accuracy, and this is an area of highly active investigation. Much of this chapter will focus on the role of various diagnostic modalities in answering this question.

Size and Growth Characteristics of Untreated SRMs

Independent of diagnostic modality, tumor size and growth rate have been shown to be predictors of malignant potential, and understanding these relationships is critical for risk stratifying and managing patients presenting with small renal masses. SRMs are most commonly discovered as incidental findings on cross-sectional imaging, and so tumor size—which is easily measured and generally translatable across modalities—has been extensively evaluated as a prognostic factor.

Several large series have been published examining the correlation between tumor size and malignancy risk [28, 33, 36–38]. For every 1 cm increase in tumor size, the odds of malignancy increase by 16%–43%. The proportion of malignancy is 78–85% for tumors <3 cm, compared to 93–94% for tumors >7 cm. A 2016 meta-analysis by Pierorazio et al. reinforced these findings, estimating a 33% increased odds of malignancy per centimeter increase in tumor size [34]. For tumor histology, increasing size is predictive of both high-grade and clear cell pathology [30, 32, 33, 36, 37, 39, 40]. Finally, tumor size has been correlated with risk of synchronous metastasis, with rates varying from 0 to 5% for tumors <1 cm, to 1.4–13% for tumors 3–4 cm, to 17–65% for tumors >7 cm [36, 41–43]. Kunkle et al. created a logistic regression model from institutional data which showed that the odds of synchronous metastasis increased by 22% for each 1 cm increase in tumor size [41].

Growth rate has also been shown to be a predictor of malignancy in SRMs. Most notably, in masses under observation, the risk of metastatic spread is virtually zero in tumors demonstrating no interval growth [31, 44]. However, the rate of tumor growth is poorly predictive of tumor histology. Kawaguchi et al. showed that 80% of oncocytomas under surveillance demonstrate interval growth, with an average estimated growth rate of 0.19 cm/year [45]. Finelli et al. conducted a pooled analysis of 136 SRMs that were biopsy-proven RCC [46]. They found that masses with clear cell histology had significantly higher average growth rates versus masses with papillary type I histology (0.28 cm/year vs. 0.0017 cm/year, $p < 0.001$), with papillary type II and chromophobe tumors falling in between. However, they also noted significant variations in growth rates among clear cell RCCs, with some tumors staying stable or even shrinking over time while a small subset (15%) grew more rapidly, >5 mm/year.

Several studies have used pooled analytic methods to consolidate institutional data and characterize the growth trends of SRMs. Chawla et al. combined data from nine single institution retrospective series and identified 234 masses followed for a mean duration of 34 months (Table 8.1) [48]. Average initial tumor diameter was 2.6 cm (range 1.73–4.08 cm), and the mean linear growth rate was 0.28 cm/year. Pathologic confirmation was available in 46%, of which 92% were RCC or RCC variants. The overall rate of metastatic disease in the entire cohort was 1.1%.

Smaldone et al. performed a pooled analysis of six studies with 259 patients (284 SRMs) undergoing AS (Table 8.2) and reported similar findings [31]. Average initial tumor diameter was 2.3 cm, with an average calculated linear growth

Table 8.1 Meta-analysis of the natural history of observed masses

References	Year	Mean age, years (range)	Number of patients/ number of SRMs	Initial mean tumor diameter (range) (cm)	Mean linear growth rate (range) (cm/year)	Mean follow-up (range) (months)	No. of metastatic events (timing of event)
Fujimoto et al. [8]	1995	59.7 (47–70)	6/6	2.47 (1.7–3.4)	0.47 (0.39–0.74)	29 (9.7–7.1)	0
Bosniak et al. [7]	1995	65.5	40/40	1.73 (all <3.5)	0.36 (0.1–1)	39 (1.8–8.5)	0
Oda et al. [10]	2001	54 (med.) (28–78)	16	2.0 (median) (1.0–4.5)	0.54 (median) (0.1–1.35)	2.1 (median) (12–72)	0
Kassouf et al. [47]	2004	68.3 (29–83)	20/26	3.27 (0.9–1.0)	0.09 (0.13–1.2)	32 (8–86)	0
Volpe et al. [22]	2004	71 (27–84)	29/32	2.48 (0.9–3.4)	0.1	35 (5.3–143)	0
Wehle et al. [23]	2004	70.5 (51–88)	29/29	1.83 (0.4–3.5)	0.12 (n/a)	32 (10–89)	0
Kato et al. [9]	2004	56.5 (37–71)	18/18	1.98 (37–71)	0.42 (0.08–1.6)	27 (12–63)	0
Sowery and Siemens [21]	2004	77 (60–92)	22/22	4.08 (2–8.8)	0.86 (0–6)	26 (1–111)	1 (timing n/a)
Chawla et al. [48]	2006	71 (42–85)	49/61	2.97 (1–12)	0.20 (−1.64–1.8)	36 (12–152)	1 (54 months)
Lamb et al. [17]	2004	76.1 (56–91)	36/36	6 (3.5–20)	n/a	n/a	1 (132 months)
Totals (median)	–		271/286	2.60 (2.48)	0.28 (0.28)	34 (32)	3/271 1.1%

Adapted from Chawla et al. [48]

Table 8.2 Pooled analysis of small renal masses managed with active surveillance

Study	Year	Median age (range) (years)	No. of patients/no of SRMs	Initial mean tumor diameter (range) (cm)	Mean linear growth rate (range) (cm/year)	Mean follow-up (range) (months)	No. of metastatic events (timing of event)
Fujimoto et al. [8]	1995	57 (47–40)	6/6	2.47 (1.7–3.4)	0.57 (0.39–0.74)	29 (9.7–71)	0
Bosniak et al. [7]	1995	65.5 (48–84)	37/40	1.73 (0.2–3.5)	0.4 (0–1.1)	43.9 (21–102)	0
Volpe et al. [22]	2004	71 (27–84)	29/32	2.48 (0.9–3.4)	0.1	35.3 (5.3–143)	3
Kato et al. [9]	2004	56.5 (37–71)	18/18	1.98 (0.8–3.4)	0.42 (0.08–1.6)	27 (12–63)	0
Matsuzaki et al. [18]	2007	72 (44–87)	15/15	2.2 (1–3.9)	0.06 (−0.09–0.28)	38 (8–91)	0
Crispen et al. [14]	2009	71 (35–88)	154/173	2.45 (0.4–12)	0.29 (−1.4–2.47)	31 (12–156)	0
Totals (range)		69 (35–88)	259/284	2.3 (0.2–12)	0.31 (−1.4–2.5)	33.5	3/259 1.1%

Adapted from Smaldone et al. [31]

rate of 0.31 cm/year. For the patients with pathology data available, 88% of masses were found to be malignant. The authors similarly found a very low rate of metastatic disease at 1.1%.

Evaluation of Small Renal Masses

Over the past several decades, a rise in utilization of cross-sectional imaging (computed tomography (CT) and MRI) has led to a dramatic increase in the number and proportion of incidentally discovered renal masses [4, 49]. Asymptomatic, small renal masses account for the majority of this increase, with fewer than 10% of renal tumors now presenting with the "classic" triad of flank pain, hematuria, and a palpable mass [2, 49–51]. Contemporary management, including patient counseling and treatment planning, is still often based solely on cross-sectional imaging characteristics without definitive pathologic confirmation of malignancy or specialized testing. The most recent AUA, NCCN, and EAU guidelines all recommend cross-sectional imaging as the core component of the initial evaluation of suspected RCC, with renal mass biopsy as an option if further pathologic characterization is desired prior to definitive management [52–55]. While conventional imaging techniques are effective in the initial characterization of SRMs, they have difficulty distinguishing RCC from certain common benign histologies, most notably oncocytomas and lipid-poor AMLs [28, 56, 57]. Recognition of these limitations has led to increased utilization of renal mass biopsy (RMB) over the years, but overall, RMB is still used in only a small proportion (10–15%) of cases [58–60]. In this section, we will review the performance of conventional imaging in the evaluation of small renal masses, explore the data surrounding renal mass biopsy, and briefly cover alternative and emerging diagnostic modalities including Tc99m-Sestamibi SPECT/CT and CA-IX-targeted positron emission tomography (PET)/CT.

Imaging

Conventional Cross-Sectional Imaging

Contrast-enhanced, multiphase cross-sectional imaging with CT or MRI remains the first-line recommendation for characterization of small renal masses [52–55]. The American College of Radiology Appropriateness Criteria for indeterminate renal masses labels both CT and MRI as "usually appropriate" when no contraindications exist [61]. Typical renal mass protocols include both noncontrast and immediate postcontrast sequences, with additional specialized sequences depending on the indication (i.e., delayed urogram phases for a urothelial lesion). On CT, lesion enhancement is defined as a change of >20 HU between noncontrast and contrast sequences, with ≤10 HU change being nonenhancing and 10–20 HU change being equivocal. On MRI, enhancement is defined as a >15% increase in signal intensity after administration of gadolinium-based contrast [62].

These modalities are adept at distinguishing most renal cystic lesions from solid masses, evaluating enhancement characteristics, estimating renal perfusion and differential function, and providing anatomic detail for treatment planning. They achieve clinical (radiographic) staging by identifying tumor size and location, involvement of other structures, and presence or absence of metastases. However, conventional imaging techniques are limited by their diagnostic accuracy in distinguishing between some benign and malignant solid tumors, and have difficulty predicting tumor histology and, most importantly, future behavior.

CT and MRI are excellent at differentiating between solid and cystic tumors, with the latter being characterized by the presence of simple, nonenhancing fluid-level signals within the mass [62, 63]. They are also the preferred imaging modalities for Bosniak classification of cystic renal masses to aid in risk stratification for malignancy (see "Classification Systems" section) [64]. Pseudoenhancement is a CT-specific artifact, most commonly seen in small lesions, where the fluid in a cyst appears to enhance on postcontrast sequences, mimicking low-enhancing solid renal tumors such as papillary RCC. In these cases, contrast-enhanced MRI or the use of dual-energy CT (DECT) can help clarify whether or not these masses are truly cystic [63, 65]. In addition, some cysts can be hyperdense due to internal hemorrhage—however, they are still easily differentiated from solid renal masses due to high density on nonenhanced CT (>66–70 HU) and lack of postcontrast enhancement [66, 67].

For separating benign and renal masses, the performance of conventional imaging is strongly dependent on tumor histology. Macroscopic fat within a tumor, measuring −15 HU or lower on CT or demonstrating signal dropout with fat suppression on MRI, is considered diagnostic for a benign AML [62, 68, 69]. However, approximately 5% of AMLs are "fat/lipid-poor"; many of these are misdiagnosed as RCC and undergo unnecessary surgical excision. The use of predictive models combining additional imaging characteristics from ultrasound, CT, or MRI can support the diagnosis of fat-poor AML over RCC, but oftentimes, renal mass biopsy is required to provide a definitive diagnosis [63, 70, 71]. Oncocytomas are another benign tumor that poses a diagnostic challenge for conventional imaging. Although classically characterized by a central scar and a characteristic enhancement pattern called segmental enhancement inversion (SEI), these findings do not reliably differentiate oncocytomas from RCC [65]. One series examining pathologically-confirmed oncocytomas found that on preoperative imaging, all tumors enhanced, and only 10.7% had a central scar [57]. Another study found no difference in the detection of SEI between oncocytomas and chromophobe tumors [72]. However, in situations where a biopsy shows an oncocytic neoplasm, the tumor:cortex peak early enhancement ratio (PEER) value on CT has been shown to have excellent accuracy in differentiating oncocytoma from chromophobe RCCs [73]. Similar to AMLs, several multivariable imaging-based models have been proposed to distinguish oncocytomas from RCC, but overall diagnostic performance has not been sufficient to gain widespread adoption at this time [63].

Some imaging differences also exist between the various RCC subtypes, which may help guide treatment decisions. On CT, clear cell RCCs demonstrate strong postcontrast enhancement and brisk contrast washout, whereas papillary RCCs tend to be hypo-enhancing with low de-enhancement [74]. On MRI, ccRCCs likewise demonstrate high postcontrast T2 signal intensity compared to pRCCs, with lower ADC values [75]. These differences are also present when comparing ccRCC to chromophobe RCCs, though to a lesser degree and with greater

Table 8.3 Traditional imaging characteristics of most common renal neoplasms

Tumor histology	Traditional imaging characteristics
Renal cell carcinoma (RCC)	
Clear cell RCC	• Heterogeneous with areas of necrosis, hemorrhage, and cysts • CT-specific – Strong postcontrast enhancement with rapid washout • MRI-specific – T2WI hyperintensity and hypervascularity postcontrast – T1-weighted dual echo microscopic/intravoxel fat
Papillary RCC	• Low-level, gradual enhancement with peak in later sequences • CT-specific – Low (<100HU) to absent (<10HU) enhancement in corticomedullary phase with peak in nephrographic phase • MRI-specific – Hypointense T2WI signal relative to normal parenchyma – Presence of hemosiderin – Low ADC values relative to ccRCC
Chromophobe RCC	• Homogeneously enhancing but less than RCC, may have central scar • Difficult to distinguish from oncocytoma • CT-specific – Lower enhancement than ccRCC but higher than pRCC, peak in corticomedullary phase – May demonstrate segmental enhancement inversion • MRI-specific – ADC values lower than ccRCC but higher than pRCC
Angiomyolipoma	
Classic AML	• Macroscopic fat without calcifications
Fat/lipid-poor AML	• No macroscopic fat • Strong, homogenous enhancement • CT-specific – Can be isoattenuating or hyperattenuating on noncontrast • MRI-specific – Low T2WI signal
Oncocytoma	• Enhancing similar to ccRCC, may have central scar • Difficult to distinguish from oncocytoma • CT-specific – May demonstrate segmental enhancement inversion • MRI-specific – T2 and ADC values similar to ccRCC

Adapted from Sasaguri and Takahashi [62] and Wang et al. [63]

potential for overlap between the two histologies. Table 8.3 summarizes some of the key CT and MRI imaging features of the most common renal mass histologies.

Compared to the evidence supporting tumor size and growth rate, the data for other CT and MRI features in predicting tumor grade are much more sporadic. CT findings significantly associated with high-grade ccRCC include low enhancement, irregular margins, calcifications, necrosis, and collecting system invasion [76, 77]. For MRI, two separate studies reported that lower parenchymal wash-in indices and lower ADC ratios are predictive of higher-grade (Fuhrman 3–4) tumors [78, 79]. They did not find any associations between MRI parameters and non-ccRCC grade. A 2015 meta-analysis of three studies found that DWI could help predict high-grade histology with an AUC of 0.83 [80].

Classification Systems and Predictive Models

Renal mass anatomy can be predictive of both underlying pathology and treatment outcomes, and several systems of standardized tumor anatomy reporting have been proposed [64, 81–85].

Of these, two have achieved widespread use in both research and clinical care settings: the Bosniak classification for cystic renal masses, and the RENAL nephrometry score [81, 82].

Proposed in 1986 by Dr. Morton A. Bosniak, MD, the Bosniak classification system seeks to guide the management of cystic renal masses by predicting the risk of malignancy based on cross-sectional imaging features [81]. It has been updated and refined several times over the years [81, 86, 87]. In its most recent form, the classic Bosniak system divides cystic renal masses into five categories [88]: Class I and II masses are thin-walled without measurable enhancement, with or without septae and/or fine calcifications. These are described as clearly benign, and no follow-up is recommended. Class IIF masses have increased the number/thickness/complexity of their walls and septations, but still lack measurable enhancement. The "F" stands for "follow," and the recommendation is for ongoing monitoring to establish and confirm stability. Class III masses have thickened walls and septae with measurable enhancement and are labeled as "indeterminate" masses with sufficient malignancy risk to justify treatment. Finally, Class IV masses are highly probable malignant masses with minor cystic components and solid-enhancing tissue outside of the walls and septae that require definitive intervention. Two recent systematic reviews have summarized the malignancy rates for each Bosniak class. Sevcenco et al. extracted data from 35 studies and calculated pooled malignancy rates for Bosniak I (3.2%), II (6%), IIF (6.7%), III (55.1%), and IV (91%) lesions [89]. Schoots et al. likewise combined data from 39 studies and calculated similar malignancy rates for Bosniak II (9%), IIF (18%), III (51%), and IV (89%) tumors [90]. The authors also found that Bosniak IIF cysts that were upgraded to class III or IV on subsequent imaging had a pooled malignancy rate of 85%, highlighting the importance of following these lesions. In 2019, an update to the Bosniak system was published, proposing several major changes, including specifically defined measurement and terms, the formal addition of MRI features, and standardized verbiage in reporting malignancy risk and management recommendations [64]. Early reviews suggest that, compared to the 2005 version, the 2019 Bosniak classification is less sensitive for malignancy but more specific, with a higher proportion of masses being classified as IIF instead of III and a resulting higher malignancy rate among IIF masses [91–93]. Interreader and intermodal agreement appear to be high for both versions and does not appear to differ significantly between the two [93].

In 2009, Kutikov and Uzzo proposed the RENAL nephrometry score to report the complexity of solid renal masses and guide surgical decision-making [82]. The five components of the nephrometry score are **r**adius, **e**xophytic/endophytic property, *n*earness to the collecting system, *a*nterior/posterior location, and *l*ocation relative to polar lines; together, they form the RENAL acronym. Each component is assigned a score of 1–3 based on increasing complexity, except for the anterior/posterior location, which is simply labeled "*a*" (anterior), "*p*" (posterior), or "*x*" (neither). An "*h*" (hilar) modifier is added if the tumor abuts the main artery or vein (Fig. 8.1). Using a large prospectively maintained institutional cohort, Kutikov et al. then evaluated the relationship between RENAL nephrometry score and tumor histology following surgical resection [94]. Total nephrometry score as well as all individual components (except degree of endophytic ness) were significantly associated with high-grade histology. Total nephrometry score and all individual components significantly differed between tumor histology groups with the exception of the anterior/posterior designation. Nephrometry scores were generally low for benign, papillary, and chromophobe tumors and high for clear cell and rare aggressive subtypes (collecting duct, sarcomatoid). Using these data, the authors constructed a nomogram that predicted malignancy with an AUC of 0.76 and high-grade histology with an AUC of 0.73, which remained consistent upon validation with an external dataset [95]. For patients undergoing partial nephrectomy, a higher RENAL nephrometry score is associated with an open approach [96, 97], postoperative urine leak [96], tumor upstaging [98], increased length of hospital stay

	1pt	2pts	3 pts
(R)adius (maximal diameter in cm)	≤4	>4 but <7	≥7
(E)xophytic/endophytic properties	≥ 50%	<50%	Entirely endophytic
(N)earness of the tumor to the collecting system or sinus (mm)	≥ 7	>4 but <7	≤4
(A)nterior/Posterior	No points given. Mass assigned a descriptor of a, p, or x		
(L)ocation relative to the polar lines* *suffix "h" assigned if the tumor touches the main renal artery or vein	Entirely above the upper or below the lower polar line	Lesion crosses polar line	>50% of mass is across polar line (a) or mass crosses the axial renal midline (b) or mass is entirely between the polar lines (c)

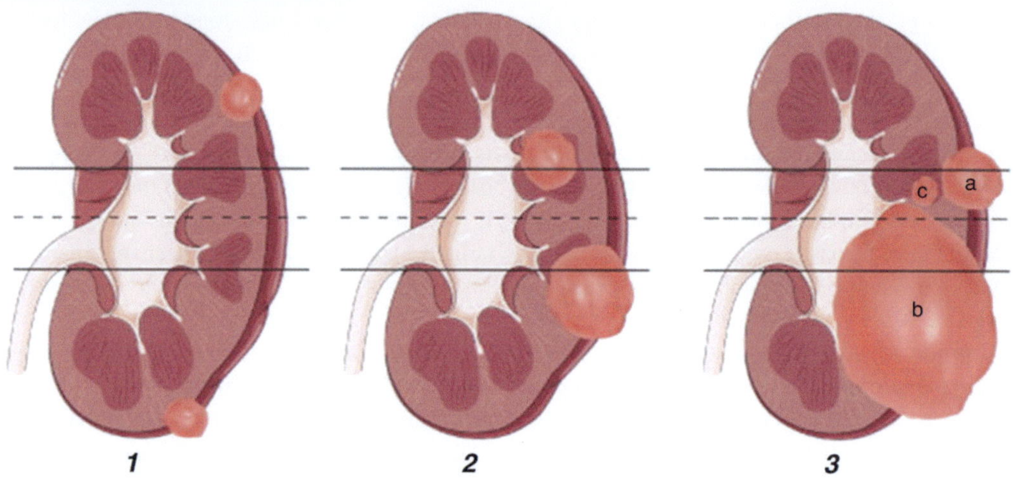

Fig. 8.1 The RENAL nephrometry score (from Kutikov and Uzzo [82])

[99, 100], higher estimated blood loss [99, 100], and longer warm ischemia time [99, 100]. A high nephrometry score is also associated with an increased likelihood of radical nephrectomy and surgical complications in all approaches [101, 102].

Contrast-Enhanced Ultrasound

Contrast-enhanced ultrasound (CEUS) is a novel imaging technique that involves ultrasonography of the kidneys before and after injection of an intravenous microbubble contrast agent [103]. These contrast agents contain microscopically encased low-solubility gasses that oscillate in response to ultrasonic waves, generating a signal that is then also detectable by a specially configured ultrasound system. The microbubble particles are small enough to pass through the pulmonary capillaries but are not filtered by the glomerulus, and so when injected intravenously, there is a rapid renal arterial enhancement phase followed by a cortical and then a parenchymal phase, without an excretory phase [104]. Uses for CEUS include differentiation between cystic and solid renal masses, characterization of complex renal masses, and differentiation between solid tumor subtypes. A systematic review and meta-analysis by Furrer et al. (2020) pooled data from

16 studies comparing CEUS to MRI and/or CT performance in characterizing renal masses [105]. The authors found that overall, CEUS performed as well or slightly better than CT and MRI in characterizing solid renal masses and especially well at characterizing cystic renal masses. However, overall adoption has been limited by the need for specialized equipment, time, and expertise in performing and interpreting these studies.

Nuclear Medicine Imaging

Whereas traditional imaging techniques provide excellent anatomic detail, nuclear medicine modalities such as positron emission tomography (PET) have the potential to noninvasively characterize biologic processes at the cellular and subcellular level. The use of ^{18}F fluorodeoxyglucose positron emission tomography (FDG-PET) to functionally image malignancies is based on the anticipated altered glycolytic pathway in malignant cells [106]. However, renal excretion of the nuclear medicine tracer significantly limits its accuracy in the evaluation of renal masses. For the detection of primary renal lesions, estimates of FDG-PET sensitivity range from 45 to 60%, and estimates of specificity range from 65 to 100%, with FDG-PET underperforming CT scans in studies comparing the two [107–110].

More recently, antibody-based molecular imaging, or immuno-PET, has been investigated as a clinically relevant strategy to improve molecular/biologic imaging in RCC. Using radiolabeled antibodies with high affinity for cancer-specific antigens as a means of identifying radiographically recognizable molecular targets, immuno-PET offers an exciting strategy to image all types of cancers. One such promising molecular target for immuno-PET is carbonic anhydrase IX (CA IX), which is produced by normal tissues in response to hypoxia along the VEGF/HIF pathway. The frequent loss of VHL in both familial and sporadic clear cell RCCs leads to a dramatic increase in CA IX expression in these tumors, with >95% of ccRCC showing high levels of CA IX [111]. Chimeric-G250 (girentuximab) is a monoclonal antibody that was discovered to bind to ccRCC, later found to be targeting CA IX. In a phase I study imaging 26 patients with renal masses prior to surgery, radiolabeled cG250 immuno-PET (^{124}I-cG250 PET/CT) was able to discriminate between ccRCC and non-ccRCC with a 94% sensitivity and 100% specificity, no serious drug-related adverse events [112]. A subsequent multi-institutional phase III study ("REDECT") enrolled 195 patients scheduled for tumor resection [113]. The authors found that, compared to conventional multiphase CT imaging, ^{124}I-cG250 PET/CT accurately discriminated ccRCC from non-ccRCC with a much higher sensitivity (86% vs 76%) and specificity (87% vs 47%). The positive predictive value for clear cell RCC for ^{124}I-G250-PET/CT was 95%, and it was well tolerated with no associated serious adverse events. More recently, the ZIRCON trial reported the performance of a different cG250 radiotracer conjugate [^{89}Zr] Zr-girentuximab PET/CET in 300 patients prior to scheduled partial nephrectomy [114]. Sensitivity and specificity for ccRCC were 85.5% and 87%, respectively, with a positive predictive value (PPV) of 92.9% and no significant complications attributable to the tracer.

Finally, data are maturing for the use of technetium-99m sestamibi single-photon emission computed tomography/X-ray computed tomography (^{99m}Tc-sestamibi SPECT/CT) for the differentiation of oncocytomas and hybrid oncocytic/chromophobe tumors (HOCTs) from other renal tumor histologies. First described in 1996, ^{99m}Tc-sestamibi SPECT/CT for renal tumor characterization relies on preferential uptake of the tracer in mitochondria, which are highly abundant in the cells of oncocytoma and chromophobe RCCs [115, 116]. In an early prospective evaluation of ^{99m}Tc-sestamibi SPECT/CT, 50 patients with a solid clinical T1 renal mass were imaged prior to surgery, with six oncocytomas and two HOCTs identified after resection [117]. ^{99m}Tc-sestamibi SPECT/CT correctly identified 5/6 oncocytomas and 2/2 HOCTs, with two false positive cases of ccRCC with high tracer uptake. Basile et al. conducted a meta-analysis of eight studies (501 renal masses) investigating ^{99m}Tc-sestamibi SPECT/CT performance and calculated overall 89% sensitivity and specificity for separating oncocytoma and HOCT from all other renal lesions and 98% sensitivity and specificity for separating oncocytoma and HOCT from clear cell and papillary RCCs [118]. However, a recent series of ^{99m}Tc-sestamibi SPECT/CT performance in a real-world practice setting with results influencing decision-making found that still approximately 20% of tumors labeled as having a "negative" ^{99m}Tc-sestamibi scan (likely RCC) still were revealed to be oncocytomas after resection [119, 120].

Renal Mass Biopsy

Traditional Role of Renal Mass Biopsy

Prior to the 2000s, renal mass biopsy (RMB) was generally viewed as having limited perceived benefit and subsequent impact on the management of SRMs. The common standard practice was to treat all SRMs as RCC, with biopsy reserved for the infrequent cases with suspicion of non-RCC pathology (such as lymphoma or infection) or concern for metastasis from another organ to the kidney. Concerns regarding limited diagnostic accuracy [121, 122] and case reports of biopsy tract seeding by viable tumor [123–125] limited its use in the standard evaluation of most renal masses.

However, since the turn of the century, there has been increasing recognition of the potential for renal mass biopsy to influence management decisions for patients with SRMs [126–128]. In particular, RMB has found utility in the differentiation between benign and malignant masses [129, 130], and refinement of biopsy techniques have brought the sensitivity and specificity of core needle RMB to above 95% with histological concordance estimates ranging from 77.5% to 100% [131].

Modern Biopsy Technique and Results

The most recent AUA and EAU guidelines recommend an 18-G core needle biopsy with a coaxial technique as the preferred method for performing renal mass biopsy [53, 55]. Both guidelines recognize fine needle aspiration (FNA) as an alternative but less accurate technique, though the EAU guidelines highlight that the addition of FNA to core needle biopsy may offer additional diagnostic benefits.

Two modern systematic reviews provide a comprehensive summary of the data regarding the diagnostic accuracy of renal mass biopsy:

Marconi et al. conducted a systematic review and meta-analysis of 57 studies encompassing 5228 patients who underwent RMB from 1967 to 2011 [132]. Overall median diagnostic rate was 92%, with nondiagnostic rates ranging from 0 to 22.6% for core biopsy and 0–36% for FNA. For cancer detection, estimated sensitivity and specificity for core biopsy were 99.1% (95% CI 96.4–99.8) and 99.7% (95% CI 93.7–100), and for FNA were 93.2% (95% CI 83–97.5) and 89.8% (95% CI 78.6–95.4), respectively. Sensitivity of RMB was higher for solid tumors (99.7%) versus cystic masses (83.6%), while specificity was high for both (98.2% vs 98%). For the identification of tumor histology, the median concordance between RMB and surgical pathology was 90.3% (IQR 84–94.45). For the classification of tumor grade, median concordance rates were 62.5% (IQR 52.1–72.1%) using the four-tier Fuhrman grading system and 87% (IQR: 71–98%) using a high/low grading system. One study comparing core biopsy to FNA found a similar ability to predict tumor histology (91% vs. 86% concordance) but much higher accuracy of core biopsy in predicting Furhman grade (76% vs. 28% concordance) [133].

Patel et al. published a systematic review of 20 RMB studies encompassing 2979 patients from 1997 to 2015 [131]. Of these, only one study evaluated FNA, while the rest examined core needle biopsy. For core needle biopsy, the average nondiagnostic rate was 13.9%. Cancer detection sensitivity was 97.5% (95% CI 78–100), specificity was 96.2% (95% CI 75–100), positive predictive value (PPV) was 99.8% (95% CI 97–100), and negative predictive value (NPV) was 68.5% (95% CI 13–100). Reported histologic concordance rates ranged from 77.5% to 100%, while grade concordance ranged from 51.5% to 75.9%, with 16% of cases upgraded by surgical pathology. The one FNA study included 25 patients who prospectively underwent FNA prior to definitive surgical management [122]. All 25 were found to have RCC; FNA was positive in 10 (40%), suspicious in 9 (36%), and negative in 6 (25%). Grade concordance in the positive FNAs was 80%. The authors concluded that FNA did not have sufficient diagnostic accuracy to justify its use in preoperative renal mass evaluation.

The AUA conducted its own meta-analysis as part of its updated renal mass guidelines, with very similar findings. Of the seven included studies, two had been included in the previous systematic reviews, while five were newly published since then [55]. The guideline authors found that core needle biopsy had a pooled sensitivity of 96.7% (95% CI 93.8–98.2), specificity of 94.5% (95% CI 71.9–99.1), PPV of 98.8% (95% CI 97.0–99.5), and NPV of 80.8% (95% CI 70.1–88.3).

Limitations of Renal Mass Biopsy

From a diagnostic accuracy standpoint, RMB has excellent sensitivity and specificity, and a positive biopsy is a near-certainty for the presence of malignancy. However, three major limitations of renal mass biopsy are highlighted by the above data: A nondiagnostic rate of ~15%, a histologic upgrading rate of ~15%, and a negative predictive value of 70–80%, meaning that 20–30% of tumors deemed benign by biopsy are proven malignant upon resection. Additionally, cystic renal masses and tumors with hybrid histology pose special diagnostic challenges to RMB.

Multiple solutions have been proposed to address the nondiagnostic rate. The simplest solution is a repeat biopsy: when an initial biopsy is nondiagnostic, a second attempt is diagnostic in 80–83% of cases [131, 134, 135]. However, in these series, only ~20% of nondiagnostic biopsies were re-biopsied, with the majority proceeding to surveillance instead. Two studies compared the diagnostic yield of FNA plus core biopsy to each component individually [136, 137]. Both found that the diagnostic rate of the combined approach (92–93%) was higher than that of FNA (63–72%) and core biopsy (76–87%) alone but that the difference was only significant in the former. Finally, the American Society of Cytopathology supports the use of rapid on-site evaluation (ROSE) to improve the diagnostic yield of biopsies through real-time assessment of specimen adequacy [138]. Diagnostic accuracy of ROSE ranges from 85–95%, depending on the biopsy modality and target characteristics [130]. The AUA recognizes the potential benefits of ROSE but also that workflow and personnel challenges may limit its adoption [55].

A study by Ball et al. showed that small renal masses exhibit significant grade heterogeneity, suggesting that the histologic upgrading rate may be an intrinsic limitation of renal mass biopsy rather than a technique issue [139]. The authors examined pathology slides from 32 small renal masses and found that 81.3% of tumors were heterogeneous (demonstrating >1 Fuhrman grade per specimen) and 31.3% were discordant (highest grade present in <50% of the specimen). For high-grade specimens (Furhman 3–4), heterogeneity and discordance rates were 93.8% and 25%, respectively. These findings suggest that while RMB may have good utility in diagnosing malignancy, it is much more limited in predicting its behavior.

Regarding the low NPV of RMB, it should be acknowledged that there is an inherent selection bias surrounding the data: negative biopsies are less likely to undergo surgery and have pathologic confirmation. Conversely, biopsy-negative tumors that proceed to surgery likely demonstrated other clinical signs of malignancy. Therefore, the lower negative predictive value of RMB should be interpreted with caution, as the cases with pathology available are likely enriched with false negatives.

Cystic renal masses are challenging to biopsy due to the lack of solid targetable tissue relative to liquid tumor components. Both the AUA and EAU generally recommend against biopsy of cystic renal masses due to concerns for tumor rupture and low diagnostic yield, though the EAU makes allowances for those with a targetable solid component [53, 55]. Nonetheless, a combination of core needle biopsy and FNA can lead to accurate diagnosis in up to 85% of cystic renal masses [140], and a limited series of aspiration and biopsy for Bosniak III ± IIF masses found that RMB allowed patients to avoid surgery in

~30% of cases [141, 142]. Of note, biopsy is also not recommended in patients with acquired polycystic disease from dialysis or adult polycystic disease because of the risk of misdiagnosing the papillary hyperplasia that frequently occurs in these cysts with RCC [143].

Oncocytomas pose another diagnostic challenge to RMB as they can be mimicked by chromophobe or hybrid oncocytoma/chromophobe tumors (HOCTs) [144]. However, this concern may be over-emphasized. A 2017 meta-analysis found that one out of four tumors diagnosed as oncocytoma on biopsy were later found to be RCC on surgical pathology [145]. However, only 22.4% of biopsied specimens proceeded to biopsy, once again suggesting a strong selection bias and a likely underestimation of the negative predictive value of RMB in these cases. In a review of 147 patients with benign resected renal masses, only 4 (2.7%) were found to have HOCT pathology, none of which experienced recurrence or progression after a median follow-up of 44 months [146].

Complications of Biopsy

Renal mass biopsy is a very safe procedure, with overall complication rates <10%. The most common complications are renal hematoma (0.1–5.5%), gross hematuria (0.5–5.2%), clinically significant pain (0.5–3.0%), bleeding requiring intervention (0.4–0.7%), and pneumothorax (0.6–1.7%) [60, 131, 132, 147]. Vascular and visceral organ injuries are exceedingly rare [60], and none of the studies reported any deaths associated with RMB.

While tumor tract seeding has been historically cited as a reason for the limited adoption of RMB, only 16 cases have been reported [148]. While the small numbers preclude any meaningful statistical analysis, it should be noted that 15/16 cases involved the use of a ≥20 G needle, and 2/2 cases omitted a coaxial sheath. 14/16 cases involved papillary histology. These data suggest that the very small risk of tumor tract seeding can be further mitigated by using a contemporary biopsy technique (18 G needle with coaxial sheath) and avoiding RMB in tumors with imaging characteristics suggestive of papillary histology.

Impact on Care

Utilization of renal mass biopsy has more than doubled over the last two decades, but overall adoption has been low, and practice patterns are highly variable. A review of 338,252 patients with clinically localized (T1-T3N0M0) RCC from the National Cancer Database found that from 2004 to 2015, rates of RMB increased from 7.6% to 16.2% [58]. A similar review of the Premier Hospital Database found the annual number of RMB increased from 7196 cases in 2006 to 11,528 cases in 2017 [60]. Practice variations are highlighted in a 2018 survey of 1131 members of the AUA, where 19.3% of academic urologists versus 36.1% of nonacademic urologists stated they would never biopsy a renal mass ≤4 cm in size [149]. The predominant cited rationale for omitting biopsy was that it would not change patient management. An increasing number of patients with SRMs seen annually correlated with willingness to consider biopsy, from 42.2% for urologists seeing 0–5 SRMs/year, to 74.6% for those seeing 20+ SRMs/year. A 2021 review of data for T1 renal masses from the Michigan Urologic Surgery Improvement Collaborative (MUSIC-KIDNEY) found that while the overall RMB rate was 15.5% across the state, median practice-level utilization was 11.3% with a range of 0–100% and IQR of 2–24% [59].

Evidence suggests that RMB has the potential to change management for a significant proportion of patients. A common predictor for biopsy across studies was a higher Charlson Comorbidity Index, indicating the increasing use of biopsy as a way to potentially avoid treatment in poor surgical candidates [58–60, 150]. In one study of 115,511 patients who had RMB performed, 74.3% had not undergone any form of treatment within 90 days, 15.0% had thermal ablation, and only 10.7% underwent surgery [60]. For patients that do proceed with surgery, RMB also appears to significantly decrease the benign resection rate at both the institutional (5% for routine-biopsy institutions vs. 16% for selective-biopsy institutions, $p < 0.001$) [151] and the individual (5.0% with biopsy vs. 13.5% without, $p = 0.01$) levels [59]. Halverson et al. developed a biopsy-directed management algorithm to assign patients with T1a masses to either treatment or surveillance, which was then retrospectively applied to 151 patients who had RMB followed by surgical resection [152]. In all 25 patients with favorable (benign or low-grade RCC) final pathology, the algorithm would have recommended active surveillance, avoiding unnecessary surgery. A follow-up study of 1175 partial nephrectomy cases found that the algorithm could have swayed management away from surgery in 52% of cases [153].

Active Surveillance

The Rationale for Active Surveillance

In 2024, the American Cancer Society estimated that 81,610 Americans would be diagnosed with kidney cancer and that 14,390 would die from it [154]. In comparison, the 2016 ACS estimates of kidney cancer incidence and mortality were 62,700 and 14,240, respectively [155]. These numbers reflect a pattern of RCC stage migration that has been occurring over the past several decades, with increasing use of cross-sectional imaging leading to increasing incidental detection of small renal masses. In 1993, stage I RCC was 43% of new kidney cancer diagnoses; in 2004, it was 57% [2]. By 2014, that proportion was 70% [3]. The estimated proportion of RCC discovered incidentally increased from 7–13% in the early 1970s to 48–66% in the late 2000s [156].

Incidental tumors are most commonly found in patients older than 65 years—a group more prone to the adverse effects of surgery due to the increased presence of comorbidities [51, 156]. A 2007 population-based study of 26,618 individuals who underwent surgery for kidney cancer found that nearly one-third of patients aged 70 years or older died of unrelated comorbid disease within 5 years of surgery [157]. For patients in this cohort treated for renal masses <4 cm, the 5-year disease-specific mortality was just 5%. Combined with natural history data showing that small renal masses rarely metastasize [31, 48], and are more often low-grade or benign [30, 33, 36], these findings suggest that many early-stage I RCCs are often clinically indolent and may not require upfront management.

Active surveillance (AS) is an approach to SRM management that centers around disease monitoring and delaying intervention until there is increased concern for progression or metastasis. Longitudinal cross-sectional imaging forms the core of AS, with the most common indications for the intervention being significant interval growth or reaching a target size threshold. Renal mass biopsy and symptom evaluation also factor into whether or not to continue surveillance. The goal of AS is to avoid treatment of benign or indolent SRMs while maintaining a window of opportunity for intervention for those that may harbor more aggressive cancers. AS should be distinguished from watchful waiting (WW), which similarly starts with nonintervention but is focused on treating symptoms as they arise rather than active monitoring to prevent disease progression.

Indications for Active Surveillance

Paramount to the evaluation of a patient with a newly diagnosed SRM is an assessment of the patient's comorbid conditions with the goal of stratifying the risk of treatment prior to choosing a treatment strategy. As with nephron-sparing surgery, reasons to elect for AS fall into absolute, relative, and elective indications. Patients with severe comorbidities in which surgical treatment would impart an immediate and unacceptable risk of mortality are considered to have an absolute indication for AS. Those with a second and potentially more aggressive malignancy, the potential need for renal replacement therapy, and other significant medical comorbidities that make surgery high-risk but not intolerable are considered to have relative indications for surveillance.

Elective indications include low-risk surgical candidates that choose to pursue AS as an alternative to active treatment. In a review of contemporary AS series, indications for surveillance were elective (60.9%), relative (12.5%), and absolute (26.6%) in the eight studies (*n* = 312 patients) reporting the reason for AS enrollment [31]. In general, patients who elect for AS over primary intervention tend to be older and with higher measures of comorbidity [158].

When patients are considering AS overactive treatment, in-depth counseling as to the limitations of radiologic surveillance and growth kinetics and the possibility of disease progression including metastases and death is critical. Patients must understand and accept the estimated risk of different outcomes due to the occasionally unpredictable behavior of RCC prior to proceeding with AS. Several calculators and nomograms have been developed to help quantify these risks. As previously described, the RENAL nephrometry score, when combined with patient age and sex, can be used to estimate the risk of renal mass malignancy and the risk of high-grade pathology if malignant (Fig. 8.2) [94]. Using this nomogram, an 80-year-old male with a nephrometry 7a mass has a 26% chance of malignancy and, if malignant, a 30% chance of it being high-grade. In contrast, an 80-year-old female with a nephrometry score of 9ah has a 92% of harboring cancer with a 59% chance of it being a high-grade disease if malignant. For more broader risk stratification, Kutikov et al. used SEER data to develop another nomogram incorporating race, gender, age, tumor size, and Charlson Comorbidity Index score to estimate the risk of death from kidney

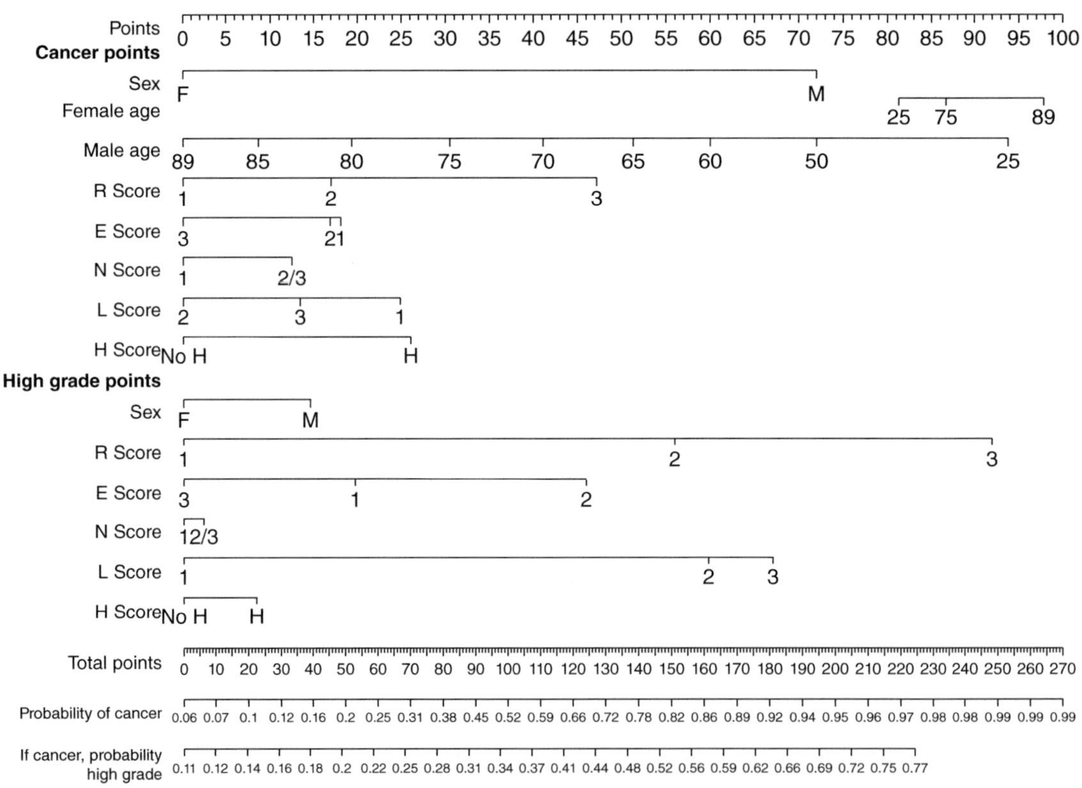

Fig. 8.2 Nomogram evaluating risks of an enhancing renal mass being malignant and high grade. Total point values are independently calculated for the cancer and the high-grade models and then applied to the corresponding probability scale at the bottom of the figure. (Modified from Kutikov et al. [94]; European Association of Urology by Elsevier, Inc.)

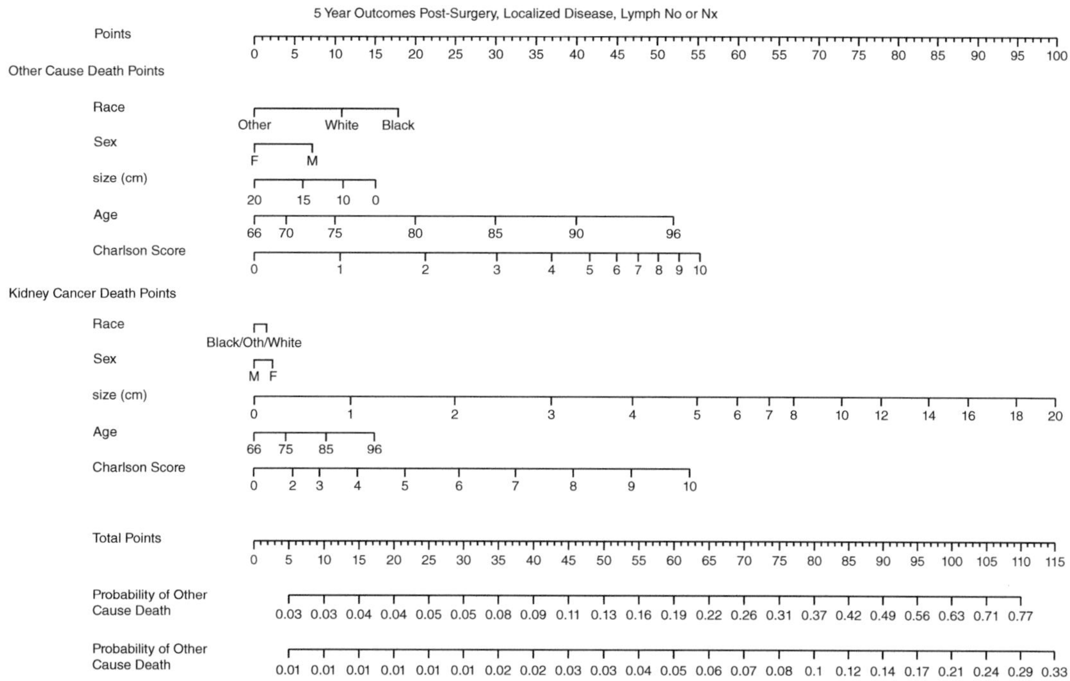

Fig. 8.3 Nomogram evaluating 5-year competing risks of death in patients with localized renal cell carcinoma. Total point values are independently calculated for each cause of death and then applied to the corresponding probability scale at the bottom of the figure. (Modified from Kutikov et al. [159]; American Urological Society by Elsevier, Inc.)

cancer versus the risk of death from other causes (Fig. 8.3) [159]. For those choosing between surgery and surveillance, the American College of Surgeons National Surgical Quality Improvement Program offers predictions of perioperative risk for a variety of surgical procedures through its website (risk calculator.facs.org), including for radical and partial nephrectomy [160]. Huynh et al. also published a partial nephrectomy-specific nomogram predicting the risk of major complications based on age, sex, and comorbidities [161]. Digital versions of these nomograms have been collated online and can be found at www.cancernomograms.com (except the ACS NSQIP calculator, which has its own website).

From a guidelines perspective, the AUA 2021 guidelines on localized renal cancer note that clinicians may recommend AS for solid renal masses <2 cm, or for complex but predominantly cystic renal masses [55]. The NCCN guidelines for kidney cancer present AS as an option for T1a and select T1b renal masses [162]. The EAU guidelines suggest offering AS to frail and/or comorbid patients with small renal masses [53].

Active Surveillance Protocols and Indications for Intervention

Currently, no randomized trials exist comparing the different AS protocols, or comparing AS with delayed intervention to upfront surgery or tumor ablation. Given the inherent unpredictability of RCC and the strong need for careful patient selection and close follow-up for AS, developing such randomized trials would require overcoming significant logistical, ethical, and methodological challenges. As such, after the decision is made to initiate AS, frequency of imaging, and reasons to intervene should be tailored to the patient health status, tolerance of risk, and disease characteristics.

From a guidelines perspective, the most recent EAU, NCCN, and AUA all recommend at least considering renal mass biopsy at the initiation of AS for additional risk stratification, recognizing its limitations in ruling out higher-risk disease [53–55]. All three also agree on using CT, MRI, or ultrasound for serial imaging. For imaging frequency, the AUA suggests every 3–6 months, while the NCCN recommends within 6 months of initiation and then annually afterward; the EAU does not specify a recommended interval. Only the AUA specifies potential triggers for change in management, those being an increase in tumor size >3 cm, stage progression, growth >5 mm/year, new biopsy results suggesting higher-risk disease, and clinical changes in patient/tumor factors [55].

Our recommendation is a risk-adapted approach with indications for treatment similar to that of the AUA guidelines (Fig. 8.4) [163]. Initial surveillance imaging is obtained at 3- to 6-month

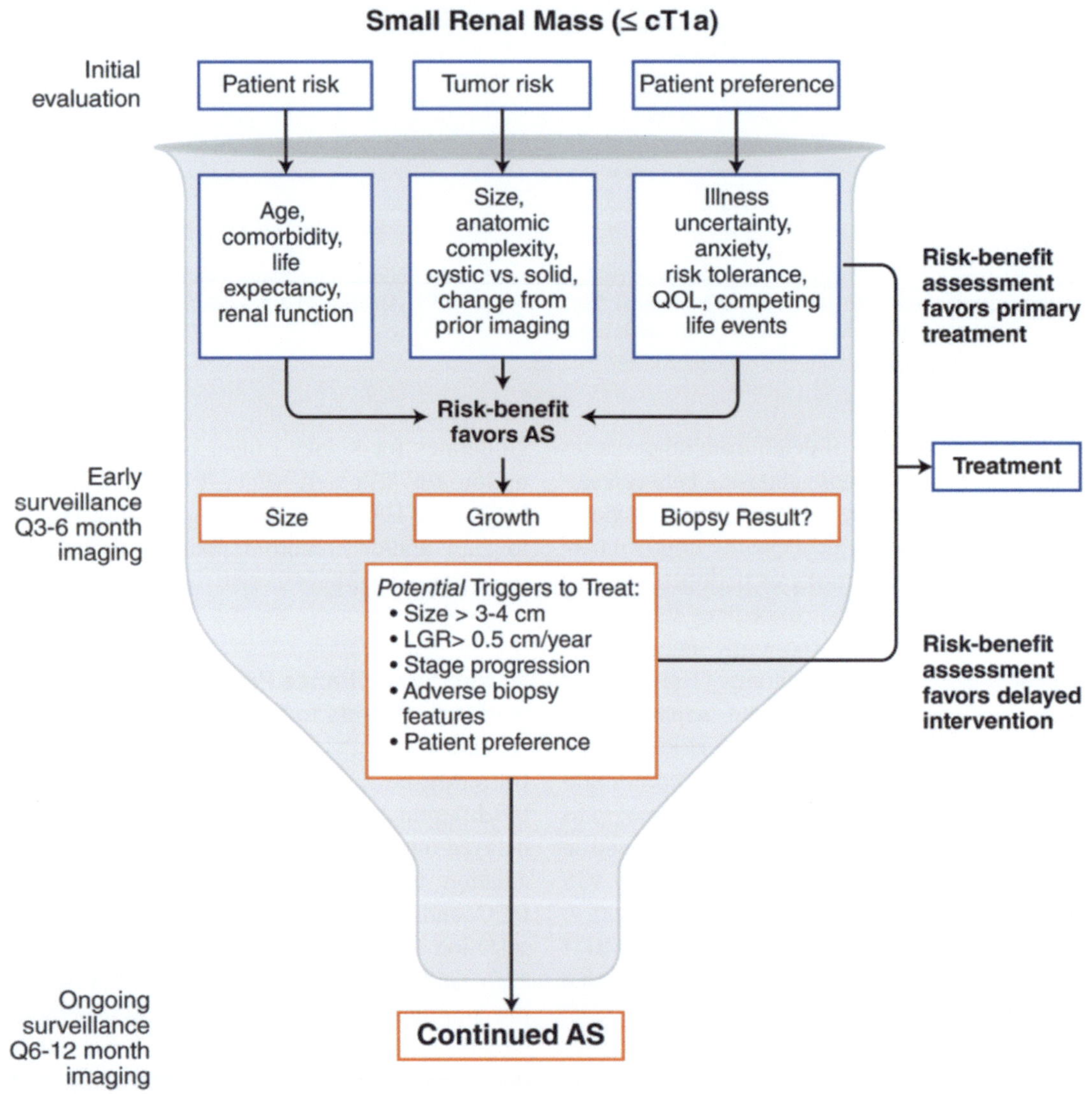

Fig. 8.4 Shared decision-making model for patients with SRMs on active surveillance. *QOL* quality of life, *AS* active surveillance, *LGR* linear growth rate. (Modified from Ristau et al. [163])

intervals following the start of AS with the goal of establishing baseline growth kinetics. Tumors demonstrating short-term stability can have subsequent imaging studies spaced further out, while those with accelerated growth may be placed on a more frequent surveillance schedule or proceed to intervention. Renal mass biopsy can be utilized for initial risk stratification or for further evaluation if intervention is being considered. Tumor size comparisons should be performed using the same lesion characteristics (e.g., maximum tumor diameter or estimated tumor volume) obtained from consistent imaging modalities measured at the same tumor level [14]. Potential triggers for treatment are based on the natural history data reviewed at the start of this chapter and include growth to >3–4 cm, growth rate > 0.5 cm/year, stage progression, new symptoms, or biopsy findings indicating adverse pathology. When these potential triggers are discovered, it is critical that patients are appropriately counseled regarding the risks of continued AS versus immediate intervention.

Outcomes of Active Surveillance

When examining the data for active surveillance, the primary measures of concern are growth rate, likelihood of delayed intervention, oncologic outcomes, and functional outcomes. To date, no randomized controlled trials have compared active surveillance to primary intervention, and the majority of published AS series have been retrospective in nature. However, data from two prospective studies have also been reported: the Renal Cell Carcinoma Consortium of Canada (RCCCC) cohort and the Delayed Intervention and Surveillance for Small Renal Masses (DISSRM) registry. The RCCCC study was a phase 2 trial of initial AS with treatment delayed until disease progression, with 178 patients (209 SRMs) enrolled across eight sites [164]. Notably, all patients in this cohort underwent percutaneous renal mass biopsy prior to surveillance. The DISSRM registry is an ongoing multi-institutional, prospectively maintained database started in 2009 tracking the disease characteristics and outcomes of adults with SRMs ≤4 cm [158]. Patients enrolled in this registry are offered primary intervention (PI) versus AS for their SRMs per standard of care and followed longitudinally.

Growth Rate

In pooled analyses of retrospective series, the average linear growth rate of small renal masses during AS is approximately 0.3 cm/year, with estimates ranging from 0.06 to 0.86 cm/year, depending on the study [31, 48, 163]. In the largest retrospective series published to date, McIntosh et al. reported on AS data from 457 patients (544 masses) with a median follow-up of 67 months and found the median growth rate to be 0.19 cm/year [27]. From the prospective series, the mean linear growth rate during AS was 0.13 cm/year in the RCCCC cohort and 0.09 cm/year in the DISSRM cohort [26, 164]. The DISSRM data also showed that the average tumor growth rate significantly decreases once fast-growing masses are selected out for intervention: Average tumor growth rate decreased from 0.54 cm/year for masses under surveillance for <180 days to 0.03 cm/year for masses surveilled for >180 days.

Delayed Intervention

Gupta et al. conducted a pooled analysis of 1245 patients from 14 active surveillance series (including the initial data from the RCCC and DISSRM cohorts), specifically examining the rates and timing of patients undergoing delayed intervention [165]. 34% of all patients underwent delayed intervention, with an average time on surveillance of 28 ± 11 months. Patients undergoing delayed intervention were generally younger (average 64 vs. 72 years old) and had more rapidly-growing tumors (average 0.70 cm/year vs. 0.28 cm/year). Triggers for intervention were tumor growth rate in 41%, patient/physician preference in 52%, and symptomatic progression in the rest. Of those undergoing intervention, 30% underwent radical nephrectomy, and 70% underwent partial nephrectomy or thermal ablation.

Oncologic Outcomes

Risk of Metastasis

Fortunately, progression to metastatic disease during active surveillance is rare. Of 880 patients with SRMs under AS identified in a systematic review, only 18 (2.0%) patients progressed to metastatic disease [31]. The mean time to detection of metastasis was 40.2 months (range 12–132 months), supporting the safety of an initial period of active surveillance to determine growth kinetics. The same study compared patients who progressed to metastatic disease to those who did not, and found that progressors were significantly older and had larger tumors that demonstrated more rapid growth (Table 8.4). In the RCCCC cohort, only 2 of 178 patients (1.1%) progressed to metastatic disease at a median follow-up of 29 months [164]. In the DISSRM cohort, 0 of 244 patients on surveillance developed metastatic disease at a median follow-up of 25 months [158].

Approximately 20–40% of masses under active surveillance exhibit zero or negative net growth [26, 27, 31, 44, 164]. While these tumors do not have a significantly lower risk of malignancy compared to those that demonstrate interval growth, their risk of metastasis is virtually zero [31]. Additionally, data from the DISSRM registry showed that about 5% of small renal masses "disappear" on follow-up imaging while on active surveillance [166]. About half reappear on subsequent imaging. These masses tend to be small (<1 cm) and have excellent overall prognosis with 100% survival at 5 years.

Survival and Mortality

Following the low rate of metastatic disease, cancer-specific survival (CSS) for patients on active surveillance is excellent. In retrospective series, reported CSS rates in short-term follow-up (typically 2–4 years) range from 92 to 100%, with the majority of studies reporting no cancer-related deaths [163]. However, overall survival (OS) rates in the same series range from 43–97%, highlighting the average greater age and comorbidity of patients electing for AS but also the significant heterogeneity of this patient population. In a study specifically focusing on older patients (≥75 years), AS was not associated with lower overall survival compared to active treatment [167].

The best long-term oncologic outcomes data for AS come from the DISSRM registry, which also provides comparisons between AS and primary intervention: At 5 years, cancer-specific survival for AS ($n = 244$) versus PI ($n = 274$) was 100% and 99% ($p = 0.003$) and overall survival was 92% and 85% ($p = 0.06$), respectively [158]. In the AS cohort, 14% of patients experienced tumor growth >0.5 cm/year, 0.8% had growth to >4 cm, 0 developed metastatic disease, and 8.5% underwent delayed intervention. Overall progression-free survival at 5 years was 67%. At 7 years, CSS for AS was 100% and no different ($p = 0.5$) from partial nephrectomy (98.8%), radical nephrectomy (100%), or ablation (100%) [168]. OS for AS was 66.1% and significantly lower ($p = 0.005$) than that of partial nephrectomy (87.9%), radical nephrectomy (90.2%), or ablation (83.5%). Recently presented 15-year data on 377 PI and 581 AS patients reported a delayed intervention rate of 15% with no difference in recurrence-free survival between DI and PI ($p = 0.24$). At 12 years, CSS for AS versus PI was 99.8% versus 99.3% ($p = 0.43$), and OS was 57.9% versus 41.6% ($p < 0.001$) [169].

Other Outcomes

Renal Function

One of the primary benefits of surveillance over primary intervention is avoidance of renal function loss. Lane et al. retrospectively reviewed renal function outcomes by management strategy in 537 patients ≥75 years [167]. As expected, the median estimated GFR loss was lower on AS compared after nephron-sparing intervention or radical nephrectomy (0 vs. 18 vs. 34 mL/min/1.73 m^2, respectively, $p < 0.0001$). Rate of CKD ≥3 was also lower with AS versus other interventions (59 vs 69 vs 86% respectively, $p < 0.0001$). Two other studies compared renal functional outcomes AS versus intervention using data from the patients in the DISSRM registry. One found that patients undergoing radical

Table 8.4 Comparison of clinical and cross-sectional imaging characteristics in patients who did not progress to metastasis (pooled cohort series data) and patients who demonstrated evidence of progression (case series data) during periods of observation

	Nonprogressors		Progressors		
Characteristic	No.	Mean ± SD: median (range)	No.	Mean ± SD: median (range)	*P*
Age (year)	230	66. ± 12.3: 69 (35–88)	9	75.1 ± 9.1: 78.0 (54. 0–84.0)	0.03
Initial MTD (cm)	281	2.3 ± 1.3: 2.0 (0.2–12.0)	16	4.3 ± 2.1: 3.1 (2.0–8.8)	<0.001
Initial ETV (cm^3)	281	15.1 ± 60.3: 4.3 (0.004–903.7)	16	66.3 ± 100.0: 15.2 (4.3–363.0)	<0.001
Final MTD (cm)	249	3.0 ± 1.6: 2.7 (0.9–15.0)	14	5.9 ± 2.1: 5.9 (3.1–10.7)	<0.001
Final ETV (cm^3)	281	29.0 ± 109.8: 10.3 (0.3–1765.1)	14	132.1 ± 170.9: 87.9 (13.4–653.0)	<0.001
Linear growth rate (cm/year)	249	0.4 ± 0.3: 0.25 (−1.4–2.47)	13	0.80 ± 0.7: 0.65 (0.1–2.72)	<0.001
Volumetric growth rate (cm^3/year)	281	6.2 ± 27.5: 1.6 (−20.0–430.7)	14	27.1 ± 24.9: 19.1 (4.8–84.4)	<0.001
Time under AS (months)	281	33.3 ± 22.6: 27.0 (5.3–156.0)	17	40.2 ± 31.2: 29.0 (9.0–132.0)	0.47

Reproduced from Smaldone et al. [31]
AS active surveillance, *ETV* estimated tumor volume, *MTD* maximum linear tumor dimension, *SD* standard deviation

nephrectomy had a higher average eGFR change (−9.2 vs. −0.5 ml/min/1.73 m^2, $p = 0.001$) and rate of CKD upstaging (40% vs. 16%, $p = 0.007$) compared to AS [170]. The authors did not find any differences in renal outcomes comparing AS to partial nephrectomy or thermal ablation. The other similarly found no differences in eGFR change between AS, partial nephrectomy, or ablation, all of which were superior to radical nephrectomy [168].

Quality of Life

As previously noted, over half of patients crossing over from active surveillance to treatment do so out of personal or physician preference as opposed to disease progression. Goldberg et al. reviewed their institutional database of 477 patients with SRMs who completed a validated cancer symptom questionnaire over the course of their disease management [171]. In general, patients on AS had similar psychological distress subscores compared to those managed with surgery or ablation, with one exception: following renal mass biopsy showing malignancy, patients who continued on AS experienced significantly higher psychological distress than those who underwent intervention. Patients enrolled in the DISSRM registry were also asked to regularly complete a different quality of life questionnaire that separately measured physical and mental well-being [168, 172]. Patients in the AS cohort were found to have significantly lower physical component subscores compared to those treated with partial nephrectomy up to 5 years of follow-up. No differences were seen between AS and any form of primary intervention in the mental well-being subscores.

Cost-Effectiveness

Cost of care has become an increasingly important consideration in clinical decision-making, especially when intervention may not significantly alter disease trajectory. Using a hypothetical case of an SRM in a healthy 65-year-old male to evaluate the cost-effectiveness of various nephron-sparing treatment approaches, Chang et al. found that immediate laparoscopic partial nephrectomy was the most cost-effective approach with an incremental cost-effectiveness ratio of $36,645 per quality-adjusted life-year (QALY) gained [173]. It should be noted that laparoscopic partial nephrectomy has largely been supplanted by the more expensive robotic-assisted approach and that addition of an initial period of surveillance decreased total costs of management by $7679–$12,430 while decreasing total QALYs by only 0.07–0.23 years. Heilbrun et al. analyzed different management strategies in a hypothetical cohort of 60-year-old healthy men with 2 cm renal masses [174]. Like the previous study, AS, percutaneous biopsy, and immediate treatment all provided very close benefits in terms of total QALYs (10.97 vs. 11.45 vs. 11.08, respectively) but had notable differences in estimated cost ($33k vs. $49.5k vs. $41.4k, respectively). An inherent limitation to all decision analytic models is that they are limited by the data used to develop them. With data on surveillance and ablation strategies limited to short- and intermediate-term follow-up, estimates of lifetime costs and treatment effects should be viewed with caution.

Conclusion

Incidental detection of small, clinically localized renal masses <4 cm (SRMs) has risen dramatically over the last several decades, in part due to the increased utilization of cross-sectional imaging. These masses present a unique clinical challenge in terms of diagnosis and management. While up to 80–85% are malignant, they tend to grow slowly—on average 0.3 cm/year, with 20–40% staying the same size or even shrinking over time. The risk of malignancy and high-grade pathology increases with tumor size and growth rate, but no single metric accurately distinguishes between benign and malignant masses. The overall risk of developing metastatic disease is low and virtually zero in masses that do not demonstrate interval growth.

Evaluation of small renal masses focuses on the question of tumor histology and behavior. Outside of surgical excision, no single imaging study, laboratory test, or procedure can predict tumor histology with diagnostic accuracy. Contrast-enhanced multiphase CT or MRI are first-line imaging for SRMs and provide good initial characterization and risk stratification, especially for masses that are cystic or those with diagnostic imaging features such as AMLs. However, they struggle to reliably differentiate between oncocytoma and RCC and between different RCC histologies. Predictive models and classification systems such as the Bosniak scale and RENAL nephrometry score have been created to augment the diagnostic accuracy of CT and MRI. Contrast-enhanced ultrasound and nuclear medicine imaging tests are newer modalities that can help noninvasively answer specific questions about SRMs but have not yet achieved broader adoption for a variety of reasons.

Renal mass biopsy is an important tool in the evaluation of SRMs, bringing greater diagnostic accuracy than noninvasive imaging but with less comorbidity than surgical excision. Using modern large-bore coaxial core needle biopsy techniques, RMB has greater than 95% sensitivity, specificity, and positive predictive value for differentiating between benign and malignant masses. It is hindered by a low (~15%) rate of nondiagnostic biopsy and tumor under-grading, as well as by a low negative predictive value of 70–80%. Cystic masses and hybrid tumors are also not well-evaluated by biopsy. Strategies to increase the diagnostic accuracy of RMB include repeat biopsy, addition of fine needle aspiration, and on-site pathologic evaluation. However, these add additional cost and complexity to the procedure and may be challenging to implement logistically.

Though SRM detection rates have increased over the years, mortality from kidney cancer has not, implying that many of these incidentally discovered masses are indolent tumors that may not require or benefit from immediate intervention. Active surveillance is an approach to SRM management focused on separating tumors requiring upfront intervention from those that do not. It starts with a period of initial monitoring to establish tumor growth kinetics, potentially augmented by renal mass biopsy. This is then followed by scheduled interval imaging that is gradually spaced out until indicators of aggressive pathology appear, at which point definitive treatment may be pursued or until the patient decides to stop surveillance. Long-term data are now available showing that active surveillance is oncologically safe while allowing for the preservation of renal function and avoiding the morbidity of intervention in a subset of patients. It has become a cornerstone of management for small renal masses alongside thermal ablation, partial nephrectomy, and radical nephrectomy.

References

1. Amin MB, Greene FL, Edge SB, et al. The eighth edition AJCC cancer staging manual: continuing to build a bridge from a population-based to a more "personalized" approach to cancer staging. CA Cancer J Clin. 2017;67(2):93–9. https://doi.org/10.3322/caac.21388.
2. Kane CJ, Mallin K, Ritchey J, Cooperberg MR, Carroll PR. Renal cell cancer stage migration: analysis of the National Cancer Data Base. Cancer. 2008;113(1):78–83. https://doi.org/10.1002/cncr.23518.
3. Patel HD, Gupta M, Joice GA, et al. Clinical stage migration and survival for renal cell carcinoma in the United States. Eur Urol Oncol. 2019;2(4):343–8. https://doi.org/10.1016/j.euo.2018.08.023.
4. Bukavina L, Bensalah K, Bray F, et al. Epidemiology of renal cell carcinoma: 2022 update. Eur Urol. 2022;82(5):529–42. https://doi.org/10.1016/j.eururo.2022.08.019.
5. Partin AW, Mangold LA, Lamm DM, Walsh PC, Epstein JI, Pearson JD. Contemporary update of prostate cancer staging nomograms (Partin tables) for the new millennium. Urology. 2001;58(6):843–8. https://doi.org/10.1016/S0090-4295(01)01441-8.
6. Cooperberg MR, Carroll PR, Klotz L. Active surveillance for prostate cancer: progress and promise. J Clin Oncol. 2011;29(27):3669–76. https://doi.org/10.1200/JCO.2011.34.9738.
7. Bosniak MA, Birnbaum BA, Krinsky GA, Waisman J. Small renal parenchymal neoplasms: further observations on growth. Radiology. 1995;197(3):589–97. https://doi.org/10.1148/radiology.197.3.7480724.
8. Fujimoto N, Sugita A, Terasawa Y, Kato M. Observations on the growth rate of renal cell carcinoma. Int J Urol. 1995;2(2):71–6. https://doi.org/10.1111/j.1442-2042.1995.tb00427.x.
9. Kato M, Suzuki T, Suzuki Y, Terasawa Y, Sasano H, Arai Y. Natural history of small renal cell carcinoma: evaluation of growth rate, histological grade, cell proliferation and apoptosis. J Urol.

2004;172(3):863–6. https://doi.org/10.1097/01.ju.0000136315.80057.99.
10. Oda T, Miyao N, Takahashi A, et al. Growth rates of primary and metastatic lesions of renal cell carcinoma. Int J Urol. 2001;8(9):473–7. https://doi.org/10.1046/j.1442-2042.2001.00353.x.
11. Abou Youssif T, Kassouf W, Steinberg J, Aprikian AG, Laplante MP, Tanguay S. Active surveillance for selected patients with renal masses: updated results with long-term follow-up. Cancer. 2007;110(5):1010–4. https://doi.org/10.1002/cncr.22871.
12. Abouassaly R, Lane BR, Novick AC. Active surveillance of renal masses in elderly patients. J Urol. 2008;180(2):505–9. https://doi.org/10.1016/j.juro.2008.04.033.
13. Beisland C, Hjelle KM, Reisæter LAR, Bostad L. Observation should be considered as an alternative in management of renal masses in older and comorbid patients. Eur Urol. 2009;55(6):1419–29. https://doi.org/10.1016/j.eururo.2008.12.031.
14. Crispen PL, Viterbo R, Boorjian SA, Greenberg RE, Chen DYT, Uzzo RG. Natural history, growth kinetics and outcomes of untreated clinically localized renal tumors under active surveillance. Cancer. 2009;115(13):2844–52. https://doi.org/10.1002/cncr.24338.
15. Fernando HS, Duvuru S, Hawkyard SJ. Conservative management of renal masses in the elderly: our experience. Int Urol Nephrol. 2007;39(1):203–7.
16. Kouba E, Smith A, McRackan D, Wallen EM, Pruthi RS. Watchful waiting for solid renal masses: insight into the natural history and results of delayed intervention. J Urol. 2007;177(2):466–70. https://doi.org/10.1016/j.juro.2006.09.064.
17. Lamb GWA, Bromwich EJ, Vasey P, Aitchison M. Management of renal masses in patients medically unsuitable for nephrectomy—natural history, complications, and outcome. Urology. 2004;64(5):909–13. https://doi.org/10.1016/j.urology.2004.05.039.
18. Matsuzaki M, Kawano Y, Morikawa H, Shiga Y, Murata H, Komatsu H. Conservative management of small renal tumors. Hinyokika Kiyo. 2007;53(4):207–11.
19. Rosales JC, Haramis G, Moreno J, et al. Active surveillance for renal cortical neoplasms. J Urol. 2010;183(5):1698–702. https://doi.org/10.1016/j.juro.2010.01.024.
20. Siu W, Hafez KS, Johnston WK, Wolf JS. Growth rates of renal cell carcinoma and oncocytoma under surveillance are similar. Urol Oncol Semin Orig Investig. 2007;25(2):115–9. https://doi.org/10.1016/j.urolonc.2006.07.018.
21. Sowery RD, Siemens DR. Growth characteristics of renal cortical tumors in patients managed by watchful waiting. Can J Urol. 2004;11(5):2407–10.
22. Volpe A, Panzarella T, Rendon RA, Haider MA, Kondylis FI, Jewett MAS. The natural history of incidentally detected small renal masses. Cancer. 2004;100(4):738–45. https://doi.org/10.1002/cncr.20025.
23. Wehle MJ, Thiel DD, Petrou SP, Young PR, Frank I, Karsteadt N. Conservative management of incidental contrast-enhancing renal masses as safe alternative to invasive therapy. Urology. 2004;64(1):49–52. https://doi.org/10.1016/j.urology.2004.02.026.
24. Wong JA, Rendon RA. Progression to metastatic disease from a small renal cell carcinoma prospectively followed with an active surveillance protocol. Can Urol Assoc J. 2007;1(2):120–2.
25. Organ M, Jewett M, Basiuk J, et al. Growth kinetics of small renal masses: a prospective analysis from the renal cell carcinoma consortium of Canada. Can Urol Assoc J. 2014;8(1–2):24–7. https://doi.org/10.5489/cuaj.1483.
26. Uzosike AC, Patel HD, Alam R, et al. Growth kinetics of small renal masses on active surveillance: variability and results from the DISSRM registry. J Urol. 2018;199(3):641–8. https://doi.org/10.1016/j.juro.2017.09.087.
27. McIntosh AG, Ristau BT, Ruth K, et al. Active surveillance for localized renal masses: tumor growth, delayed intervention rates, and >5-yr clinical outcomes. Eur Urol. 2018;74(2):157–64. https://doi.org/10.1016/j.eururo.2018.03.011.
28. Kutikov A, Fossett LK, Ramchandani P, et al. Incidence of benign pathologic findings at partial nephrectomy for solitary renal mass presumed to be renal cell carcinoma on preoperative imaging. Urology. 2006;68(4):737–40. https://doi.org/10.1016/j.urology.2006.04.011.
29. Lane BR, Babineau D, Kattan MW, et al. A preoperative prognostic nomogram for solid enhancing renal tumors 7 cm or less amenable to partial nephrectomy. J Urol. 2007;178(2):429–34. https://doi.org/10.1016/j.juro.2007.03.106.
30. Corcoran AT, Russo P, Lowrance WT, et al. A review of contemporary data on surgically resected renal masses—benign or malignant? Urology. 2013;81(4):707–13. https://doi.org/10.1016/j.urology.2013.01.009.
31. Smaldone MC, Kutikov A, Egleston BL, et al. Small renal masses progressing to metastases under active surveillance. Cancer. 2012;118(4):997–1006. https://doi.org/10.1002/cncr.26369.
32. Pahernik S, Ziegler S, Roos F, Melchior SW, Thüroff JW. Small renal tumors: correlation of clinical and pathological features with tumor size. J Urol. 2007;178(2):414–7. https://doi.org/10.1016/j.juro.2007.03.129.
33. Frank I, Blute ML, Cheville JC, Lohse CM, Weaver AL, Zincke H. Solid renal tumors: an analysis of pathological features related to tumor size. J Urol. 2003;170:2217–20. https://doi.org/10.1097/01.ju.0000095475.12515.5e.
34. Pierorazio PM, Patel HD, Johnson MH, et al. Distinguishing malignant and benign renal masses with composite models and nomograms: a systematic review and meta-analysis of clinically localized

renal masses suspicious for malignancy. Cancer. 2016;122(21):3267–76. https://doi.org/10.1002/cncr.30268.

35. Hunt JD, van der Hel OL, McMillan GP, Boffetta P, Brennan P. Renal cell carcinoma in relation to cigarette smoking: meta-analysis of 24 studies. Int J Cancer. 2005;114(1):101–8. https://doi.org/10.1002/ijc.20618.
36. Thompson RH, Kurta JM, Kaag M, et al. Tumor size is associated with malignant potential in renal cell carcinoma cases. J Urol. 2009;181(5):2033–6. https://doi.org/10.1016/j.juro.2009.01.027.
37. Ball MW, Gorin MA, Bhayani SB, et al. Preoperative predictors of malignancy and unfavorable pathology for clinical T1a tumors treated with partial nephrectomy: a multi-institutional analysis. Urol Oncol Semin Orig Investig. 2015;33(3):112.e9–112.e14. https://doi.org/10.1016/j.urolonc.2014.11.003.
38. Johnson DC, Vukina J, Smith AB, et al. Preoperatively misclassified, surgically removed benign renal masses: a systematic review of surgical series and United States population level burden estimate. J Urol. 2015;193(1):30–5. https://doi.org/10.1016/j.juro.2014.07.102.
39. Remzi M, Özsoy M, Klingler HC, et al. Are small renal tumors harmless? Analysis of histopathological features according to tumors 4 cm or less in diameter. J Urol. 2006;176(3):896–9. https://doi.org/10.1016/j.juro.2006.04.047.
40. Rothman J, Egleston B, Wong YN, Iffrig K, Lebovitch S, Uzzo RG. Histopathological characteristics of localized renal cell carcinoma correlate with tumor size: a SEER analysis. J Urol. 2009;181(1):29–34. https://doi.org/10.1016/j.juro.2008.09.009.
41. Kunkle DA, Crispen PL, Li T, Uzzo RG. Tumor size predicts synchronous metastatic renal cell carcinoma: implications for surveillance of small renal masses. J Urol. 2007;177(5):1692–7. https://doi.org/10.1016/j.juro.2007.01.029.
42. Lee H, Lee JK, Kim K, et al. Risk of metastasis for T1a renal cell carcinoma. World J Urol. 2016;34(4):553–9. https://doi.org/10.1007/s00345-015-1659-4.
43. Lughezzani G, Jeldres C, Isbarn H, et al. Tumor size is a determinant of the rate of stage T1 renal cell cancer synchronous metastasis. J Urol. 2009;182(4):1287–93. https://doi.org/10.1016/j.juro.2009.06.018.
44. Kunkle DA, Crispen PL, Chen DYT, Greenberg RE, Uzzo RG. Enhancing renal masses with zero net growth during active surveillance. J Urol. 2007;177(3):849–54. https://doi.org/10.1016/j.juro.2006.10.073.
45. Kawaguchi S, Fernandes KA, Finelli A, Robinette M, Fleshner N, Jewett MAS. Most renal oncocytomas appear to grow: observations of tumor kinetics with active surveillance. J Urol. 2011;186(4):1218–22. https://doi.org/10.1016/j.juro.2011.05.080.
46. Finelli A, Cheung DC, Al-Matar A, et al. Small renal mass surveillance: histology-specific growth rates in a biopsy-characterized cohort. Eur Urol. 2020;78(3):460–7. https://doi.org/10.1016/j.eururo.2020.06.053.
47. Kassouf W, Aprikian AG, Laplante M, Tanguay S. Natural history of renal masses followed expectantly. J Urol. 2004;171(1):111–3. https://doi.org/10.1097/01.ju.0000102409.69570.f5.
48. Chawla SN, Crispen PL, Hanlon AL, Greenberg RE, Chen DYT, Uzzo RG. The natural history of observed enhancing renal masses: meta-analysis and review of the world literature. J Urol. 2006;175(2):425–31. https://doi.org/10.1016/S0022-5347(05)00148-5.
49. Turner RM, Morgan TM, Jacobs BL. Epidemiology of the small renal mass and the treatment disconnect phenomenon. Urol Clin North Am. 2017;44(2):147–54. https://doi.org/10.1016/j.ucl.2016.12.001.
50. Hollingsworth JM, Miller DC, Daignault S, Hollenbeck BK. Rising incidence of small renal masses: a need to reassess treatment effect. JNCI J Natl Cancer Inst. 2006;98(18):1331–4. https://doi.org/10.1093/jnci/djj362.
51. Saad AM, Gad MM, Al-Husseini MJ, Ruhban IA, Sonbol MB, Ho TH. Trends in renal-cell carcinoma incidence and mortality in the United States in the last 2 decades: a SEER-based study. Clin Genitourin Cancer. 2019;17(1):46–57. https://doi.org/10.1016/j.clgc.2018.10.002.
52. Campbell SC, Uzzo RG, Karam JA, Chang SS, Clark PE, Souter L. Renal mass and localized renal cancer: evaluation, management, and follow-up: AUA guideline: part II. J Urol. 2021;206(2):209–18. https://doi.org/10.1097/JU.0000000000001912.
53. Ljungberg B, Bex A, Albiges L, et al. EAU guidelines on RCC. Uroweb - European Association of Urology 2024. https://uroweb.org/guidelines/renal-cell-carcinoma. Accessed 27 August 2024.
54. Motzer RJ, Jonasch E, Agarwal N, et al. Kidney cancer, version 3.2022, NCCN clinical practice guidelines in oncology. J Natl Compr Cancer Netw. 2022;20(1):71–90. https://doi.org/10.6004/jnccn.2022.0001.
55. Campbell SC, Clark PE, Chang SS, Karam JA, Souter L, Uzzo RG. Renal mass and localized renal cancer: evaluation, management, and follow-up: AUA guideline: part I. J Urol. 2021;206(2):199–208. https://doi.org/10.1097/JU.0000000000001911.
56. Kay FU, Canvasser NE, Xi Y, et al. Diagnostic performance and interreader agreement of a standardized MR imaging approach in the prediction of small renal mass histology. Radiology. 2018;287(2):543–53. https://doi.org/10.1148/radiol.2018171557.
57. Choudhary S, Rajesh A, Mayer NJ, Mulcahy KA, Haroon A. Renal oncocytoma: CT features cannot reliably distinguish oncocytoma from other renal neoplasms. Clin Radiol. 2009;64(5):517–22. https://doi.org/10.1016/j.crad.2008.12.011.
58. Patel DN, Ghali F, Meagher MF, et al. Utilization of renal mass biopsy in patients with localized renal cell

carcinoma: a population-based study utilizing the National Cancer Database. Urol Oncol Semin Orig Investig. 2021;39(1):79. https://doi.org/10.1016/j.urolonc.2020.10.015.
59. Patel AK, Lane BR, Chintalapati P, et al. Utilization of renal mass biopsy for T1 renal lesions across Michigan: results from music-kidney, a statewide quality improvement collaborative. Eur Urol Open Sci. 2021;30:37–43. https://doi.org/10.1016/j.euros.2021.06.004.
60. Ozambela M, Wang Y, Leow JJ, Silverman SG, Chung BI, Chang SL. Contemporary trends in percutaneous renal mass biopsy utilization in the United States. Urol Oncol Semin Orig Investig. 2020;38(11):835–43. https://doi.org/10.1016/j.urolonc.2020.07.022.
61. Wang ZJ, Nikolaidis P, Khatri G, et al. ACR Appropriateness criteria® indeterminate renal mass. J Am Coll Radiol. 2020;17(11):S415–28. https://doi.org/10.1016/j.jacr.2020.09.010.
62. Wang ZJ, Westphalen AC, Zagoria RJ. CT and MRI of small renal masses. Br J Radiol. 2018;2018:20180131. https://doi.org/10.1259/bjr.20180131.
63. Sasaguri K, Takahashi N. CT and MR imaging for solid renal mass characterization. Eur J Radiol. 2018;99:40–54. https://doi.org/10.1016/j.ejrad.2017.12.008.
64. Silverman SG, Pedrosa I, Ellis JH, et al. Bosniak classification of cystic renal masses, version 2019: an update proposal and needs assessment. Radiology. 2019;292(2):475–88. https://doi.org/10.1148/radiol.2019182646.
65. Krishna S, Murray CA, McInnes MD, et al. CT imaging of solid renal masses: pitfalls and solutions. Clin Radiol. 2017;72(9):708–21. https://doi.org/10.1016/j.crad.2017.05.003.
66. Davarpanah AH, Spektor M, Mathur M, Israel GM. Homogeneous T1 hyperintense renal lesions with smooth borders: is contrast-enhanced MR imaging needed? Radiology. 2016;280(1):128–36. https://doi.org/10.1148/radiol.16151240.
67. Jonisch AI, Rubinowitz AN, Mutalik PG, Israel GM. Can high-attenuation renal cysts be differentiated from renal cell carcinoma at unenhanced CT? Radiology. 2007;243(2):445–50. https://doi.org/10.1148/radiol.2432060559.
68. Flum AS, Hamoui N, Said MA, et al. Update on the diagnosis and management of renal angiomyolipoma. J Urol. 2016;195(4):834–46. https://doi.org/10.1016/j.juro.2015.07.126.
69. Davenport MS, Neville AM, Ellis JH, Cohan RH, Chaudhry HS, Leder RA. Diagnosis of renal angiomyolipoma with hounsfield unit thresholds: effect of size of region of interest and nephrographic phase imaging. Radiology. 2011;260(1):158–65. https://doi.org/10.1148/radiol.11102476.
70. Farrell C, Noyes SL, Tourojman M, Lane BR. Renal angiomyolipoma: preoperative identification of atypical fat-poor AML. Curr Urol Rep. 2015;16(3):12. https://doi.org/10.1007/s11934-015-0484-z.
71. Jeong IG, Khandwala YS, Kim JH, et al. Association of robotic-assisted vs laparoscopic radical nephrectomy with perioperative outcomes and health care costs, 2003 to 2015. JAMA. 2017;318(16):1561–8. https://doi.org/10.1001/jama.2017.14586.
72. Schieda N, Al-Subhi M, Flood TA, El-Khodary M, McInnes MDF. Diagnostic accuracy of segmental enhancement inversion for the diagnosis of renal oncocytoma using biphasic computed tomography (CT) and multiphase contrast-enhanced magnetic resonance imaging (MRI). Eur Radiol. 2014;24(11):2787–94. https://doi.org/10.1007/s00330-014-3310-y.
73. Amin J, Xu B, Badkhshan S, et al. Identification and validation of radiographic enhancement for reliable differentiation of CD117(+) benign renal oncocytoma and chromophobe renal cell carcinoma. Clin Cancer Res. 2018;24(16):3898–907. https://doi.org/10.1158/1078-0432.CCR-18-0252.
74. Lee-Felker SA, Felker ER, Tan N, et al. Qualitative and quantitative MDCT features for differentiating clear cell renal cell carcinoma from other solid renal cortical masses. Am J Roentgenol. 2014;203(5):W516–24. https://doi.org/10.2214/AJR.14.12460.
75. Young JR, Coy H, Kim HJ, et al. Performance of relative enhancement on multiphasic MRI for the differentiation of clear cell renal cell carcinoma (RCC) from papillary and chromophobe RCC subtypes and oncocytoma. Am J Roentgenol. 2017;208(4):812–9. https://doi.org/10.2214/AJR.16.17152.
76. Coy H, Young JR, Douek ML, et al. Association of qualitative and quantitative imaging features on multiphasic multidetector CT with tumor grade in clear cell renal cell carcinoma. Abdom Radiol. 2019;44(1):180–9. https://doi.org/10.1007/s00261-018-1688-8.
77. Zhu YH, Wang X, Zhang J, Chen YH, Kong W, Huang YR. Low enhancement on multiphase contrast-enhanced CT images: an independent predictor of the presence of high tumor grade of clear cell renal cell carcinoma. Am J Roentgenol. 2014;203(3):W295–300. https://doi.org/10.2214/AJR.13.12297.
78. Cornelis F, Tricaud E, Lasserre AS, et al. Multiparametric magnetic resonance imaging for the differentiation of low and high grade clear cell renal carcinoma. Eur Radiol. 2015;25(1):24–31. https://doi.org/10.1007/s00330-014-3380-x.
79. Moran K, Abreu-Gomez J, Krishna S, et al. Can MRI be used to diagnose histologic grade in T1a (<4 cm) clear cell renal cell carcinomas? Abdom Radiol. 2019;44(8):2841–51. https://doi.org/10.1007/s00261-019-02018-y.
80. Kang SK, Zhang A, Pandharipande PV, Chandarana H, Braithwaite RS, Littenberg B. DWI for renal mass characterization: systematic review and

meta-analysis of diagnostic test performance. Am J Roentgenol. 2015;205(2):317–24. https://doi.org/10.2214/AJR.14.13930.
81. Bosniak MA. The Bosniak renal cyst classification: 25 years later. Radiology. 2012;262(3):781–5. https://doi.org/10.1148/radiol.11111595.
82. Kutikov A, Uzzo RG. The R.E.N.A.L. nephrometry score: a comprehensive standardized system for quantitating renal tumor size, location and depth. J Urol. 2009;182(3):844–53. https://doi.org/10.1016/j.juro.2009.05.035.
83. Simmons MN, Ching CB, Samplaski MK, Park CH, Gill IS. Kidney tumor location measurement using the C index method. J Urol. https://doi.org/10.1016/j.juro.2010.01.005.
84. Ficarra V, Novara G, Secco S, et al. Preoperative aspects and dimensions used for an anatomical (PADUA) classification of renal tumours in patients who are candidates for nephron-sparing surgery. Eur Urol. 2009;56(5):786–93. https://doi.org/10.1016/j.eururo.2009.07.040.
85. Simmons MN, Hillyer SP, Lee BH, Fergany AF, Kaouk J, Campbell SC. Diameter-axial-polar nephrometry: integration and optimization of R.E.N.A.L. and centrality index scoring systems. J Urol. 2012. https://doi.org/10.1016/j.juro.2012.03.123.
86. Bosniak MA. Difficulties in classifying cystic lesions of the kidney. Urol Radiol. 1991;13(1):91–3. https://doi.org/10.1007/BF02924597.
87. Israel GM, Bosniak MA. An update of the Bosniak renal cyst classification system. Urology. 2005;66(3):484–8. https://doi.org/10.1016/j.urology.2005.04.003.
88. Silverman SG, Israel GM, Herts BR, Richie JP. Management of the incidental renal mass. Radiology. 2008;249(1):16–31. https://doi.org/10.1148/radiol.2491070783.
89. Sevcenco S, Spick C, Helbich TH, et al. Malignancy rates and diagnostic performance of the Bosniak classification for the diagnosis of cystic renal lesions in computed tomography—a systematic review and meta-analysis. Eur Radiol. 2017;27(6):2239–47. https://doi.org/10.1007/s00330-016-4631-9.
90. Schoots IG, Zaccai K, Hunink MG, Verhagen PCMS. Bosniak classification for complex renal cysts reevaluated: a systematic review. J Urol. 2017;198(1):12–21. https://doi.org/10.1016/j.juro.2016.09.160.
91. McGrath TA, Bai X, Kamaya A, et al. Proportion of malignancy in Bosniak classification of cystic renal masses version 2019 (v2019) classes: systematic review and meta-analysis. Eur Radiol. 2023;33(2):1307–17. https://doi.org/10.1007/s00330-022-09102-w.
92. Zhang Q, Dai X, Li W. Diagnostic performance of the Bosniak classification, version 2019 for cystic renal masses: a systematic review and meta-analysis. Front Oncol. 2022;12:931592. https://doi.org/10.3389/fonc.2022.931592.
93. Park MY, Park KJ, Kim MH, Kim JK. Bosniak classification of cystic renal masses version 2019: comparison with version 2005 for class distribution, diagnostic performance, and interreader agreement using CT and MRI. Am J Roentgenol. 2021;217(6):1367–76. https://doi.org/10.2214/AJR.21.25796.
94. Kutikov A, Smaldone MC, Egleston BL, et al. Anatomic features of enhancing renal masses predict malignant and high-grade pathology: a preoperative nomogram using the RENAL Nephrometry score. Eur Urol. 2011;60(2):241–8. https://doi.org/10.1016/j.eururo.2011.03.029.
95. Wang HK, Zhu Y, Yao XD, et al. External validation of a nomogram using RENAL nephrometry score to predict high grade renal cell carcinoma. J Urol. 2012;187(5):1555–60. https://doi.org/10.1016/j.juro.2011.12.099.
96. Stroup SP, Palazzi K, Kopp RP, et al. RENAL nephrometry score is associated with operative approach for partial nephrectomy and urine leak. Urology. 2012;80(1):151–6. https://doi.org/10.1016/j.urology.2012.04.026.
97. Canter D, Kutikov A, Manley B, et al. Utility of the R.E.N.A.L. nephrometry scoring system in objectifying treatment decision-making of the enhancing renal mass. Urology. 2011;78(5):1089–94. https://doi.org/10.1016/j.urology.2011.04.035.
98. Gorin MA, Ball MW, Pierorazio PM, et al. Outcomes and predictors of clinical T1 to pathological T3a tumor up-staging after robotic partial nephrectomy: a multi-institutional analysis. J Urol. 2013;190(5):1907–11. https://doi.org/10.1016/j.juro.2013.06.014.
99. Ellison JS, Montgomery JS, Hafez KS, et al. Association of RENAL nephrometry score with outcomes of minimally invasive partial nephrectomy. Int J Urol. 2013;20(6):564–70. https://doi.org/10.1111/j.1442-2042.2012.03222.x.
100. Hayn MH, Schwaab T, Underwood W, Kim HL. RENAL nephrometry score predicts surgical outcomes of laparoscopic partial nephrectomy. BJU Int. 2011;108(6):876–81. https://doi.org/10.1111/j.1464-410X.2010.09940.x.
101. Rosevear HM, Gellhaus PT, Lightfoot AJ, Kresowik TP, Joudi FN, Tracy CR. Utility of the RENAL nephrometry scoring system in the real world: predicting surgeon operative preference and complication risk. BJU Int. 2012;109(5):700–5. https://doi.org/10.1111/j.1464-410X.2011.10452.x.
102. Simhan J, Smaldone MC, Tsai KJ, et al. Objective measures of renal mass anatomic complexity predict rates of major complications following partial nephrectomy. Eur Urol. 2011;60(4):724–30. https://doi.org/10.1016/j.eururo.2011.05.030.
103. Bertolotto M, Catalano O. Contrast-enhanced ultrasound: past, present, and future. Ultrasound Clin. 2009;4(3):339–67. https://doi.org/10.1016/j.cult.2009.10.011.

104. Bertolotto M, Bucci S, Valentino M, Currò F, Sachs C, Cova MA. Contrast-enhanced ultrasound for characterizing renal masses. Eur J Radiol. 2018;105:41–8. https://doi.org/10.1016/j.ejrad.2018.05.015.
105. Furrer MA, Spycher SCJ, Büttiker SM, et al. Comparison of the diagnostic performance of contrast-enhanced ultrasound with that of contrast-enhanced computed tomography and contrast-enhanced magnetic resonance imaging in the evaluation of renal masses: a systematic review and meta-analysis. Eur Urol Oncol. 2020;3(4):464–73. https://doi.org/10.1016/j.euo.2019.08.013.
106. Hicks RJ, Ware RE, Lau EWF. PET/CT: will it change the way that we use CT in cancer imaging? Cancer Imaging. 2006;6:S52–62. https://doi.org/10.1102/1470-7330.2006.9012.
107. Kang DE, White RL, Zuger JH, Sasser HC, Teigland CM. Clinical use of fluorodeoxyglucose F18 positron emission tomography for detection of renal cell carcinoma. J Urol. 2004;171(5):1806–9. https://doi.org/10.1097/01.ju.0000120241.50061.e4.
108. Wang HY, Ding HJ, Chen JH, et al. Meta-analysis of the diagnostic performance of [18F] FDG-PET and PET/CT in renal cell carcinoma. Cancer Imaging. 2012;12(3):464–74. https://doi.org/10.1102/1470-7330.2012.0042.
109. Aide N, Cappele O, Bottet P, et al. Efficiency of [18 F] FDG PET in characterising renal cancer and detecting distant metastases: a comparison with CT. Eur J Nucl Med Mol Imaging. 2003;30(9):1236–45. https://doi.org/10.1007/s00259-003-1211-4.
110. Özülker T, Özülker F, Özbek E, Özpaçaci T. A prospective diagnostic accuracy study of F-18 fluorodeoxyglucose-positron emission tomography/computed tomography in the evaluation of indeterminate renal masses. Nucl Med Commun. 2011;32(4):265. https://doi.org/10.1097/MNM.0b013e3283442e3b.
111. Stillebroer AB, Mulders PFA, Boerman OC, Oyen WJG, Oosterwijk E. Carbonic anhydrase IX in renal cell carcinoma: implications for prognosis, diagnosis, and therapy. Eur Urol. 2010;58(1):75–83. https://doi.org/10.1016/j.eururo.2010.03.015.
112. Divgi CR, Pandit-Taskar N, Jungbluth AA, et al. Preoperative characterisation of clear-cell renal carcinoma using iodine-124-labelled antibody chimeric G250 (124I-cG250) and PET in patients with renal masses: a phase I trial. Lancet Oncol. 2007;8(4):304–10. https://doi.org/10.1016/S1470-2045(07)70044-X.
113. Divgi CR, Uzzo RG, Gatsonis C, et al. Positron emission tomography/computed tomography identification of clear cell renal cell carcinoma: results from the REDECT trial. J Clin Oncol. 2013;31(2):187–94. https://doi.org/10.1200/JCO.2011.41.2445.
114. Shuch B, Pantuck AJ, Bernhard JC, et al. [89Zr] Zr-girentuximab for PET–CT imaging of clear-cell renal cell carcinoma: a prospective, open-label, multicentre, phase 3 trial. Lancet Oncol. 2024;25(10):1277–87. https://doi.org/10.1016/S1470-2045(24)00402-9.
115. Gormley TS, Van Every MJ, Moreno AJ. Renal oncocytoma: preoperative diagnosis using technetium 99m sestamibi imaging. Urology. 1996;48(1):33–9. https://doi.org/10.1016/s0090-4295(96)00095-7.
116. Rowe SP, Gorin MA, Gordetsky J, et al. Initial experience using 99mTc-MIBI SPECT/CT for the differentiation of oncocytoma from renal cell carcinoma. Clin Nucl Med. 2015;40(4):309–13. https://doi.org/10.1097/RLU.0000000000000670.
117. Gorin MA, Rowe SP, Baras AS, et al. Prospective evaluation of 99mTc-sestamibi SPECT/CT for the diagnosis of renal oncocytomas and hybrid oncocytic/chromophobe tumors. Eur Urol. 2016;69(3):413–6. https://doi.org/10.1016/j.eururo.2015.08.056.
118. Basile G, Fallara G, Verri P, et al. The role of 99mTc-sestamibi single-photon emission computed tomography/computed tomography in the diagnostic pathway for renal masses: a systematic review and meta-analysis. Eur Urol. 2024;85(1):63–71. https://doi.org/10.1016/j.eururo.2023.07.013.
119. Schober JP, Braun A, Ginsburg KB, et al. Clinical performance of technetium-99m–Sestamibi SPECT/CT imaging in differentiating oncocytic tumors from renal cell carcinoma in routine clinical practice. J Urol. 2023. https://doi.org/10.1097/JU.0000000000003557.
120. Wang RS, Yu JQ, Schober J, et al. Limited utility of quantitative thresholds on 99mTc-sestamibi single-photon emission computed tomography/computed tomography for distinguishing renal cell carcinoma from oncocytic renal masses. JU Open Plus. 2024;2(9):194. https://doi.org/10.1097/JU9.0000000000000194.
121. Wolf JS. Evaluation and management of solid and cystic renal masses. J Urol. 1998;159(4):1120–33. https://doi.org/10.1016/S0022-5347(01)63529-8.
122. Campbell SC, Novick AC, Herts B, et al. Prospective evaluation of fine needle aspiration of small, solid renal masses: accuracy and morbidity. Urology. 1997;50(1):25–9. https://doi.org/10.1016/S0090-4295(97)00111-8.
123. Gibbons RP, Bush WH, Burnett LL. Needle tract seeding following aspiration of renal cell carcinoma. J Urol. 1977;118(5):865–7. https://doi.org/10.1016/S0022-5347(17)58226-9.
124. Kiser GC, Totonchy M, Barry JM. Needle tract seeding after percutaneous renal adenocarcinoma aspiration. J Urol. 1986;136(6):1292–3. https://doi.org/10.1016/S0022-5347(17)45318-3.
125. Wehle MJ, Grabstald H. Contraindications to needle aspiration of a solid renal mass: tumor dissemination by renal needle aspiration. J Urol. 1986;136(2):446–8. https://doi.org/10.1016/S0022-5347(17)44900-7.
126. Lane BR, Samplaski MK, Herts BR, Zhou M, Novick AC, Campbell SC. Renal mass biopsy—a renaissance? J Urol. 2008;179(1):20–7. https://doi.org/10.1016/j.juro.2007.08.124.

127. Wood BJ, Khan MA, McGovern F, Harisinghani M, Hahn PF, Mueller PR. Imaging guided biopsy of renal masses: indications, accuracy and impact on clinical management. J Urol. 1999. https://doi.org/10.1016/S0022-5347(05)68929-X.
128. Lim CS, Schieda N, Silverman SG. Update on indications for percutaneous renal mass biopsy in the era of advanced CT and MRI. Am J Roentgenol. 2019;212(6):1187–96. https://doi.org/10.2214/AJR.19.21093.
129. Haifler M, Kutikov A. Current role of renal biopsy in urologic practice. Urol Clin North Am. 2017;44(2):203–11. https://doi.org/10.1016/j.ucl.2016.12.006.
130. Choy B, Nayar R, Lin X. Role of renal mass biopsy for diagnosis and management: review of current trends and future directions. Cancer Cytopathol. 2023;131(8):480–94. https://doi.org/10.1002/cncy.22697.
131. Patel HD, Johnson MH, Pierorazio PM, et al. Diagnostic accuracy and risks of biopsy in the diagnosis of a renal mass suspicious for localized renal cell carcinoma: systematic review of the literature. J Urol. 2016;195(5):1340–7. https://doi.org/10.1016/j.juro.2015.11.029.
132. Marconi L, Dabestani S, Lam TB, et al. Systematic review and meta-analysis of diagnostic accuracy of percutaneous renal tumour biopsy. Eur Urol. 2016;69(4):660–73. https://doi.org/10.1016/j.eururo.2015.07.072.
133. Schmidbauer J, Remzi M, Memarsadeghi M, et al. Diagnostic accuracy of computed tomography-guided percutaneous biopsy of renal masses. Eur Urol. 2008;53(5):1003–12. https://doi.org/10.1016/j.eururo.2007.11.041.
134. Richard PO, Jewett MAS, Bhatt JR, et al. Renal tumor biopsy for small renal masses: a single-center 13-year experience. Eur Urol. 2015;68(6):1007–13. https://doi.org/10.1016/j.eururo.2015.04.004.
135. Leveridge MJ, Finelli A, Kachura JR, et al. Outcomes of small renal mass needle core biopsy, nondiagnostic percutaneous biopsy, and the role of repeat biopsy. Eur Urol. 2011;60(3):578–84. https://doi.org/10.1016/j.eururo.2011.06.021.
136. Yang CS, Choi E, Idrees MT, Chen S, Wu HH. Percutaneous biopsy of the renal mass: FNA or core needle biopsy? Cancer Cytopathol. 2017;125(6):407–15. https://doi.org/10.1002/cncy.21852.
137. Li G, Cuilleron M, Zhao A, et al. Combination of core biopsy and fine-needle aspiration increases diagnostic rate for small solid renal tumors. Anticancer Res. 2012;32(8):3463–6.
138. ASC Guidelines and Position Statements - American Society of Cytopathology. https://cytopathology.org/general/custom.asp?page=ASCGuidelines&DGPCrPg=1&DGPCrSrt=6A. Accessed 23 September 2024.
139. Ball MW, Bezerra SM, Gorin MA, et al. Grade heterogeneity in small renal masses: potential implications for renal mass biopsy. J Urol. 2015;193(1):36–40. https://doi.org/10.1016/j.juro.2014.06.067.
140. Richter F, Kasabian NG, Irwin RJ, Watson RA, Lang EK. Accuracy of diagnosis by guided biopsy of renal mass lesions classified indeterminate by imaging studies. Urology. 2000;55(3):348–52. https://doi.org/10.1016/S0090-4295(99)00468-9.
141. Harisinghani MG, Maher MM, Gervais DA, et al. Incidence of malignancy in complex cystic renal masses (Bosniak category III): should imaging-guided biopsy precede surgery? Am J Roentgenol. 2003;180(3):755–8. https://doi.org/10.2214/ajr.180.3.1800755.
142. Lang EK, Macchia RJ, Gayle B, et al. CT-guided biopsy of indeterminate renal cystic masses (Bosniak 3 and 2F): accuracy and impact on clinical management. Eur Radiol. 2002;12(10):2518–24. https://doi.org/10.1007/s00330-001-1292-z.
143. Volpe A, Kachura JR, Geddie WR, et al. Techniques, safety and accuracy of sampling of renal tumors by fine needle aspiration and core biopsy. J Urol. 2007. https://doi.org/10.1016/j.juro.2007.03.131.
144. Williamson SR, Gadde R, Trpkov K, et al. Diagnostic criteria for oncocytic renal neoplasms: a survey of urologic pathologists. Hum Pathol. 2017;63:149–56. https://doi.org/10.1016/j.humpath.2017.03.004.
145. Patel HD, Druskin SC, Rowe SP, Pierorazio PM, Gorin MA, Allaf ME. Surgical histopathology for suspected oncocytoma on renal mass biopsy: a systematic review and meta-analysis. BJU Int. 2017;119(5):661–6. https://doi.org/10.1111/bju.13763.
146. Ginzburg S, Uzzo R, Al-Saleem T, et al. Coexisting hybrid malignancy in a solitary sporadic solid benign renal mass: implications for managing patients following renal biopsy. J Urol. 2014;191(2):296–300. https://doi.org/10.1016/j.juro.2013.07.059.
147. Alle N, Tan N, Huss J, Huang J, Pantuck A, Raman SS. Percutaneous image-guided core biopsy of solid renal masses: analysis of safety, efficacy, pathologic interpretation, and clinical significance. Abdom Radiol. 2018;43(7):1813–9. https://doi.org/10.1007/s00261-017-1337-7.
148. Renshaw AA, Powell A, Caso J, Gould EW. Needle track seeding in renal mass biopsies. Cancer Cytopathol. 2019;127(6):358–61. https://doi.org/10.1002/cncy.22147.
149. Patel RM, Safiullah S, Okhunov Z, et al. Pretreatment diagnosis of the small renal mass: status of renal biopsy in The United States of America. J Endourol. 2018;32(9):884–90. https://doi.org/10.1089/end.2018.0175.
150. Maurice MJ, Zhu H, Kiechle JE, Kim SP, Abouassaly R. Increasing biopsy utilization for renal cell carcinoma is closely associated with treatment. Urology. 2015;86(5):906–13. https://doi.org/10.1016/j.urology.2015.08.020.
151. Richard PO, Lavallée LT, Pouliot F, et al. Is routine renal tumor biopsy associated with lower rates of benign histology following nephrectomy for small

renal masses? J Urol. 2018;200(4):731–6. https://doi.org/10.1016/j.juro.2018.04.015.
152. Halverson SJ, Kunju LP, Bhalla R, et al. Accuracy of determining small renal mass management with risk stratified biopsies: confirmation by final pathology. J Urol. 2013;189(2):441–6. https://doi.org/10.1016/j.juro.2012.09.032.
153. Rahbar H, Bhayani S, Stifelman M, et al. Evaluation of renal mass biopsy risk stratification algorithm for robotic partial nephrectomy—could a biopsy have guided management? J Urol. 2014;192(5):1337–42. https://doi.org/10.1016/j.juro.2014.06.028.
154. Siegel RL, Giaquinto AN, Jemal A. Cancer statistics, 2024. CA Cancer J Clin. 2024;74(1):12–49. https://doi.org/10.3322/caac.21820.
155. Siegel RL, Miller KD, Jemal A. Cancer statistics, 2016. CA Cancer J Clin. 2016;66(1):7–30. https://doi.org/10.3322/caac.21332.
156. Jewett M, Zuniga A. Renal tumor natural history: the rationale and role for active surveillance. Urol Clin North Am. 2008;35(4):627–34.
157. Hollingsworth JM, Miller DC, Daignault S, Hollenbeck BK. Five-year survival after surgical treatment for kidney cancer: a population-based competing risk analysis. Cancer. 2007;109(9):1763–8. https://doi.org/10.1002/cncr.22600.
158. Pierorazio PM, Johnson MH, Ball MW, et al. Five-year analysis of a multi-institutional prospective clinical trial of delayed intervention and surveillance for small renal masses: the DISSRM registry. Eur Urol. 2015;68(3):408–15. https://doi.org/10.1016/j.eururo.2015.02.001.
159. Kutikov A, Egleston BL, Canter D, Smaldone MC, Wong YN, Uzzo RG. Competing risks of death in patients with localized renal cell carcinoma: a comorbidity based model. J Urol. 2012;188(6):2077–83. https://doi.org/10.1016/j.juro.2012.07.100.
160. American College of Surgeons National Surgical Quality Improvement Program. ACS NSQIP surgical risk calculator. https://riskcalculator.facs.org/RiskCalculator/index.jsp. Accessed 29 October 2024.
161. Huynh MJ, Wang Y, Joshi M, et al. Patient factors predict complications after partial nephrectomy: validation and calibration of the preoperative risk evaluation for partial nephrectomy (PREP) score. BJU Int. 2021;127(3):369–74. https://doi.org/10.1111/bju.15240.
162. NCCN Clinical Practice Guidelines in Oncology (NCCN Guidelines®) for Kidney Cancer V.1.2025. © National Comprehensive Cancer Network, Inc. 2024. All rights reserved. https://www.nccn.org/guidelines/guidelines-detail?category=1&id=1440. Accessed 30 August 2024.
163. Ristau BT, Kutikov A, Uzzo RG, Smaldone MC. Active surveillance for small renal masses: when less is more. Eur Urol Focus. 2017;2(6):660–8. https://doi.org/10.1016/j.euf.2017.04.004.
164. Jewett MAS, Mattar K, Basiuk J, et al. Active surveillance of small renal masses: progression patterns of early stage kidney cancer. Eur Urol. 2011;60(1):39–44. https://doi.org/10.1016/j.eururo.2011.03.030.
165. Gupta M, Blute ML Jr, Su LM, Crispen PL. Delayed intervention of small renal masses on active surveillance. J Kidney Cancer. 2017;4(2):24–30. https://doi.org/10.15586/jkcvhl.2017.75.
166. Srivastava A, Patel HD, Gupta M, et al. The incidence, predictors, and survival of disappearing small renal masses on active surveillance. Urol Oncol Semin Orig Investig. 2020;38(2):42. https://doi.org/10.1016/j.urolonc.2019.10.005.
167. Lane BR, Abouassaly R, Gao T, et al. Active treatment of localized renal tumors may not impact overall survival in patients aged 75 years or older. Cancer. 2010;116(13):3119–26. https://doi.org/10.1002/cncr.25184.
168. Alam R, Patel HD, Osumah T, et al. Comparative effectiveness of management options for patients with small renal masses: a prospective cohort study. BJU Int. 2019;123(1):42–50. https://doi.org/10.1111/bju.14490.
169. Alkhatib KY, Harmatz IM, Wlajnitz T, et al. PD58-05 active surveillance versus primary intervention for clinical t1a kidney tumors: how does renal biopsies modulate management plan? Contemporary results the fifteen-year DISSRM prospective comparative study. J Urol. 2024;211(5S):e1215. https://doi.org/10.1097/01.JU.0001008868.74763.2c.05.
170. Danzig MR, Ghandour RA, Chang P, et al. Active surveillance is superior to radical nephrectomy and equivalent to partial nephrectomy for preserving renal function in patients with small renal masses: results from the DISSRM registry. J Urol. 2015;194(4):903–9. https://doi.org/10.1016/j.juro.2015.03.093.
171. Goldberg H, Ajaj R, Cáceres JOH, et al. Psychological distress associated with active surveillance in patients younger than 70 with a small renal mass. Urol Oncol Semin Orig Investig. 2020;38(6):603. https://doi.org/10.1016/j.urolonc.2020.02.015.
172. Patel HD, Riffon MF, Joice GA, et al. A prospective, comparative study of quality of life among patients with small renal masses choosing active surveillance and primary intervention. J Urol. 2016;196(5):1356–62. https://doi.org/10.1016/j.juro.2016.04.073.
173. Chang SL, Cipriano LE, Harshman LC, Garber AM, Chung BI. Cost-effectiveness analysis of nephron sparing options for the management of small renal masses. J Urol. 2011;185(5):1591–7. https://doi.org/10.1016/j.juro.2010.12.100.
174. Heilbrun ME, Yu J, Smith KJ, Dechet CB, Zagoria RJ, Roberts MS. The cost-effectiveness of immediate treatment, percutaneous biopsy and active surveillance for the diagnosis of the small solid renal mass: evidence from a markov model. J Urol. 2012;187(1):39–43. https://doi.org/10.1016/j.juro.2011.09.055.

Rationale for Partial Nephrectomy, Current Practice Patterns

9

Jesse B. Persily and William C. Huang

Abbreviations

AS	Active surveillance
ASCO	American Society for Clinical Oncology
AUA	American Urological Association
CKD	Chronic kidney disease
EAU	European Association of Urology
EORTC-GU	European Organization for Research and Treatment of Cancer Genito Urinary Group
ESRD	End-stage renal disease
LPN	Laparoscopic partial nephrectomy
LRN	Laparoscopic radical nephrectomy
MDRD	Modification of Diet in Renal Disease
MSKCC	Memorial Sloan-Kettering Cancer Center
NCCN	National Comprehensive Cancer Network
NSS	Nephron-sparing surgery
OPN	Open partial nephrectomy
ORN	Open radical nephrectomy
PN	Partial nephrectomy
QOL	Quality of life
RCTs	Renal cortical tumors
RMS	Renal mass sampling (RMS)
RN	Radical nephrectomy
RPN	Robotic partial nephrectomy
SEER	Surveillance epidemiology and end results
SRMs	Small renal masses

J. B. Persily
Department of Urology, NYU Langone Medical Center, New York, NY, USA

W. C. Huang (✉)
Division of Urologic Oncology, Department of Urology, NYU Langone Medical Center, New York, NY, USA
e-mail: William.huang@nyumc.org

Introduction

The oncologic and medical rationale for PN has evolved over the past two decades and is built upon the convergence of epidemiologic, histologic, oncologic, and renal functional data, which point to PN as an ideal strategy for maximizing oncologic control of malignant RCTs, while preserving renal function and minimizing the long-term risks associated with decreased renal function. Historically, localized solid renal masses were treated with RN, stemming from the recognition that systemic medical therapy is rarely curative for kidney cancer. PN, while described as early as 1887, was traditionally limited to patients with a solitary kidney, bilateral tumors, or patients with underlying chronic kidney disease (CKD), because of its surgical complexity, increased rate of complications, and less recognition of the potential morbidity associated with removal of functioning, healthy nephrons.

J. A. Libertino, J. R. Gee (eds.), *Renal Cancer*, https://doi.org/10.1007/978-3-031-97599-8_9

This paradigm began to shift in the early 1990s, driven by a host of new radiologic, pathologic, oncologic, and cardiovascular developments and discoveries. The increasing use of cross-sectional imaging meant greater numbers of small, asymptomatic lesions were being diagnosed incidentally, resulting in an overall downward stage migration in kidney cancer. Evolving surgical techniques and experience led to increasing numbers of urologists comfortable performing partial nephrectomy. There was also increasing recognition that a nontrivial proportion of these small, asymptomatic solid renal lesions were in fact benign, meaning that a nontrivial proportion of patients were undergoing RN for benign lesions and were thus losing significant renal function despite the lesions having no metastatic potential or mortality threat. Concurrent with these observations was newly available long-term follow-up data of a large series of patients undergoing PN for small renal lesions that demonstrated oncologic equivalency between PN and RN. Finally, retrospective studies of large cohorts of patients with modestly decreased renal function from a variety of causes demonstrated an increased risk of cardiovascular disease and death with mild renal dysfunction. The convergence of these considerations increased the utilization of PN for the treatment of SRMs in both the United States and abroad. However, despite the strong retrospective data in favor of PN, the single prospective randomized trial evaluating PN versus RN failed to demonstrate an overall survival benefit in those undergoing PN compared with RN. Various possible explanations have been posited to explain this finding, with some arguing that the decreased renal function resulting from loss of nephrons during renal surgery may carry fewer long-term risks than decreased renal function from medical renal disease, thus diminishing the theoretical potential benefit of PN in certain patients. Despite this result, PN remains the preferred treatment for SRMs and is reflected in the 2021 American Urological Association Guideline for Renal Mass and Localized Renal Cancer. This chapter will outline the evidence and rationale for PN as a treatment for renal cortical tumors.

Epidemiology of Renal Masses

Kidney cancer accounts for over 4% of all adult malignant neoplasms, 2.4% of all cancer deaths, and is the third most commonly diagnosed genitourinary malignancy. In 2023, there are predicted to be 81,800 incident cases and 14,890 deaths from kidney cancer in the United States, with an approximately 3:2 male-to-female predominance [1]. The annual incidence of kidney cancer has increased at a rate of approximately 3–4% annually over the past three decades. The vast majority of this increase is represented by clinically localized disease. Simard et al. demonstrated the annual rate of localized disease increased from 7.6 per 100,000 in 1999 to 12.2 per 100,000 in 2008 [2]. Furthermore, several population-based studies have demonstrated that the majority of this increase in localized disease can be accounted for by an increase in the diagnosis of clinical stage T1a lesions (<4 cm diameter [2–5]), often referred to as small renal masses (SRMs) (see Fig. 9.1).

Today, the majority of newly diagnosed renal tumors are SRMs, and SRMs account for the majority, if not all, of the increasing incidence of renal tumors [6–8]. The gradual increase in the number and proportion of SRMs has been met with a parallel increase in the number of renal surgeries, meaning that an increasing number of patients now undergo surgery for small, asymptomatic RCTs [9].

The increasing incidence of small renal lesions in the past three decades has been attributed at least partially to the advent and growing clinical use of modern imaging procedures such as computed tomography (CT), magnetic resonance imaging (MRI), and ultrasound (US). Beginning in the 1970s, these new technologies revolutionized the diagnosis of kidney cancer. The classically taught triad of flank pain, hematuria, and abdominal mass is rarely encountered in modern clinical practice and has given way to the asymptomatic mass found incidentally on imaging performed for a variety of signs and symptoms, most often unrelated to the renal lesion itself. Indeed, it has been estimated that at least 48–66% of RCC diagnoses in the modern era occur as a result of

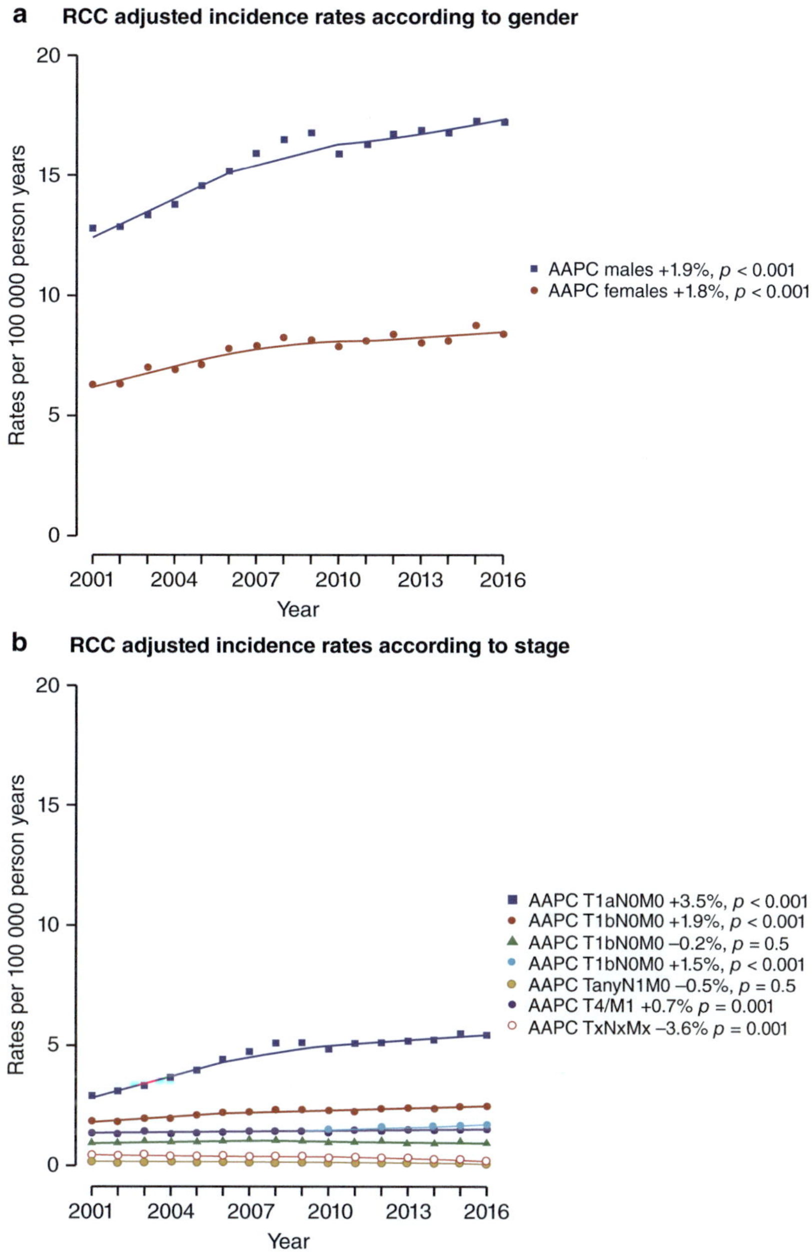

Fig. 9.1 Age-adjusted incidence of kidney cancer stratified by gender (**a**) and disease stage (**b**), Surveillance, Epidemiology, and End Results (SEER), 2001–2016. (Adapted from Palumbo et al. [5])

cross-sectional imaging in an otherwise asymptomatic patient [10]. Recent SEER data suggests that the increasing incidence seen over the preceding 30 years has plateaued [11]. Consistent with this trend is the observation that the number of renal masses, both benign and malignant, discovered at autopsy has been observed to be declining, possibly due to increased detection and treatment before death [12].

Given that smaller renal masses are associated with a decreased risk of malignancy, as well as increased survival rates, one would expect mortality from kidney cancer to decrease as greater proportions of renal masses are diagnosed at <4 cm. This phenomenon, however, has not been clearly demonstrated in the epidemiological data. A 2006 study by Hollingsworth et al. of Surveillance Epidemiology and End Results

(SEER) cancer registry data demonstrated that from 1983 to 2002, despite the increasing proportions of renal masses that were <4 cm and detected incidentally on cross-sectional imaging, overall mortality for patients with kidney cancer rose to 15.5% [9]. This effect persisted despite a virtually identical increase in renal tumor surgery to match the observed increase in renal tumors, suggesting that the trend of increased mortality could not be attributed to inadequate numbers of surgeries being performed to treat these masses. Additionally, when investigators stratified the lesions by tumor size, the proportional increase in the overall mortality rate for lesions 2–4 cm (from 0.2 to 1.5 deaths per 100,000) was in fact slightly greater than for lesions >7 cm in size (0.4–2.2 deaths per 100,000). These findings, which utilize a data set spanning 1983–2002, suggested that early detection of renal tumors and treatment at a lower stage did not provide an overall survival benefit during this era. Through 2015, SEER analyses began to suggest that mortality from kidney cancer has been decreasing at a rate of approximately 0.7% per year from 2006 to 2015 [13]. Despite these modest gains in the more recent data, it is unknown why the observed downward stage migration of kidney cancer and seemingly appropriate increase in treatment of small renal lesions has not resulted in greater decreases in mortality from kidney cancer. Some have shown that missing data in the SEER database may at least in part explain some of this apparent discrepancy, but further work is needed to understand the mortality trend [14].

Heterogeneity of Renal Cortical Tumors

RCTs represent a diverse group of biological entities with varying cytogenetic defects, histologies, and biological aggressiveness. While any RCT, benign, indolent, or malignant, can display growth over time, any given lesion's metastatic potential is intrinsically related to the lesion's histological subtype. Several large series have demonstrated the prognostic relevance of histologic type in univariate analysis models, with papillary and chromophobe subtypes thought to display favorable biological behavior and clear cell, collecting duct, and unclassified subtypes thought to display more aggressive behavior [15, 16]. As such, knowing the histology of the lesion may help to determine which patients with small, localized RCTs are at risk for metastatic disease. This scenario, however, presents a clinical problem because at present, reliable methods for determining the histologic identity of a renal lesion prior to surgical excision are limited. Researchers have investigated the sensitivity and specificity of percutaneous biopsy, or renal mass sampling (RMS), and while diagnostic yields are improving with time at several specialized centers, the robust clinical utility of RMS is limited at this time [17, 18]. Determining the malignant potential of RCTs, particularly small RCTs, from cross-sectional imaging is also limited due to the significant overlap in imaging characteristics of benign and malignant lesions in traditional cross-sectional imaging. Work is ongoing to develop functional imaging modalities able to better differentiate benign from malignant lesions [19, 20]. Sestamibi SPECT/CT imaging has been utilized for the diagnosis of renal oncocytomas, benign entities that do not require treatment. In addition, The phase 3 study of PET-CT with radiolabeled girentuximab demonstrated reasonable sensitivity (86.2%) and specificity (85.9%), but further work and more widespread dissemination and availability of these radiotracers is needed. As a result of these limitations, a considerable number of patients with RCTs undergo nephrectomy for masses ultimately found to be benign. Contemporary series of patients undergoing nephrectomy for RCTs have demonstrated that 10–20% of lesions are in fact benign [21–25]. Clearly, techniques that could reliably determine a lesion's histologic identity prior to surgery could significantly alter the management of SRMs.

History of Partial Nephrectomy

The modern era of renal surgery began on August 2, 1869, in Heidelberg, Germany, when Gustav Simon performed a planned RN on a 46-year-old female with persistent urinary fistula [26]. The procedure was performed in front of 50 observers and took 40 min, with an estimated blood loss of 50 cc. The patient survived her procedure and was cured of her disease. Eighteen years later, in 1887, Vincenz Czerny performed the first PN to remove an angiosarcoma in a 30-year-old gardener, who also recovered from his procedure. Since these initial descriptions, renal surgery has evolved substantially, with modifications and improvements in surgical approach, antisepsis measures, and mortality rates. In 1969, Robson published the results from his landmark series of 88 patients with solid renal masses who underwent RN, a new and more aggressive approach to surgery for solid renal masses that included removal of perinephric fat, the ipsilateral adrenal, overlying peritoneum, and regional lymph nodes. In this series, he demonstrated improved rates of survival over historical standards and a 3% mortality rate [27]. His radical procedure would become the surgical gold-standard treatment for localized and locally advanced renal tumors for the next 40 years. The next major milestone in renal surgery occurred in 1991 when Clayman published the initial case report of a laparoscopic RN (LRN) [28]. From the early 1990s onward, there was progressive adoption of both LRN and open PN (OPN) as literature grew revealing equivalent intermediate and longer-term oncologic outcomes between these modalities and the gold standard of open RN (ORN) for renal masses up to 7 cm.

Despite early descriptions of PN, along with clinical and experimental evidence of its technical feasibility as early as the 1800s, its use during the first half of the twentieth century remained limited, likely due to its increased technical demands and surgeon reticence for fear of complications. Textbooks published between 1937 and 1970, almost 100 years after the first PN was successfully performed, rarely mention the procedure [26]. PN was utilized during this time period, albeit infrequently, in cases of a tumor in a solitary kidney, bilateral tumors, or in patients with significant underlying medical renal disease or renal insufficiency. Several surgeons who had successfully performed PN for renal masses advocated the procedure in cases of modest-sized tumors limited to the poles of the kidney [29].

By the mid-twentieth century, the limited role of PN began to yield to a greater interest in performing the procedure in broader groups of patients, including those with normal contralateral kidneys. In 1950, Vermooten was the first to suggest that PN may be undertaken in certain appropriately selected patients with normal contralateral kidneys [30]. Herr and Licht are credited as the first to publish follow-up data on a large series of patients with suspected malignant renal masses undergoing PN. In 1976 Herr began performing planned PN on patients with normal contralateral kidneys and in 1994 published a landmark case series of 230 patients, 41 of whom underwent PN, in which he reported no complications and 95% freedom from disease [26]. Moreover, while Herr conceded in his publication "the best available data indicate no functional advantage to PN when the opposite kidney is normal," he concluded that the sacrifice of uninvolved renal parenchyma might be unnecessary if local tumor control can be achieved by a partial excision.

Since these initial cohorts, interest in PN for the treatment of SRMs grew, driven by a variety of factors. The aforementioned downward size and stage migration of newly diagnosed renal cortical tumors meant increasing numbers of patients were presenting with small masses that were technically amenable to PN. Technical concerns about tumor multifocality, endophytic location, and nearness to the collecting system and major vessels could be routinely overcome by a variety of techniques developed over subsequent decades. Intraoperative ultrasound allowed for the determination of tumor multifocality, depth of invasion, and location respective to critical structures. Nearness to vessels and the collecting system were managed with suture repair, adjunct hemostatic agents, and modern renorrhaphy techniques, which are effective in achieving hemostasis and maintaining the integrity of the collecting system [31]. Complication rates for PN are now comparable with RN and can usually be managed conservatively [32]. Previously, the desire for a 1-cm surgical margin, deemed necessary for adequate oncologic control, meant many tumors with a central or hilar location were not considered candidates for PN. However, it has since been demonstrated that gross tumor resection with only a microscopically negative margin is adequate for effective oncologic control [33, 34]. There are even some studies that suggest that margin status does not have an impact on OS, though this is a subject for debate [35]. As such, greater numbers of tumors are now considered technically and oncologically amenable to PN.

Minimally invasive PN is now effectively performed both laparoscopically and robotically, with oncologic results equivalent to OPN and with low complication rates. The shift to MIS PN was most apparent with the uptake of the robotic-assisted approach, which tended to present a shorter learning curve compared to the laparoscopic approach [36]. More recently, adoption of the single-port robotic surgery system, as well as totally retroperitoneal approaches to PN have served to further minimize the morbidity of the procedure, but further long-term data is needed to better understand the advantages and disadvantages to these specific approaches in specific cases [37].

Oncologic Outcomes in Partial Nephrectomy

Oncologic outcomes following surgery for localized RCC are dependent on several clinicopathologic factors, including stage, tumor size, nuclear grade, and histologic subtype, with pathologic stage being the single most important factor. Data from one randomized prospective trial, as well as multiple large institution and population-based studies, have consistently demonstrated that PN provides equivalent oncologic outcomes to RN for the treatment of cT1a and cT1b tumors, with 5-year cancer-specific survival rates following surgery for clinically localized disease exceeding 90% [38–44]. Lee et al. published follow-up results of a retrospective analysis of 262 nephrectomies, 30% of which were PN, performed for pT1a RCC [38]. In this study, with an overall median follow-up of 40 months, there was no difference in disease-specific, disease-free, or overall survival between patients who underwent PN versus RN. While patients undergoing PN were slightly younger (mean 61 vs. 64) and the tumors excised by PN were slightly smaller (mean 2.5 vs. 3.0), there were no differences in tumor histologic type or pathologic stage. At approximately the same time, Lau et al. published a matched comparison of RN versus PN in 164 pairs of patients matched for tumor grade, pathologic stage, tumor diameter, age, gender, and year of surgery [39]. At 15-year follow-up, they found no significant difference in overall survival, cancer-specific survival, metastasis-free survival, or local-recurrence free survival. In addition, Soputro et al. recently published oncologic outcomes from 15 years of follow-up specifically after robotic PN (N = 769) and RN (N = 142). The group found equivalent cancer-specific mortality rates of 1.1% between the two groups, with no statistical difference in local recurrence, metastatic, and disease-specific survival [45]. Results of these studies, both of which utilize data from specialized tertiary-care centers, have been corroborated in population-based cohorts, from which results may be more generalizable [40].

Additional studies have shown similar results for stage pT1b masses. A collaborative study between the Mayo Clinic and Memorial Sloan-Kettering Cancer Center of 1159 patients who underwent surgery for sporadic spontaneous unilateral renal masses 4.1–7 cm demonstrated no difference in overall survival or cancer-specific survival when comparing patients undergoing PN versus RN [41]. While the risk of death from RCC was increased for patients undergoing RN compared with PN, the results did not achieve significance—HR 1.97 (0.92–4.20)—and patients undergoing RN were on average older and were more likely to have larger tumors with perinephric or renal sinus fat invasion than patients treated with PN. The oncologic equivalency between PN and RN for pT1b masses has been demonstrated by other investigators in multiple patient cohorts, both in American and European centers [41–44]. Finally, in 2011, the European Organization for Research and Treatment of Cancer Genito-Urinary Group

(EORTC-GU) published results of a randomized phase 3 clinical trial comparing RN to PN for the treatment of a solitary renal mass ≤5 cm. This trial, designed as a noninferiority trial, found nearly equivalent 10-year CSS rates of 75.2% for PN versus 79.4% for RN ($p = 0.07$) [46]. This is the only prospective randomized study comparing PN to RN and helps to confirm the results of the various retrospective studies with regard to CSS. Finally, in more recent years, studies have begun to emerge assessing the safety and efficacy of PN for the management of cT2 tumors. These results are highlighted in a 2019 meta-analysis by Li et al., which found better postoperative renal function but slightly higher postoperative complication rate for PN compared to RN, with results that suggested that PN is noninferior to RN in terms of recurrence rates, tumor-specific mortality, and all-cause mortality [47].

A central tenet of PN is the goal of complete excision of the mass with a margin that is devoid of tumor. The precise amount of normal parenchyma that needs to be excised along with the tumor to achieve adequate cancer control is not fully agreed upon. For experienced surgeons, a positive margin during PN is relatively rare, with published rates of approximately 2.4–5.5% [48, 49]. The effect of a positive surgical margin on oncologic outcome has been examined, and at present, the best available evidence demonstrates that a microscopic-positive surgical margin does not adversely affect cancer-specific or overall survival. In a bi-institutional retrospective study, Yossepowitch et al. examined the effect of a positive margin on survival and recurrence in 77 patients who had positive surgical margins following PN [48]. With a median follow-up of 3.4 years, including 5-year follow-up in 33% of the cohort and 10-year follow-up in 10% of the cohort, there was no difference between the 5- and 10-year freedom from local disease recurrence or metastatic progression when comparing patients with positive and negative surgical margins. In a multivariable analysis, positive margin status did not predict the likelihood of local recurrence or development of metastatic disease. In a retrospective study of multiple European centers, 111 patients with positive surgical margins following PN were compared with a cohort matched for tumor size, indication for PN (imperative vs. elective), and age [50]. They found that while rates of recurrence were greater for patients with a positive surgical margin (10.9% vs. 2.9%, $p = 0.03$), rates of cancer-specific survival and overall survival were the same among patients with positive and negative surgical margins. Multivariable modeling showed that positive surgical margins did not predict recurrence. Similar results have been found in other studies [51]. Despite these findings, the risk of recurrence likely remains greater in instances where residual tumor tissue is left behind in the resection bed. Some have suggested that what are read to be positive margins on pathology may in fact be the result of a tissue-processing artifact, which distorts the tumor and causes margins that are in fact negative to appear positive on pathology, thus making the true positive margin rate lower [52]. These false positives could theoretically wash out what may in fact be an increased risk of recurrence and progression in patients with positive margins. Persistence of these uncertainties means that a negative surgical margin remains a key goal during PN.

As elective PN is increasingly being performed for clinically localized T1 disease and even T2 disease, as stated previously, there exists a concern that PN may be inadvertently performed for more aggressive pathologic T3a disease than traditionally mandated RN. Several investigators have examined the outcomes of PN for clinical T1a lesions that were ultimately found to be pT3a (venous involvement) on final pathology [53]. Investigators from Columbia University Medical Center revealed no evidence of disease recurrence in their cohort of patients with incidental pT3a disease following NSS, with good preservation of kidney function [54]. More recently, a meta-analysis was conducted that compared outcomes between RN and PN for pT3a tumors, ultimately analyzing nine articles with a total of 2113 RN and 1278 PN. The group found no significant difference in cancer-specific survival, overall survival, relapse-free survival, and complication rates, suggesting, fortunately, that PN may not significantly impact outcomes in these patients [55]. While venous invasion on pathologic analysis portends a worse prognosis, these studies indicate that it is still unclear whether or not performing NSS for incidental pathologic T3a disease compromises oncologic outcomes [56].

Renal Functional Outcomes in Partial Nephrectomy

The central concept driving contemporary interest in nephron-sparing approaches for the treatment of RCTs is the appreciation of the potentially deleterious long-term effects that radical extirpative renal surgery has on non-oncologic morbidity and mortality in the population of patients with RCTs. Historically, it was believed that RN, although likely to cause a detectable and permanent rise in serum creatinine because of the sacrifice of normal renal parenchyma not involved by tumor, would not contribute to serious long-term morbidity unless the patient were to develop renal replacement therapy such as dialysis or transplantation. This assumption was rooted in clinical outcomes data from renal transplant literature, in which patients undergoing donor nephrectomy were not reported to have higher rates of kidney failure requiring dialysis or resulting in death [57, 58]. However, key differences between the population of patients undergoing donor nephrectomy and the population of patients with renal masses make these assumptions invalid. Kidney donors tend to be younger (<40 years), carefully selected, and screened for medical comorbidities. In contrast, patients with spontaneous renal tumors are older (mean age 61) and often have systemic comorbidities known to affect renal function (e.g., hypertension, diabetes, vascular disease, and metabolic syndrome). The known and predictable decline in renal function over time, as nephrons atrophy and glomerular filtration rate (GFR) falls, means that patients with RCTs, by the mere fact of their age alone, are likely to harbor significantly depressed baseline renal function in the non-neoplastic parenchyma of their kidneys. Indeed, both clinical and pathologic studies have demonstrated that a substantial proportion of patients undergoing surgery for small RCTs have significant baseline underlying chronic kidney disease (CKD). Huang et al. found a 26% rate of Stage 3 CKD in a cohort of 662 patients with a solitary RCT <4 cm and a serum creatinine in the normal range [59]. A pathologic study from Harvard Medical School evaluated nonneoplastic normal tissue adjacent to the tumor in nephrectomy specimens from patients who underwent PN or RN [60]. These investigators found that only 10% of patients who underwent surgery had completely normal adjacent renal tissue. Twenty-eight percent were found to have histologic evidence of vascular sclerotic changes, and the remaining 62% demonstrated evidence of significant intrinsic renal abnormalities, including diabetic nephropathy, glomerular hypertrophy, mesangial expansion, and diffuse glomerulosclerosis. These studies provide clinical and pathologic evidence to suggest that a significant proportion of patients who undergo surgical treatment for RCTs have underlying, and potentially unrecognized, renal disease.

A substantial body of retrospective evidence from numerous large institution and population-based studies has demonstrated that renal volume loss during RN adversely affects long-term renal function and is a risk factor for the development and progression of CKD. In 1995, Butler et al. published results from a series of 88 patients undergoing RN or PN for pT1a unilateral RCC [61]. At a mean follow-up of 48 months, they found no significant difference between preoperative and postoperative creatinine in the PN group (1.3 ± 0.4 vs. 1.3 ± 0.6 mg/dL) but a significant increase in postoperative creatinine in the RN group (1.1 ± 0.3 vs. 1.5 ± 0.4 mg/dL, $p < 0.001$). This initial report was followed several years later by studies from the Mayo Clinic in 2000 and Memorial Sloan-Kettering Cancer Center (MSKCC) in 2002, both of which demonstrated a detrimental effect of RN on renal function. In the Mayo Clinic study, Lau et al. retrospectively compared matched cohorts of patients who underwent RN or PN for a single sporadic unilateral RCC with a normal contralateral kidney and serum cr <1.5 mg/dL [39].

Patients were matched for age at surgery, sex, tumor size, pathologic T stage and grade, and year of surgery. While median preoperative serum creatinine was 1.1 in both the PN and RN groups, at a median follow-up of 3.8 years, the cumulative incidence of chronic renal insufficiency (arbitrarily defined in this study as creatinine >2.0 mg/dL) was 22.4% in the RN group versus 11.6% in the PN group (risk ratio 3.7; 95% CI, 1.2–11.2; $p < 0.01$). These investigators also looked at a subset of patients for whom 10-year follow-up data was available and found the cumulative 10-year incidence in chronic renal insufficiency was almost twice as high in RN versus PN (20.2 vs. 10.5, RR; 5.5, 95% CI 1.2–25.0). In the study from MSKCC, McKiernan et al. retrospectively identified 290 patients with normal preoperative serum creatinine and normal contralateral kidney undergoing PN or RN for a single spontaneous unilateral pT1a renal mass [62]. With a mean follow-up of 26 months, they demonstrated a significantly higher postoperative creatinine in the RN group versus the PN group (1.5 mg/dL vs. 1.0 mg/dL) despite having no difference between groups in preoperative creatinine. Nine percent of the patients in the RN group achieved a creatinine level > 2.0, versus none in the PN group, and Kaplan-Meier analysis demonstrated the chance of developing a creatinine >2.0 was significantly higher in the RN group ($p = 0.008$).

These early reports were corroborated in 2006 in a landmark study in Lancet Oncology in which Huang et al. clearly demonstrated the measurable detrimental effect RN can have on long-term postoperative renal function in patients undergoing surgery for RCTs [59]. This study from MSKCC included 662 patients who underwent RN or PN for a unilateral RCT <4 cm and who had a normal preoperative serum creatinine concentration and a normal contralateral kidney on imaging. Rather than using serum creatinine concentration as an estimate of renal function, this study utilized the Modification of Diet in Renal Disease (MDRD) equation to calculate the estimated glomerular filtration rate (eGFR). This equation, which estimates GFR using serum creatinine, age, race, and gender, was developed in a group of over 1500 patients and has since been validated in larger, diverse groups of patients and has proved to be a more accurate estimate of kidney function than measured serum creatinine [63–65]. Using this equation, Huang et al. made several novel observations. First, as mentioned previously, in this group of 662 patients with normal preoperative serum creatinine levels, the use of the MDRD equation revealed a 26% rate of Stage 3 CKD (eGFR <60 mL/min/1.73 m^2), demonstrating a high level of baseline renal insufficiency in this population of patients with normal serum creatinine and normal contralateral kidneys. Additionally, after surgery, the 3-year probability of freedom from new onset of eGFR lower than 60 mL/min/1.73 m^2 was 80% (95% CI 73–85) after PN and only 35% (28–43; $p < 0.0001$) after RN; corresponding values for GFRs lower than 45 mL/min/1.73 m^2 were 95% and 64% ($p < 0.0001$), respectively (see Fig. 9.2).

Multivariable analysis showed that RN remained an independent risk factor for patients developing new onset of eGFR lower than 60 mL/min/1.73 m^2 (hazard ratio 3.82 [95% CI 2.75–5.32]) and 45 mL/min/1.73 m^2 (11.8 [95% CI 6.24–22.4]; both $p < 0.0001$). These trends were similarly demonstrated in a cohort of 510 patients with cT1b renal masses from the Cleveland Clinic [66] as well as a US population-based cohort from the SEER program [13]. In addition, in contrast to the traditional paradigm mentioned at the start of this section, a recent study comparing a donor nephrectomy population to a partial nephrectomy population found significantly higher rates of CKD development among donor nephrectomy patients, despite younger age and higher preoperative eGFR [67]. Finally, a more recent propensity score-matched analysis of a US VA population found that partial nephrectomy was associated with a significantly lower relative risk of new-onset CKD stage 4, further cementing the risk for meaningful renal function decline [68]. At present, all available data have clearly demonstrated that the loss of normal, functioning nephrons during RN has a measurable detrimental effect on postoperative renal function and puts patients at risk for new-onset CKD when compared with PN.

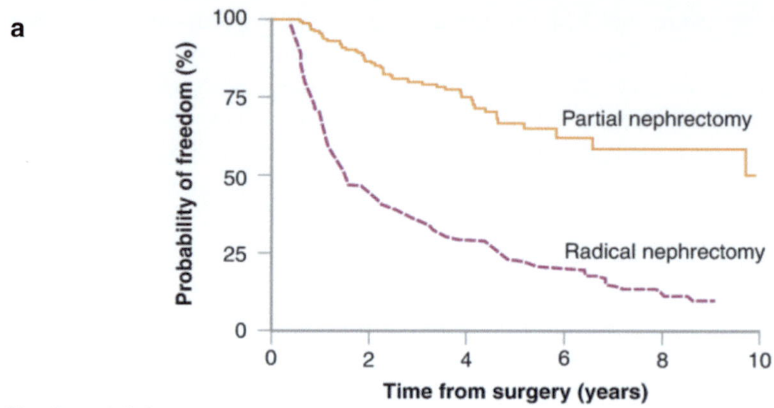

Number at risk

Partial nephrectomy	287	134	62	23	11	6
Radical nephrectomy	204	69	43	20	12	0

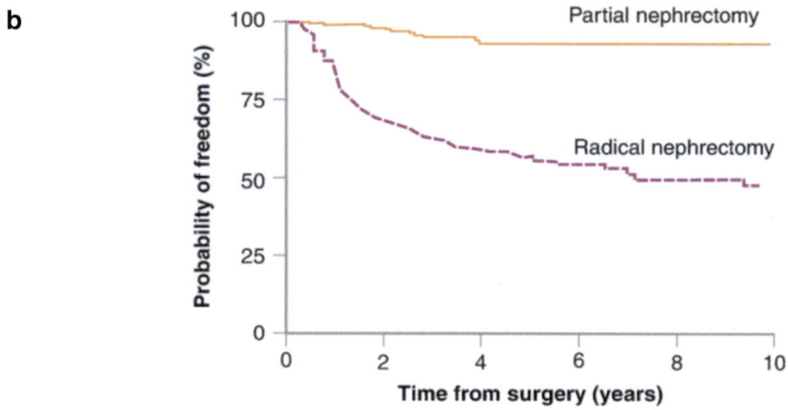

Number at risk

Partial nephrectomy	385	187	84	33	13	6
Radical nephrectomy	262	130	86	56	33	21

Fig. 9.2 Probability of freedom from new-onset GFR lower than 60 mL/min/1.72 m^2 (panel **a**) and 45 mL/min/1.72 m^2 (panel **b**), by operation type. (Adapted from Huang et al. [59])

Chronic Kidney Disease, Morbidity, and Mortality

Chronic kidney disease is a significant public health concern in the United States and is recognized as one of the leading causes of mortality. Currently, it is estimated that CKD affects over 37 million, or 1 in 7, United States adults [69–71] (see Fig. 9.3).

The prevalence and incidence of CKD rose progressively during the end of the twentieth century, but in the last decade, more advanced stages of the disease appear to be leveling off [72, 73]. Despite this, a person today is over five times more likely to be diagnosed with CKD than they were 20 years ago. In addition, some studies suggest that the prevalence may begin to rise again in the coming decades [74]. Because of the effects of aging on renal function, the disease disproportionately affects older persons, and it is estimated that 47% of persons over the age of 70 have early stages of the disease [75]. The human and financial toll of this disease is tremendous. Once hemodialysis is initiated, the expected remaining life span is 8 years for patients aged 40–44 and 4.5 years for those 60–64 years of age. Treatment costs for patients with CKD are more than double that of those without CKD and can reach up to $23,000 per person annually [70]. The high prevalence of conditions that contribute to CKD, such as diabe-

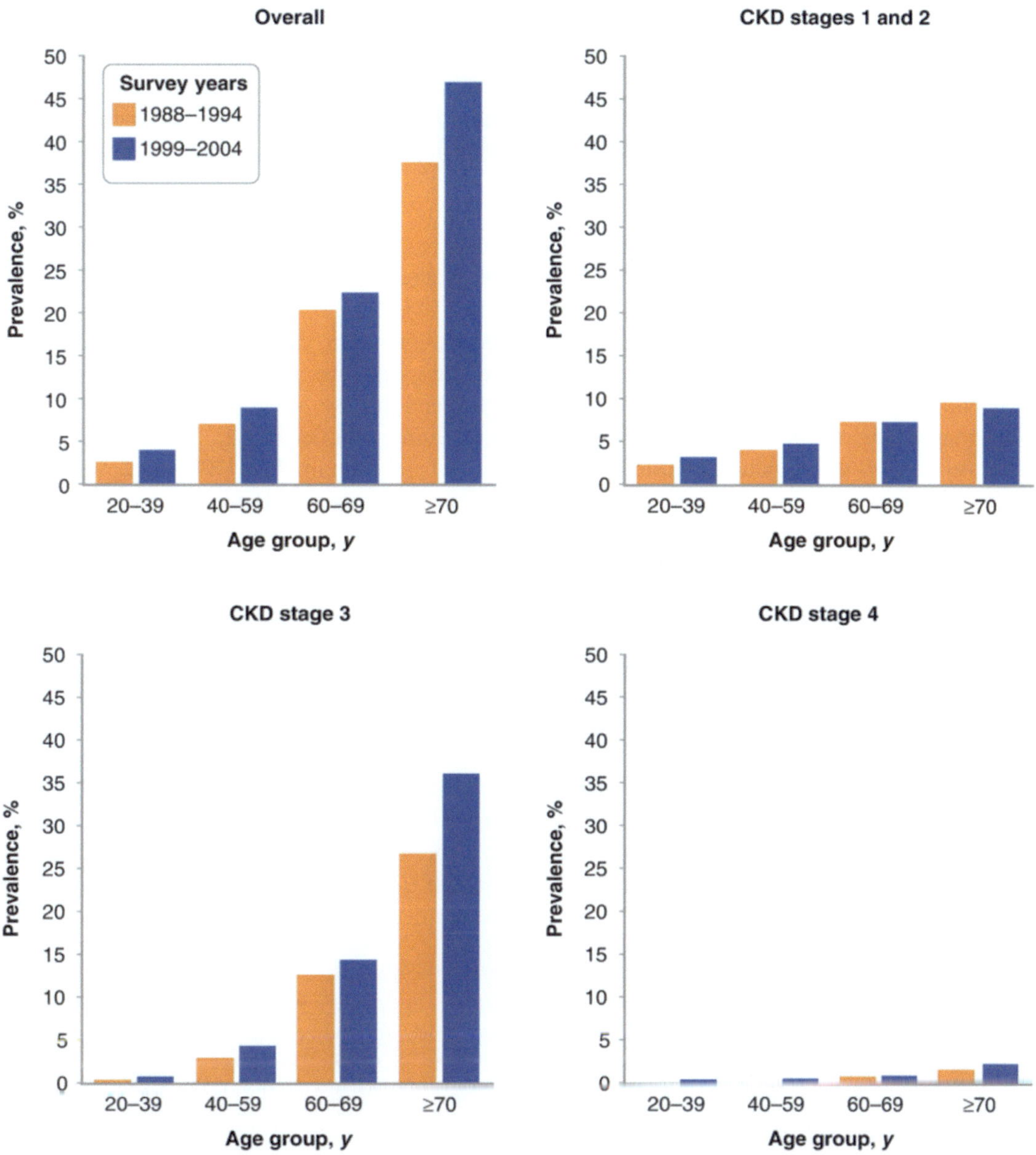

Fig. 9.3 Prevalence of chronic kidney disease (CKD) stages by age group in NHANES 1988–1994 and 1999–2004. (Adapted from Coresh et al. [69])

tes, obesity, and hypertension, means that CKD will continue to be a significant US public health issue, and even if prevalence rates have stabilized, increasing population size means a rise in the absolute number of people with CKD over time.

Beginning in 1999, the National Kidney Foundation began to recognize that a significant number of patients in the United States had underlying, undiagnosed early stages of kidney disease and that, if detected early, could be treated and potentially prevented from progressing to more severe stages of renal dysfunction. In response, they launched the Kidney Disease Outcomes Quality Initiative (KDOQI), which aimed to increase the detection of early stages of CKD, improve the treatment of kidney disease in these patients, and hopefully slow the progression of their kidney disease and prevent progression to ESRD. The prior Kidney Disease Improving Global Outcomes (KDIGO) guidelines, which were published in 2012, define CKD as abnormalities of kidney structure or function, present for >3 months, with implications for health, and is classified into one of four risk groups based on etiology of CKD, eGFR category, and albuminuria category [76]. The eGFR in the initial guideline was calculated using one of several Chronic Kidney Disease Epidemiology Collaboration (CKD-EPI) equations, which use gender, age, race, and either serum creatinine or serum cystatin C to estimate the GFR [77, 78]. The risk groups (e.g., low, moderate, high, and very high) are aimed at predicting the risk of concurrent and future complications from CKD. With the update of the KDIGO guidelines in 2024 came a shift to the 2021 CKD-EPI equation for eGFR prediction, which notably no longer includes race as a component [79]. This change was predicated on a large body of literature that suggested that the use of the race component may have adversely affected minority populations [80]. However, widespread implantation and the long-term implications of such a change are not yet fully known but will be an area of active research in the coming years.

It has been known since the 1970s that the risk of adverse cardiovascular events is dramatically increased in patients who are on renal replacement therapy [81]. Mortality rates for patients requiring maintenance hemodialysis approach 20%, with more than 50% of deaths attributable to cardiovascular disease. However, until relatively recently, little was known about the risk of death among patients living with more modest levels of CKD. In 2004, Go et al. published their seminal work in the *New England Journal of Medicine* demonstrating the association between CKD and the risk of cardiovascular events, hospitalization, and death [82]. These investigators estimated the longitudinal GFR among 1,120,295 adults within a large healthcare delivery system in whom serum creatinine had been measured between 1996 and 2000 and who had not undergone dialysis or kidney transplantation. In this population, with a median age of 52, the risk of death increased progressively as the GFR decreased below 60 mL/min/1.73 m^2. The adjusted hazard ratio for cardiovascular events also increased inversely in a dose-dependent fashion, as did the risk of hospitalization (see Fig. 9.4).

This study was groundbreaking because it was the first to demonstrate a significantly increased risk of death in patients whose eGFR was only

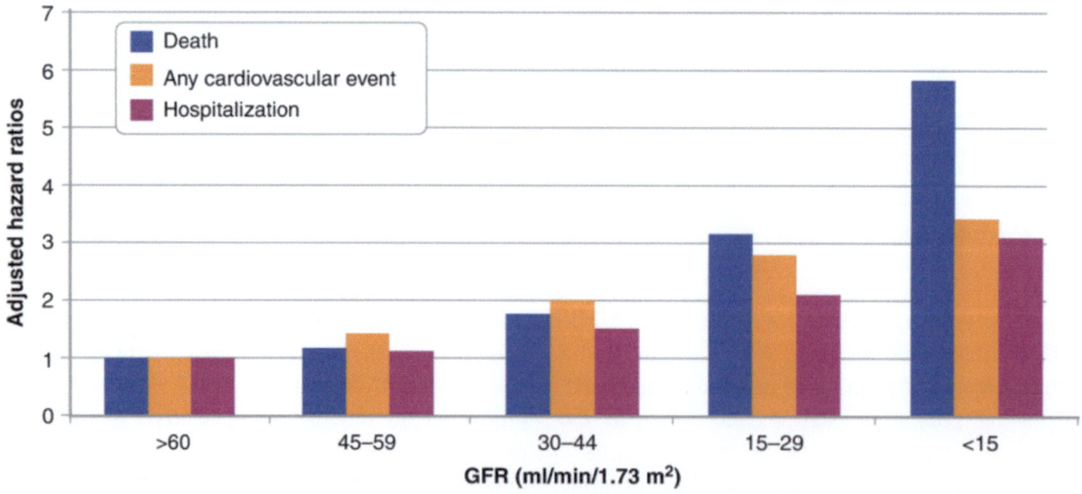

Fig. 9.4 Adjusted hazard ratio for death from any cause, cardiovascular events, and hospitalization among 1,120,295 ambulatory adults, according to estimated GFR. (Adapted from Go et al. [82])

moderately decreased (<60 mL/min/1.73 m^2), and that risk increased in a graded response inversely proportional to eGFR. These original findings have since been corroborated in subsequent large, longitudinal cohort studies, again demonstrating that CKD is a significant risk factor for poor cardiovascular outcomes and cardiovascular death [83–86]. Other researchers have found an eGFR <60 mL/min/1.73 m^2 to be a risk factor for morbidity and death from other noncardiovascular causes in elderly populations [87].

The connection between renal dysfunction and cardiovascular disease has been an active area of research since it was first observed over 30 years ago, and while the mechanisms behind the association are incompletely characterized at present, some associations have been established [88]. Increased rates of atherogenesis in patients with CKD have been observed and are thought to be one of the major contributors to increased cardiovascular morbidity and mortality among patients with CKD [89]. Evidence for this phenomenon was noted in a retrospective case-control study evaluating pre- and post-nephrectomy aortic calcium volume scores (ACS) [90]. In this study, 739 patients who underwent RN were compared with an age and gender-matched control cohort. Investigators found that patients who underwent nephrectomy had greater postoperative ACS compared with controls and that age, postoperative GFR, and time since nephrectomy were independent predictors of ACS on multivariate regression. It has since been shown that the extent and rate of progression of vascular classifications portends a poor prognosis in CKD patients, suggesting the continued importance of this association [91]. As a cause or consequence of this atherogenesis, evidence of oxidative stress and a state of microinflammation is usually found in patients with CKD. Investigators have since studied the use of anti-inflammatory cytokine inhibitors to combat the deleterious effects of inflammation on the cardiovascular system and saw a greater benefit in those with a decreased eGFR compared to those with normal eGFR [92]. In addition, other well-established risk factors for cardiovascular disease, such as hypertension and left ventricular dysfunction, have been demonstrated to be increased in patients with intrinsic renal disease, even in patients with a normal GFR [93]. Both experimental and clinical studies have demonstrated increased sympathetic output in patients with even minor degrees of CKD, possibly due to activation of intrarenal chemoreceptors and baroreceptors that send activating signals to the hypothalamus, where catecholamine turnover is increased [94, 95]. Other serum abnormalities such as altered apolipoprotein patterns with increased Lp(a) have been found in patients with renal disease even when inulin clearance was still normal [96]. Finally, there is a known association between CKD, cardiac arrhythmias, and sudden cardiac death, with more than two-thirds of deaths in patients with advanced CKD attributable to sudden cardiac death [97].

As our understanding of the connection between CKD and cardiovascular disease improves, we have been working toward treatments specifically targeted to improve outcomes in these patients, though many of these interventions still require large-scale validation. Born out of the diabetes literature, SGLT2 inhibitors have shown both cardiovascular and renoprotective effects. Specifically, two of these agents have been shown to reduce the progression of albuminuria and to preserve eGFR, even in patients with more advanced stages of CKD [98, 99]. More recently, the CREDENCE trial specifically assessed the use of SGLT2 inhibitors in CKD patients and demonstrated a significant reduction in the risk of renal replacement therapy and death caused by renal insufficiency [100]. Additionally, selective mineralocorticoid receptive antagonists, including a novel agent called Finerenone, have been studied specifically in patients with CKD and diabetes for their potential anti-fibrotic and vascular remodeling effects and have been found to decrease the risk of CKD progression and to improve cardiovascular outcomes, specifically in patients with higher stage CKD or even early CKD with significant albuminuria [101]. These studies highlight advances in the field, but more work is needed to improve outcomes for these patients.

Renal Surgery, Morbidity, and Mortality

Increasing awareness of the association between CKD and cardiovascular disease and mortality as well as the recognition of the deleterious effects that nephron loss during kidney surgery can have on postoperative renal function has prompted interest in examining the impact of renal surgery on cardiovascular outcomes, as well as overall mortality. While the previously cited studies demonstrate an association between RN and an increased risk of new-onset CKD, there exists some uncertainty over whether the CKD resulting from surgically induced loss of nephrons leads to an increased risk of adverse cardiovascular events and death.

A number of early retrospective studies examined the relationship between surgery and non-oncologic morbidity and mortality and demonstrated that RN is a risk factor for adverse cardiovascular events and worsened overall survival. The first of such papers was published using data from 648 patients who underwent either RN or PN at the Mayo Clinic between 1989 and 2003 [102]. When analyzed as a whole, investigators found no significant association between the type of surgery (RN vs. PN) and overall mortality. However, during multivariate analysis, they found a significant interaction between age and mortality, leading them to stratify their cohort by the median age of 65. In doing so, they found that in patients <65 years old, RN was associated with an increased risk of death from any cause when compared with PN (RR 2.16, 95% CI 1.12–4.19, $p = 0.022$). As an aside, this stratification based on age highlights another ongoing debate within the CKD community, which is that some have argued that different "meaningful" eGFR thresholds should be used for younger and older individuals, respectively [103]. This is predicated on the theory that younger patients with any decrease in their eGFR have a longer potential lead time for adverse outcomes, while older individuals may not be at a significant lifetime risk of complications until their eGFR passes a lower threshold. The 2024 KDIGO guidelines refute this claim, citing the relative risk scores generated by the guidelines committee as evidence to suggest that vigilant use of the current CKD groups should adequately address all potential adverse outcomes.

The initial report of increased mortality from RN was followed soon thereafter by researchers analyzing data from the SEER cancer registry linked to Medicare claims, who demonstrated an association between RN, overall mortality, and postoperative adverse cardiovascular events [104]. In this study, 2991 patients older than 66 years were identified who were treated with RN or PN for renal tumors 4 cm or less between 1995 and 2002. Multivariate and Kaplan-Meier analysis demonstrated that RN was associated with an increased risk of overall mortality (HR 1.38, $p < 0.01$) and a 1.4 times greater number of cardiovascular events after surgery ($p < 0.05$) (see Fig. 9.5).

Several subsequent studies have demonstrated similar findings. Using SEER data from 1998 to 2004 for T1a lesions, Zini et al. reported that RN was significantly associated with increased overall mortality (RR 1.23, $p = 0.001$) as well as noncancer-related mortality as compared with PN for cT1a masses [105]. Research published in JAMA using SEER-Medicare data as recent as 2007 demonstrated that for cT1a lesions, PN resulted in a predicted survival increase of 5.6 (95% CI, 1.9–9.3), 11.8 (95% CI, 3.9–19.7), and 15.5 (95% CI, 5.0–26.0) percentage points at 2, 5, and 8 years posttreatment ($p < 0.001$) when compared with RN [106]. This finding corresponded to a number-needed-to-treat of 7 at the 8-year time point. In other words, treating seven patients with PN rather than RN would result in one life saved during 8 years of follow-up. Investigators have demonstrated similar trends in patients with tumors greater than cT1a. In a study of data from 1004 patients who underwent surgery at the Cleveland Clinic for cT1b renal masses, Weight et al. demonstrated that RN resulted in a greater averaged decrease in postoperative eGFR (23.5% vs. 16.6%) when compared to PN and that postoperative eGFR was associated with overall survival and cardiovascular survival in an independent and graded fashion [66, 107]. The paradigm suggested by these studies—

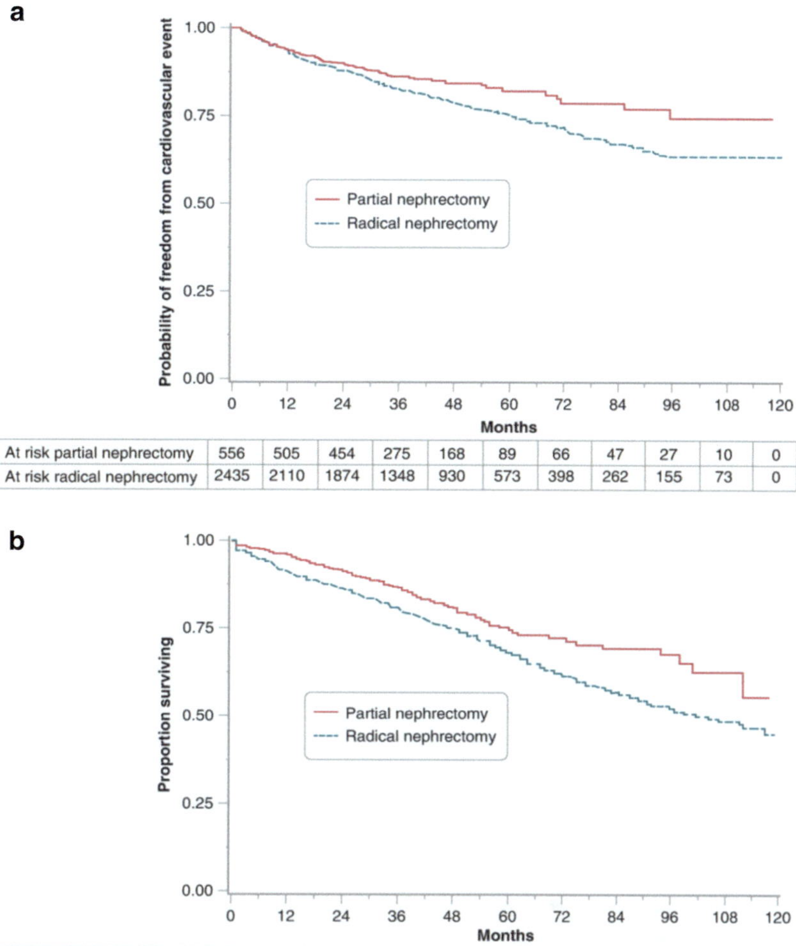

Panel a:

At risk partial nephrectomy	556	505	454	275	168	89	66	47	27	10	0
At risk radical nephrectomy	2435	2110	1874	1348	930	573	398	262	155	73	0

Panel b:

At risk partial nephrectomy	556	534	492	324	198	106	78	56	33	12	0
At risk radical nephrectomy	2435	2217	2077	1544	1099	711	522	363	233	105	0

Fig. 9.5 Probability of freedom from cardiovascular events (panel **a**) and freedom from death (panel **b**) by surgery type. (Adapted from Huang et al. [104])

that PN saves nephrons and that greater numbers of nephrons and higher eGFR (irrespective of absolute level of eGFR and irrespective of baseline underlying renal disease) translates into lower cardiovascular disease and death—was widely adopted by the urologic community and prompted some to promote partial nephrectomy virtually "at all costs" when technically feasible.

However, this paradigm, which was widely accepted and promoted by the urologic community based on the retrospective studies, was called into question in 2011 when the EORTC-GU published the results of the only randomized prospective clinical trial comparing RN with PN for the treatment of a solitary renal mass. The study compared RN with PN for patients with a solitary renal mass ≤5 cm and a normal contralateral kidney [46]. The study was initially designed as a noninferiority trial intended to detect a 10% difference in overall survival. However, after 5 years, the decision was made to redesign the trial to detect a more modest 3% difference, and the trial would ultimately close early due to poor accrual after randomizing 541 patients. The two groups were well-balanced with regard to preoperative characteristics. The primary outcome of the study was overall survival, and in the intention-to-treat analysis, investigators found, unexpectedly, that RN had a slightly higher 10-year overall survival rate when compared with PN 81.1% versus 75.7%. With a hazard ratio of 1.50 (95% CI 1.03–2.16), the statistical test of noninferiority for OS was not significant ($p = 0.77$), while the test for superiority was significant ($p = 0.03$). When considering only the clinically and pathologically eligible patients, the hazard ratios were more modest, and the findings were no longer significant, but the results trended similarly—there was no overall survival benefit to PN. There were only 12 deaths from RCC, with no difference between treatment groups, and there was no difference in progression rates. Interestingly, rates of cardiovascular deaths were higher in the PN group compared with the RN group (9.3% vs. 7.3%), and the authors were at a loss to explain this observation. This study is, at present, the only prospective randomized trial comparing PN with RN, and also the only study to find an overall survival benefit for RN. It has caused some to reevaluate the previously accepted paradigm, which holds that PN should produce a survival benefit compared with RN. This will be discussed below.

The findings of the EORTC randomized trial have been questioned by some. The questioning is not only because its findings are inconsistent with the large body of retrospective data but also because of concerns about the study design and methodology. First, the study was closed prematurely because of poor accrual and was thus statistically underpowered to detect small differences. Second, while designed as a noninferiority trial, the finding of an overall survival benefit in the intention-to-treat analysis for RN over PN was based on a test of superiority. Additionally, there was no standardization of surgical technique (surgeries were carried out at over 60 centers), and there was unequal crossover between arms. The authors themselves acknowledge that their findings are perplexing, inconsistent with the existing observational data, and continue to recommend PN when feasible.

However, more recently, a reappraisal of retrospective data has led to a newfound perspective on the surgical effect of nephrectomy on renal functional outcomes and its downstream effects and allows for a reconciliation of the prospective and retrospective data. The paradigm in which PN produces overall survival benefits over RN owing to its improved postoperative renal functional outcomes relies on several assumptions which have more recently been called into question. These assumptions and the data suggesting they may not be appropriately applied to patients undergoing surgery for renal masses are described below.

Flawed Assumption #1: The entirety of the increase in cardiovascular and mortality risk conferred by CKD can be determined by the eGFR. This assumption was largely adopted by the urologic community during the emergence of PN and formed the backbone of the foundation of the support for the potential benefits of PN over RN in improving overall survival. However, this assumption has never been consistent with the nephrologic literature, which has long recognized that, in addition to eGFR, both the cause of the CKD and the degree of albuminuria have a significant impact with regard to the prognosis and potential future complications from CKD. This entity is a recognized component of the KDIGO clinical practice guidelines, which classify CKD, not only by eGFR but also by the cause of the CKD and albuminuria category, with management recommendations directed at patients based on CKD cause. The significance of proteinuria in the calculation of the risk of adverse events from CKD has largely been ignored by the urologic community, which has relied almost entirely on eGFR in calculations of risk. In fact, the albumin-to-creatinine ratio is known to be an independent predictor of both all-cause and cardiovascular mortality, suggesting that intrinsic renal disease, in addition to a decrease in the number of functioning, is a critical determinant in the evaluation of risk attributable to CKD.

Causes of CKD include renal volume loss (cystic kidney disease, trauma, *kidney cancer surgery*), intrinsic renal disease (glomerulonephritis), and systemic diseases affecting the kidney (DM, HTN). The differing etiologies of chronic kidney disease produce different clinical outcomes, and as such, the cause of CKD has clear implications for the clinical outcome of the disease. This idea is also a recognized concept in nephrologic literature and reflected in KDIGO guidelines, which advocate classifying CKD by its cause (renal volume loss vs. intrinsic renal disease vs. medical diseases affecting the kidney). Consistent with this have been recent observations that CKD from renal volume loss, as can occur following nephrectomy, appears to have a lower risk of progressive loss in GFR and lower risk of mortality when compared with CKD caused by systemic or intrinsic renal disease. Lane et al. investigated this consideration in a very large cohort of >4000 patients undergoing nephrectomy for renal masses from the Cleveland Clinic [108]. They compared the patients who had decreased preoperative eGFR (CKD from intrinsic renal diseases or medical diseases affecting the kidney) versus those who had normal renal function preoperatively but developed an eGFR <60 following surgery (CKD from renal volume loss). They found that a low preoperative eGFR (from medical renal disease) was a strong predictor of overall survival when compared with those with a normal preoperative eGFR. However, interestingly, they found that neither surgically induced chronic kidney disease (CKD from renal volume loss) nor postoperative glomerular filtration rate was a significant predictor of survival in patients without pre-existing CKD. This scenario suggests that patients with CKD attributable entirely to renal volume loss from surgery may not be at greater mortality risk. They also found that annual renal functional decline was 4.7% and 0.7% for patients with CKD from medical renal disease and CKD from renal volume loss, respectively, suggesting that CKD from renal volume loss may not result in a further progressive loss of eGFR over time. The same group of researchers published a second study using the same cohort of patients in which they compared patients with postoperative eGFR >60 (no CKD), patients with normal preoperative eGFR but postoperative eGFR <60 (CKD from renal volume loss), and those with both pre- and postoperative eGFR <60 (CKD from both medical renal disease and renal volume loss) [109]. They made several interesting observations. First, they found no difference in the rate of progressive renal decline or the need for dialysis between those with no postoperative CKD and those with CKD from renal volume loss. This scenario again suggests that CKD attributable solely to loss of nephrons during surgery may not result in further declines in eGFR after surgery. Second, they found all-cause and nonrenal-cancer-cause mortality was highest in those with CKD from both medical renal disease and renal volume loss, followed by those with CKD from renal volume loss and then those with no CKD. This finding was again consistent with their first study and suggested that those with decreased eGFR exclusively from surgery may not be at increased mortality risk. Finally, they found that the probability of various adverse outcomes, including a 50% drop in eGFR, need for dialysis, and 5-year all-cause mortality, did not begin to increase until the postoperative eGFR reached a level of approximately 45 mL/min/1.73 m^2 (see Fig. 9.6).

This observation was interesting and suggested that the commonly used cutoff of <60 mL/min/1.73 m^2—widely discussed in urologic literature—for determining who may be at risk of the consequences of postoperative CKD may have been too stringent, and in fact, the risk of cardiovascular disease and death may not begin to rise until a much lower level of eGFR—45 mL/min/1.73 m^2—is reached. These observations led the authors to conclude that CKD from renal volume loss is associated with better renal functional outcomes and overall survival than CKD from medical renal disease and that the probability of adverse events does not truly begin to rise until the postoperative eGFR falls below 45 mL/min/1.73 m^2. This scenario led the authors to further conclude that in patients without pre-existing CKD, and in whom the postoperative eGFR is expected to be >45, RN is an appropriate choice, particularly in cT1b and cT2 tumors, and in those in whom PN could be technically challenging.

Flawed Assumption #2: Inverse linear relationship exists between eGFR and cardiovascular mortality risk at all levels of eGFR. As described above, data from the Cleveland Clinic cohort suggests that the increase in cardiovascular risk may not begin at an eGFR <60 mL/min/m^2 but rather at lower levels of eGFR, perhaps <45 mL/min/m^2 (see Fig. 9.6). Interestingly, a similar finding is present in the seminal work of Go et al. They found that while rates of death, cardiovascular events, and hospitalization all

Fig. 9.6 The 5-year probability of all-cause mortality according to the new baseline GFR (*CKD-M/S* chronic kidney disease attributable to medical renal disease and loss of nephrons from surgery, *CKD-S* chronic kidney disease attributable to loss of nephrons from surgery). (Adapted from Lane et al. [109])

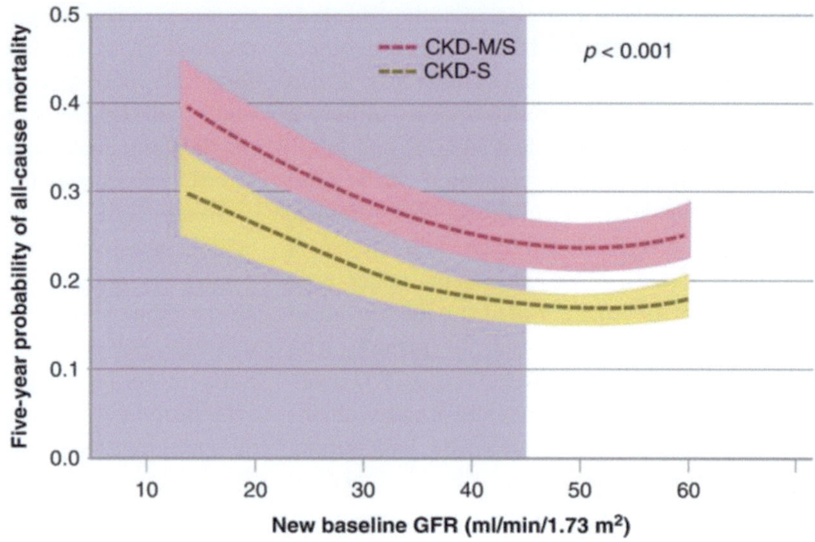

began to increase at an eGFR of <60 mL/min/m^2, the increases in risk at this level of eGFR are relatively minimal. However, these risks increase in a much more dramatic fashion at an eGFR <45 mL/min/m^2 (see Fig. 9.4). This observation has not been widely adopted by the urologic community, in which the majority of publications use an eGFR cutoff of 60 mL/min/m^2 as the meaningful cutoff for determining CKD. And interestingly, it is this point that may help explain why PN did not produce overall survival benefits in the EORTC randomized trial. In a manuscript by Scosyrev et al., the EORTC investigators reported the renal functional outcomes of the two trial groups [110]. With a median follow-up of 6.7 years, they reported that, as expected, modest postoperative renal dysfunction (eGFR <60 mL/min/1.73 m^2) was significantly more common in the RN group versus the PN group (85.7% vs. 64.7%, $p < 0.001$). However, more advanced renal dysfunction (eGFR <30 mL/min/1.73 m^2) was similar between the two groups (10.0% vs. 6.3%, nonsignificant), and very advanced renal dysfunction (eGFR <15 mL/min/1.73 m^2) was almost identical between the two groups (1.5% vs. 1.6%, nonsignificant). Given the appreciation that the increased risks of cardiovascular events, hospitalization, and death may not truly begin to increase until eGFR falls below 45 mL/min/1.73 m^2 and that the rates of these levels of more severe renal dysfunction were relatively similar between the two treatment arms in the EORTC trial, it is not surprising that PN failed to improve overall survival compared to RN. This result is further supported when considering that the postoperative renal dysfunction in this cohort is largely attributable to CKD from renal volume loss (preoperative eGFR was similar between the treatment arms) and that, as the studies from the Cleveland Clinic suggest, this form of CKD tends not to result in progressive renal decline and does not carry with it the same risk of cardiovascular disease or death as medical renal disease. Even more recently, a large scale study using South Korean insurance data specifically compared surgically induced CKD with nonsurgical CKD, and found that medical CKD patients had a high risk of progression to ESRD and higher risk of developing cardiovascular disease, corroborating the prior studies [111].

With these findings in mind, one important ongoing area of research, both by investigators at our institution and several others, is the development of preoperative nomograms and calculators to predict postoperative renal function after both partial and radical nephrectomy. There is an ever-growing body of tools that have been developed, each with unique inputs, including clinical, oncologic, and radiographic characteristics, but no tool to date can perfectly predict postoperative

GFR [112]. It will be important as the field progresses to ensure that investigators design models that predict not just any decline in GFR, but meaningful declines with thresholds below an eGFR of 60 to adequately inform clinicians and patients of postoperative risks to aid in decision making. Along these lines, one group recently published a nomogram to predict the development of significant renal functional decline at 2 years after PN, using a threshold of 25% decline in baseline renal function instead of a threshold of eGFR <60 [113]. Whether this represents a clinically meaningful cut will require further investigation.

While RN may not put patients at the increased risk of cardiovascular complication originally believed, there is some evidence that RN may be a risk factor for other adverse outcomes, including increased rates of osteoporosis and poor postoperative quality of life metrics when compared with PN. A retrospective analysis of 905 patients undergoing either RN or PN with a mean follow-up of 6.4 years evaluated the primary outcomes of the development of osteoporosis and non-pathologic fractures. While the two groups were comparable preoperatively with respect to the prevalence of osteoporosis and fractures, postoperatively, a significantly greater proportion of patients in the RN group had developed osteoporosis (22.6% vs. 12.5%, $p < 0.001$) and postoperative fractures (9.8% vs. 4.4%, $p = 0.007$). Several studies have attempted to evaluate the impact that surgical approach for localized renal masses has on overall postoperative quality of life. Poulakis et al. utilized quality of life (QOL) questionnaires to retrospectively evaluate 416 patients and prospectively evaluate 51 patients, all of whom underwent RN or PN for localized RCTs [114]. Using three validated QOL questionnaires along with two sets of questions designed to address the fear of recurrence and attitudes associated with having less than two functional kidneys, they found that at the 12-month postoperative mark, patients after elective NSS showed significantly better scores on physical functioning, role functioning, fatigue, and bodily pain than those who underwent RN ($p < 0.05$). There was no statistically significant difference in the fear of recurrence between patients who underwent PN versus RN. Similar results were found by Novaro et al., who prospectively evaluated 129 patients undergoing RN or PN and demonstrated that patients undergoing elective PN had significantly higher chances of returning to baseline physical functioning scores 6 months after surgery and significantly higher probability of returning to baseline social function scores 12 months after surgery compared with those undergoing mandatory NSS [115]. One possible explanation for this finding is that patients who underwent mandatory NSS, presumably for either bilateral tumors, a tumor in a solitary kidney, or CKD, may have a heightened awareness and sensitivity to the potential deleterious effects kidney surgery may have on their overall kidney functioning. This hypothesis is supported by findings by Clark et al., who demonstrated that a patient's self-reported perception of the amount of remaining kidney tissue after their surgery was directly and highly correlated with their overall physical quality of life [116]. Clark also found that patients with more remaining parenchyma were less apt to worry about cancer recurrence or to believe that renal cancer had negatively impacted their overall health.

Complications of Partial Nephrectomy

PN is an inherently technically demanding procedure. Control of segmental blood vessels, repair of the collecting system, excision of the tumor with an adequate margin, and performing satisfactory renorrhaphy all contribute to the difficulty of the operation. Despite these challenges, the majority of procedures are completed without complications, and when they do arise, complications are generally minor. Reported rates of complication in the literature vary somewhat widely, from 10 to 36% [117, 118], likely based in part on inconsistent criteria and reporting. Contemporary series using more standardized grading criteria demonstrate complication rates of approximately 20%, with equivalency between open and laparoscopic approaches. In two large studies of complications graded using a standardized 5-tiered scale, investigators from the Cleveland Clinic and MSKCC found overall rates of complications for PN were less than 20% and that over 70% of these complications were relatively minor and could be successfully managed conservatively [31, 32]. When interventional procedures were necessary, the vast majority were either endoscopic (placement of a ureteral stent) or percutaneous (drainage of urinoma or angioembolization). The most common complications are hemorrhage and urine leak, with both reported to occur in approximately 2–5% of patients in most contemporary series from high-volume centers [31, 32, 118]. Hemorrhage is generally managed expectantly with observation, bed rest, and transfusion as needed. Bleeding that cannot be controlled with these modalities prompts angioembolization or, rarely, re-exploration. Urine leak is treated with percutaneous image-guided drainage and ureteral stent placement, as indicated. Prolonged fistula is rare and requires long-term percutaneous drainage. Death was extremely uncommon, occurring in only 0.2% of cases. In the study from MSKCC, there was no significant difference in overall complication rates between PN and RN; however, PN did result in higher rates of procedural complications (9% vs. 3%) and need for intervention (2.5% vs. 0.6%) [32].

Investigators have evaluated the factors associated with complications following PN. Patient age, tumor stage, operative time, and surgery on a solitary kidney have been shown to be independent predictors of postoperative complications following PN. Some of these variables, such as tumor size, operative time, and tumor in a solitary kidney, may function as surrogates for the technical difficulty of the procedure, in which case higher rates of complication might be inferred. An early study comparing complication rates in 1800 laparoscopic PN (LPN) and open PN (OPN) demonstrated that LPN was independently predictive of greater rates of postoperative complications, hemorrhage, and need for reintervention [119]. A follow-up study from the same group, however, demonstrated that complication rates for LPN have decreased over time and that contemporary rates for LPN are equivalent to OPN [31]. This improvement is presumably due to technical improvements and increased surgical experience. Over time, investigators were able to show that, on average, complication rates after PN are lower at high-volume centers when compared with centers that perform fewer PNs, again suggesting that experience and volume contribute to lower rates of complications [120].

One potential way to improve surgical complications and outcomes after LPN is through the utilization of robot-assisted LPN or robotic PN (RPN). LPN is technically challenging, thus limiting its use to a few experienced laparoscopic surgeons. With articulating, wristed arms, magnified visualization, and more precise control, RPN may allow for more facile tumor excision and renorrhaphy than LPN and thus broaden the potential utilization of minimally invasive NSS to a larger urologic community. In contrast to the estimated learning curve of over 100 cases to master LPN, studies have suggested that the learning curve for RPN is on the order of two dozen cases [121]. Literature examining the initial experience with RPN revealed similar complication rates as LPN, while an early meta-analysis demonstrated favorable rates of conversion to RN and possible even postoperative renal function benefits [122]. In a large multi-institutional review of RPN versus LPN, Benway et al. demonstrated that morbidity after RPN was equivalent to LPN [123]. Our own institutional data suggests exceedingly low vascular and urine leak complication rates of 2% [124].

Two additional technical considerations that have theoretical benefits are the retroperitoneal PN approach, and the use of the newer single-port robotic surgical platform. The retroperitoneal PN has gained traction in recent years, with early technical reports suggesting that the approach was comparable to the traditional transperitoneal approach, but with the benefit of avoiding the peritoneal cavity while offering more direct access to posterior tumors [125]. Early papers suggested that the retroperitoneal approach may offer shorter operative times, lower EBL, and comparable warm ischemia time [126]. In a meta-analysis of several retrospective studies, the authors also found lower operative time, lower EBL, and shorter length of stay, with no difference in complication rates [127]. Thus, at this time, the data does not suggest improved complication rates with this approach, but the theoretical benefit of avoiding a hostile abdomen should still be taken into consideration when thinking about potential complications. Along the same lines, some groups have begun using the Da Vinci single-port robotic surgery platform to perform both transperitoneal and retroperitoneal partial [128, 129]. Though early syntheses of available data suggest only similar outcomes compared to the multiport platform, the approach offers several potential benefits, including decreased incisional morbidity and a wider variety of patient positioning options that may minimize potential nerve injuries, but this has not been born out in the data as of yet.

Utilization of Partial Nephrectomy

The growing awareness of the potential functional benefits of PN, the diffusion of technology allowing for more rapid and widespread adoption of PN, growing surgical experience, and publication of guidelines for the management of renal masses has resulted in a progressive decrease in the number of RNs being performed in the United States, in favor of NSS. This finding is particularly true for the small renal mass. The trend away from RN and toward PN has been ongoing for decades. Multiple investigators have reported slowly increasing annual rates of PN over the last two decades. Based on SEER data abstracted between 1988 and 2001, Miller et al. demonstrated that the use of PN progressively increased for all tumors less than 7 cm in size, and a patient diagnosed in 2001 was nearly five times more likely to undergo PN than those diagnosed in 1988 [130]. Follow-up studies capturing data through 2008 demonstrated a 49% increase in the PN as a proportion of all renal surgeries [131, 132]. By 2009, the number of patients who underwent a nephron-sparing procedure as treatment for SRM in the United States eclipsed those who underwent radical nephrectomy [133]. Despite this, there is evidence that PN may remain underutilized in the management of surgically amenable RCTs [134]. While in high-volume tertiary-care centers, approximately 90% of pT1a lesions are treated with PN [135, 136], population-based studies suggest PN is likely utilized less frequently outside these centers [130, 137]. A more recent analysis of the national inpatient sample database, currently published only as an AUA abstract, highlighted a similar trend toward underutilization of PN outside urban areas, and found that PN utilization did not increase between 2014 and 2019 [138]. In addition, a recent SEER analysis looked at small renal mass management more broadly, and found that urologist preference and local practice patterns were major drivers of utilization of the various acceptable strategies for managing T1a tumors [139]. Thus, interventions directed at providers may be needed to influence management strategies.

The reasons for the underutilization of PN are unknown, but a number of factors have been identified that appear to predict the likelihood of a patient receiving PN. Size has been clearly demonstrated to be associated with a probability of receiving PN, with larger tumors treated less frequently with PN than smaller ones [130, 137]. This finding may be unsurprising given that size may serve as a surrogate for increased perceived technical difficulty in performing PN on the part of the surgeon. Along these lines, nephrometry score, a standardized scoring system developed to capture a tumor's complexity based on size, location, and endophytic or exophytic position, has also been found in single-institution studies to predict the likelihood of receiving PN [21, 140]. In theory, increased utilization of local ablative therapies and active surveillance for small renal masses, which may offset any potential increases in utilization of PN, but data confirming or denying this claim has yet to fully mature (see Fig. 9.7) [141, 142].

Older age has been found in multiple studies of both US and European populations to predict a decreased likelihood of undergoing PN [136, 137]. One speculative explanation for this age bias toward RN is the result of surgeon preference, as RN is believed to carry fewer periopera-

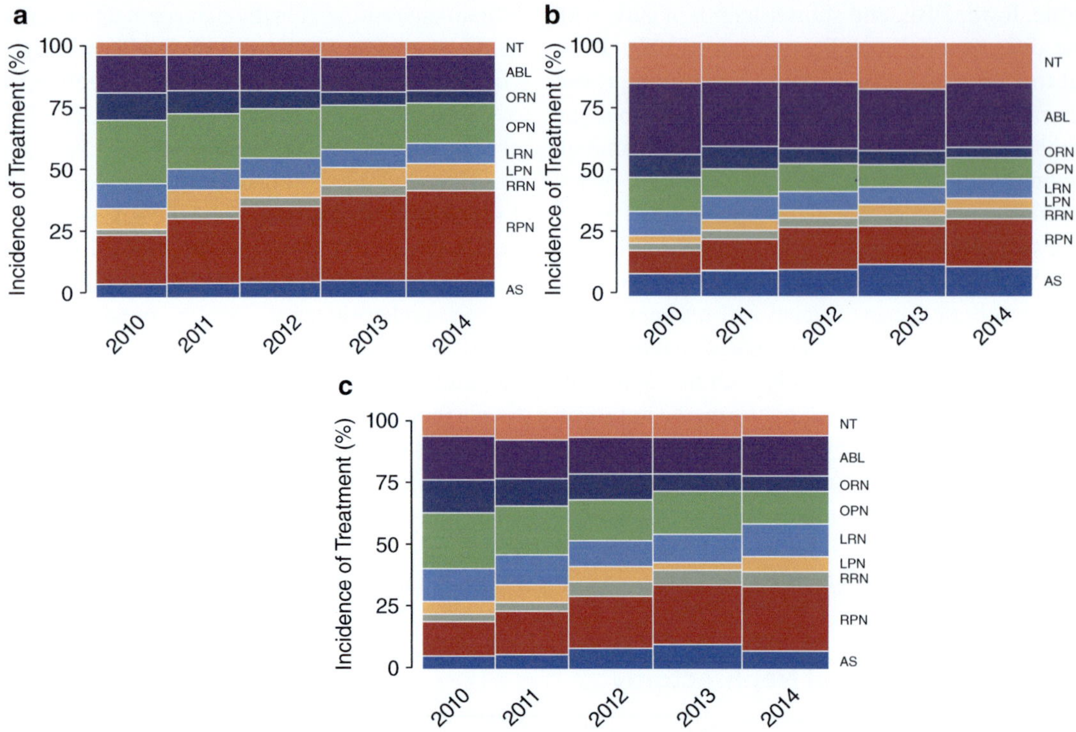

Fig. 9.7 Temporal trends in small renal mass management strategies, 2010–2014. (Adapted from Shah et al. [141])

tive complications than PN. Another possible explanation is the surgeon perception of a decreased benefit of preserved renal function in older patients. However, given the age-dependent decrease in GFR, older patients may be the most likely to benefit from aggressive preservation of renal parenchyma and renal function, especially in patients with other comorbidities that may result in a decline of GFR [143, 144]. Female gender has also been demonstrated to be significantly associated with a decreased likelihood of receiving PN [136, 137]. One postulated explanation for this phenomenon includes physician underestimation of the risk of CKD in women due to lower preoperative serum creatinine values as a result of lesser muscle mass in females rather than improved renal function. This phenomenon is especially troubling, given that women are more likely to have a benign renal mass [145]. The presence of comorbidities has been shown to be associated with a decreased risk of being treated with PN [131]. Again, the reasons for this assumption are unknown, but one potential explanation is surgeon preference to perform the less-complex RN in patients in whom perioperative complications may be poorly tolerated. This logic, however, fails to appreciate that patients with multiple comorbidities and preoperative intrinsic renal disease may be those at the highest risk for the potential morbidity and mortality that may result from post-RN renal dysfunction. As a result, patients with multiple comorbidities may be those who stand to benefit most from the aggressive pursuit of a nephron-sparing approach.

Some have postulated that the increasing use of laparoscopy and specifically LRN led to underuse of PN. This hypothesis is based on the premise that PN, particularly LPN, is an inherently more complex procedure with higher rates of perioperative complications. Thus, surgeons faced with a choice between LRN and PN (open or lap) may be preferentially performing LRN, for which they have an increased level of experience and comfort. While evidence for this phenomenon has been observed in one population-based study, data supporting this conjecture remains limited

[134, 146]. With the wider spread dissemination of the robotic-assisted PN, with the shorter perceived learning curve, time will tell as to whether technical considerations continue to drive underutilization, or if the robot levels the playing field in terms of overall access to PN.

Candidate Selection

The absolute indications for PN, many of which have been recognized as early as the 1800s [29], include tumors in a solitary kidney, bilateral tumors, or patients with preexisting renal disease for whom RN would likely result in the need for hemodialysis. In addition, multifocal tumors, frequently associated with genetic syndromes, should also be strongly considered for excision by PN, given that these patients are at high risk for developing subsequent ipsilateral and contralateral tumors, requiring additional surgeries and further loss of renal parenchyma and function. Relative indications for PN include pre-existing medical renal disease or conditions that predispose to CKD such as hypertension, diabetes, or atherosclerotic vascular disease in whom RN would potentially lead to significant acceleration or worsening of kidney function. As mentioned previously, while there appears to be a tendency for surgeons to preferentially perform RN in more elderly patients or in patients with greater burdens of comorbidity, careful consideration should be taken in these instances because these patients may be at highest risk for postoperative CKD and its associated morbidity and mortality, particularly if their postoperative eGFR is anticipated to be <45 mL/min/1.73 m^2. Unfortunately, there is also some recent evidence to suggest that age is an independent risk factor for long-term renal functional decline even after robotic partial nephrectomy, and studies aimed at assessing treatment efficacy specifically in older patients may help elucidate the need to emphasize or deemphasize NSS in these patients [147].

For patients without absolute indications, tumor stage is paramount when considering PN. At present, given the strong evidence for the oncologic efficacy, safety, and superior renal functional outcomes provided by PN for cT1 lesions, only the location of the tumor and complexity of the resection should be considered contraindications to the procedure. However, it must be remembered that PN is, first and foremost, a procedure performed for suspected malignancy, and as such, any procedure must be undertaken with the goal of complete excision of the tumor with a pathologically negative surgical margin. Surgeons should be familiar with anatomic complexity scoring systems such as the RENAL score and should plan procedures with the aim of complete tumor resection as the primary goal, with preservation of functional parenchyma as secondary.

While surgical excision is the mainstay in the treatment of any enhancing renal mass suspected to be malignant, the potentially indolent nature of a significant portion of SRMs must be appreciated. As detailed in the next section, both thermal ablation and active surveillance have emerged as alternative management strategies for SRMs. Thermal ablation, which includes both microwave ablation and cryoablation, has been utilized for some time, but series have now begun to mature, and we have a better understanding of oncologic outcomes. Generally recommended for masses <3 cm given evidence of worse oncologic outcomes for T1b tumors, thermal ablation appears to have similar metastasis-free survival compared to PN for small masses [148, 149]. After a single thermal ablative procedure, meta-analyses have found a higher risk of local recurrence compared with PN, but this can be mitigated with a salvage or secondary ablation [149]. Thus, for those who are poor surgical candidates, including older or comorbid patients, thermal ablation is a reasonable alternative that should be discussed.

Additionally, it should be mentioned that there has been increasing interest in the use of active surveillance for the management of SRMs, driven largely by the discovery of the indolent (and at times benign) nature of some SRMs as with prostate cancer active surveillance, clinicians should engage in shared decision making, patient on both patient and SRM factors. Key to this discussion is the importance of serial imaging and follow-up, as surveillance series to date highlight a cross-over to active treatment rate ranging from 10 to 30% [150, 151]. Tumor factors that should prompt consideration for treatment include tumor size >3 cm, median growth rate >5 mm per year, infiltrative appearance, clinical stage migration, or aggressive histology on RMB.

The oncologic efficacy and safety of PN in the treatment of clinical T2, T3, and locally advanced tumors remains largely unproven at this time. There is some limited data, however, to suggest that PN may be oncologically equivalent to RN in these larger tumors. Breau et al. compared the outcomes of 69 patients who underwent PN for pT2, pT3a, and pT3b spontaneous unilateral renal tumors with a matched cohort of 207 patients who had undergone RN [152]. They found no significant difference in recurrence, metastasis, or cancer-specific survival at a mean follow-up of 3.2 years. In a single-institution retrospective study of 213 patients undergoing nephrectomy for cT1 who were upstaged to pT2 disease or greater, PN demonstrated at least equivalent cancer control and overall survival outcomes when compared with RN, a finding that held when tumors were stratified stage for stage [153]. On multivariate analysis, the type of nephrectomy did not predict overall survival. A single-institution study of eight patients in whom PN was performed for tumors presumed preoperative to be cT1a but who were ultimately pathologically upstaged to pT3b (renal vein involvement) demonstrated high rates of negative surgical margins and no recurrences at a median of 20 months [54]. It must be remembered that the aforementioned findings were in cohorts of patients who were cT1 and then subsequently upstaged intraoperatively or on final pathology. As a result, these results may not be generalizable to patients who present with >cT1 disease. While these promising oncologic findings suggest that PN may ultimately be proven to be a viable option for the treatment of renal masses >cT1, researchers have noted higher rates of complications in these larger masses, likely due to more difficult resection and more complicated reconstruction. Early studies presenting this concern were corroborated by a more recent meta-analysis, which found an RR of 1.96 for postoperative complications, as well as, in this case, a higher positive margin rate. One more recent study specifically compared robotic PN to minimally invasive radical nephrectomy in complex renal masses (defined as RENAL score 10–12) and did not find an increased risk of complications or inferior oncologic outcomes [154]. Thus, given discrepancies in the literature, there is more to learn when it comes to the safety and efficacy of PN in larger, more complex renal masses.

Small Renal Masses and Partial Nephrectomy in Clinical Practice Guidelines

The American Urological Association (AUA) [155], American Society for Clinical Oncology (ASCO) [156], European Association of Urology (EAU) [157], and the National Comprehensive Cancer Network (NCCN) [158] all have published and widely available guidelines which provide recommendations and guidance in the management of renal tumors, though it should be noted that several of these guidelines have not been updated in some time, with the most recent ASCO guideline published in 2017 and the most recent AUA guideline published in 2021. The majority of recommendations provided across these multiple guidelines are congruent, with some notable, albeit subtle, differences. It should be noted that these guidelines are limited by a paucity of level 1 evidence in the field, particularly with regard to active surveillance and ablative treatment of masses. The retrospective design of most studies makes them subject to selection bias and heterogeneous practice patterns. All guidelines emphasize that management recommendations be based on a comprehensive evaluation of both disease (tumor size, location, multifocality) and host (age, comorbid status, baseline renal function, life expectancy) characteristics. Active surveillance is an option in the elderly and comorbid with small masses in all guidelines, despite no prospective comparative data evaluating its effectiveness versus active treatment. AUA guidelines are somewhat unique in specifying a particular size (<2 cm) in which active surveillance is a particular option for patients with both solid and cystic masses. All guidelines list PN as the preferred treatment of choice in patients in whom the intervention is indicated for a cT1a renal mass, in whom PN is technically feasible, and all guidelines recommend radical nephrectomy when partial is not feasible based on tumor characteristics (central location, complexity). AUA guidelines, however, go further in specifying that RN is preferred when tumor is complex AND no preexisting CKD AND postop eGFR expected to be >45 mL/min/1.73 m^2, perhaps reflecting the increasing appreciation that moderately decreased eGFR resulting from surgery may not be a significant risk factor for mortality or cardiovascular disease.

Conclusion

The widespread use of cross-sectional abdominal imaging means that significant numbers of patients in the United States and abroad are diagnosed with asymptomatic, early-stage renal cancers. At present, given the limitations in determining the biological identity and aggressiveness of a lesion preoperatively, as well as a paucity of data regarding the natural history of kidney tumors, surgery remains the reference standard for curative treatment of these lesions. While RN has traditionally been the procedure of choice for renal tumors, data has consistently demonstrated that PN provides oncologically equivalent control to RN, with comparative rates of complication when performed by experienced surgeons. There is a substantial body of evidence demonstrating that RN may put patients at an increased risk for CKD and its attendant morbidity when compared with PN. However, the single prospective study aimed at evaluating this question found no difference in overall survival between those receiving RN and PN, calling this paradigm into question. Closer evaluation of retrospective data suggests that the potential benefits may apply only to those with a significantly diminished postoperative eGFR. Despite this, PN is recognized, in the United States and abroad, as the current standard by which other treatments must be compared. As our understanding of small RCTs and their treatments evolves, so too may future treatment options for these tumors.

References

1. Siegel RL, Miller KD, Wagle NS, Jemal A. Cancer statistics, 2023. CA Cancer J Clin. 2023;73(1):17–48. https://doi.org/10.3322/caac.21763. PMID: 36633525.
2. Simard EP, Ward EM, Siegel R, Jemal A. Cancers with increasing incidence trends in the United States: 1999 through 2008. CA Cancer J Clin. 2012;62(2):118–28.
3. Chow W-H, Devesa SS, Warren JL, Joseph F, Fraumeni J. Rising incidence of renal cell cancer in the United States. JAMA. 1999;281(17):1628–31.
4. Decastro GJ, McKiernan JM. Epidemiology, clinical staging, and presentation of renal cell carcinoma. Urol Clin North Am. 2008;35(4):581–92; vi.
5. Palumbo C, Pecoraro A, Knipper S, Rosiello G, Luzzago S, Deuker M, Tian Z, Shariat SF, Simeone C, Briganti A, Saad F, Berruti A, Antonelli A, Karakiewicz PI. Contemporary age-adjusted incidence and mortality rates of renal cell carcinoma: analysis according to gender, race, stage, grade, and histology. Eur Urol Focus. 2021;7(3):644–52. https://doi.org/10.1016/j.euf.2020.05.003. Epub 2020 May 23. PMID: 32456993.
6. Hock LM, Lynch J, Balaji KC. Increasing incidence of all stages of kidney cancer in the last 2 decades in the United States: an analysis of surveillance, epidemiology and end results program data. J Urol. 2002;167(1):57–60.
7. Gandaglia G, Ravi P, Abdollah F, Abd-El-Barr A-E-RM, Becker A, Popa I, et al. Contemporary incidence and mortality rates of kidney cancer in the United States. Can Urol Assoc J. 2014;8(7–8):247–52.
8. Kane CJ, Mallin K, Ritchey J, Cooperberg MR, Carroll PR. Renal cell cancer stage migration: analysis of the National Cancer Data Base. Cancer. 2008;113(1):78–83.
9. Hollingsworth JM, Miller DC, Daignault S, Hollenbeck BK. Rising incidence of small renal masses: a need to reassess treatment effect. J Natl Cancer Inst. 2006;98(18):1331–4.
10. Hollenbeck BK, Taub DA, Miller DC, Dunn RL, Wei JT. National utilization trends of partial nephrectomy for renal cell carcinoma: a case of underutilization? Urology. 2006;67(2):254–9.
11. Saad AM, Gad MM, Al-Husseini MJ, Ruhban IA, Sonbol MB, Ho TH. Trends in renal-cell carci-

noma incidence and mortality in the United States in the last 2 decades: a SEER-based study. Clin Genitourin Cancer. 2019;17(1):46–57.e5. https://doi.org/10.1016/j.clgc.2018.10.002. Epub 2018 Oct 11. PMID: 30391138; PMCID: PMC6348014.
12. Mindrup SR, Pierre JS, Dahmoush L, Konety BR. The prevalence of renal cell carcinoma diagnosed at autopsy. BJU Int. 2005;95(1):31–3.
13. Surveillance Epidemiology and End Results Program. seer.cancer.gov.
14. Smaldone MC, Egleston B, Hollingsworth JM, Hollenbeck BK, Miller DC, Morgan TM, Kim SP, Malhotra A, Handorf E, Wong YN, Uzzo RG, Kutikov A. Understanding treatment disconnect and mortality trends in renal cell carcinoma using tumor registry data. Med Care. 2017;55(4):398–404. https://doi.org/10.1097/MLR.0000000000000657. PMID: 27820596; PMCID: PMC5352513.
15. Linehan WM. The genetic basis of kidney cancer: implications for management and use of targeted therapeutic approaches. Eur Urol. 2012;61(5):896–8.
16. Deng F-M, Melamed J. Histologic variants of renal cell carcinoma: does tumor type influence outcome? Urol Clin North Am. 2012;39(2):119–32, v.
17. Schmidbauer J, Remzi M, Memarsadeghi M, Haitel A, Klingler HC, Katzenbeisser D, et al. Diagnostic accuracy of computed tomography-guided percutaneous biopsy of renal masses. Eur Urol. 2008;53(5):1003–11.
18. Barwari K, de la Rosette JJ, Laguna MP. The penetration of renal mass biopsy in daily practice: a survey among urologists. J Endourol. 2012;26(6):737–47.
19. Uzzo R, Russo P, Chen D, et al. Multicenter phase 3 REDECT trial with iodine I 124 Girentuximab-PET/CT for the presurgical detection of clear cell renal cell carcinoma (ccRCC) [abstract]. Kidney Cancer J. 2010;8:79, 85.
20. Rowe SP, Gorin MA, Hammers HJ, Javadi MS, Hawasli H, Szabo Z, et al. Imaging of metastatic clear cell renal cell carcinoma with PSMA-targeted 18F-DCFPyL PET/CT. Ann Nucl Med. 2015;29(10):877–82.
21. Kutikov A, Fossett LK, Ramchandani P, Tomaszewski JE, Siegelman ES, Banner MP, et al. Incidence of benign pathologic findings at partial nephrectomy for solitary renal mass presumed to be renal cell carcinoma on preoperative imaging. Urology. 2006;68(4):737–40.
22. Frank I, Blute ML, Cheville JC, Lohse CM, Weaver AL, Zincke H. Solid renal tumors: an analysis of pathological features related to tumor size. J Urol. 2003;170(6 Pt 1):2217–20.
23. Fujii Y, Komai Y, Saito K, Iimura Y, Yonese J, Kawakami S, et al. Incidence of benign pathologic lesions at partial nephrectomy for presumed RCC renal masses: Japanese dual-center experience with 176 consecutive patients. Urology. 2008;72(3):598–602.
24. Johnson DC, Vukina J, Smith AB, et al. Preoperatively misclassified, surgically removed benign renal masses: a systematic review of surgical series and United States population level burden estimate. J Urol. 2015;193:30.
25. Vijay V, Vokshi FH, Smigelski M, Nagpal S, Huang WC. Incidence of benign renal masses in a contemporary cohort of patients receiving partial nephrectomy for presumed renal cell carcinoma. Clin Genitourin Cancer. 2023;21(3):e114–8. https://doi.org/10.1016/j.clgc.2022.11.006. Epub 2022 Nov 18. PMID: 36535809.
26. Herr H. Surgical management of renal tumors: a historical perspective. Urol Clin North Am. 2008;35:543–9; v.
27. Robson CJ, Churchill BM, Anderson W. The results of radical nephrectomy for renal cell carcinoma. J Urol. 1969;101(3):297–301.
28. Clayman RV, Kavoussi LR, Soper NJ, Dierks SM, Meretyk S, Darcy MD, et al. Laparoscopic nephrectomy: initial case report. J Urol. 1991;146(2):278–82.
29. Goldstein AE, Abeshouse BS. Partial resections of the kidney. J Urol. 1937;38(1):15–42.
30. Vermooten V. Indications for conservative surgery in certain renal tumors: a study based on the growth pattern of the cell carcinoma. J Urol. 1950;64(2):200–8. PubMed – NCBI [Internet]. [cited 2018 Jun 16]. https://www.ncbi.nlm.nih.gov/pubmed/15429181.
31. Simmons MN, Gill IS. Decreased complications of contemporary laparoscopic partial nephrectomy: use of a standardized reporting system. J Urol. 2007;177(6):2067–73; discussion 2073.
32. Stephenson AJ, Hakimi AA, Snyder ME, Russo P. Complications of radical and partial nephrectomy in a large contemporary cohort. J Urol. 2004;171(1):130–4.
33. Sutherland SE, Resnick MI, Maclennan GT, Goldman HB. Does the size of the surgical margin in partial nephrectomy for renal cell cancer really matter? J Urol. 2002;167(1):61–4.
34. Timsit M-O, Bazin J-P, Thiounn N, Fontaine E, Chrétien Y, Dufour B, et al. Prospective study of safety margins in partial nephrectomy: intraoperative assessment and contribution of frozen section analysis. Urology. 2006;67(5):923–6.
35. Carvalho JAM, Nunes P, Tavares-da-Silva E, Parada B, Jarimba R, Moreira P, Retroz E, Caetano R, Sousa V, Cipriano A, Figueiredo A. Impact of positive surgical margins after partial nephrectomy. Eur Urol Open Sci. 2020;21:41–6. https://doi.org/10.1016/j.euros.2020.08.006. PMID: 34337467; PMCID: PMC8317835.
36. Shah PH, Alom MA, Leibovich BC, et al. The temporal association of robotic surgical diffusion with overtreatment of the small renal mass. J Urol. 2018;200(5):981–8.
37. Porpiglia F, Mari A, Amparore D, Fiori C, Antonelli A, Artibani W, Bove P, Brunocilla E, Capitanio U, Da Pozzo L, Di Maida F, Gontero P, Longo N, Marra G, Rocco B, Schiavina R, Simeone C, Siracusano S, Tellini R, Terrone C, Villari D, Ficarra V, Carini M, Minervini A, RECORD 2 Project. Transperitoneal vs

retroperitoneal minimally invasive partial nephrectomy: comparison of perioperative outcomes and functional follow-up in a large multi-institutional cohort (The RECORD 2 Project). Surg Endosc. 2021;35(8):4295–304. https://doi.org/10.1007/s00464-020-07919-4. Epub 2020 Aug 27. PMID: 32856156; PMCID: PMC8263535.
38. Lee CT, Katz J, Shi W, Thaler HT, Reuter VE, Russo P. Surgical management of renal tumors 4 cm or less in a contemporary cohort. J Urol. 2000;163(3):730–6.
39. Lau WK, Blute ML, Weaver AL, Torres VE, Zincke H. Matched comparison of radical nephrectomy vs nephron-sparing surgery in patients with unilateral renal cell carcinoma and a normal contralateral kidney. Mayo Clin Proc. 2000;75(12):1236–42.
40. Crépel M, Jeldres C, Sun M, Lughezzani G, Isbarn H, Alasker A, et al. A population-based comparison of cancer-control rates between radical and partial nephrectomy for T1A renal cell carcinoma. Urology. 2010;76(4):883–8.
41. Thompson RH, Siddiqui S, Lohse CM, Leibovich BC, Russo P, Blute ML. Partial versus radical nephrectomy for 4 to 7 cm renal cortical tumors. J Urol. 2009;182(6):2601–6.
42. Leibovich BC, Blute ML, Cheville JC, Lohse CM, Weaver AL, Zincke H. Nephron sparing surgery for appropriately selected renal cell carcinoma between 4 and 7 cm results in outcome similar to radical nephrectomy. J Urol. 2004;171(3):1066–70.
43. Dash A, Vickers AJ, Schachter LR, Bach AM, Snyder ME, Russo P. Comparison of outcomes in elective partial vs radical nephrectomy for clear cell renal cell carcinoma of 4-7 cm. BJU Int. 2006;97(5):939–45.
44. Patard J-J, Shvarts O, Lam JS, Pantuck AJ, Kim HL, Ficarra V, et al. Safety and efficacy of partial nephrectomy for all T1 tumors based on an international multicenter experience. J Urol. 2004;171(6 Pt 1):2181–5, quiz 2435.
45. Soputro NA, Ferguson EL, Ramos-Carpinteyro R, Chavali JS, Geskin A, Fareed K, Berglund R, Fergany AF, Stein RJ, Haber GP, Campbell SC, Weight CJ, Kaouk JH. Long-term functional and oncologic outcomes following robotic partial and radical nephrectomy: a report from a single institution with up to 15 years of follow-up. J Endourol. 2024;38(6):573–83. https://doi.org/10.1089/end.2023.0543. PMID: 38568897.
46. Van Poppel H, Da Pozzo L, Albrecht W, Matveev V, Bono A, Borkowski A, et al. A prospective, randomised EORTC intergroup phase 3 study comparing the oncologic outcome of elective nephron-sparing surgery and radical nephrectomy for low-stage renal cell carcinoma. Eur Urol. 2011;59(4):543–52.
47. Li J, Zhang Y, Teng Z, Han Z. Partial nephrectomy versus radical nephrectomy for cT2 or greater renal tumors: a systematic review and meta-analysis. Minerva Urol Nefrol. 2019;71(5):435–44. https://doi.org/10.23736/S0393-2249.19.03470-2. Epub 2019 Jul 8. PMID: 31287256.
48. Yossepowitch O, Thompson RH, Leibovich BC, Eggener SE, Pettus JA, Kwon ED, et al. Positive surgical margins at partial nephrectomy: predictors and oncological outcomes. J Urol. 2008;179(6):2158–63.
49. Breda A, Stepanian SV, Liao J, Lam JS, Guazzoni G, Stifelman M, et al. Positive margins in laparoscopic partial nephrectomy in 855 cases: a multi-institutional survey from the United States and Europe. J Urol. 2007;178(1):47–50; discussion 50.
50. Bensalah K, Pantuck AJ, Rioux-Leclercq N, Thuret R, Montorsi F, Karakiewicz PI, et al. Positive surgical margin appears to have negligible impact on survival of renal cell carcinomas treated by nephron-sparing surgery. Eur Urol. 2010;57(3):466–71.
51. Kwon EO, Carver BS, Snyder ME, Russo P. Impact of positive surgical margins in patients undergoing partial nephrectomy for renal cortical tumours. BJU Int. 2007;99(2):286–9.
52. Kheterpal E, Taneja SS. Partial nephrectomy: contemporary outcomes, candidate selection, and surgical approach. Urol Clin North Am. 2012;39(2):199–210, vii.
53. Fergany AF, Hafez KS, Novick AC. Long-term results of nephron sparing surgery for localized renal cell carcinoma: 10-year followup. J Urol. 2000;163(2):442–5.
54. Woldu SL, Barlow LJ, Patel T, Hruby GW, Benson MC, McKiernan JM. Single institutional experience with nephron-sparing surgery for pathologic stage T3bNxM0 renal cell carcinoma confined to the renal vein. Urology. 2010;76(3):639–42.
55. Liu H, Kong QF, Li J, Wu YQ, Pan KH, Xu B, Wang YL, Chen M. A meta-analysis for comparison of partial nephrectomy vs. radical nephrectomy in patients with pT3a renal cell carcinoma. Transl Androl Urol. 2021;10(3):1170–8. https://doi.org/10.21037/tau--20-1262. PMID: 33850752; PMCID: PMC8039616.
56. Ramaswamy K, Kheterpal E, Pham H, Mohan S, Stifelman M, Taneja S, et al. Significance of pathologic T3a upstaging in clinical T1 renal masses undergoing nephrectomy. Clin Genitourin Cancer. 2015;13(4):344–9.
57. Najarian JS, Chavers BM, McHugh LE, Matas AJ. 20 years or more of follow-up of living kidney donors. Lancet. 1992;340(8823):807–10.
58. Fehrman-Ekholm I, Dunér F, Brink B, Tydén G, Elinder CG. No evidence of accelerated loss of kidney function in living kidney donors: results from a cross-sectional follow-up. Transplantation. 2001;72(3):444–9.
59. Huang WC, Levey AS, Serio AM, Snyder M, Vickers AJ, Raj GV, et al. Chronic kidney disease after nephrectomy in patients with renal cortical tumours: a retrospective cohort study. Lancet Oncol. 2006;7(9):735–40.
60. Bijol V, Mendez GP, Hurwitz S, Rennke HG, Nosé V. Evaluation of the nonneoplastic pathology in tumor nephrectomy specimens: predicting the risk of progressive renal failure. Am J Surg Pathol. 2006;30(5):575–84.

61. Butler BP, Novick AC, Miller DP, Campbell SA, Licht MR. Management of small unilateral renal cell carcinomas: radical versus nephron-sparing surgery. Urology. 1995;45(1):34–40, 41.
62. McKiernan J, Simmons R, Katz J, Russo P. Natural history of chronic renal insufficiency after partial and radical nephrectomy. Urology. 2002;59(6):816–20.
63. Levey AS, Bosch JP, Lewis JB, Greene T, Rogers N, Roth D. A more accurate method to estimate glomerular filtration rate from serum creatinine: a new prediction equation. Modification of Diet in Renal Disease Study Group. Ann Intern Med. 1999;130(6):461–70.
64. Stevens LA, Coresh J, Feldman HI, Greene T, Lash JP, Nelson RG, et al. Evaluation of the modification of diet in renal disease study equation in a large diverse population. J Am Soc Nephrol. 2007;18(10):2749–57.
65. Levey AS, Coresh J, Greene T, Stevens LA, Zhang YL, Hendriksen S, et al. Using standardized serum creatinine values in the modification of diet in renal disease study equation for estimating glomerular filtration rate. Ann Intern Med. 2006;145(4):247–54.
66. Weight CJ, Larson BT, Gao T, Campbell SC, Lane BR, Kaouk JH, et al. Elective partial nephrectomy in patients with clinical T1b renal tumors is associated with improved overall survival. Urology. 2010;76(3):631–7.
67. Shen J, Ruckle D, Li R, Keheila M, Alsyouf M, Schober J, Tryon D, Stokes P, Ruckle HC, Baron P, De Vera M, Baldwin DD. How a donor nephrectomy population can help give perspective to the effects of renal parenchymal preservation during partial nephrectomy. J Endourol. 2019;33(5):417–22. https://doi.org/10.1089/end.2018.0654. Epub 2019 Apr 8. PMID: 30838888.
68. Leppert JT, Lamberts RW, Thomas IC, Chung BI, Sonn GA, Skinner EC, Wagner TH, Chertow GM, Brooks JD. Incident CKD after radical or partial nephrectomy. J Am Soc Nephrol. 2018;29(1):207–16. https://doi.org/10.1681/ASN.2017020136. Epub 2017 Oct 10. PMID: 29018140; PMCID: PMC5748903.
69. Coresh J, Selvin E, Stevens LA, Manzi J, Kusek JW, Eggers P, et al. Prevalence of chronic kidney disease in the United States. JAMA. 2007;298(17):2038–47.
70. United States Renal Data System. 2017 annual data report [Internet]. [cited 2018 Jun 16]. https://www.usrds.org/adr.aspx.
71. Centers for Disease Control and Prevention. Chronic kidney disease in the United States, 2021. Centers for Disease Control and Prevention, US Department of Health and Human Services; 2021.
72. Murphy D, McCulloch CE, Lin F, Banerjee T, Bragg-Gresham JL, Eberhardt MS, et al. Trends in prevalence of chronic kidney disease in the United States. Ann Intern Med. 2016;165(7):473–81.
73. Kibria GMA, Crispen R. Prevalence and trends of chronic kidney disease and its risk factors among US adults: an analysis of NHANES 2003-18. Prev Med Rep. 2020;20:101193. https://doi.org/10.1016/j.pmedr.2020.101193. PMID: 33101883; PMCID: PMC7578737.
74. Chen TK, Knicely DH, Grams ME. Chronic kidney disease diagnosis and management: a review. JAMA. 2019;322(13):1294–304. https://doi.org/10.1001/jama.2019.14745. PMID: 31573641; PMCID: PMC7015670.
75. Levey AS, Coresh J. Chronic kidney disease. Lancet. 2012;379(9811):165–80.
76. Kidney Disease: Improving Global Outcomes (KDIGO) CKD Work Group. KDIGO 2012 clinical practice guideline for the evaluation and management of chronic kidney disease. Kidney Int Suppl. 2013;3:1–150.
77. Lane BR, Demirjian S, Weight CJ, Larson BT, Poggio ED, Campbell SC. Performance of the chronic kidney disease-epidemiology study equations for estimating glomerular filtration rate before and after nephrectomy. J Urol. 2010;183(3):896–901.
78. Matsushita K, Mahmoodi BK, Woodward M, Emberson JR, Jafar TH, Jee SH, et al. Comparison of risk prediction using the CKD-EPI equation and the MDRD study equation for estimated glomerular filtration rate. JAMA. 2012;307(18):1941–51.
79. Kidney Disease: Improving Global Outcomes (KDIGO) CKD Work Group. KDIGO 2024 clinical practice guideline for the evaluation and management of chronic kidney disease. Kidney Int. 2024;105(4S):S117–314. https://doi.org/10.1016/j.kint.2023.10.018. PMID: 38490803.
80. Charles K, Lewis MJ, Montgomery E, Reid M. The 2021 chronic kidney disease epidemiology collaboration race-free estimated glomerular filtration rate equations in kidney disease: leading the way in ending disparities. Health Equity. 2024;8(1):39–45. https://doi.org/10.1089/heq.2023.0038. PMID: 38250300; PMCID: PMC10797164.
81. Lindner A, Charra B, Sherrard DJ, Scribner BH. Accelerated atherosclerosis in prolonged maintenance hemodialysis. N Engl J Med. 1974;290(13):697–701.
82. Go AS, Chertow GM, Fan D, McCulloch CE, Hsu C. Chronic kidney disease and the risks of death, cardiovascular events, and hospitalization. N Engl J Med. 2004;351(13):1296–305.
83. Shlipak MG, Fried LF, Cushman M, Manolio TA, Peterson D, Stehman-Breen C, et al. Cardiovascular mortality risk in chronic kidney disease: comparison of traditional and novel risk factors. JAMA. 2005;293(14):1737–45.
84. Pun PH, Smarz TR, Honeycutt EF, Shaw LK, Al-Khatib SM, Middleton JP. Chronic kidney disease is associated with increased risk of sudden cardiac death among patients with coronary artery disease. Kidney Int. 2009;76(6):652–8.
85. Bae EH, Lim SY, Cho KH, Choi JS, Kim CS, Park JW, et al. GFR and cardiovascular outcomes after acute myocardial infarction: results from the Korea

Acute Myocardial Infarction Registry. Am J Kidney Dis. 2012;59(6):795–802.
86. Weiner DE, Tighiouart H, Stark PC, Amin MG, MacLeod B, Griffith JL, et al. Kidney disease as a risk factor for recurrent cardiovascular disease and mortality. Am J Kidney Dis. 2004;44(2):198–206.
87. Fried LF, Katz R, Sarnak MJ, Shlipak MG, Chaves PHM, Jenny NS, et al. Kidney function as a predictor of noncardiovascular mortality. J Am Soc Nephrol. 2005;16(12):3728–35.
88. Jankowski J, Floege J, Fliser D, Böhm M, Marx N. Cardiovascular disease in chronic kidney disease: pathophysiological insights and therapeutic options. Circulation. 2021;143(11):1157–72. https://doi.org/10.1161/CIRCULATIONAHA.120.050686. Epub 2021 Mar 15. PMID: 33720773; PMCID: PMC7969169.
89. Buzello M, Törnig J, Faulhaber J, Ehmke H, Ritz E, Amann K. The apolipoprotein e knockout mouse: a model documenting accelerated atherogenesis in uremia. J Am Soc Nephrol. 2003;14(2):311–6.
90. Glodny B, Nasseri P, Rehder P, Unterholzner V, Plaikner M, Koppelstätter C, et al. Reduced glomerular filtration rate due to loss of nephron mass may be an independent risk factor for atherosclerosis. Nephrol Dial Transplant. 2011;26(6):1882–7.
91. Raggi P. Cardiovascular disease: coronary artery calcification predicts risk of CVD in patients with CKD. Nat Rev Nephrol. 2017;13:324–6. https://doi.org/10.1038/nrneph.2017.61.
92. Ridker PM, MacFadyen JG, Glynn RJ, Koenig W, Libby P, Everett BM, Lefkowitz M, Thuren T, Cornel JH. Inhibition of interleukin-1β by canakinumab and cardiovascular outcomes in patients with chronic kidney disease. J Am Coll Cardiol. 2018;71:2405–14. https://doi.org/10.1016/j.jacc.2018.03.490.
93. Stefanski A, Schmidt KG, Waldherr R, Ritz E. Early increase in blood pressure and diastolic left ventricular malfunction in patients with glomerulonephritis. Kidney Int. 1996;50(4):1321–6.
94. Converse RL Jr, Jacobsen TN, Toto RD, Jost CM, Cosentino F, Fouad-Tarazi F, et al. Sympathetic overactivity in patients with chronic renal failure. N Engl J Med. 1992;327:1912–8. [Internet]. [cited 2018 Jun 16]. https://www.nejm.org/doi/full/10.1056/NEJM199212313272704.
95. Campese VM, Kogosov E. Renal afferent denervation prevents hypertension in rats with chronic renal failure. Hypertension. 1995;25(4 Pt 2):878–82.
96. Kronenberg F, Kuen E, Ritz E, Junker R, König P, Kraatz G, et al. Lipoprotein(a) serum concentrations and apolipoprotein(a) phenotypes in mild and moderate renal failure. J Am Soc Nephrol. 2000;11(1):105–15.
97. Genovesi S, Boriani G, Covic A, Vernooij RWM, Combe C, Burlacu A, Davenport A, Kanbay M, Kirmizis D, Schneditz D, et al. Sudden cardiac death in dialysis patients: different causes and management strategies. Nephrol Dial Transplant. 2019;1:1–10. https://doi.org/10.1093/ndt/gfz182.
98. Neal B, Perkovic V, Mahaffey KW, de Zeeuw D, Fulcher G, Erondu N, Shaw W, Law G, Desai M, Matthews DR, CANVAS Program Collaborative Group. Canagliflozin and cardiovascular and renal events in type 2 diabetes. N Engl J Med. 2017;377:644–57. https://doi.org/10.1056/NEJMoa1611925.
99. Zinman B, Wanner C, Lachin JM, Fitchett D, Bluhmki E, Hantel S, Mattheus M, Devins T, Johansen OE, Woerle HJ, et al.; EMPA-REG OUTCOME Investigators. Empagliflozin, cardiovascular outcomes, and mortality in type 2 diabetes. N Engl J Med. 2015;373:2117–2128. https://doi.org/10.1056/NEJMoa1504720.
100. Perkovic V, Jardine MJ, Neal B, Bompoint S, Heerspink HJL, Charytan DM, Edwards R, Agarwal R, Bakris G, Bull S, Cannon CP, Capuano G, Chu PL, de Zeeuw D, Greene T, Levin A, Pollock C, Wheeler DC, Yavin Y, Zhang H, Zinman B, Meininger G, Brenner BM, Mahaffey KW, CREDENCE Trial Investigators. Canagliflozin and renal outcomes in type 2 diabetes and nephropathy. N Engl J Med. 2019;380(24):2295–306. https://doi.org/10.1056/NEJMoa1811744. Epub 2019 Apr 14. PMID: 30990260.
101. Pitt B, Filippatos G, Agarwal R, Anker SD, Bakris GL, Rossing P, Joseph A, Kolkhof P, Nowack C, Schloemer P, Ruilope LM, FIGARO-DKD Investigators. Cardiovascular events with finerenone in kidney disease and type 2 diabetes. N Engl J Med. 2021;385(24):2252–63. https://doi.org/10.1056/NEJMoa2110956. Epub 2021 Aug 28. PMID: 34449181.
102. Thompson RH, Boorjian SA, Lohse CM, Leibovich BC, Kwon ED, Cheville JC, et al. Radical nephrectomy for pT1a renal masses may be associated with decreased overall survival compared with partial nephrectomy. J Urol. 2008;179(2):468–71; discussion 472–3.
103. Delanaye P, Glassock RJ, Pottel H, Rule AD. An age calibrated definition of chronic kidney disease: rationale and benefits. Clin Biochem Rev. 2016;37(1):17–26. PMID: 27057075; PMCID: PMC4810758.
104. Huang WC, Elkin EB, Levey AS, Jang TL, Russo P. Partial nephrectomy versus radical nephrectomy in patients with small renal tumors—is there a difference in mortality and cardiovascular outcomes? J Urol. 2009;181(1):55–61; discussion 61–2.
105. Zini L, Perrotte P, Capitanio U, Jeldres C, Shariat SF, Antebi E, et al. Radical versus partial nephrectomy: effect on overall and noncancer mortality. Cancer. 2009;115(7):1465–71.
106. Tan H-J, Norton EC, Ye Z, Hafez KS, Gore JL, Miller DC. Long-term survival following partial vs radical nephrectomy among older patients with early-stage kidney cancer. JAMA. 2012;307(15):1629–35.
107. Weight CJ, Larson BT, Fergany AF, Gao T, Lane BR, Campbell SC, et al. Nephrectomy induced chronic renal insufficiency is associated with increased risk

of cardiovascular death and death from any cause in patients with localized cT1b renal masses. J Urol. 2010;183(4):1317–23.
108. Lane BR, Campbell SC, Demirjian S, Fergany AF. Surgically induced chronic kidney disease may be associated with a lower risk of progression and mortality than medical chronic kidney disease. J Urol. 2013;189(5):1649–55.
109. Lane BR, Demirjian S, Derweesh IH, Takagi T, Zhang Z, Velet L, et al. Survival and functional stability in chronic kidney disease due to surgical removal of nephrons: importance of the new baseline glomerular filtration rate. Eur Urol. 2015;68(6):996–1003.
110. Scosyrev E, Messing EM, Sylvester R, Campbell S, Van Poppel H. Renal function after nephron-sparing surgery versus radical nephrectomy: results from EORTC randomized trial 30904. Eur Urol. 2014;65(2):372–7.
111. Jung G, Park S, Kim H, Lee J, Jeong CW. Comparative analysis of mortality and progression to end-stage renal disease between surgically induced and medical chronic kidney disease: A study using the National Health Insurance customized database. Investig Clin Urol. 2023;64(4):338–45. https://doi.org/10.4111/icu.20230095. PMID: 37417558; PMCID: PMC10330416.
112. Pecoraro A, Campi R, Bertolo R, Mir MC, Marchioni M, Serni S, Joniau S, Van Poppel H, Albersen M, Roussel E. Estimating postoperative renal function after surgery for nonmetastatic renal masses: a systematic review of available prediction models. Eur Urol Oncol. 2023;6(2):137–47. https://doi.org/10.1016/j.euo.2022.11.007. Epub 2023 Jan 9. PMID: 36631353.
113. Mari A, Tellini R, Antonelli A, Porpiglia F, Schiavina R, Amparore D, Bertini R, Brunocilla E, Capitanio U, Checcucci E, Da Pozzo L, Di Maida F, Fiori C, Furlan M, Gontero P, Longo N, Roscigno M, Simeone C, Siracusano S, Ficarra V, Carini M, Minervini A. A nomogram for the prediction of intermediate significant renal function loss after robot-assisted partial nephrectomy for localized renal tumors: a prospective multicenter observational study (RECORd2 project). Eur Urol Focus. 2022;8(4):980–7. https://doi.org/10.1016/j.euf.2021.09.012. Epub 2021 Sep 21. PMID: 34561199.
114. Poulakis V, Witzsch U, de Vries R, Moeckel M, Becht E. Quality of life after surgery for localized renal cell carcinoma: comparison between radical nephrectomy and nephron-sparing surgery. Urology. 2003;62(5):814–20.
115. Novara G, Secco S, Botteri M, De Marco V, Artibani W, Ficarra V. Factors predicting health-related quality of life recovery in patients undergoing surgical treatment for renal tumors: prospective evaluation using the RAND SF-36 health survey. Eur Urol. 2010;57(1):112–20.
116. Clark PE, Schover LR, Uzzo RG, Hafez KS, Rybicki LA, Novick AC. Quality of life and psychological adaptation after surgical treatment for localized renal cell carcinoma: impact of the amount of remaining renal tissue. Urology. 2001;57(2):252–6.
117. Link RE, Bhayani SB, Allaf ME, Varkarakis I, Inagaki T, Rogers C, et al. Exploring the learning curve, pathological outcomes and perioperative morbidity of laparoscopic partial nephrectomy performed for renal mass. J Urol. 2005;173(5):1690–4.
118. Ray ER, Turney BW, Singh R, Chandra A, Cranston DW, O'Brien TS. Open partial nephrectomy: outcomes from two UK centres. BJU Int. 2006;97(6):1211–5.
119. Gill IS, Kavoussi LR, Lane BR, Blute ML, Babineau D, Colombo JR, et al. Comparison of 1,800 laparoscopic and open partial nephrectomies for single renal tumors. J Urol. 2007;178(1):41–6.
120. Sun M, Bianchi M, Trinh QD, Abdollah F, Schmitges J, Jeldres C, Shariat SF, Graefen M, Montorsi F, Perrotte P, Karakiewicz PI. Hospital volume is a determinant of postoperative complications, blood transfusion and length of stay after radical or partial nephrectomy. J Urol. 2012;187(2):405–10. https://doi.org/10.1016/j.juro.2011.10.025. Epub 2011 Dec 15.
121. Haseebuddin M, Benway BM, Cabello JM, Bhayani SB. Robot-assisted partial nephrectomy: evaluation of learning curve for an experienced renal surgeon. J Endourol. 2010;24(1):57–61.
122. Choi JE, You JH, Kim DK, Rha KH, Lee SH. Comparison of perioperative outcomes between robotic and laparoscopic partial nephrectomy: a systematic review and meta-analysis. Eur Urol. 2015;67(5):891–901. https://doi.org/10.1016/j.eururo.2014.12.028. Epub 2015 Jan 6. PMID: 25572825.
123. Benway BM, Bhayani SB, Rogers CG, Dulabon LM, Patel MN, Lipkin M, et al. Robot assisted partial nephrectomy versus laparoscopic partial nephrectomy for renal tumors: a multi-institutional analysis of perioperative outcomes. J Urol. 2009;182(3):866–72.
124. Kola O, Smigelski M, Nagpal S, Gogaj R, Taneja SS, Wysock JS, Huang WC. Urine leak and vascular complications following robotic partial nephrectomy: a contemporary single-center experience. J Robot Surg. 2024;18(1):387. https://doi.org/10.1007/s11701-024-02096-1. PMID: 39470887.
125. Strauss DM, Lee R, Maffucci F, Abbott D, Masic S, Kutikov A. The future of "Retro" robotic partial nephrectomy. Transl Androl Urol. 2021;10(5):2199–208. https://doi.org/10.21037/tau.2019.12.09. PMID: 34159103; PMCID: PMC8185662.
126. Hughes-Hallett A, Patki P, Patel N, et al. Robot-assisted partial nephrectomy: a comparison of the transperitoneal and retroperitoneal approaches. J Endourol. 2013;27:869–74. https://doi.org/10.1089/end.2013.0023.
127. Pavan N, Derweesh I, Hampton L, et al. Retroperitoneal robotic partial nephrectomy: sys-

tematic review and cumulative analysis of comparative outcomes. J Endourol. 2018;32:591–6.
128. Carbonara U, Amparore D, Borregales LD, Caliò A, Ciccarese C, Diana P, Erdem S, Marandino L, Marchioni M, Muselaers CHJ, Palumbo C, Pavan N, Pecoraro A, Roussel E, Warren H, Wu ZJ, Campi R, Bertolo R. Single-port robotic partial nephrectomy: impact on perioperative outcomes and hospital stay. Ther Adv Urol. 2023;15:17562872231172834. https://doi.org/10.1177/17562872231172834. PMID: 37325290; PMCID: PMC10265377.
129. Mehrazin R, Ranti D, Altschuler J. Early perioperative outcomes of single-port compared to multi-port robot-assisted laparoscopic partial nephrectomy. J Robot Surg. 2023;17(5):2409–14. https://doi.org/10.1007/s11701-023-01617-8. Epub 2023 Jul 11. PMID: 37432590.
130. Miller DC, Hollingsworth JM, Hafez KS, Daignault S, Hollenbeck BK. Partial nephrectomy for small renal masses: an emerging quality of care concern? J Urol. 2006;175(3 Pt 1):853–7; discussion 858.
131. Kim SP, Shah ND, Weight CJ, Thompson RH, Moriarty JP, Shippee ND, et al. Contemporary trends in nephrectomy for renal cell carcinoma in the United States: results from a population based cohort. J Urol. 2011;186(5):1779–85.
132. Patel SG, Penson DF, Pabla B, Clark PE, Cookson MS, Chang SS, et al. National trends in the use of partial nephrectomy: a rising tide that has not lifted all boats. J Urol. 2012;187(3):816–21.
133. Huang WC, Atoria CL, Bjurlin M, Pinheiro LC, Russo P, Lowrance WT, et al. Management of small kidney cancers in the new millennium: contemporary trends and outcomes in a population-based cohort. JAMA Surg. 2015;150(7):664–72.
134. Sivarajan G, Huang WC. Current practice patterns in the surgical management of renal cancer in the United States. Urol Clin North Am. 2012;39(2):149–60, v.
135. Thompson RH, Kaag M, Vickers A, Kundu S, Bernstein M, Lowrance W, et al. Contemporary use of partial nephrectomy at a tertiary care center in the United States. J Urol. 2009;181(3):993–7.
136. Zini L, Patard JJ, Capitanio U, Mejean A, Villers A, de La Taille A, et al. The use of partial nephrectomy in European tertiary care centers. Eur J Surg Oncol. 2009;35(6):636–42.
137. Dulabon LM, Lowrance WT, Russo P, Huang WC. Trends in renal tumor surgery delivery within the United States. Cancer. 2010;116(10):2316–21.
138. Ranganathan S, Riveros C, Xu J, Chang C, Geng M, Klaassen Z, et al. MP47-06 Contemporary national trends in partial nephrectomy utilization for renal cancer: a real-world study using the National Inpatient Sample Database. J Urol [Internet]. 2023 [cited 2024 Aug 11];209(Supplement 4):e645. https://doi.org/10.1097/JU.0000000000003293.06.
139. Cheaib JG, Talwar R, Roberson DS, Alam R, Lee DJ, Gupta M, Patel SH, Singla N, Pavlovich CP, Patel HD, Pierorazio PM. Urologist-level variation in the management of T1a renal cell carcinoma: a population-based cohort study. Urol Oncol. 2024;42(3):71.e9–71.e18. https://doi.org/10.1016/j.urolonc.2024.01.011. Epub 2024 Jan 26. PMID: 38278631.
140. Satasivam P, Rajarubendra N, Chia PH, Munshey A, Sengupta S, Bolton D. Trends in the use of nephron-sparing surgery (NSS) at an Australian tertiary referral centre: an analysis of surgical decision-making using the R.E.N.A.L. nephrometry scoring system. BJU Int. 2012;109(9):1341–4.
141. Shah PH, Alom MA, Leibovich BC, Thompson RH, Uzzo RG, Kavoussi LR, Richstone L, Bhindi B, Habermann EB, Joshi V, Boorjian SA. The temporal association of robotic surgical diffusion with overtreatment of the small renal mass. J Urol. 2018;200(5):981–8. https://doi.org/10.1016/j.juro.2018.05.081. Epub 2018 May 22. PMID: 29792881.
142. Kiechle JE, Abouassaly R, Smaldone MC, Shah ND, Dong S, Cherullo EE, Nakamoto D, Zhu H, Cooney MM, Kim SP. National trends of local ablative therapy among young patients with small renal masses in the United States. Urology. 2015;86(5):962–7. issn:0090-4295.
143. Rifkin DE, Shlipak MG, Katz R, Fried LF, Siscovick D, Chonchol M, et al. Rapid kidney function decline and mortality risk in older adults. Arch Intern Med. 2008;168(20):2212–8.
144. Shlipak MG, Katz R, Kestenbaum B, Siscovick D, Fried L, Newman A, et al. Rapid decline of kidney function increases cardiovascular risk in the elderly. J Am Soc Nephrol. 2009;20(12):2625–30.
145. Snyder ME, Bach A, Kattan MW, Raj GV, Reuter VE, Russo P. Incidence of benign lesions for clinically localized renal masses smaller than 7 cm in radiological diameter: influence of sex. J Urol. 2006;176(6 Pt 1):2391–5, 2396.
146. Abouassaly R, Alibhai SMH, Tomlinson G, Timilshina N, Finelli A. Unintended consequences of laparoscopic surgery on partial nephrectomy for kidney cancer. J Urol. 2010;183(2):467–72.
147. Saitta C, Garofano G, Lughezzani G, Meagher MF, Yuen KL, Fasulo V, Diana P, Uleri A, Piccolini A, Mancon S, Arena P, Sordelli F, Mantovani M, Avolio PP, Beatrici E, Hurle RF, Lazzeri M, Saita A, Casale P, Derweesh IH, Paciotti M, Buffi NM. Preoperative age and its impact on long-term renal functional decline after robotic-assisted partial nephrectomy: insights from a Tertiary Referral Center. Medicina (Kaunas). 2024;60(3):463. https://doi.org/10.3390/medicina60030463. PMID: 38541189; PMCID: PMC10971873.
148. Andrews JR, Atwell T, Schmit G, Lohse CM, Kurup AN, Weisbrod A, Callstrom MR, Cheville JC, Boorjian SA, Leibovich BC, Thompson RH. Oncologic outcomes following partial nephrectomy and percutaneous ablation for cT1 renal masses. Eur Urol. 2019;76(2):244–51. https://doi.org/10.1016/j.eururo.2019.04.026. Epub 2019 May 3. PMID: 31060824.

149. Pierorazio PM, Johnson MH, Patel HD, Sozio SM, Sharma R, Iyoha E, Bass EB, Allaf ME. Management of renal masses and localized renal cancer: systematic review and meta-analysis. J Urol. 2016;196(4):989–99. https://doi.org/10.1016/j.juro.2016.04.081. Epub 2016 May 6. PMID: 27157369; PMCID: PMC5593254.
150. Pierorazio PM, Johnson MH, Ball MW, Gorin MA, Trock BJ, Chang P, Wagner AA, McKiernan JM, Allaf ME. Five-year analysis of a multi-institutional prospective clinical trial of delayed intervention and surveillance for small renal masses: the DISSRM registry. Eur Urol. 2015;68(3):408–15. https://doi.org/10.1016/j.eururo.2015.02.001. Epub 2015 Feb 16. PMID: 25698065.
151. Metcalf MR, Cheaib JG, Biles MJ, Patel HD, Peña VN, Chang P, Wagner AA, McKiernan JM, Pierorazio PM. Outcomes of active surveillance for young patients with small renal masses: prospective data from the DISSRM registry. J Urol. 2021;205(5):1286–93. https://doi.org/10.1097/JU.0000000000001575. Epub 2020 Dec 24. PMID: 33356478.
152. Breau RH, Crispen PL, Jimenez RE, Lohse CM, Blute ML, Leibovich BC. Outcome of stage T2 or greater renal cell cancer treated with partial nephrectomy. J Urol. 2010;183(3):903–8.
153. Weight CJ, Lythgoe C, Unnikrishnan R, Lane BR, Campbell SC, Fergany AF. Partial nephrectomy does not compromise survival in patients with pathologic upstaging to pT2/pT3 or high-grade renal tumors compared with radical nephrectomy. Urology. 2011;77(5):1142–6.
154. Cerrato C, Patel D, Autorino R, Simone G, Yang B, Uzzo R, Porpiglia F, Capitanio U, Porter J, Beksac AT, Minervini A, Antonelli A, Cerruto MA, Lau C, Ashrafi A, Eun D, Mottrie A, Mir C, Meagher MF, Puri D, Nguyen M, Dhanji S, Liu F, Pandolfo SD, Kutikov A, Montorsi F, Gill IS, Sundaram C, Kaouk J, Derweesh IH. Partial or radical nephrectomy for complex renal mass: a comparative analysis of oncological outcomes and complications from the ROSULA (Robotic Surgery for Large Renal Mass) Collaborative Group. World J Urol. 2023;41(3):747–55. https://doi.org/10.1007/s00345-023-04279-1. Epub 2023 Mar 1. PMID: 36856832.
155. Campbell SC, Uzzo RG, Allaf ME, et al. Renal mass and localized renal cancer: AUA guideline. J Urol. 2017;198(3):520–9.
156. Finelli A, Ismaila N, Bro B, et al. Management of small renal masses: American Society of Clinical Oncology clinical practice guideline. J Clin Oncol. 2017;35(6):668–80.
157. Ljungberg B, Bensalah K, Canfield S, Dabestani S, Hofmann F, Hora M, et al. EAU guidelines on renal cell carcinoma: 2014 update. Eur Urol. 2015;67(5):913–24.
158. NCCN clinical practice guidelines in oncology (NCCN Guidelines®) kidney cancer. Version 1.2018 [Internet]. https://www.nccn.org/professionals/physician_gls/pdf/kidney.pdf.

Objectifying Complexity of Kidney Cancers: Relationship of Tumor Anatomy and Outcomes

10

Jason R. Gee, Alexander Kutikov, Joseph Izes, and John A. Libertino

Kidney cancer is an aggressive disease with incidence on the rise. In 2024, in the United States, 81,610 new kidney cancers were detected, and 14,390 patients died from this malignancy [1]. The highest rise in incidence is noted for localized tumors and is widely believed to be due to the ubiquitous utilization of cross-sectional imaging [2–4]. Management options for localized kidney cancer continue to evolve and move away from the former gold standard, open radical nephrectomy [5, 6]. Open and minimally invasive nephron-sparing approaches are being applied as alternatives to complete renal unit removal and have been endorsed by the American Urologic Association and the European Association of Urology [7, 8]. Despite being on the rise at high volume tertiary care centers, diffusion of nephron-sparing approaches nationally remains limited [9]. While ablative techniques have gained significant clinical traction over the years, tumor resection in appropriate surgical candidates remains the gold standard [10]. Evidence demonstrating oncologic non-inferiority of nephron-sparing approaches relative to radical nephrectomy continues to accumulate. Thus, given a plethora of treatment options, clinical treatment decisions for a localized renal mass are increasingly complex [4, 11]. Despite the rise in incidence of small renal masses, resulting in a rise in interventions, the proportional impact on mortality has yet to be documented, suggesting that ideal target populations for intervention remain imperfectly defined [12, 13]. The incidence of benign tumors may range between 15 and 30% in the localized renal mass population, depending on size. Meanwhile, a majority of histologically malignant tumors are low grade and/or potentially destined for a more indolent course [14, 15]. Even patients with localized disease and high-grade pathology may exhibit a protracted clinical course [16]. In fact, active surveillance has emerged as a viable option for a select population with localized kidney cancer, recognizing issues of overtreatment and appreciating competing death risks [17].

With ablation, active surveillance, or a number of surgical approaches being available to the patient or

J. R. Gee (✉)
Associate Professor of Urology, Tufts University School of Medicine, Department of Urology, Tufts University Medical Center, Boston, MA, USA

Department of Urology, MGH Cancer Center, Emerson Hospital, Concord, MA, USA
e-mail: JGee@emersonhosp.org

A. Kutikov
Division of Urology and Urologic Oncology, Department of Surgery, Fox Chase Cancer Center, Temple University School of Medicine, Philadelphia, PA, USA

J. Izes
Department of Urology, Tufts University School of Medicine, Department of Urology Tufts University Medical Center, Boston, MA, USA

J. A. Libertino
Professor of Urology, Tufts University School of Medicine, Department of Urology Tufts University Medical Center, Boston, MA, USA

J. A. Libertino, J. R. Gee (eds.), *Renal Cancer*, https://doi.org/10.1007/978-3-031-97599-8_10

the physician, appropriate patient selection is paramount. While the choice of which intervention to pursue is multifactorial, unfortunately these treatment decisions are rarely objectified by the physician [18, 19]. A patient's clinicodemographic characteristics and medical/surgical comorbid risks have an obvious impact on treatment choice; intangibles such as physician biases stemming from training, ability, and available technology may also affect critical clinical decision-making [18, 19]. Furthermore, anatomic attributes and tumor location play a critical role in the selection of treatment choice for patients with small renal masses. Yet, until recently, anatomic attributes of a renal tumor that reflect its surgical complexity, and thereby risk, have neither been quantified nor compared. This lack of a standardized objectification system has made published treatment outcomes difficult to interpret [20]. In recent years, a flurry of manuscripts describing and validating a common language to communicate renal tumor anatomy and location has emerged.

Basis of Anatomic Classification System Development

In the general surgery literature, the Couinaud classification, adopted by the hepatobiliary surgeons and radiologists for decades, has allowed for standardized reporting of the location of liver lesions and for a more meaningful comparison of surgical outcomes [21, 22]. The urologic literature is replete with large case series and multi-institutional studies reporting surgery on renal masses of variable and often unreported anatomic complexity, yielding surgical outcomes that are difficult to interpret or compare.

Tumor size, location, and depth have classically been described as the anatomic features that play a role in surgical decision-making [23]. As such, these attributes largely form the basis for modern renal tumor anatomic classification strategies.

Tumor Size

It was recognized early that tumor size is an important prognosticator of both surgical and oncologic outcomes. While the early staging systems by Kadesky and Robson underappreciated tumor size as a prognostic factor, the TNM staging system was thought to be a major improvement [5, 24–27]. Not only did size correlate with oncologic prognosis, but it was also suggestive of the likelihood of complications and postoperative renal function [24, 28, 29]. Increased size and complexity of renal tumors can also lead to increased warm ischemia times, as renal artery clamping during partial nephrectomy was a universally accepted technique at that time, resulting in postoperative renal insufficiency. This was clearly illustrated by Libertino et al. who initially described the non-clamping partial nephrectomy technique, effectively establishing a new paradigm in addressing this issue [30–32]. This important technique, as well as its role in addressing renal ischemic injury, is described in detail in Chaps. 12 and 13 of this text. In this important research, the deleterious effects of renal artery clamping were exposed in patients with either preoperative renal insufficiency or a solitary kidney, in which even brief warm ischemia times were associated with a decline in renal function following partial nephrectomy [33, 34]. In subsequent confirmatory studies, other investigators similarly reported the significant role ischemic injury plays in postoperative renal function [35–37].

In exploring an alternate hypothesis, Campbell et al. were able to correlate tumor size with the likelihood of postoperative urinary leak and acute renal failure [38]. Although tumor size may correlate with residual renal function, they concluded that preoperative renal function and the volume of the residual parenchyma may have a higher impact on functional outcomes [35, 39]. However, these findings need to be interpreted in light of the sentinel studies by Libertino noted above, which established the significant negative impact effect of ischemia on renal function [30–34]. Afterall, the function of any residual renal parenchyma ultimately depends on its overall health and the extent of any ischemic damage following partial nephrectomy due to the clamping of renal hilar vessels.

Tumor Location

Tumor location is defined in relation to the renal topography and vascular system. Anterior versus posterior location may be important in preoperative planning when minimally invasive transperitoneal or retroperitoneoscopic approaches are being considered, as additional kidney mobilization may be required [40, 41]. Tumor polarity, upper versus middle (mesonephric) versus lower pole location, adds additional complexity, as lesions at the tips of upper and lower poles may be easier to excise [42]. The "hilar" designation has been inconsistently defined and used in the literature, sometimes interchangeably with a description of a central location, and other times describing a spectrum of lesions, from those that abut the hilar vessels to lesions >5 mm from the hilum [43, 44]. Some authors have suggested that hilar location is the most influential factor in deciding between an open and minimally invasive approach for nephron-sparing surgery (NSS) [45].

Tumor Depth

Tumor depth is defined as the tumor's relation to structures, such as the renal sinus or collecting system as well as the relative degree of the exophytic component. Tumor depth relative to the renal capsule can determine the need for hilar clamping during a nephron-sparing surgery (NSS), impacts the complexity and feasibility of NSS, and has been correlated with surgical complications [42, 46]. The depth of a renal tumor can range from nearly completely exophytic to entirely intrarenal. Earlier literature inconsistently attempted to characterize lesions as central, peripheral, cortical, exophytic, endophytic, or mesophytic [42]. It is often difficult to localize and map to the surface of the kidney an entirely endophytic lesion, which may present significant barriers to using some minimally invasive surgical techniques.

Contemporary Classification Systems for Renal Masses

Lack of standardization in description and in means of comparison of renal lesions persisted until recently, when several scoring and classification systems emerged. The first such system, the RENAL nephrometry score (NS), was developed in 2008 by the team at the Fox Chase Cancer Center [23, 47]. The proposed objective scoring system was designed to standardize reporting and facilitate decision-making in a simple, reproducible manner. It is based on the five most surgically relevant, commonly available, and radiographically measurable anatomic features of renal masses. It requires only the availability of cross-sectional imaging. In developing the system, the investigators hoped to design not only a reproducible but also a simple means of objectifying salient anatomic attributes of renal tumors. The components that follow the acronym RENAL include *(R)adius—size (albeit measured by the tumor's maximum diameter), (E) endophytic/exophytic characteristics, (N)earness to the collecting system or renal sinus, and (L)ocation relative to the polar lines, with each component scored on a 1–3 point scale. Qualitative descriptors correspond to the designator (A) and include (a)nterior, (p)osterior, or (x) indeterminable location descriptors with relationship to the renal axis* (Fig. 10.1). *An additional suffix (h) captures hilar location of tumors and is reserved for tumors that abut the main artery or vein,* thereby potentially making hilar dissection more complex. Following the TNM staging size cutoffs, tumor size (R) is given one point for lesions <4 cm, two points for tumors 4–7 cm, and three points for masses >7 cm. The exophycity attribute (E) is assigned one point if the tumor is >50% exophytic, two points for those tumors with >50% of their diameter surrounded by normal renal parenchyma, and three points for entirely endophytic masses. The nearness (N) descriptor of the RENAL nephrometry score designates proximity of the mass to the sinus or the collecting system. (N) is assigned one point if the closest portion of the mass is >7 mm from the renal sinus or the collecting system, two points if 4–7 mm, and three points if <4 mm. Albeit the 4 and 7 mm cutoff distances are arbitrary, the values were chosen for simplicity to parallel the values in the R component of the score. Polar lines have been developed to define three relative zones—the upper pole, the interpolar region, and the lower pole—each separated by a polar line. Each renal unit has two polar lines that border the

	1pt	2pts	3 pts
(R)adius (maximal diameter in cm)	≤4	>4 but <7	≥7
(E)xophytic/endophytic properties	≥ 50%	<50%	Entirely endophytic
(N)earness of the tumor to the collecting system or sinus (mm)	≥ 7	>4 but <7	≤4
(A)nterior/Posterior	No points given. Mass assigned a descriptor of a, p, or x		
(L)ocation relative to the polar lines* *suffix "h" assigned if the tumor touches the main renal artery or vein	Entirely above the upper or below the lower polar line	Lesion crosses polar line	>50% of mass is across polar line (a) or mass crosses the axial renal midline (b) or mass is entirely between the polar lines (c)

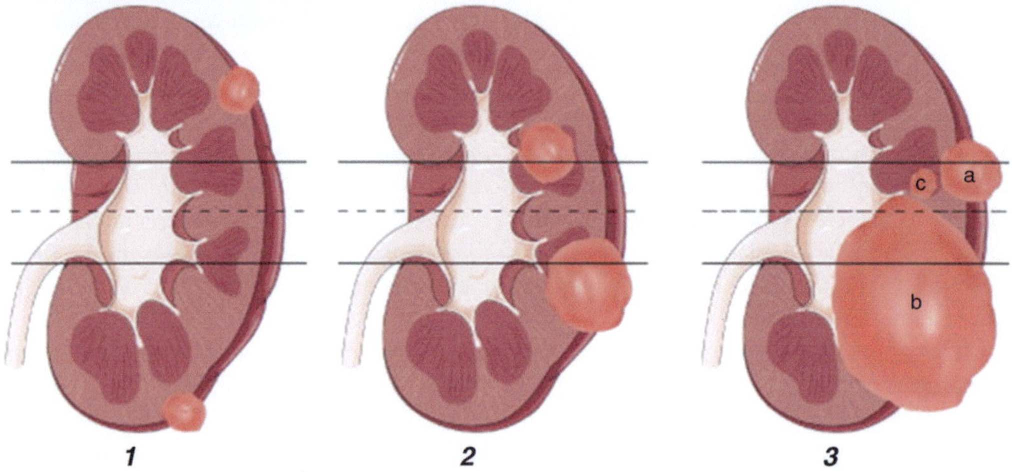

Fig. 10.1 RENAL nephrometry score with scoring of (L)ocation component. Polar lines (*solid lines*) and axial renal midline (*broken line*) are depicted on each sagittal view of kidney. Numbers 1–3 represent points attributed to each category of tumor [23]

interpolar region. Polar lines are defined by the axial cuts on cross-sectional imaging as the transition where the concentric rim of parenchyma is interrupted by the renal sinus/vessels (Fig. 10.1). Polar (L)ocation score assignments relate the tumor's position relative to the polar lines. Several authors have criticized the RENAL NS for necessitating coronal reconstructions [20, 48]; however, while polar assignment can be made on coronal imaging, it is *best to do so on the axial images*, as the mass is often out of plane with the polar line on coronal views. As such, lesions that are entirely above or below a given polar line are assigned one point. Two points are given if <50% of a tumor crosses into the interpolar region. Tumors with >50% of volume crossing the polar line or large tumors that cross the renal interpolar axis are assigned three points (Fig. 10.1). The interpolar axis is the plane halfway between the polar lines.

The nephrometry sum is the combination of individual RENAL nephrometry components and may be used for broad comparisons, with sums between 4 and 6 (inclusive) considered as low complexity, 7–9 as moderate, and greater than 9 as high complexity renal masses (Fig. 10.2). Qualitative descriptors *a*, *p*, *x*, and *h* provide additional information. Nevertheless, reporting of the nephrometry sum alone without individual components is of less value, since masses with different individual nephrometry components may vary significantly in complexity but are associated with the same nephrometry sum. The RENAL NS system has been operationalized and can be accessed via a web-based tool at www.nephrometry.com [49].

Another classification system, developed after the RENAL NS, was the preoperative aspects and dimensions used for an anatomical (PADUA) classification of renal tumors. PADUA is very similar to nephrometry, although in its initial report, the stated intention was to predict the overall perioperative complication risk of open nephron-sparing surgery [48]. This system assigned a score based on the following anatomic characteristics: longitudinal location (polarity), rim location (lateral vs. medial), relations to renal sinus and collecting system, percentage of tumor that is endophytic, and maximum diameter. Similar to the RENAL NS, an anterior/posterior qualifier was used. Points were assigned for each characteristic. One point is given for upper/lower and two for interpolar location. Depth is scored by assigning one point if the tumor is >50% exophytic, two if <50%, and three if entirely endophytic. Lateral tumor location incurred one point, whereas medial location was given two points. Involvement of the renal sinus and urinary collecting system were assigned two points each, whereas one point was given to each if invasion was absent. Tumor size was scored similar to the RENAL NS system. Complexity was categorized into low, moderate, and high, corresponding to PADUA scores of 6–7, 8–9, and >10, respectively. The major differences between the PADUA classification and the RENAL NS include the radiologic definition of renal sinus and polar locations, as well as the PADUA's more detailed assessment of tumor involvement with the sinus and the collecting system, possibly at the expense of ease of use and reproducibility. The focus of PADUA's classification on collecting system invasion may warrant merit, as the prognostic value of collecting system invasion has been documented before [50]. RENAL NS and PADUA are compared in Table 10.1 [51].

A third classification system, known as the centrality (C) index, also emerged recently, focusing on tumor location relative to the renal central sinus [52]. Using the Pythagorean theorem, the distance between the tumor center and the renal sinus center is calculated and divided *by*

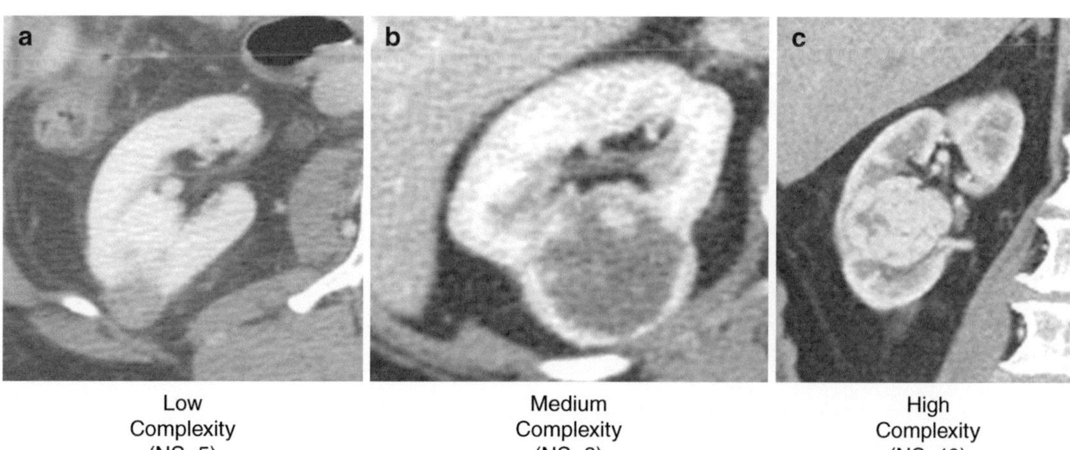

Fig. 10.2 Examples of tumor complexity based on RENAL nephrometry score [23]. (**a**) Low complexity mass, treated with robotic-assisted partial nephrectomy; (**b**) medium complexity mass, treated with robotic-assisted partial nephrectomy; (**c**) high complexity mass, treated with open partial nephrectomy

Table 10.1 RENAL nephrometry and PADUA classification scoring systems

	1 pt	2 pts	3 pts
RENAL nephrometry score [23]			
(R)adius (maximal diameter in cm)	≤4	>4 but <7	≥7
(E)xophytic/endophytic properties	≥50%	<50%	Entirely endophytic
(N)earness of the tumor to the collecting system or sinus (mm)	≥7	>4 but <7	≤4
(A)nterior/posterior[a]	No points given. Mass assigned a descriptor of a, p, or x		
(L)ocation relative to the polar lines[b]	Entirely above the upper or below the lower pole line	Lesion crosses polar line	>50% of mass is across polar line or mass crosses the axial renal midline or mass is entirely between the polar lines
Preoperative aspects and dimensions used for an anatomic (PADUA) classification [48]			
Longitudinal (polar) location	Superior/inferior	Middle	–
Exophytic rate	≥50%	<50%	Endophytic
Renal rim	Lateral	Medial	–
Renal sinus	Not involved	Involved	–
Urinary collecting system	Not involved	Dislocated/ infiltrated	–
Tumor size (cm)	≤4	>4 but ≤7	>7

Adapted from [51]

[a] Anterior or posterior face can be indicated with a letter ("a" or "p") following the score

[b] Suffix "h" assigned if the tumor touches the main renal artery or vein

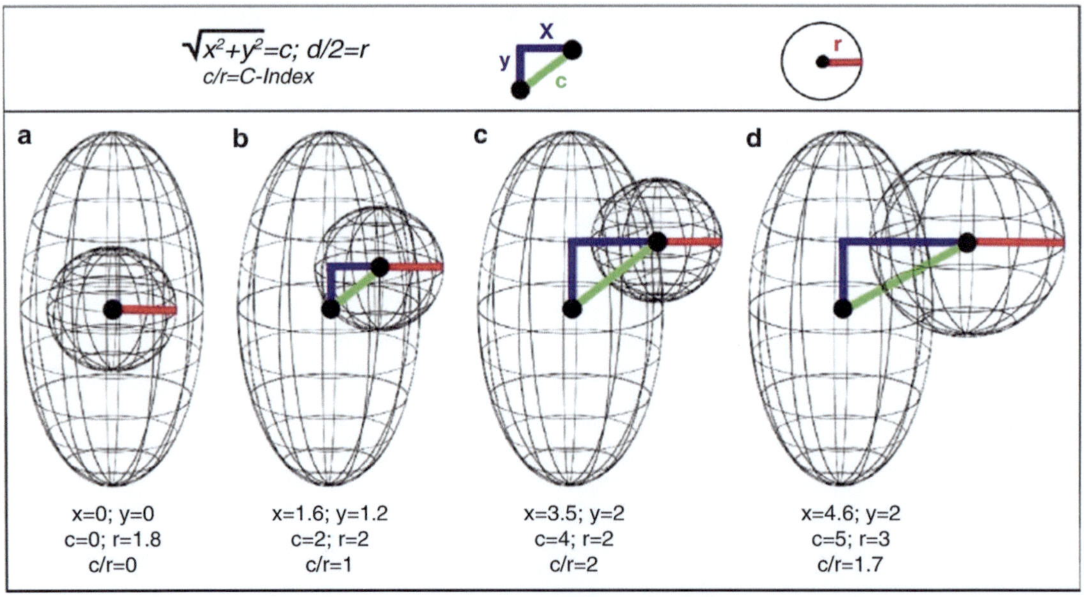

Fig. 10.3 (**a–d**), in a C-Index model *c* (*green lines*) is hypotenuse of triangle formed by sides *x* and *y* (*blue lines*). C-Index is calculated by dividing *c* by *r* (*red lines*) [52]

the tumor radius, yielding a C-Index value. A C-Index of 0 corresponds to a tumor concentric with the renal center, and C-Index of 1 corresponds to a tumor that abuts the renal center (Fig. 10.3). This system was initially reported in the context of a laparoscopic NSS cohort, focusing on its ability to predict intraoperative outcomes and perioperative complications.

Validation of Current Classification Systems

The clinical applications of these anatomic classification systems depend on their validity, reliability, and reproducibility. In recent years, multiple publications have focused on external validation of the existing classification systems. Interobserver reliability, a necessary characteristic of any robust classification system, has been assessed in numerous studies and demonstrated excellence for all three classification systems after a relatively short learning curve [53–56]. Inter-reviewer agreement has been demonstrated to be high for RENAL NS across a spectrum of training levels and specialties; however, scoring of large tumors may be less reproducible [57]. Kolla et al. found the RENAL NS to have substantial to almost perfect interobserver reliability for all components, with the (L)ocation component being the least reliable, with a 54% frequency of concordance (Kappa 0.73) [54]. This phenomenon is somewhat surprising, as appropriate scoring of the L component is objective and requires identification of the polar line (the axial cut where the parenchyma opens) and quantification of the number of cuts on which the tumor appears above and below this polar line. Validation of the PADUA system has also been described, with some reporting that it is the involvement of and the proximity to the urinary system that were more difficult to reproduce [53, 58].

Surrogate metrics to assess tumor complexity, such as perioperative outcomes and complications, are often used in these analyses. Following the initial reports by Libertino et al. in 2005 and 2008 in establishing the non-clamping partial nephrectomy technique as the new standard of care [30–34], thereby effectively addressing the deleterious effects of warm ischemia on renal injury, other investigators subsequently also noted the importance of minimizing renal injury secondary to warm ischemia [35, 36]. Early in 2009, Lifshitz et al. published a nomogram to predict warm ischemia time of >30 min, based on tumor size, location (central vs. peripheral), and patient's BMI [46]. Later, in a multivariable analysis, RENAL NS >9 and PADUA >10 were shown to be independent predictors of relative total ischemia time and perioperative complications, with RENAL NS predicting the need for any ischemia [53, 58]. Ficarra et al. demonstrated the ability of the PADUA to predict longer warm ischemia time and overall complication rates in a robotic-assisted nephron-sparing surgical cohort, even when controlling for tumor size, and others have shown similar results using the RENAL NS and C-Index [37, 59, 60]. Samplaski et al. correlated C-Index with short-term postoperative renal function, estimated by GFR via MDRD formula, demonstrating >30% decrease in GFR for lesions with C-Index of 2.5 or less [60].

Application of Standardized Classifications

Since their inception, the classification systems have been actively applied for standardized comparisons, prognostication of perioperative outcomes, surgical complications, and beyond [18, 37, 59, 61–63]. For example, according to a large multi-institutional series, without stratification, a patient undergoing a minimally invasive partial nephrectomy may be informed of a 19% risk of incurring a complication [64]. When stratified by RENAL NS, patient counseling, including major, minor, overall, and organ-specific complications, can be individualized [62]. RENAL NS has been shown to risk-stratify for specific urologic complications, such as a urine leak, which in itself can be as high as 20% for complex lesions [62, 65, 66].

Studies suggest that RENAL NS also has predictive value with respect to long-term survival, metastatic potential, and cancer-specific survival, independent of tumor size [57]. Additionally, based on a large retrospective cohort, Kutikov et al. developed a nomogram to establish a relation between RENAL NS and tumor pathology, benign versus malignant, histology, and grade (high vs. low) [61]. This concept was further confirmed and externally validated in Australian and Chinese cohorts [67, 68]. Nephrometry scores were correlated with surgical treatment preferences, where higher complexity tumors were preferentially addressed via radical nephrectomy or open approaches [18, 69].

Limitations of Current Classification Systems

Current classification systems are not without limitations. As described, none account for multifocality of renal masses which can dramatically alter treatment decisions. Also, the complexity of renal vasculature with respect to the tumor is not reflected. While anterior and posterior location qualifiers in the RENAL NS and PADUA scoring systems are used, currently no score is assigned to this descriptor, yet anterior (a) versus posterior (p) locations can potentially affect or complicate treatment choices. For example, posterior lesions may require near-complete mobilization of the kidney with additional dissection of adjacent organs, including the liver, adrenal gland, spleen, or pancreas. For larger tumors, anatomy may be distorted, making it difficult to estimate individual E and N components of the RENAL NS [57].

The Role of Nephrometry Score in Partial Nephrectomy: Lahey Experience

As has been pointed out earlier in this chapter, there are a multitude of treatment options available for the management of localized renal tumors. Clinical treatment decisions are increasingly complex and multifactorial. The complexity of the lesion, the preoperative renal function, and the general medical condition of the patient are but to name a few. The proportional impact on mortality and renal function has not been completely elucidated, suggesting that the ideal procedure for various lesions and their clinical settings is not clearly defined. As we have come to appreciate, the choice for intervention is multifactorial, and the treatment decisions are rarely objectified by physicians who are biased by their surgical skill set. One can imagine that a patient who has a complex lesion, with a high nephrometry score, and marginal renal function might have a radical nephrectomy rather than a partial nephrectomy because of the surgeon's skill set or lack thereof. Clearly, the nephrometry score can help objectify this decision-making process, knowing that 60% of radical nephrectomy specimens have evidence of histologic medical renal disease in addition to the renal tumor for which the kidney was removed (Chap. 24).

With this in mind, we reviewed a large series of patients who underwent partial nephrectomy at the Lahey Clinic Medical Center [70]. It was our aim to evaluate the role of nephrometry scores in directing the surgical approach for partial nephrectomy, open versus minimally invasive. Nephrometry scores and the surgical approaches' impact on the ultimate postoperative renal function (see Chap. 24) formed the basis for this analysis of unpublished data and the type of partial nephrectomy chosen, open versus minimally invasive.

A retrospective analysis of perioperative outcomes was performed on a prospectively collected database of 838 patients who underwent laparoscopic, robotic, or open partial nephrectomy from 2003 to 2012 at a single institution. Various preoperative, intraoperative, and postoperative characteristics and outcomes were compared between the OPN and MIPN groups. These characteristics and outcomes included preoperative Charlson comorbidity indices and postoperative complications as categorized by the Clavien–Dindo classification of surgical complications. The nephrometry scoring system was used to stratify patients into low (4–6), moderate (7–9), and high (10–12) tumor complexity groups (Fig. 10.4).

Five hundred patients were included for the analysis; 376 (75%) underwent OPN, and 124 (25%) underwent MIPN, which included laparoscopic and robotic techniques. Moreover, 153 patients (52% OPN) were stratified in the low tumor complexity group, 275 patients (83% OPN) in the moderately complex group, and 68 patients (97% OPN) in the highly complex group. An overall comparison showed no difference in age, gender, BMI, tumor stage, margin positivity, recurrence, or death. There was a statistically significant difference in OPN cases with higher preoperative Charlson comorbidity scores (2.0 vs. 1.2) and larger tumor size (3.5 vs. 2.5 cm) than

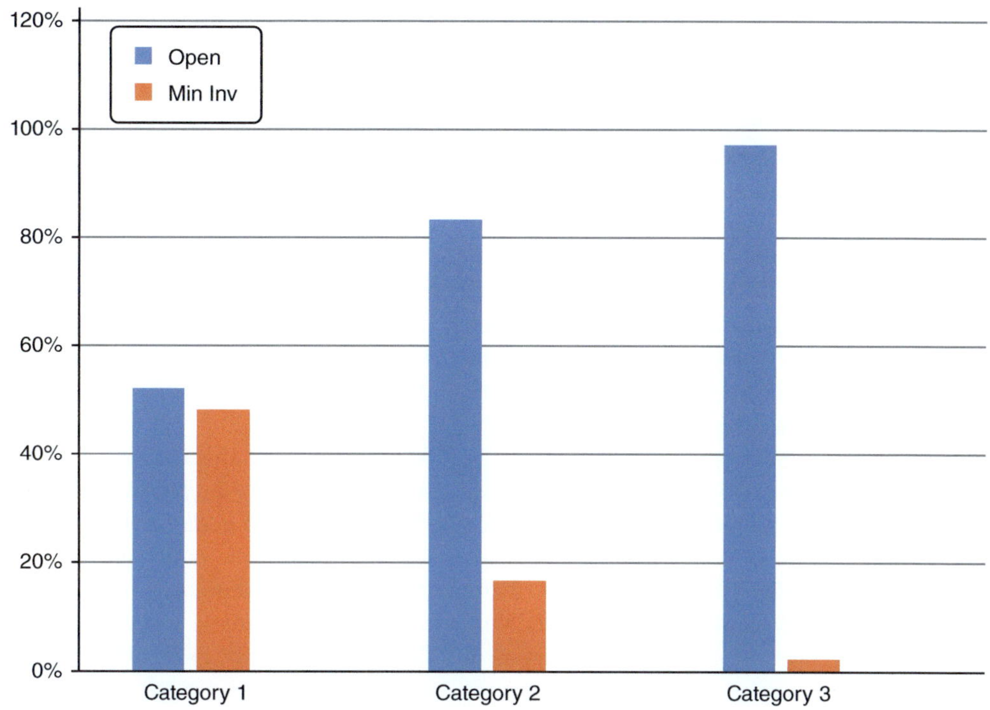

Nephrometry score	(4,5,6)	(7,8,9)	(10,11,12)
N=	153 pts	275 pts	68 pts

Fig. 10.4 Surgical approach by nephrometry score

MIPN cases. Overall and in every nephrometry complexity subgroup, the MIPN cohort had significantly less blood loss (211 vs. 696 cc), shorter lengths of hospital stay (3.2 vs. 5.6 days), and fewer Clavien I complications (17% vs. 37%). Incidences of Clavien II–V complications and blood transfusion requirement did not differ between OPN and MIPN in any of the tumor complexity strata. The open cohort had shorter operative times (216 vs. 247 min) and used the non-clamping technique, which accounts for the greater blood loss and better preservation of renal function. Statistical analysis was not performed in the high tumor complexity strata due to the limited number of cases by MIPN.

Our observations based on nephrometry score demonstrated that minimally invasive partial nephrectomy shows similar perioperative outcomes with the advantage of decreased blood loss, shorter length of hospital stay, and fewer minor complications in patients with smaller and less complex tumors. Among patients with higher complexity lesions and multiple comorbidities, there was a propensity to use the open approach, indicating the recognized advantage of the open, non-clamping, non-ischemic approach in more complex, azotemic patients with larger tumors and increased incidence of medical comorbidities [70].

The initial nephrometry classification systems have addressed the need for a method of characterizing renal tumors for surgical planning and prognosis, and have undergone external validation as noted above, as well as by more recent studies [71–73]. And the utility of nephrometry scoring has probably been best summarized in a recent meta-analysis by Veccia et al. [74]. In this meta-analysis of 51 clinical studies of mostly the RENAL and PADUA scoring systems, significant correlation of scores were noted with perioperative complications as well as warm ischemia time. The RENAL nephrometry score was also found to correlate significantly with estimated glomerular filtration rate. Additionally, malignancy on final surgical pathology could be predicted by RENAL scores R = 3, E = 2, and hilar location [74].

However, despite the advantages of these nephrometry scoring systems, important limitations were also recognized. For instance, interobserver variability has led to inconsistency in scoring. This has been thought perhaps to vary with experience of the clinician [75, 76]. Furthermore, inconsistent association with surgical outcomes, in conjunction with partial characterization of pertinent anatomic features, has resulted in a need for a more reliable method of describing surgically relevant complexity of renal tumors [77].

Furthermore, other limitations of the RENAL and PADUA classification system that have been noted relate to ease of use, which in turn lends toward reproducibility [78]. For instance, Arora et al. found significant variability in the RENAL nephrometry system. In particular, determination of polar lines and nearness to the collecting system were parameters found to be most inconsistent among even the most experienced clinicians [79].

In response to these issues with the early nephrometry scoring systems, other methods have been described. These include the arterial-based complexity (ABC) system, the diameter-axial-polar (DAP) nephrometry scoring system and a method incorporating tumor contact surface area (CSA), among others [80–82]. However, these newer systems were neither simpler nor more effective than the RENAL or PADUA methods [77].

With the goal of designing a simpler and yet equally effective nephrometry system, this ultimately led to a modification of the PADUA system known as the SPARE (Simplified PAdua REnal) classification. This was first described by Ficarra et al. in 2019 [77]. In this original study, 531 patients who underwent partial nephrectomy were classified by the parameters of the PADUA system, including polar location, rim score, renal sinus involvement, collecting system involvement, exophytic rate, and tumor size. In determining which of these variables would comprise the SPARE classification, only those factors that demonstrated a statistically significant correlation with predicted complications were utilized. These were found to include rim score, renal sinus involvement, exophytic rate, and tumor size. Table 10.2 illustrates the comparison of the

Table 10.2 The PADUA versus SPARE nephrometry scoring systems [77]

Variables	Original PADUA score	SPARE score
Polar location		
Upper/Lower	1	Not included
Medium	2	
Rim location		
Lateral	10	
Medial	2	2
Renal sinus involvement		
Absent	1	0
Present	2	3
UCS involvement		
Absent	1	Not included
Present	2	
Exophytic rate, %		
≥50%	1	0
<50%	2	1
Endophytic	3	2
Maximum tumor size, cm		
≤4 cm	1	0
4.1–7 cm	2	2
>7 cm	3	4

UCS urinary collecting system

PADUA and the more recent SPARE nephrometry scoring systems [77].

The SPARE nephrometry system has already been validated by multiple investigators. In a retrospective analysis of 202 patients that had undergone partial nephrectomy, Weprin et al. established that SPARE was as effective as the RENAL and PADUA nephrometry scoring systems in predicting perioperative complications [83]. Diana et al. corroborated these results in a larger cohort of 536 patients who underwent robotic partial nephrectomy, in determining that SPARE, PADUA, and RENAL were all effective in predicting surgical outcomes. In this study, surgical success was defined according to surgical margins, warm ischemia time, and complications. In their statistical analysis, patients with low-risk SPARE scores (0–3) had significantly better outcomes than either those patients with intermediate-risk (4–7) scores ($p < 0.001$) or high-risk (8–10) scores ($p < 0.001$). Furthermore, SPARE was actually found to have higher accuracy based on a higher receiver operating characteristic (ROC) area under the curve (AUC) of 0.73 as compared to 0.68 for RENAL and 0.65 for PADUA nephrometry scoring [78].

Conclusion

Standardized anatomic classification of renal lesions offers the potential to objectify clinical decision-making by quantifying previously qualitative variables that influence clinical treatments of patients with localized renal tumors. With further clinical validation, newer nephrometry scoring systems featuring simpler methodology may facilitate this strategy. Using these systems may help standardize patient selection, individualize risk, and objectify quality of care outcomes.

References

1. Siegel RL, Giaquinto AN, Jemal A. Cancer statistics, 2024. CA Cancer J Clin. 2024;74(1):12–49.
2. Simard EP, Ward EM, Siegel R, Jemal A. Cancers with increasing incidence trends in the United States: 1999 through 2008. CA Cancer J Clin. 2012;62:118–28.
3. Parsons JK, Schoenberg MS, Carter HB. Incidental renal tumors: casting doubt on the efficacy of early intervention. Urology. 2001;57(6):1013–5.
4. Cooperberg MR, Mallin K, Kane CJ, Carroll PR. Treatment trends for stage I renal cell carcinoma. J Urol. 2011;186(2):394–9.
5. Robson CJ, Churchill BM, Anderson W. The results of radical nephrectomy for renal cell carcinoma. J Urol. 1969;101(3):297–301.
6. Volpe A, Cadeddu JA, Cestari A, et al. Contemporary management of small renal masses. Eur Urol. 2011;60(3):501–15.
7. Campbell SC, Novick AC, Belldegrun A, et al. Guideline for management of the clinical T1 renal mass. J Urol. 2009;182(4):1271–9.
8. Ljungberg B, Cowan NC, Hanbury DC, et al. EAU guidelines on renal cell carcinoma: the 2010 update. Eur Urol. 2010;58(3):398–406.
9. Patel SG, Penson DF, Pabla B, et al. National trends in the use of partial nephrectomy: a rising tide that has not lifted all boats. J Urol. 2012;187(3):816–21.
10. Kunkle DA, Egleston BL, Uzzo RG. Excise, ablate or observe: the small renal mass dilemma-a meta-analysis and review. J Urol. 2008;179(4):1227–33; discussion 1233–4.
11. Van Poppel H, Da Pozzo L, Albrecht W, et al. A prospective, randomised EORTC intergroup phase 3 study comparing the oncologic outcome of elective nephron-sparing surgery and radical nephrectomy for low-stage renal cell carcinoma. Eur Urol. 2011;59(4):543–52.
12. Chow WH, Devesa SS, Warren JL, Fraumeni JF Jr. Rising incidence of renal cell cancer in the United States. JAMA. 1999;281(17):1628–31.
13. Hollingsworth JM, Miller DC, Daignault S, Hollenbeck BK. Rising incidence of small renal masses: a need to reassess treatment effect. J Natl Cancer Inst. 2006;98(18):1331–4.
14. Snyder ME, Bach A, Kattan MW, Raj GV, Reuter VE, Russo P. Incidence of benign lesions for clinically localized renal masses smaller than 7 cm in radiological diameter: influence of sex. J Urol. 2006;176(6 Pt 1):2391–5; discussion 2395–6.
15. McKiernan J, Yossepowitch O, Kattan MW, et al. Partial nephrectomy for renal cortical tumors: pathologic findings and impact on outcome. Urology. 2002;60(6):1003–9.
16. Smaldone MC, Kutikov A, Egleston BL, et al. Small renal masses progressing to metastases under active surveillance: a systematic review and pooled analysis. Cancer. 2012;118(4):997–1006.
17. Smaldone MC, Uzzo RG. Active surveillance: a potential strategy for select patients with small renal masses. Future Oncol. 2011;7(10):1133–47.
18. Canter D, Kutikov A, Manley B, et al. Utility of the R.E.N.A.L. nephrometry scoring system in objectifying treatment decision-making of the enhancing renal mass. Urology. 2011;78(5):1089–94.
19. Weight CJ, Crispen PL, Breau RH, et al. Practice-setting and surgeon characteristics heavily influence

the decision to perform partial nephrectomy among American urologic association surgeons. BJU Int. 2013;111(5):731–8.
20. Volpe A, Terrone C. Anatomic classification systems of renal tumors: new, useful tools in renal surgical oncology. Eur Urol. 2011;60(4):731–3.
21. Buechter KJ, Zeppa R, Gomez G. The use of segmental anatomy for an operative classification of liver injuries. Ann Surg. 1990;211(6):669–73; discussion 673–5.
22. Couinaud C. Liver anatomy: portal (and suprahepatic) or biliary segmentation. Dig Surg. 1999;16(6):459–67.
23. Kutikov A, Uzzo RG. The R.E.N.A.L. nephrometry score: a comprehensive standardized system for quantitating renal tumor size, location and depth. J Urol. 2009;182(3):844–53.
24. Flocks RH, Kadesky MC. Malignant neoplasms of the kidney; an analysis of 353 patients followed five years or more. J Urol. 1958;79(2):196–201.
25. Nguyen CT, Campbell SC. Staging of renal cell carcinoma: past, present, and future. Clin Genitourin Cancer. 2006;5(3):190–7.
26. Guinan P, Sobin LH, Algaba F, et al. TNM staging of renal cell carcinoma: workgroup no. 3. Union International Contre le Cancer (UICC) and the American Joint Committee on Cancer (AJCC). Cancer. 1997;80(5):992–3.
27. Elmore JM, Kadesky KT, Koeneman KS, Sagalowsky AI. Reassessment of the 1997 TNM classification system for renal cell carcinoma. Cancer. 2003;98(11):2329–34.
28. Patard JJ, Pantuck AJ, Crepel M, et al. Morbidity and clinical outcome of nephron-sparing surgery in relation to tumour size and indication. Eur Urol. 2007;52(1):148–54.
29. Crispen PL, Boorjian SA, Lohse CM, et al. Outcomes following partial nephrectomy by tumor size. J Urol. 2008;180(5):1912–7.
30. Triaca V, Zagha R, Libertino JA. Does thrombin sealant allow nephron sparing surgery (NSS) without renal artery occlusion? Description of technique and initial results. J Urol. 2005;171(4):Supplement Abstract #1338.
31. Smith G, Cohen M, Kurteva T, Libertino JA. Non-clamped, non ischemia partial nephrectomy in patients with compromised preoperative renal function or with a solitary kidney. J Urol. 2008;179(4):Supplement Abstract #1096.
32. Kurteva T, Cohen M, Smith G, Libertino JA. Non-clamped, non-ischemic partial nephrectomy: the new gold standard. J Urol. 2008;179(4):Supplement Abstract #1392.
33. Smith G, Kenney P, Lee Y, Libertino JA. Non-clamped partial nephrectomy: techniques and surgical outcomes. BJU Int. 2011;107(7):1054–8. https://doi.org/10.1111/j.1464-410X.2010.09798.x. Epub 2010 Oct 29.
34. Wszolek M, Kenney P, Lee Y, Libertino JA. Comparison of hilar clamping and non-hilar clamping partial nephrectomy for tumors involving a solitary kidney. BJU Int. 2011;107(12):1886–92. https://doi.org/10.1111/j.1464-410X.2010.09713.x. Epub 2010 Nov 11.
35. Lane BR, Russo P, Uzzo RG, et al. Comparison of cold and warm ischemia during partial nephrectomy in 660 solitary kidneys reveals predominant role of nonmodifiable factors in determining ultimate renal function. J Urol. 2011;185(2):421–7.
36. Thompson RH, Lane BR, Lohse CM, et al. Every minute counts when the renal hilum is clamped during partial nephrectomy. Eur Urol. 2010;58(3):340–5.
37. Ficarra V, Bhayani S, Porter J, et al. Predictors of warm ischemia time and perioperative complications in a multicenter, international series of robot-assisted partial nephrectomy. Eur Urol. 2012;61(2):395–402.
38. Campbell SC, Novick AC, Streem SB, Klein E, Licht M. Complications of nephron sparing surgery for renal tumors. J Urol. 1994;151(5):1177–80.
39. Simmons MN, Fergany AF, Campbell SC. Effect of parenchymal volume preservation on kidney function after partial nephrectomy. J Urol. 2011;186(2):405–10.
40. Wright JL, Porter JR. Laparoscopic partial nephrectomy: comparison of transperitoneal and retroperitoneal approaches. J Urol. 2005;174(3):841–5.
41. Ng CS, Gill IS, Ramani AP, et al. Transperitoneal versus retroperitoneal laparoscopic partial nephrectomy: patient selection and perioperative outcomes. J Urol. 2005;174(3):846–9.
42. Porpiglia F, Volpe A, Billia M, Renard J, Scarpa RM. Assessment of risk factors for complications of laparoscopic partial nephrectomy. Eur Urol. 2008;53(3):590–6.
43. Reisiger K, Venkatesh R, Figenshau RS, Bae KT, Landman J. Complex laparoscopic partial nephrectomy for renal hilar tumors. Urology. 2005;65(5):888 91.
44. Hruby G, Reisiger K, Venkatesh R, Yan Y, Landman J. Comparison of laparoscopic partial nephrectomy and laparoscopic cryoablation for renal hilar tumors. Urology. 2006;67(1):50–4.
45. Raman JD, Smith B, Messer J, Rohner TJ, Harpster LE, Reese CT. Preoperative predictors of surgical approach for partial nephrectomy. Can J Urol. 2011;18(5):5896–902.
46. Lifshitz DA, Shikanov S, Jeldres C, et al. Laparoscopic partial nephrectomy: predictors of prolonged warm ischemia. J Urol. 2009;182(3):860–5.
47. Kutikov ACP, Uzzo RG. The fox chase R.E.N.A.L. nephrometry score: a comprehensive standardized scoring system for assessing renal tumor size, location and depth. J Urol. 2009;181(suppl 1):354.
48. Ficarra V, Novara G, Secco S, et al. Preoperative aspects and dimensions used for an anatomical (PADUA) classification of renal tumours in patients who are candidates for nephron-sparing surgery. Eur Urol. 2009;56(5):786–93.
49. http://nephrometry.com/.
50. Uzzo RG, Cherullo EE, Myles J, Novick AC. Renal cell carcinoma invading the urinary collecting system: implications for staging. J Urol. 2002;167(6):2392–6.

51. Cha EK, Ng CK, Jeun B, et al. Preoperative radiographic parameters predict long-term renal impairment following partial nephrectomy. World J Urol. 2013;31(4):817–22.
52. Simmons MN, Ching CB, Samplaski MK, Park CH, Gill IS. Kidney tumor location measurement using the C index method. J Urol. 2010;183(5):1708–13.
53. Hew MN, Baseskioglu B, Barwari K, et al. Critical appraisal of the PADUA classification and assessment of the R.E.N.A.L. nephrometry score in patients undergoing partial nephrectomy. J Urol. 2011;186(1):42–6.
54. Kolla SB, Spiess PE, Sexton WJ. Interobserver reliability of the RENAL nephrometry scoring system. Urology. 2011;78(3):592–4.
55. Montag S, Waingankar N, Sadek MA, Rais-Bahrami S, Kavoussi LR, Vira MA, et al. Reproducibility and fidelity of the R.E.N.A.L. nephrometry score. J Endourol. 2011;25(12):1925–8.
56. Okhunov Z, Rais-Bahrami S, George AK, et al. The comparison of three renal tumor scoring systems: C-index, P.A.D.U.A., and R.E.N.A.L. nephrometry scores. J Endourol. 2011;25(12):1921–4.
57. Weight CJ, Atwell TD, Fazzio RT, et al. A multidisciplinary evaluation of inter-reviewer agreement of the nephrometry score and the prediction of long-term outcomes. J Urol. 2011;186(4):1223–8.
58. Waldert M, Waalkes S, Klatte T, et al. External validation of the preoperative anatomical classification for prediction of complications related to nephron-sparing surgery. World J Urol. 2010;28(4):531–5.
59. White MA, Haber GP, Autorino R, et al. Outcomes of robotic partial nephrectomy for renal masses with nephrometry score of ≥7. Urology. 2011;77(4):809–13.
60. Samplaski MK, Hernandez A, Gill IS, Simmons MN. C-index is associated with functional outcomes after laparoscopic partial nephrectomy. J Urol. 2010;184(6):2259–63.
61. Kutikov A, Smaldone MC, Egleston BL, et al. Anatomic features of enhancing renal masses predict malignant and high-grade pathology: a preoperative nomogram using the RENAL nephrometry score. Eur Urol. 2011;60(2):241–8.
62. Simhan J, Smaldone MC, Tsai KJ, et al. Objective measures of renal mass anatomic complexity predict rates of major complications following partial nephrectomy. Eur Urol. 2011;60(4):724–30.
63. Novak R, Mulligan D, Abaza R. Robotic partial nephrectomy without renal ischemia. Urology. 2012;79(6):1296–301.
64. Gill IS, Kavoussi LR, Lane BR, et al. Comparison of 1,800 laparoscopic and open partial nephrectomies for single renal tumors. J Urol. 2007;178(1):41–6.
65. Bruner B, Breau RH, Lohse CM, Leibovich BC, Blute ML. Renal nephrometry score is associated with urine leak after partial nephrectomy. BJU Int. 2011;108(1):67–72.
66. Breau RH, Crispen PL, Jimenez RE, Lohse CM, Blute ML, Leibovich BC. Outcome of stage T2 or greater renal cell cancer treated with partial nephrectomy. J Urol. 2010;183(3):903–8.
67. Wang HK, Zhu Y, Yao XD, et al. External validation of a nomogram using RENAL nephrometry score to predict high grade renal cell carcinoma. J Urol. 2012;187(5):1555–60.
68. Satasivam P, Sengupta S, Rajarubendra N, Chia PH, Munshey A, Bolton D. Renal lesions with low R.E.N.A.L nephrometry score are associated with more indolent renal cell carcinomas (RCCs) or benign histology: findings in an Australian cohort. BJU Int. 2012;109(3):44–7.
69. Rosevear HM, Gellhaus PT, Lightfoot AJ, Kresowik TP, Joudi FN, Tracy CR. Utility of the RENAL nephrometry scoring system in the real world: predicting surgeon operative preference and complication risk. BJU Int. 2012;109(5):700–5.
70. Ginzburg S, Kutikov A, Uzzo R, Schloss S. Objectifying complexity of kidney cancers: relationship of tumor anatomy and outcomes. In: Libertino JA, Gee JR, co-editors. Renal cancer: contemporary management, 2nd ed. Springer; 2020.
71. Schiavina R, Novara G, Borghesi M, et al. PADUA and R.E.N.A.L. nephrometry scores correlate with perioperative outcomes of robot-assisted partial nephrectomy: analysis of the Vattikuti Global Quality Initiative in Robotic Urologic Surgery (GQI-RUS) database. BJU Int. 2017;119:456–63.
72. Gupta R, Tori M, Babitz SK, et al. Comparison of RENAL, PADUA, CSA, and PAVP nephrometry scores in predicting functional outcomes after partial nephrectomy. Urology. 2019;124:160–7.
73. Sterzik A, Solyanik O, Eichelberg C, et al. Improved prediction of nephron-sparing surgery versus radical nephrectomy by the optimized R.E.N.A.L. score in patients undergoing surgery for renal masses. Minerva Urol Nefrol. 2019;71:249–57.
74. Veccia A, Antonelli A, Uzzo RG, Novara G, Kutikov A, Ficarra V, Simeone C, Mirone V, Hampton LJ, Derweesh I, Porpiglia F, Autorino R. Predictive value of nephrometry scores in nephron-sparing surgery: a systematic review and meta-analysis. Eur Urol Focus. 2020;6(3):490–504. https://doi.org/10.1016/j.euf.2019.11.004. Epub 2019 Nov 24.
75. Benadiba S, Verin AL, Pignot G, et al. Are urologists and radiologists equally effective in determining the RENAL nephrometry score? Ann Surg Oncol. 2015;22:1618–24.
76. Monn MF, Gellhaus PT, Masterson TA, et al. R.E.N.A.L. nephrometry scoring: how well correlated are urologist, radiologist, and collaborator scores? J Endourol. 2014;28:1006–10.
77. Ficarra V, Porpiglia F, Crestani A, Minervini A, Antonelli A, Longo N, Novara G, Giannarini G, Fiori C, Simeone C, Carini M, Mirone V. The Simplified PADUA REnal (SPARE) nephrometry system: a novel classification of parenchymal renal tumours suitable for partial nephrectomy. BJU Int. 2019;124(4):621–8. https://doi.org/10.1111/bju.14772. Epub 2019 May 7.

78. Diana P, Lughezzani G, Uleri A, Casale P, Saita A, Hurle R, Lazzeri M, Mottrie A, De Naeyer G, De Groote R, Porter J, Buffi N. Multi-institutional retrospective validation and comparison of the Simplified PADUA REnal nephrometry system for the prediction of surgical success of robot-assisted partial nephrectomy. Eur Urol Focus. 2021;7(5):1100–6. https://doi.org/10.1016/j.euf.2020.11.003. Epub 2020 Dec 4.
79. Arora M, Randhawa LS, Lakhera D, Thakker V, Abhishek KA, Singh D, Chaudhary R, Azad RK. Interobserver reproducibility of RENAL nephrometry score in comparison to simplified PADUA Renal nephrometry score. Urol Ann. 2023;15(4):373–82. https://doi.org/10.4103/ua.ua_37_23. Epub 2023 Aug 3.
80. Simmons MN, Hillyer SP, Lee BH, Fergany AF, Kaouk J, Campbell SC. Diameter-axial polar nephrometry: integration and optimization of R.E.N.A.L. and centrality index scoring systems. J Urol. 2012;188:384–90.
81. Spaliviero M, Poon BY, Karlo CA, et al. An arterial based complexity (ABC) scoring system to assess the morbidity profile of partial nephrectomy. Eur Urol. 2016;69:72–9.
82. Leslie S, Gill IS, de Castro A, et al. Renal tumor contact surface area: a novel parameter for predicting complexity and outcomes of partial nephrectomy. Eur Urol. 2014;66:884–93.
83. Weprin S, Falagario U, Veccia A, Nandanan N, Emerson D, Ovanez C, Albuquerque EV, Zukovski EB, Clayton R, Hampton L, Autorino R. Simplified PADUA REnal (SPARE) nephrometry scoring system: external validation, interobserver variability, and comparison with RENAL and PADUA in a single-center robotic partial nephrectomy series. Eur Urol Focus. 2021;7(3):591–7. https://doi.org/10.1016/j.euf.2020.05.016. Epub 2020 Jun 23.

11 History of Renal Surgery for Cancer

Samuel Donnenfeld and Brendan M. Browne

History of Renal Surgery

The late nineteenth century was when the first documented nephrectomy took place. In 1861, Wolcott mistakenly removed a kidney when operating for liver cysts. It weighed 2 ½ pounds and was described by Stoddard who assisted Wolcott. Subsequently, Speigelberg in 1867 performed a nephrectomy while excising an echinococcus cyst. This was an inauspicious beginning as both patients expired shortly postoperatively, and this procedure was not readily accepted. Theodor Kocher carried out a transperitoneal nephrectomy for carcinoma in 1876 in two patients, both of whom died of peritonitis following surgery. The first successful planned nephrectomy was completed by Gustav Simon in 1869 for a persistent urinary fistula and hydronephrosis [1] at the University of Heidelberg. This patient survived, and two important factors were discovered. First, that a patient could survive elective removal of a kidney, and secondly, could live with only one kidney. Gilmore successfully performed the first elective nephrectomy in the United States in 1870 for the treatment of pyelonephritis and persistent urinary tract infection.

The diagnosis of renal cell cancer was readily made during the early 1900s. The kidneys were visualized using intravenous pyelography and retrograde pyelogram. A filling defect combined with a palpable mass would give ample assurance of the tumor's existence. The extent and degree of fixation could be assessed. Arteriography [2] as well as retroperitoneal coccygeal air insufflation [3] were techniques used to further characterize kidney tumors. Parke Smith et al. [4] used arteriography not just to define the arterial structure but also to differentiate benign from malignant lesions.

The end of the nineteenth century also introduced advances in surgical technique that allowed improvement in the survival of patients undergoing nephrectomy. Joseph Lister, in Edinburgh, introduced antiseptic techniques. Hand washing and disinfection of instruments as well as steam sterilization resulted in a significant reduction in peri-operative complications and mortality from nephrectomy. These discoveries helped gain a greater acceptance of kidney surgery. By the end of the 19th century, more than 300 radical nephrectomies were performed both in America and Europe.

Era of Radical Nephrectomy: Gold Standard

Once the diagnosis was made, the surgical approach for malignant disease was a total (or radical) nephrectomy. The retroperitoneal

S. Donnenfeld
Department of Urology, Brown University, Providence, RI, USA

B. M. Browne (✉)
Department of Urology, Emory University School of Medicine, Atlanta, GA, USA

J. A. Libertino, J. R. Gee (eds.), *Renal Cancer*, https://doi.org/10.1007/978-3-031-97599-8_11

approach was favored by most urologists in this era; however, Emil Kocher removed a kidney via the transperitoneal approach in 1878 [5]. Dr. Atle Berg modified his technique, utilizing the lateral incision and mobilization of the colon to improve visualization of the renal pedicle. Additionally, during the late 1940s, Chute et al. [6] performed a thoracoabdominal approach. This technique gave excellent exposure of the tumor and renal pedicle as well as neighboring structures that may be involved. Radical nephrectomy for kidney cancer was subsequently adopted by numerous surgeons both in the United States as well as Europe. Vernon Dick and others from the Lahey Clinic described a series of 280 cases of renal cell carcinoma over 20 years. The technique described by Foley et al. [7] was recommended as it removes all perirenal fat as well as sampling of local lymph nodes. Three-year survival rates of 88% and 80% were described by Robson and Somerset and provided encouraging results for renal cell cancer [8]. Solitary metastases were also successfully removed from various organs, including the lungs, brain, and bones, with reasonable success. It has also been demonstrated that spontaneous regression of metastatic disease may follow excision of the primary tumor [9]. As time went on, a larger number of nephrectomy series were published. Several hundred cases, many of them for malignant disease, were evaluated both in the United States and Europe. With these promising result, radical nephrectomy became the gold standard for tumors of the kidney.

With greater acceptance of this surgical technique came the ability to examine these tumors histologically. In the mid 1800s, Robson [8] evaluated solid renal tumors and concluded that renal cell carcinoma arose from renal tubular epithelium. Other pathologists suggested that these tumors were derived from adrenal rests within the kidney. This idea persisted throughout the early 1900s. The term hypernephroid tumor was used extensively during this time and was first used to describe the origin of renal tumors above the kidney. However, there were many who objected to this concept. Hugh Hampton Young in his book [10] *Practice of Urology* reinforces the idea that the term, hypernephroma, should be abandoned as it assumes that the tumor arises from adrenal tissue.

The classification of kidney tumors also allowed for better stratification of this disease and more improved selection of those who could undergo renal sparing surgery. Glenn [11] provided a simple pathologic outline of renal tumors. Benign disease, including oncocytomas and cystic disease, were categorized, as well as malignant and embryonic lesions. Prior to this, Deming and Harvard [12] had proposed a more complex and comprehensive system based on all known cellular subtypes. This system has 11 categories with multiple subtypes that cover most renal lesions. It, however, was felt to be a difficult way of looking at kidney pathology. Ideally, classification based on simple clinical and radiographic criteria would become more appealing to the surgeon. In 1994, Barbaric approached this concern by suggesting that renal masses be categorized into three large pathologic groups: benign, malignant, or inflammatory. This provided surgeons with pathologic guidance for selecting the best treatment. More recently, the category of renal cell carcinoma has been sub-divided, identifying different subtypes using genetic markers and tumor biology.

The Rise of Nephron-Sparing Surgery (Partial Nephrectomy)

> Few procedures provide the urologist with more satisfaction than those that preserve renal function
> —Abeshouse, 1950

Although there was always interest in renal-sparing surgery, the complications were much too significant to adopt this technique. Many patients died because of sepsis, uremia, and shock from early attempts at partial nephrectomy. Massive hemorrhage, urinary fistula formation, and poor patient selection all contributed to the preferential use of radical nephrectomy for both benign and malignant disease.

In the early stages of kidney surgery, partial nephrectomy was a procedure used only in very narrow circumstances. This procedure was first performed by Czerny in 1887 for an angiosarcoma [13]. As mentioned above, the early experience with partial nephrectomy was abandoned quickly due to the injudicious use of this technique and the high rate of complications. With the improvement in preoperative evaluation of patients as well as the postoperative management, more conservative operations for benign disease gained acceptance [14]. It was, however, the pioneering ideas of Vermooten [15] in the 1950s that led to the modern era of partial nephrectomy for renal neoplasms. His observations were based on the pathological studies showing that clear cell carcinomas were locally advancing and grew by expansion. Few lesions under 3 cm were found to be metastatic, and some tumors could safely be excised with a 1 cm margin, with little fear of local recurrence. Collectively, 321 procedures were done safely by these surgeons; however, partial nephrectomy was still reserved for patients with a functional contralateral kidney [16].

It was unfortunate that few urologists initially believed Dr. Vermooten's ideas and observations. As mentioned, the majority felt that radical nephrectomy was the procedure of choice for renal cancers, especially in patients with two functional kidneys. Partial nephrectomy was reserved for cases of solitary kidneys, marginal renal function, or bilateral tumors. Zinman and Dowd [17] collected a series of partial nephrectomy between 1950 and 1967. They described the feasibility of this technique but reinforced the use of radical nephrectomy with excision of adipose tissue and lymphatics in all cases with a normal contralateral kidney. Semb [18] performed the removal of a carcinoma in a solitary kidney. However, most surgeons of that era rarely, if ever, published on partial nephrectomy, and radical nephrectomy would remain the gold standard for the next several decades.

It was during the later part of the twentieth century that multiple centers worldwide began to publish their experience with partial nephrectomy. Renal hypothermia allowed longer and more complicated reconstruction of the kidney. Back bench surgery gained acceptance in some centers, but many prominent surgeons realized that most cases could be done in situ. The 1980s would see some groups who favored partial nephrectomy for certain patients with a normal, contralateral kidney. Criteria were developed that allowed for the accurate prediction of survival in this patient population. The major concern among the urological community was recurrence after partial nephrectomy, which was amplified by Mukamel et al. [19] when they reported evidence of occult multifocal renal tumors in 30% of nephrectomy specimens, which might recur if only the primary tumor was removed. However, in 1993, Licht and Novick [20] reported only 2 recurrences and 95% survival in a series of 241 partial nephrectomy cases collected from literature (1967 to 1991). Their follow-up was only 3 years. Herr [21] and Fergany et al. [22] later showed a rare local recurrence and almost 100% survival on patients undergoing partial nephrectomy especially in those tumors less than 4 cm. Dr. Herr states that this survival can be explained by the fact that a majority of these tumors were less than 4 cm and had benign characteristics or favorable pathology [23].

As surgical techniques improved, so did imaging of the patient, both preoperatively as well as intraoperatively. Three-dimensional imaging using CT scan and MRI is standard and imperative for surgical planning of partial nephrectomy. Intraoperative imaging, using ultrasound, is helpful and at times essential for these cases. Although there was a time that many groups remained skeptical about the merits of partial nephrectomy in patients with a contralateral normal kidney, the results demonstrated equivalent long-term oncologic outcomes to radical nephrectomy in specific patient populations. For most patients with a clinical T1 tumor who are surgical candidates, partial nephrectomy has become the accepted gold standard.

Twenty-First Century and the Future

The advent of minimally invasive techniques allowed urologists to perform nephrectomy with less blood loss, lower narcotic requirements, shorter hospitalization, and faster return to normal activity. Ralph Clayman [24] from Washington University in St. Louis was the first urologist to remove a kidney through 11 mm incisions. Hand-assisted radical nephrectomy (HALN) was introduced by Stephen Nakada in 1997 [25]. This technique allowed minimally invasive surgery to provide similar steps performed in classic open surgery. Debates ensued regarding optimal various technique but focus always should remain on the patients' best interest.

Further advancements in open surgical technology have also limited morbidity. In the cases of larger renal tumors or caval thrombi, whereas formerly surgical exposure would have necessitated entry into the chest and abdomen with a thoracoabdominal incision, retractors such as the Liver/Oncology system by Thompson Surgical Instruments (Traverse City, MI) have largely done away with this inherently morbid incision. Greater surgical exposure through advanced retractors improves several operative metrics, including operative time and decreases the inherent morbidity associated with entering the thorax, which can necessitate a chest tube and increase pain associated with rib removal. Furthermore, one study found that while overall contemporary operative residency training volumes have increased from a period of 2003 to 2019, the overall rate of open procedures has declined substantially in favor of laparoscopy [26].

Lastly, we have begun to understand the necessity of renal preservation. Huang et al. [27] published the first series describing the importance of maintaining renal parenchyma. He notes that chronic kidney disease may be present in 30% of patients with small renal lesions. More importantly, patients who undergo radical nephrectomy have a twofold increase in developing chronic renal insufficiency as compared to patients who underwent partial nephrectomy. Libertino [28] originally described and reported more than 800 cases of non-clamping partial nephrectomy, one of the largest experiences in the world. In his series, GFR is significantly reduced in patients who have undergone clamping during partial nephrectomy. Inderber Gill has also examined this phenomenon. He clearly states that every minute of ischemia counts during laparoscopic and robotic partial nephrectomy [29]. The increasing understanding of tumor biology, advances in radiological imaging, and surgical technology has led to expanding the indications of partial nephrectomy and nephron-sparing treatment. Minimally invasive laparoscopic and percutaneous energy ablation procedures effectively control renal tumors with far less morbidity and better quality of life than open surgery. Robotic approaches, as well as single-port surgery, and the use of natural orifice transluminal endoscopic surgery all offer the field a variety of techniques to improve surgical outcomes.

History of Renal Surgery for Cancer

Renal surgery has evolved significantly over the past 150 years; however, there is much to do and learn in this area of urology. Advancement in tumor detection and biology will more adequately stage our patients, hoping to maximize renal function and longevity. Surgical techniques will continue to improve, and the role of partial nephrectomy continues to expand with excellent results. The next 150 years will certainly bring novel approaches to maximize oncologic success and preserving renal function while minimizing morbidity. It is exciting to see what the future will hold.

References

1. Simon G. Chirurgie der Nieren, vol. II. Stuttgart: Ferdinand Enke; 1876. p. 314.
2. Wagner FB. Arteriography in renal diagnosis; preliminary report and critical evaluation. J Urol. 1946;56(6):625–35.
3. Lindblom K. Percutaneous puncture of renal cysts and tumors. Acta Radiol. 1946;27(1):66–72.

4. Smith PG, Rush TW, Evans AT. An evaluation of translumbar arteriography. J Urol. 1951;65(5):911–23.
5. Kocher T. Eine nephrotomie wegen nierensarkom. Deutsch Z Chir. 1878;9:312.
6. Chute R, Soutter L, Kerr WS. The value of the thoracoabdominal incision in the removal of kidney tumors. N Engl J Med. 1949;241(24):951–60.
7. Foley FB, Mulvaney WP, Richardson EJ, Victor I. Radical nephrectomy for neoplasms. J Urol. 1952;68(1):39–49.
8. Robson CJ. Radical nephrectomy for renal cell carcinoma. J Urol. 1963;89:37–42.
9. Ljunggren E, Holm S, Karth B, Pompeius R. Some aspects of renal tumors with special reference to spontaneous regression. J Urol. 1959;82:553–7.
10. Young HH. Neoplasms of the urogenital tract. Young's practice of urology. Philadelphia: W.B. Saunders Company; 1926.
11. Glenn JF. Renal tumors. In: Harrison JH, Gittes RF, Perlmutter AD, et al., editors. Campbell's urology. 4th ed. Philadelphia: Saunders; 1980. p. 967–1009.
12. Deming CLHB. Tumors of the kidney. In: Campbell MF, Harrison JH, editors. Urology, vol. 2. 3rd ed. Philadelphia: WB Saunders; 1970.
13. Czerny HE. Ueber nierenextirpation bietr. Klin Khirurg. 1890;6:485.
14. Goldstein AE. Polycystic renal disease with particular reference to author's surgical procedure. J Urol. 1951;66(2):163–72.
15. Vermooten V. Indications for conservative surgery in certain renal tumors: a study based on the growth pattern of the cell carcinoma. J Urol. 1950;64(2):200–8.
16. Poletajew S, Antoniewicz AA, Borowka A. Kidney removal: the past, presence, and perspectives: a historical review. Urol J. 2010;7(4):215–23.
17. Zinman L, Dowd JB. Partial nephrectomy in renal cell carcinoma. Surg Clin North Am. 1967;47(3):685–93.
18. Semb C. Conservative renal surgery. J R Coll Surg Edinb. 1964;10:9–30.
19. Mukamel E, Konichezky M, Engelstein D, Servadio C. Incidental small renal tumors accompanying clinically overt renal cell carcinoma. J Urol. 1988;140(1):22–4.
20. Licht MR, Novick AC. Nephron sparing surgery for renal cell carcinoma. J Urol. 1993;149(1):1–7.
21. Herr HW. Partial nephrectomy for unilateral renal carcinoma and a normal contralateral kidney: 10-year followup. J Urol. 1999;161(1):33–4; discussion 34-5.
22. Fergany AF, Hafez KS, Novick AC. Long-term results of nephron sparing surgery for localized renal cell carcinoma: 10-year followup. J Urol. 2000;163(2):442–5.
23. Herr HW. A history of partial nephrectomy for renal tumors. J Urol. 2005;173(3):705–8.
24. Clayman RV, Kavoussi LR, Soper NJ, et al. Laparoscopic nephrectomy: initial case report. J Urol. 1991;146(2):278–82.
25. Nakada SY, Moon TD, Gist M, Mahvi D. Use of the pneumo sleeve as an adjunct in laparoscopic nephrectomy. Urology. 1997;49(4):612–3.
26. St John A, Caturegli I, Kubicki NS, Kavic SM. The rise of minimally invasive surgery: 16 year analysis of the progressive replacement of open surgery with laparoscopy. JSLS. 2020;24(4):e2020.00076. https://doi.org/10.4293/JSLS.2020.00076. PMID: 33510568; PMCID: PMC7810432.
27. Huang WC, Levey AS, Serio AM, et al. Chronic kidney disease after nephrectomy in patients with renal cortical tumours: a retrospective cohort study. Lancet Oncol. 2006;7(9):735–40.
28. Wszolek MF, Kenney PA, Libertino JA. Nonclamping partial nephrectomy: towards improved nephron sparing. Nat Rev Urol. 2011;8(9):523–7.
29. Gill IS, Eisenberg MS, Aron M, et al. "Zero ischemia" partial nephrectomy: novel laparoscopic and robotic technique. Eur Urol. 2011;59(1):128–34.

12 The Surgical Approaches to Renal Masses and Their Impact on Postoperative Renal Function

John A. Libertino

Introduction

The data in the literature are confusing and conflicted as to the role of various surgical maneuvers and their impact on postoperative renal function. This chapter aims to review the current literature and present my personal experience regarding the role of warm ischemia and the volume of renal parenchyma preserved on the ultimate postoperative renal functional outcome following partial nephrectomy (PN).

Nephrectomy Versus Partial Nephrectomy: The Rationale for Partial Nephrectomy and Preservation of Renal Function

It is estimated that approximately 30 million Americans are living with chronic kidney disease (CKD) [1]. In addition, the increased incidence of obesity, heart disease, hypertension, and diabetes puts millions more Americans at risk for developing chronic kidney disease. It is also estimated that 30% of patients diagnosed with a renal mass already have chronic kidney disease (CKD). Chronic kidney disease (CKD) also develops in many patients who undergo a radical nephrectomy (RN) [2, 3]. Although radical nephrectomy for kidney cancer cures one disease (kidney cancer), it can often cause another disease, chronic kidney disease (CKD), that may be just as ominous.

This notion is underscored by the fact that the average 60-year-old patient is expected to live another 21 years, as opposed to a 60-year-old patient on dialysis who has an average life expectancy of 4.6 years [1]. In addition to requiring renal replacement therapy, many patients with moderate to severe chronic kidney disease have an increased incidence of cardiovascular events [4]. Patients with GFR less than 45 ml/min are 11 times more likely to experience a major cardiovascular event than those with normal renal function [4]. Therefore, radical nephrectomy, although it provides a good oncologic cure for *small renal masses*, should be avoided in these patients because of the significant possibility of their developing CKD following radical nephrectomy.

When compared with radical nephrectomy, partial nephrectomy provides better renal functional outcomes in similar patients (Table 12.1) [3].

As a result, the *AUA guidelines* recommend partial nephrectomy for tumors under four centimeters in size and up to 7 cm in size in those patients who are in need of preserving kidney function. This concept of renal preservation takes on added significance when one considers that Bijol and colleagues reviewed a series of specimens for patients undergoing radical nephrectomy, and found that apart from the tumor, 62%

J. A. Libertino (✉)
Professor of Urology, Tufts University School of Medicine, Department of Urology Tufts University Medical Center, Boston, MA, USA

J. A. Libertino, J. R. Gee (eds.), *Renal Cancer*, https://doi.org/10.1007/978-3-031-97599-8_12

Table 12.1 Summary of renal functional changes according to type of management for renal mass (numerical values in percentages)

Surgery	Ipsilateral parenchyma removed (%)	Total parenchyma preserved (%)	Median loss of renal function (%)	% Developing new-onset CKD (GFR < 45)
RN	100	Approximately 50	35	35–43
PN with extended ischemia (>30 min)	25 (15–60)	Approximately 70–90	19	19
PN with regional hypothermia	20 (15–40)	Approximately 75–92	11	10
PN with limited ischemia (<30 min)	20 (10–40)	Approximately 80–95	12	10
PN without ischemia	10 (0–20)	Approximately 90–100	5–10	7
TA	0	Approximately 90–100	0–10	NA
AS	0	100	0–5	NA

of the specimens showed microscopic signs of renal disease in the non-tumor portion of the kidney [5].

Additional factors supporting the role of partial nephrectomy rather than radical nephrectomy, were demonstrated by Huang and associates, who in a series of 662 patients with *small renal masses*, a normal contralateral kidney, and normal serum creatinine levels, found that 26% had preexisting CKD as evidenced by an eGFR of less than 60 by the MDRD method [2]. In addition, they found that chronic kidney disease develops in 50–60% of patients following radical nephrectomy.

Motivated by these observations, several series reported the successful use of partial nephrectomy in tumors even larger than 7 cm in diameter. This collective experience, fortified by my observations in a large series of patients, has led me to conclude that the preservation of normally functioning renal parenchyma that remains, and not the size of the tumor, should be the main determinant for performing partial nephrectomy, especially in solitary kidneys.

This concept is evident in the case below, where a non-clamping, nonischemic, tissue-sparing partial nephrectomy was performed on the patient's solitary kidney, rather than a radical nephrectomy, dialysis, and a renal transplant. Bench surgery and an autotransplant were also a potential option, but would have been technically difficult because of the three arteries supplying this kidney and would have exposed the kidney to ischemic injury. The partial nephrectomy provided this patient with a good functional outcome (preoperative e-GFR = 53 ml/min; postoperative eGFR of 35 ml/min), rather than the potential risks associated with the alternative approaches. This, despite a large, complex, centrally located lesion (nephrometry score of 12) (Fig. 12.1a–e).

Therefore, despite tumor size, partial nephrectomy is the treatment of choice when mandated by the clinical situation and is technically feasible. Unfortunately, in the USA currently, 54% of patients with *small renal masses* still undergo radical nephrectomy rather than partial nephrectomy [6].

The major goals of PN are as follows:

- Obtain the best possible oncologic outcome.
- Maximally preserve renal function.
- Minimize surgical complications.

There are certain factors that are modifiable and others that are not alterable when considering a partial nephrectomy. These factors are listed in Table 12.2.

The factors that influence renal function after partial nephrectomy are as follows: *lower preop GFR, solitary kidney, smaller volume of kidney*

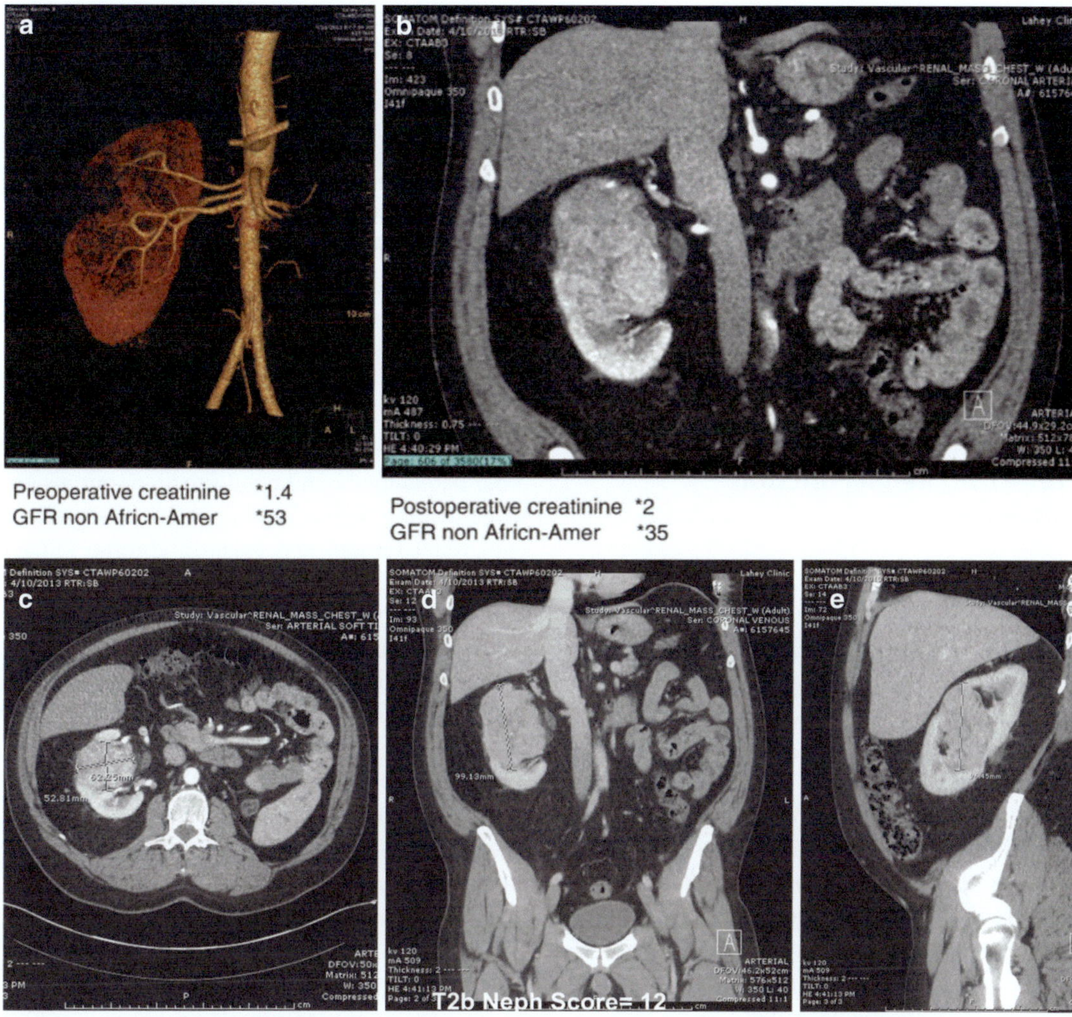

Fig. 12.1 Solitary kidney (**a**–**e**)

Table 12.2 Modifiable and nonmodifiable factors when considering a partial nephrectomy

Nonmodifiable	Modifiable
Renal tumor size	Surgical margins
Preexisting renal function	Ischemia time
	Volume of kidney tissue resected
	Or injured by the procedure itself

preserved, longer warm ischemia time (WIT), larger tumor size, and older age. These are independent predictors of reduced GFR postoperatively.

Role of Preoperative CKD on Postoperative Renal Function Following Partial Nephrectomy

Takagi and associates assessed whether adequately functioning parenchyma is preserved in patients with preexisting chronic kidney disease (CKD) who undergo a partial nephrectomy (PN) when compared to those who underwent a radical nephrectomy (RN). Ninety-five azotemic patients were analyzed, who underwent curative surgery for pathological T1a–T2 NOMO renal cell carcinoma, with a 24-month follow-up period. Moreover, 51 patients underwent RN, and 44 patients had a PN. Renal function was assessed using estimated GFR (e-GFR). These investigators demonstrated that the PN patients with a 2-year follow-up had a 64% freedom from progression of CKD class, as opposed to 22% who had freedom from progression of CKD class following radical nephrectomy [7].

This work demonstrated that, even in patients with CKD and an eGFR between 45 and 59 ml/min, there is value in preserving renal parenchyma by performing a PN as illustrated in Case 1.

Predicting Renal Function Outcomes

Predicting renal functional outcomes after radical nephrectomy or partial nephrectomy is critically important and may be helpful in choosing the type of procedure to be done: LRN, ORN, LPN, or 0PN. The prognostic risk of CKD in patients is increased when the preop GFR is less than 60 ml/min or post op GFR is less than 45 ml/min.

The ability to predict renal function is difficult. However, Bhindi et al. [8] derived a nomogram from an analysis of 3000 patients who underwent either radical nephrectomy or partial nephrectomy. The nomogram is designed to assist surgeons predict the possible renal functional outcome following either radical nephrectomy or partial nephrectomy. This information is helpful in selecting the proper surgical approach and in counseling patients about which of the various surgical options is preferable in avoiding postoperative CKD.

Another group of investigators, Krebs et al. [9], objectively assessed the loss of renal function by the type of procedure utilized. LRN caused the greatest loss of absolute renal function, followed by ORN, LPN, and OPN. OPN caused the least loss of postoperative renal function. The integration of these two studies is very important in predicting postoperative renal function following kidney surgery. These studies need to be correlated with the effects of warm ischemia and residual volume of renal tissue following renal surgery to properly predict postoperative renal function.

Role of Warm Ischemia on Postoperative Renal Function Following Partial Nephrectomy

Vincenz Czerny, from Heidelberg University, originally described the technique for partial nephrectomy in 1887. For over 100 years, the renal hilum was clamped as originally described. While the technique allowed preservation of renal parenchyma and renal function, our group, while dealing with a large population of patients with renal tumors and existing chronic kidney disease (CKD), began to question the need for routine clamping of the renal hilum. This question was stimulated by a publication in 1992 from Schumer et al., who described the morphologic, biochemical, and molecular evidence for apoptosis during the reperfusion phase, even after brief periods of renal ischemia [10]. Application of these analytical techniques to renal vascular injury has determined that brief periods of complete ischemia initiate a form of cell death (apoptosis) during a subsequent reperfusion phase that is drastically different from cellular necrosis induced by prolonged severe ischemia. Motivated by this research, I became interested in developing new methods for the non-clamping, nonischemic partial nephrectomy.

Simultaneously, in the late 1990s, our institution began working with a German company to develop 3D CT imaging. This technology allowed us to obtain 3D images of the renal vasculature in a noninvasive way, thus obviating the need for selective renal angiography prior to partial nephrectomy. This, in conjunction with the evolution of newer hemostatic agents, at about the same time, allowed us to visualize the intrarenal vascular anatomy noninvasively and carry out partial nephrectomies without hilar clamping.

From a historical perspective, the author (JAL) originated and developed the technique of the non-clamping, nonischemic partial nephrectomy in the mid-1990s and has successfully used it since that time. We reported our technique and presented our initial results at the 2005 AUA meeting entitled: "Does Thrombin Sealant Allow Nephron Surgery without Renal Artery Occlusion? Description of Technique and Initial Results" [11]. At the 2008 AUA meeting, we presented two other related reports entitled: "Non-Clamped, Non-Ischemic Partial Nephrectomy in Patients with Compromised Pre-Operative Renal Function or with a Solitary Kidney" [12] and "Non-Clamped, Non-Ischemic Partial Nephrectomy: "The New Gold Standard" [13]. These presentations resulted in two publications, one dealing with the "non-clamped partial nephrectomy: techniques and surgical outcomes" [14] and the other "the comparison of hilar clamping and non-hilar clamping for tumors involving a solitary kidney" [15]. In the initial publication, we compared clamping (116 PNs) versus non-clamping (192 PNs) and evaluated postoperative GFR after a 1-year follow-up. The clamped group had a decline in GFR of 12.3% and non-clamped group of 9.8% (p = 0.037), which did not appear to be statistically significant in the patients with two kidneys. However, in the subset of patients with a solitary kidney, we noted a 21% decrease in GFR in the clamped group as opposed to the 4% decrease in GFR in the non-clamped group [12]. This observation leads us to review our solitary kidney experience in detail. In our publication dealing with 104 patients with solitary kidneys, the non-clamping group had a significantly smaller percent decrease in late GFR 11.8% versus 27.7% in the clamped group (p = 0.01) [15]. In a subsequent review of 188 patients, from our institution, who underwent partial nephrectomies in solitary kidneys, the non-clamped group had a 13% decreased eGFR, and the clamped group had a 30% decreased eGFR® at day 200 (Fig. 12.2) (unpublished data).

After these original observations, other investigators began to carefully evaluate the role of ischemia in patients undergoing partial nephrectomy. Notably, Thompson and colleagues investigated the safe duration of warm ischemia during partial nephrectomy [16]. Their aim was to evaluate the short- and long-term renal effects of warm ischemia on renal function in patients with a solitary kidney. A total of 362 patients with a solitary kidney who underwent open (319) or laparoscopic (43) partial nephrectomy, using warm ischemia with hilar clamping, had the association of warm ischemic time (4–55 min) and renal functional outcome evaluated. Postoperative acute renal failure occurred in 70 patients (19%), including 58 patients (16%) who had a GFR of <15 ml/min within 30 days of surgery. Among 226 patients with a preoperative GFR > 30 ml/min, an additional 38 patients (17%) developed new-onset stage IV CKD. Their conclusion was that longer warm ischemia time is associated with short- and long-term renal consequences.

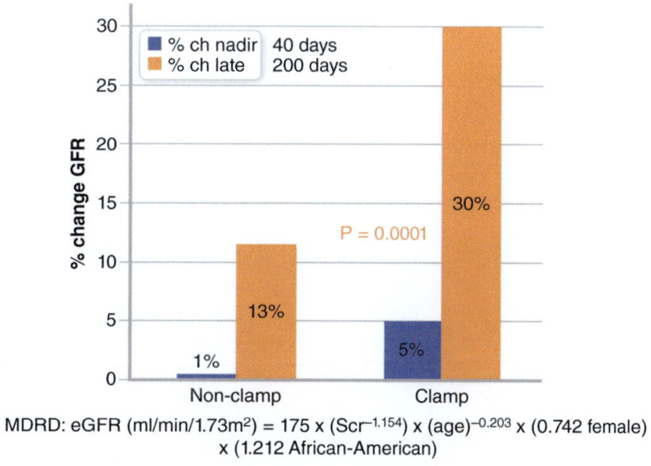

Fig. 12.2 Non-clamping vs clamping % change eGFR

These results suggested that every minute counts when the renal hilum is clamped [16].

The findings of Thompson and his group confirmed our original observations that renal ischemic injury is temporarily related to hilar clamping in solitary kidneys and damages postoperative renal function following partial nephrectomy.

Many publications have stated that in patients with two kidneys, hilar clamping versus non-clamping has minimal effect on postoperative renal function following partial nephrectomy. Unfortunately, many of these publications have only *short-term follow-up* data available. However, even in patients with two kidneys who underwent partial nephrectomy with warm ischemia, and had *long term* follow up, Mikkamalla and Assoc [17] noted in the Kaplan–Meier curves that the overall freedom from clinically significant CKD progression is 50% at 10 years (Fig. 12.3). The two most important predictive parameters are preoperative GFR values and length of warm ischemia time (Figs. 12.4 and 12.5). They reported that when warm ischemia exceeds 22 min, only 30% of patients were free of progressive CKD at 10 years. Stated another way, 70% of patients with warm ischemia >22 min had progression of CKD class at 10 years. In addition, preoperative azotemia (with GFR <79 cc/min) also compromised postoperative renal function, and 70% of these patients had progression of CKD class at 10 years.

The role of warm ischemia compromising long-term postoperative renal function following partial nephrectomy is clearly established, even in patients with two kidneys, with long-term, not short-term follow-up.

Regardless of these findings, the debate continues in the literature regarding the benefits of clamping versus non-clamping in robotic partial nephrectomy. Daniel Rosen et al. presented, at the 2018 AUA meeting, a series of 668 patients with two kidneys who underwent partial nephrectomy with hilar clamping and noted that there was a strong association between warm ischemia time (WIT) and acute kidney injury (AKI). A threshold of WIT >20 min was identified as a significant risk factor for developing AKI at the time of discharge, while 15 min WIT was identified as a cutoff for a worse e-GFR outcome with long-

Fig. 12.3 Overall freedom from progression free in CKD in all patients

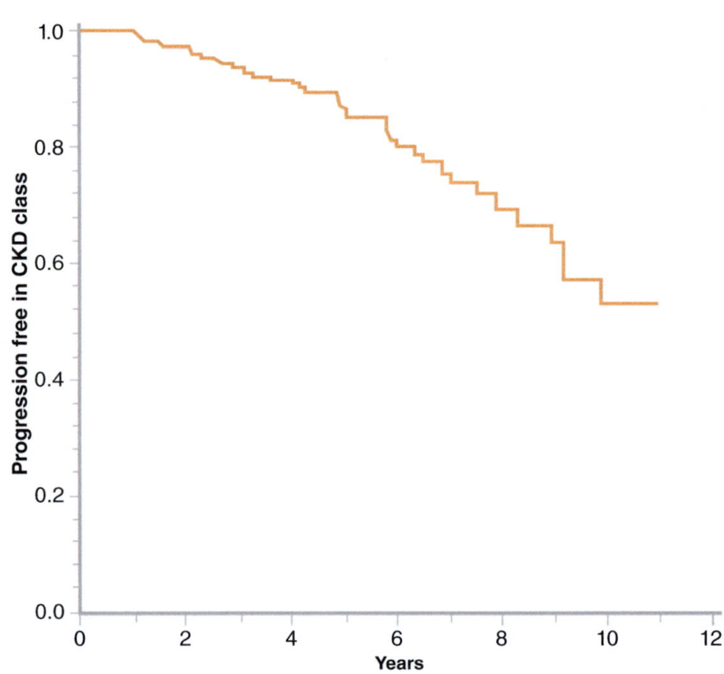

Follow up years	0	2.0	4.0	6.0	8.0	10.0
Pateiens at risk	358	263	152	78	27	12

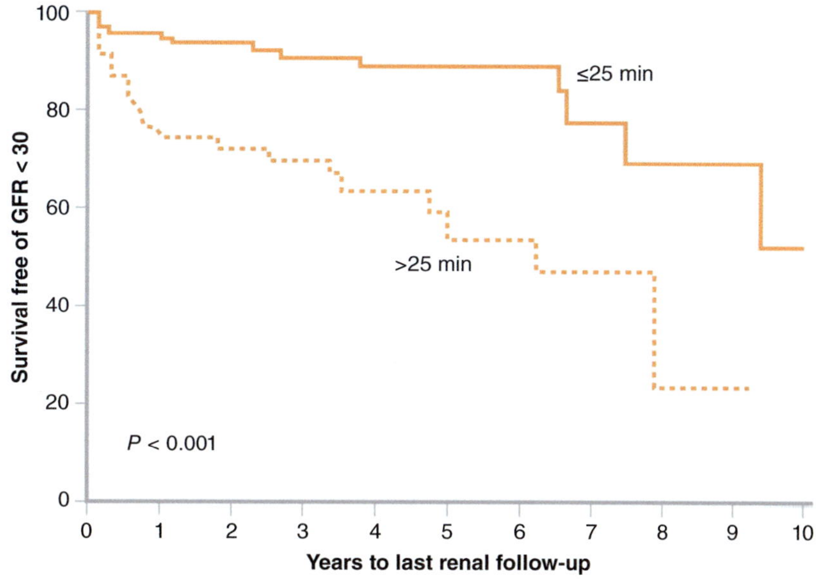

Fig. 12.4 Impact of WIT on freedom from progression of CKD class. (Modified from [17])

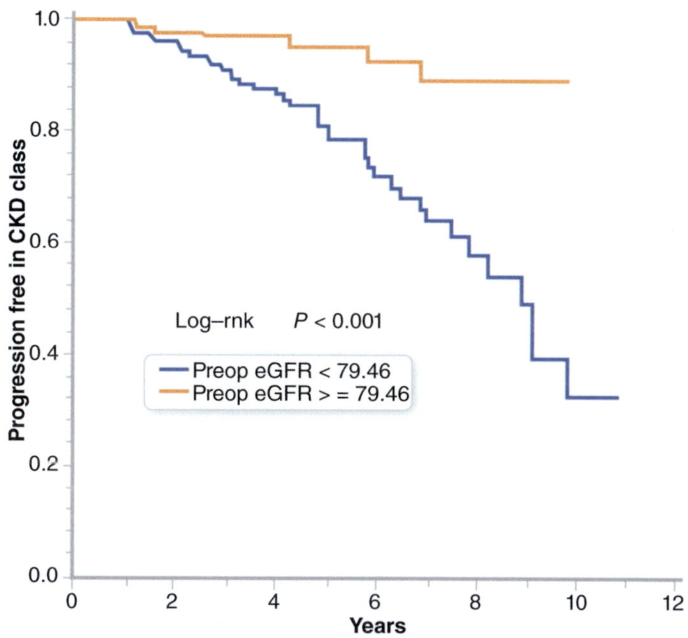

Patients at risk time	0	2.0	4.0	6.0	8.0	10.0
Below median	179	150	89	42	16	5
Above median	179	145	106	36	26	26

Fig. 12.5 Impact of pre op GFR on progression-free in CKD class

term follow-up. *These authors also agree that every effort should be made to limit every minute of warm ischemia during a robotic PN and keep the WIT® under 15 min* [18].

In 2023, Antonelli et al. [19] studied the role of warm ischemia time on the functional outcomes after robotic partial nephrectomy: a radionuclide renal scan study from the CLOCK randomized trials and found *short term* changes in renal function which correlated with a warm ischemia time of greater than 10 min (Fig. 12.6). It will be necessary to follow these patients to

Fig. 12.6 Impact of warm ischemia on renal function changes

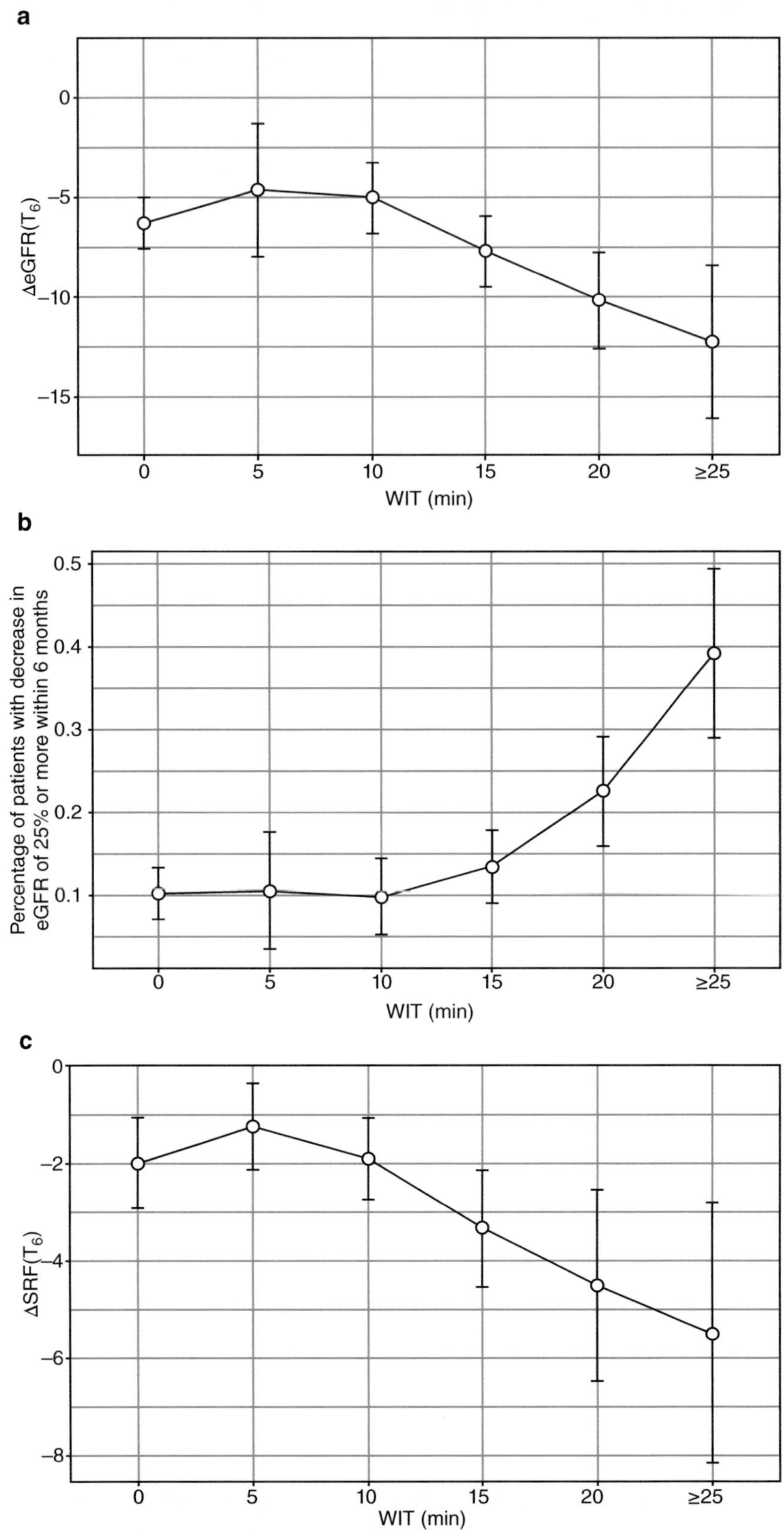

determine the *long term* effects of WIT on clinical renal function. This concept, the effect of WIT on renal function, is just as relevant in robotic and open partial nephrectomy.

There is little doubt as to the importance of renal ischemia and its short and long-term effects on postoperative renal function following partial nephrectomy, even in patients with two kidneys. The two-kidney model is not as ideal a setting to study the effect of ischemia on kidney function as is the solitary kidney model. Long-term follow-up is mandatory in analyzing the current literature regarding clamping versus non-clamping partial nephrectomy. *It is axiomatic, however, that If less WIT is better, then no ischemia is the best method of avoiding long-term renal ischemic injury in any patient undergoing a partial nephrectomy, open or minimally invasive.*

Role of Volume on Postoperative Renal Function Following Partial Nephrectomy

In addition to ischemic injury, the percentage of volume preserved is another primary determinant of the renal functional outcome following partial nephrectomy. Steve Campbell and his colleagues carried out an elegant study, of a novel method to estimate the percentage of functional volume preserved in order to assess its effect on renal functional outcomes [20]. They studied the GFR outcome based on the MDRD score in 38 patients who had normal preoperative serum creatinine and who underwent open or laparoscopic partial nephrectomy. A cylindrical volume ratio method was used to estimate the percentage of functional volume preserved on CT images obtained before and after partial nephrectomy. A model to predict the postoperative estimated GFR was based on multiplying the preoperative GFR by the percentage of volume preserved, followed by adjustment for the functional contribution of the contralateral kidney. Correlation and multiple regression analysis were done to test this model. On multivariate analysis, the preoperative glomerular filtration rate ($p < 0.001$) and ischemia time ($p = 0.02$) correlated with the nadir glomerular filtration rate, and the preoperative glomerular filtration rate ($p < 0.001$) and the percent of functional volume preservation ($p = 0.04$) correlated with the late glomerular filtration rate. These data support the notion that preoperative nephron endowment and the percentage of functional volume preserved are primary determinants of long-term functional outcome after partial nephrectomy in patients with normal preoperative kidney function and an ischemia time within acceptable limits. What is difficult to discern, from this study, is how much of the kidney tissue preserved was damaged by hilar clamping and renal ischemic injury (Fig. 12.7).

Split renal function (SRF) is another fundamentally important factor in predicting functional recovery after radical nephrectomy. As Rathi et al. have discussed in a recent publication, partial nephrectomy is generally preferred for localized renal cell carcinoma, but radical nephrectomy is occasionally required. A new baseline glomerular filtration rate (NBGFR) greater than 45 ml/min after cancer surgery is associated with favorable survival outcomes. If predicted NBGFR after radical nephrectomy will be above this threshold and the tumor has an aggressive oncological potential, radical nephrectomy may be an appropriate consideration. These investigators calculated split renal function by using a semi-automated software (Fuji Medical Systems), which provides differential parenchymal volume analysis on the basis of preoperative imaging that was retrospectively studied in 445 RN patients; and split renal function (SRF) was calculated in these patients. Based on differential volume analysis, they were able to predict the NBGFR after radical nephrectomy more accurately than five other published non-SFR-based models, and also improved the prediction of the clinically relevant threshold of NBGFR of less than 45 ml/min [21]. SRF analysis is an important adjunct in preoperatively selecting RN vs PN as the procedure of choice for each individual patient (Fig. 12.8).

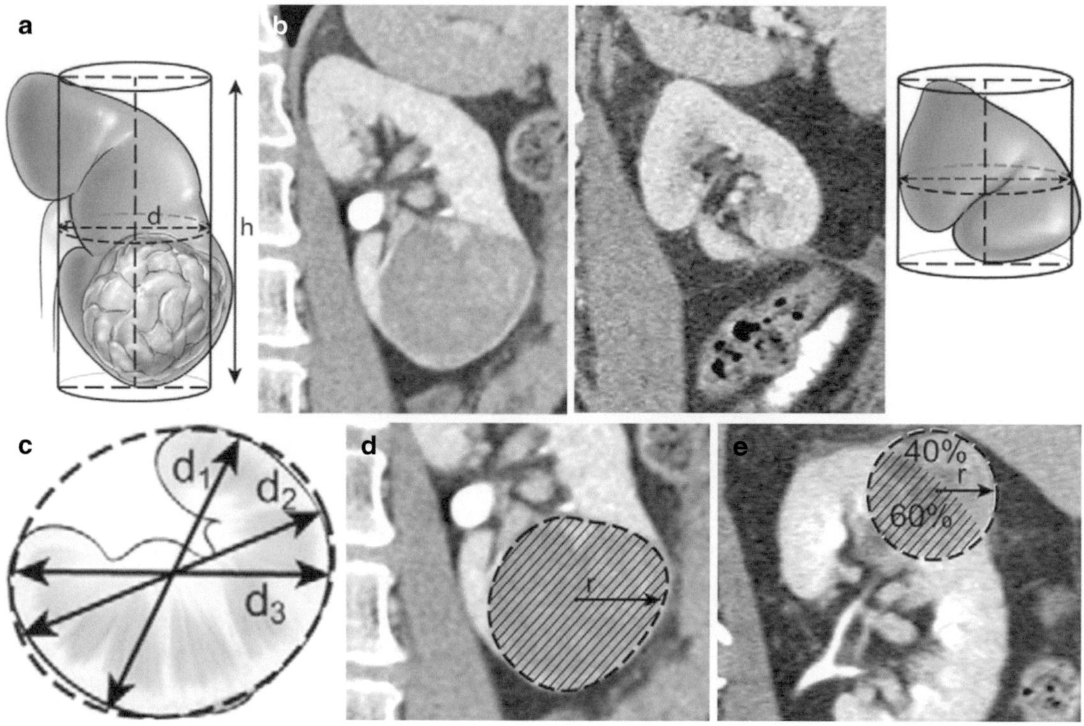

Fig. 12.7 Method for calculating residual renal parenchyma following partial nephrectomy. (Reprinted with permission from Simmons et al. [20])

It seems reasonable to conclude that warm ischemia and the volume of functioning renal tissue that remains are both critical in determining postoperative kidney function following partial nephrectomy. WIT needs to be eliminated and volume maximized to obtain the best renal functional outcome for the patient. Preserving renal parenchyma which has been damaged by warm ischemic injury does not maximally enhance renal function.

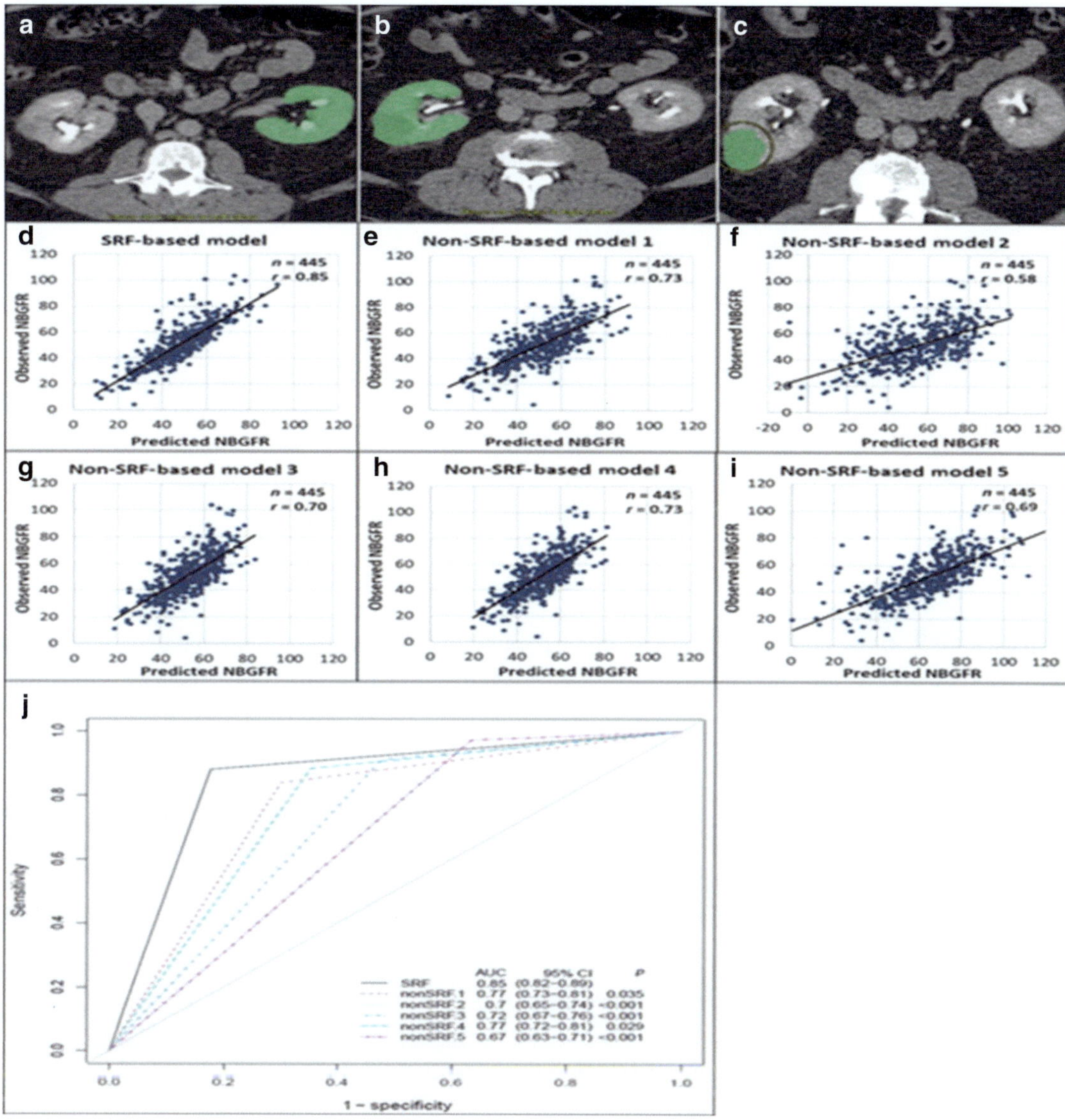

Fig. 12.8 (**a**–**j**) Calculation of split renal function [21]

Combined Role of Ischemia and Volume on Renal Function Following Partial Nephrectomy

We have demonstrated that ischemia and volume are independent factors determining renal functional outcomes following partial nephrectomy. What about the combined role of nonischemia and preservation of renal parenchymal volume (enucleation rather than wedge resection) on renal function following partial nephrectomy?

For many years, we have combined the nonclamping, nonischemic partial nephrectomy approach with renal tumor enucleation in order to maximize renal function following partial nephrectomy. We have recently reviewed our series 1422 partial nephrectomies where tumor enucleation was utilized, 434 clamped versus 988 non-clamped. As expected, there was more blood loss in the non-clamped cohort (600 cc vs. 250 cc). However, even in patients with two kidneys, long-term follow-up demonstrated a 35% decrease in renal function in the clamped group and an 18% in the non-clamped group as measured by changes in pre- and postoperative creatinine and eGFR, again clearly demonstrating better preservation of renal function in the non-clamped group (unpublished data). These results were confirmed by the University of Michigan group, who reported that even in patients with two kidneys, with long-term follow-up (10 years), approximately 50% of patients developed clinically significant progression of CKD class following robotic partial nephrectomy [17]. Our results are even clearer in patients with solitary kidneys. In our series of 188 partial nephrectomies in solitary kidneys, there was a 13% decreased GFR in the non-clamped group and a 30% decreased GFR® in the clamped group at day 200 (unpublished data).

These results underscore the value of non-clamping, nonischemic tissue-sparing technique, which I believe provides the optimal renal functional outcome following partial nephrectomy. As can be seen in this text, many other researchers have also confirmed our original observations that avoiding ischemic injury and sparing renal parenchyma are key determinants of renal function following partial nephrectomy.

One final technical point is the avoidance of large mattress sutures in both open and minimally invasive partial nephrectomy. These mattress sutures compromise residual parenchymal volume and therefore impair postoperative renal function. This observation is clearly demonstrated in a recent study of 20 patients who had a robotic partial nephrectomy [22, 23]. As seen in the illustration and chart below, after 1 year of follow-up, there is a significant (24%) reduction in the remaining renal parenchymal volume because of large mattress sutures (Fig. 12.9).

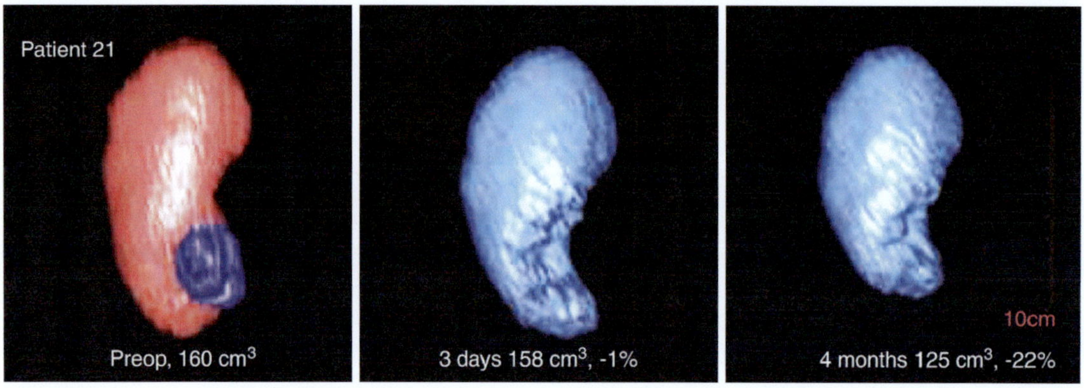

Fig. 12.9 Loss of renal parenchyma following robotic partial nephrectomy. (Adapted from AUA News December 2017)

Conclusion

Regardless of whether the partial nephrectomy is performed open or minimally invasively, the data, in my opinion, very strongly support that "The Non-Ischemic Tissue Sparing Technique" *provides the best long-term renal functional outcome, in patients with either two functioning kidneys or a solitary kidney at the time of surgery.*

Surgical Approach to Multifocal or Bilateral Renal Tumors

Managing patients with bilateral, multiple tumors or tumors in a solitary kidney adds another dimension of complexity. Many patients with hereditary renal syndromes, such as Von Hippel–Lindau, Birt–Hogg–Dube, hereditary leiomyomatosis, renal cell cancer, hereditary renal papillary carcinoma, succinate dehydrogenase deficiency, tuberous sclerosis, familial oncocytoma, and familial renal cancer, *often present with multifocal, bilateral renal tumors synchronous or asynchronous in nature*. For patients with these conditions, the surgical approach requires the cure of the cancer while maximizing renal function. These patients generally present with tumors at a younger age, and the clinician needs to be forward-thinking. The goal in these patient populations is to prevent cancer dissemination, maximize renal function, limit the number of surgeries performed, and minimize ischemia, while at the same time maximizing the remaining renal parenchyma.

Decisions on the timing of genetic testing, the order of surgery, optimal method for partial nephrectomy, and surveillance of de novo lesions are critically important in managing patients with multifocal or bilateral disease. Information obtained from nuclear scans may help more accurately delineate split renal function and help with planning of the surgical approach. For synchronous, bilateral tumors, the timing of surgery is debatable. Three major surgical options exist, they include:

1. Concomitant bilateral partial nephrectomies.
2. Staged partial nephrectomy with the larger, more complex side first.
3. Staged partial nephrectomy with the smaller, less complex side first [24].

Each surgeon or center advocates its own surgical approach. My personal preference to use is option [3], the staged open partial nephrectomy approach, doing the less complicated lesions first. This process allows the kidney containing the more complicated lesion or lesions to remain as a backup dialysis unit during the immediate postoperative period in the event that the more complex tumor may require a subsequent radical nephrectomy. If done in the opposite order, and radical nephrectomy is performed initially, ischemia in the remaining solitary kidney after the partial nephrectomy may place the patient at greater risk for renal complications.

While it is possible to carry out minimally invasive surgery on patients with multiple or bilateral tumors, ischemia becomes a significant potential problem due to the prolonged clamping time required and the need for bilateral renal artery occlusion. *That is why, I prefer a non-clamping, nonischemia, tissue sparing open partial nephrectomy as the preferred approach in patients with multiple, bilateral tumors or tumors in a solitary kidney*, as illustrated in the following case studies.

Case Study 1

The patient is a 60-year-old male who underwent a left radical nephrectomy in 2007. He developed a tumor in his solitary right kidney and underwent a right partial nephrectomy in 2011. In 2018, he was referred for surgery of two recurrent tumors in his solitary right kidney. His preoperative creatinine was 1.3. He underwent a non-clamping, tissue-sparing partial nephrectomy with removal of the two tumors in his solitary kidney, seen in the following MRI and CT scans (Fig. 12.10a–d). The vessels supplying the tumor are ligated in continuity (Fig. 12.10d). Note that the entire kidney has normal blood flow during the non-clamping partial nephrectomy. The middle pole tumor was excised initially. One can see the upper edge of the lower pole tumor through the enucleation site of the first tumor (Fig. 12.10e). After both tumors were excised,

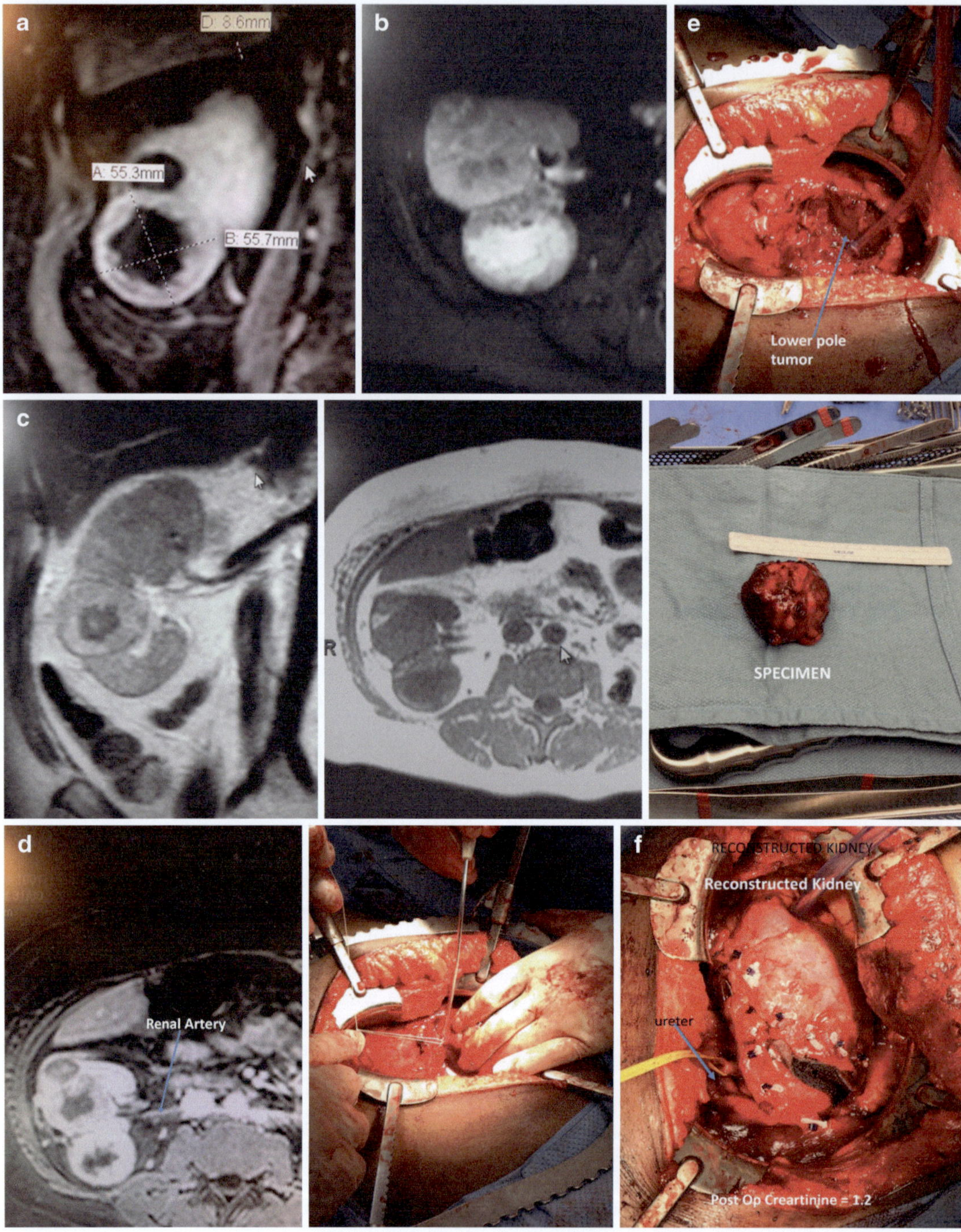

Fig. 12.10 Case study 1. (**a**) Preoperative CT scan of two recurrent tumors in a solitary kidney. (**b**) Preoperative MRI of two recurrent tumors in a solitary kidney. (**c**) MRI—2 recurrent in solitary right kidney. (**d**) Intraoperative view—ligating segmental renal artery in continuity without clamping the main renal artery. (**e**) Tumor bed after resection of the first renal tumor, arrow points to the upper border of the second renal mass before removal. (**f**) Reconstructed solitary kidney after non-clamping partial nephrectomy

the kidney was reconstructed as seen in (Fig. 12.10e). His postoperative creatinine remains 1.3.

Case Study 2

The patient is a 52-year-old female who was in good general health until she noted persistent right flank pain and gross hematuria with passage of clots. A CAT scan demonstrated a large right renal tumor and a midpolar tumor in the left kidney (Fig. 12.11a, b). She initially underwent a non-clamping, nonischemic, tissue-sparing left partial nephrectomy (Fig. 12.11c, d). Thereafter, she had a right radical nephrectomy. Her postoperative BUN is 10, creatinine 1.1, and GFR > 60. The final pathology of the left partial nephrectomy revealed a clear cell renal cell carcinoma grade 2 of 4. Stage PT 1b is with negative surgical margins and no evidence of lymphovascular invasion. The pathology of the right thoracoabdominal radical nephrectomy was clear cell carcinoma Fuhrman grade 3–4, stage PT 3a with extension into the perirenal fat, negative surgical margins, and negative for lymphovascular invasion.

Case Study 3

The patient is a 60-year-old male who was referred with bilateral renal tumors. Outside studies revealed a large tumor in the left kidney (Fig. 12.12a) and a tumor in the lower pole of the right kidney (Fig. 12.12b). He was also noted to have what was thought to be perihilar nodes in the hilum of the liver surrounding the portal vein (Fig. 12.12a). Because of the unusual nature of periportal lymph node metastasis, we evaluated this mass with a liver scintigram, which demonstrated a hemangioma of the caudate lobe of the liver. The lesions were biopsied, and the diagnosis of hemangioma of the caudate lobe was confirmed. The patient underwent sequential right lower pole non-clamping, nonischemic, tissue sparing partial nephrectomy followed 6 weeks later by a left radical nephrectomy. The postoperative image is noted in (Fig. 12.12c) His preoperative creatinine was 1.3 and GFR > 60 ml/min. His postoperative creatinine is 1.5, and his GFR equals 55 ml/min.

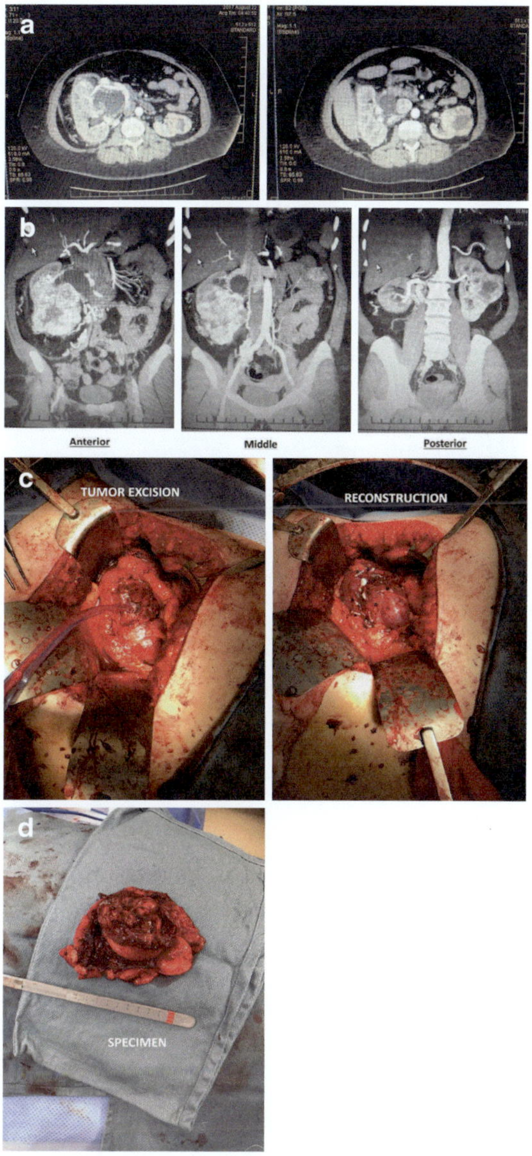

Fig. 12.11 Case study 2. (**a**) Preoperative CT scan demonstrating large right renal tumor and midpolar left renal tumor. (**b**) Preoperative CTA scan of large right renal tumor and midpolar left renal tumor, without evidence of adenopathy or venous involvement. (**c**, **d**) reconstruction of midpolar partial neph

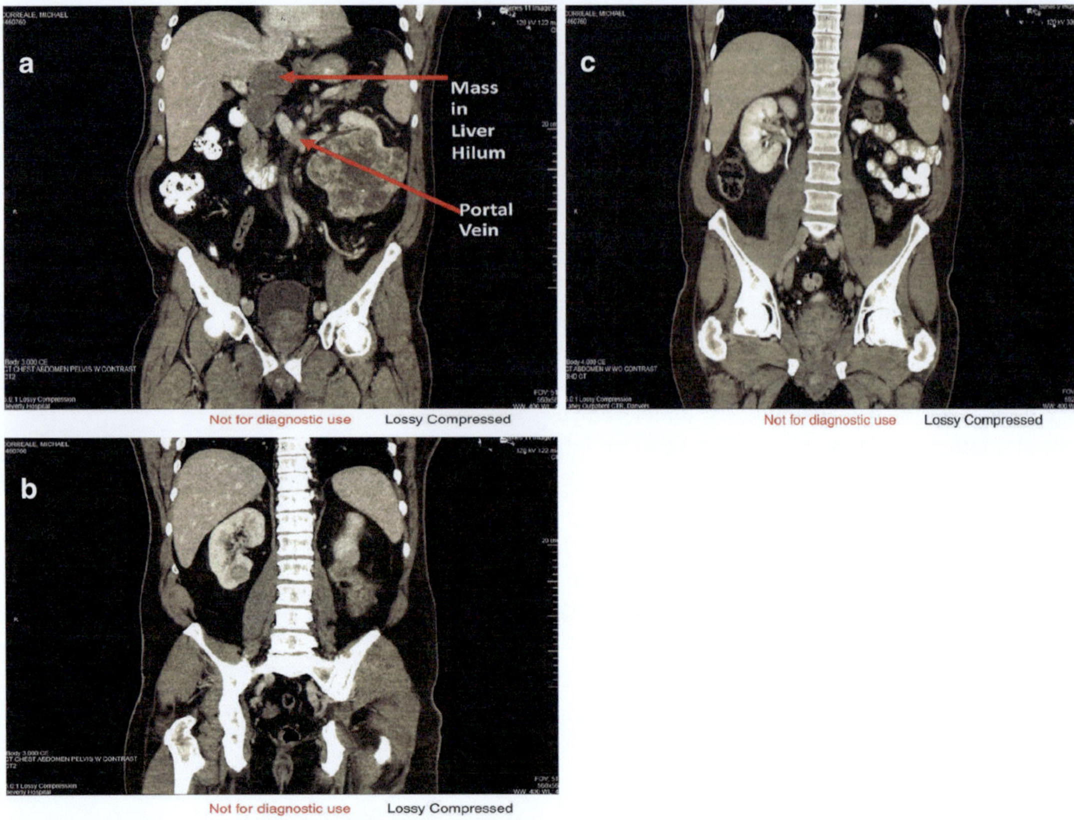

Fig. 12.12 Case study 3. (**a**) Preoperative CT scan demonstrating a large left renal tumor and an additional mass surrounding the portal vein. (**b**) Preoperative CT scan demonstrating a right lower pole tumor. (**c**) Postoperative CT scan following a left radical nephrectomy and a right lower pole partial nephrectomy

Summary

In essence, the non-clamping, nonischemic, tissue-sparing partial nephrectomy, in my experience, provides the best long-term outcome in patients with two kidneys or those with a solitary kidney, especially in those patients with multiple or bilateral synchronous tumors.

References

1. National Kidney Foundation. The facts about chronic kidney disease (CKD). 2018. Available at https://www.kidney.org/kidneydisease/CKD/index.cfm.
2. Huang WC, Levey AS, Serio AM, et al. Chronic kidney disease after nephrectomy in patients with renal cortical tumors: a retrospective cohort study. Lancet Oncol. 2006;7(9):735–40.
3. Lane BR, Fergany AF, Wright CJ, et al. Renal functional outcome after partial nephrectomy with extended ischemia intervals are better than after radical nephrectomy. J Urol. 2010;184(4):1286–90.
4. Go AS, Cherow GM, Fan D, et al. Chronic kidney disease and the risk of death, cardiovascular events and hospitalization. N Engl J Med. 2004;351(13):1296–305.
5. Bijol V, Mendez GP, Hurwitz S, et al. Evaluation of non-neoplastic pathology in tumor nephrectomy specimens: predicting the risk of progressive renal failure. Am J Surg Pathol. 2006;30(5):575–84.
6. Seer incidence Data Base, NIH National Cancer Institute, surveillance, epidemiology and end results Program 1973–2016.
7. Takagi T, Kondo T, Sizuka J, et al. Postoperative renal function after partial nephrectomy for renal cell cancer in patients with preexisting chronic kidney dis-

ease: a comparison with radical nephrectomy. Int J Urol. 2011;18:472–6.
8. Bhindi B, Lohse CM, Schulte PJ, et al. Predicting renal function outcomes after partial and radical nephrectomy. Eur Urol. 2019;75(5):766.
9. Krebs RK, Andreoni C, Ortiz V. The impact of radical and partial nephrectomy on renal function in patients with renal cancer. Urol Int. 2014;92(4):449–54.
10. Schumer M, Colomber M, Sawczuk I, Gobe G, Connor J, O'Toole K, Olsson C, Wise G, Buttyan R. Morphologic, biochemical, and molecular evidence of apoptosis during the reperfusion phase after brief periods of renal ischemia. Am J Pathol. 1992;140(4):831–8.
11. Triaca V, Zagha R, Libertino JA. Does thrombin sealant allow nephron sparing surgery (NSS) without renal artery occlusion? Description of technique and initial results. J Urol. 2005;171(4):1338.
12. Smith G, Cohen M, Kurteva T, Libertino JA. Nonclamped, non ischemia partial nephrectomy in patients with compromised preoperative renal function or with a solitary kidney. J Urol. 2008;179(4):1096.
13. Kurteva T, Cohen M, Smith G, Libertino JA. Nonclamped, non-ischemic partial nephrectomy: the new gold standard. J Urol. 2008;179(4):1392.
14. Smith G, Kenney P, Lee Y, Libertino JA. Nonclamped partial nephrectomy: techniques and surgical outcomes. BJU Int. 2011;107(7):1054–8. https://doi.org/10.1111/j.1464-410X.2010.09798.x. Epub 2010 Oct 29.
15. Wszolek M, Kenney P, Lee Y, Libertino JA. Comparison of hilar clamping and non-hilar clamping partial nephrectomy for tumors involving a solitary kidney. BJU Int. 2011;107(12):1886–92. https://doi.org/10.1111/j.1464-410X.2010.09713.x. Epub 2010 Nov 11.
16. Thompson RH, Lane BR, Lohse C, et al. Every minute counts when the renal hilum is clamped during partial nephrectomy. Eur Urol. 2010;58:340–5.
17. Mukkamalla A, Weier A, Hafez KS, et al. Long-term renal functional outcomes of minimally invasive partial nephrectomy for renal cell cancer. Urol Oncol. 2014;32(8):1247–51.
18. Rosen D, Oaulucci D, Reynolds C, Abaza R, Eun D, Bahndari A, Hemal A, Badani K, Valet LP. Reevaluating warm ischemia as a predictor of renal function outcomes in patients undergoing robotic partial nephrectomy. Urology. 2018;120:156–61.
19. Antonelli, et al. The role of warm ischemia on the functional outcomes after robotic partial nephrectomy: a radionuclide scan study from CLOCK randomized trial. World J Urol. 2023;4:1337–44.
20. Simmons MN, Fergany AF, Campbell SC. The effect of parenchymal volume preservation on kidney function after partial nephrectomy. J Urol. 2011;186(2):405–10.
21. Rathi N, et al. Split renal function is fundamentally important for predicting functional recovery after radical nephrectomy. Eur Urol Open Sci. 2022;40:112–6.
22. Bahler C, Sudaram C, Kondo T. Volume loss after partial nephrectomy-could suture renorrhaphy be a cause? AUA meeting, Boston, Best Poster Prize. 2017.
23. Bahler CD, Dube HT, Flynn KJ, et al. Feasibility of omitting cortical renorrhaphy during robot assisted partial nephrectomy: a matched analysis. J Endourol. 2015;29:548.
24. Shuch B, Singer E, Bratslavsky G. The surgical approach to multifoca; renal cancers: ipsilateral multifocality and bilateral tumors. Urol Clin N Am. 2012;39(2):133–48.

Open Partial Nephrectomy

13

Marianne M. Casilla-Lennon, Patrick A. Kenney, Matthew Wszolek, and John A. Libertino

Introduction

Despite broader acceptance of active surveillance and ablative approaches, surgical excision partial nephrectomy (PN) remains an excellent option for treatment of locally confined renal cell carcinoma (RCC). Historically, radical nephrectomy (RN) was utilized to treat locally confined RCC, regardless of tumor size and complexity. RN remains overutilized for RCC amenable to partial nephrectomy (PN) despite contemporary studies demonstrating equivocal oncologic outcomes between PN and RN for T1 RCC. Comparable oncologic outcomes coupled with contemporary studies correlating RN with increased cardiovascular morbidity, development of chronic kidney disease (CKD), and inferior overall survival have led to more widespread acceptance of nephron-sparing surgery (NSS). To this end, the 2017 American Urologic Association and 2014 European Association of Urology guidelines recommend PN for T1 RCC when technically feasible, especially when there is a need to preserve renal function [1, 2].

PN, however, remains a challenging endeavor requiring complete tumor resection with a negative margin and maximal preservation of functioning renal parenchyma. The chief advantages of PN compared to RN include avoiding the overtreatment of benign renal masses without compromising oncologic efficacy in malignant tumors and preserving renal function to minimize postoperative CKD, morbidity, and mortality. This chapter will provide a detailed discussion of the rationale for PN as well as its current indications. The importance of minimizing renal ischemia and other predictors of postoperative CKD will be discussed. The techniques of open PN will be described, as will perioperative management. Minimally invasive approaches, ablative therapies, and active surveillance will be discussed in other chapters.

Historical Perspective

In 1887, Vincenz Czerny (1842–1915) performed the first planned PN for a renal tumor (angiosarcoma) over 15 years after Gustav Simon

Supplementary Information The online version contains supplementary material available at https://doi.org/10.1007/978-3-031-97599-8_13.

M. M. Casilla-Lennon
Department of Urology, Yale New Haven Health, New Haven, CT, USA
e-mail: Marianne.casilla-lennon@yale.edu

P. A. Kenney
Department of Urology, Yale School of Medicine, Yale New Haven Hospital, New Haven, CT, USA
e-mail: Patrick.kenney@yale.edu

M. Wszolek
Department of Urology, Massachusetts General Hospital, Boston, MA, USA
e-mail: mwzolek@mgh.harvard.edu

J. A. Libertino (✉)
Professor of Urology, Tufts University School of Medicine, Department of Urology Tufts University Medical Center, Boston, MA, USA

J. A. Libertino, J. R. Gee (eds.), *Renal Cancer*, https://doi.org/10.1007/978-3-031-97599-8_13

(1824–1876), his predecessor at Heidelberg, Germany, performed both the first planned nephrectomy and PN for nonmalignant renal pathology [3]. Initial interest in PN, however, waned due to concerns about complications including intraoperative hemorrhage, delayed bleeding, and urinary fistulae [4]. The observation that a patient could survive with one functioning kidney after nephrectomy also diminished early interest in NSS [3]. In the early twentieth century, nephrectomy was considered a standard therapy for malignant renal tumors due to the technical challenges associated with advanced clinical stage at presentation and concerns about perinephric tumor extension, although PN was occasionally employed in the treatment of benign conditions such as cysts, infarcts, caruncles, calculi, or localized hydronephrosis [3]. In the late twentieth century, the necessity of radical Halstedian resections for renal cancer was questioned by pathological studies demonstrating the noninvasive, expansile local growth of renal tumors [3] as well as studies reporting a low rate of metastasis from small renal tumors [5]. In 1950, Vermooten notably questioned the necessity of RN in all cases of RCC, even in the presence of a functioning contralateral kidney, and established the basis for the modern approach of NSS for RCC [6]. For the next several decades, however, PN was rarely performed even in patients with solitary kidneys, renal dysfunction, or bilateral tumors [7]. As researched by Herr, surgical textbooks written between 1937 and 1970 do not mention PN for renal cancer [3]. Surgical advancements in the 1960s and 1970s, more specifically renal hypothermia and resection techniques based on segmental blood supply, which permitted resection and reconstruction in a bloodless field, as well as published favorable local recurrence rates (4–10%) and survival rates comparable to RN in patients with solitary kidneys and bilateral tumors stimulated interest in widespread use of PN in RCC [3, 8].

In the late 1970s and 1980s, progressive urologists increasingly questioned the rationale of removing an entire kidney for a small renal mass, leading to the modern era of routine elective PN. As mentioned previously, the concept was not novel. However, advancements in technique and anatomical knowledge, promising low local recurrence rates and favorable survival outcomes in preliminary studies of essential PN, and a downward stage migration resulting from more frequent axial imaging provided the foundation for the preliminary experiences of elective PN for patients with RCC and normal contralateral renal function. As often true for any dramatic paradigm shift, the change was not immediate or unanimous. Opponents raised concerns over inadequate excision of the primary tumor and possible occult tumors in the renal remnant. Licht and Novick in 1993 published their short-term experience of 241 PNs in patients with a normal contralateral kidney. They reported a <1% local recurrence rate and 95% survival rate [9]. Subsequent publications with longer follow-up validated these results and solidified the role of PN in the treatment of small renal masses with a normal contralateral kidney [10, 11]. With continued technical advancements, including intraoperative ultrasound and more effective hemostatic agents, urologists have expanded indications for NSS to include larger tumor size, multiple tumors in a single operation, and complex locations such as hilar, endophytic, and centrally located lesions. The role of NSS has been further solidified by the observation that RN compared to PN is associated with an increased risk of CKD and non-cancer-related morbidity and mortality [12, 13]. In recent years, urologists have focused on techniques to minimize ischemic injury and also lessen surgical morbidity by minimally invasive approaches, as well as avoidance of surgery through the use of active surveillance or ablation in appropriate cases.

Epidemiology of Small Renal Masses

Kidney cancer is the 12th most common malignancy worldwide, with 338,000 new cases in 2012 [14]. In the United States, there will be an estimated 65,340 new cases and 14,970 deaths from renal tumors (including RCC and urothelial renal pelvis tumors) in 2018 [15]. For cases with pathological confirmation in the US Surveillance,

Epidemiology, and End Results (SEER) database, over 90% of "renal tumors" were RCC, while the majority of the remaining tumors were urothelial tumors of the renal pelvis [16]. For malignant renal tumors, the clear cell (conventional) type constitutes approximately 70% of cases with papillary, chromophobe, renal medullary, and collecting duct comprising the remaining cases [17]. Established risk factors for RCC include increasing age [16, 18], male sex [14], geographic location (higher in the United States and Europe) [19], race (lower in Asian/Pacific descendent than in the United States) [16, 18], smoking [20], obesity [21–23], and hypertension [21].

Total kidney cancer incidence increased for an approximately 20-year period from the 1970s to the 1990s, but has plateaued or declined recently in many countries worldwide [19, 24]. In the United States, where histologic information is available unlike many cancer registries, the rates of renal pelvis urothelial tumors have declined, while RCC rates have continued to rise among all age classifications, tumor sizes, and racial groups [18]. The increased incidence of RCC has been attributed to the incidental diagnosis of small, asymptomatic renal masses due to more frequent usage of axial imaging. Contemporary studies support this observation. A study from the US National Cancer Database (NCDB) between 1993 and 2004 showed a significant increase in Stage I RCC with a corresponding decrease in Stage II–IV RCC [25]. Furthermore, the mean size of Stage I RCC decreased from 4.1 cm in 1993 to 3.6 cm in 2003, with a particular increase in the incidence of tumors <3 cm [25, 26]. Stage migration may account for the recent plateauing of RCC mortality rates in Europe [24] and the United States [16, 18]. Other factors are likely also contributing to this trend, as the survival of RCC patients with more advanced disease has improved recently as well. Possible explanations include early detection of all stages through incidental diagnosis and recent therapeutic advancements, including targeted therapy [16, 18].

There is a distinct relationship between tumor size and risk of malignancy. Smaller lesions are more likely to be benign tumors such as oncocytoma, angiomyolipoma, papillary adenoma, and metanephric adenoma. In the Mayo Clinic, 6.3% of tumors >7 cm were benign compared with 46.3% of tumors <1 cm [27]. Furthermore, larger tumor size was associated with an increased risk of high compared to low grade and clear cell compared to papillary RCC [27]. For renal masses <4 cm treated surgically, upstaging to T3 and advanced grade was associated with increasing tumor size, especially for tumors >3 cm [28, 29]. The relationship between tumor size and risk of metastasis at presentation has been established. Patients with tumors 1 cm or less, 1.1–2 cm, 2.1–3 cm, and 3.1–4 cm had a prevalence of metastasis at diagnosis of 1.4%, 2.5%, 4.7%, and 7.4%, respectively, in a recent SEER study [30]. The most rapid increase in both the prevalence of metastases at diagnosis and disease-specific death occurred for tumor sizes between 4 and 12 cm [30]. A similar pattern to the increased risk of metastasis at presentation with tumors >3 cm was evident in the probability of de novo asynchronous metastatic RCC in postsurgical patients [31].

Oncologic Efficacy of Partial Nephrectomy

Traditionally, RN was the treatment of choice for renal cortical tumors. PN was performed only in "essential" cases, such as patients with solitary kidneys, bilateral renal tumors, or severe chronic renal insufficiency with a goal of avoiding dialysis dependence. Consistent with trends across other surgical disciplines favoring organ preservation, the American Urological Association (1) and European Association of Urology (2) now recommend PN as a treatment for T1 (<7 cm) RCC in patients with two functioning kidneys. The rationale driving this paradigm shift was multifactorial, including concerns over the relationship between CKD and non-RCC-related mortality as well as a downward stage migration in RCC, resulting in an increased detection of renal cortical tumors amenable to PN. Since the goal of any oncologic procedure is local cancer control, the aforementioned factors would be irrelevant if PN was inferior to RN in oncologic outcomes.

There is a significant selection bias in early retrospective studies comparing the oncologic efficacy of PN versus RN as many of the PNs were performed in "essential" cases. A group from the Mayo Clinic reported a case-control study comparing PN with RN in elective cases with unilateral RCC with a normal contralateral kidney. Each group contained 164 patients and was matched for tumor size, pathological stage (97% T1), grade, age, sex, and year of surgery. The 10-year cancer-specific survival (96% RN vs. 98% PN) or metastasis-free survival (95% RN vs. 98% PN) was similar between the two groups, and no difference was noted in 10-year overall survival (74% RN vs. 73% PN) [32].

The EORTC Intergroup (EORTC 30904) conducted a non-inferiority Phase III trial comparing PN and RN for <5 cm solitary tumors suspicious for RCC in patients with normal contralateral kidneys. The study has been noted to have several shortcomings. Foremost, the analysis was underpowered due to poor accrual (541 patients enrolled with 1300 patients required), and there was a > 10% crossover rate following randomization. There was also a small number of total deaths (117) and cancer-related deaths (12), limiting meaningful comparative statistics relating to survival. In the intent-to-treat analysis, RN unexpectedly had superior overall survival compared with the PN (81.1% vs. 75.7%, $p = 0.03$). In the secondary analysis of RCC patients only, and clinically and pathologically eligible patients, the trend in overall survival was not statistically significant. The estimated risk of RCC-related death and 10-year progression rates (3.3% after RN and 4.1% after PN, $p = 0.48$) were similar between the two groups. Since only 3% of the PN patients died from RCC, this study may be interpreted as supporting the oncologic efficacy of NSS for T1 disease [33].

The remainder of this section will detail pertinent literature relating to the oncologic efficacy of PN compared with RN based on primary tumor stage (Table 13.1). Table 13.2 summarizes many of the studies reporting oncologic outcomes in T1 RCC.

Table 13.1 TNM staging of renal cancer

T1: Tumor <7 cm in greatest dimension, confined to kidney
T1a: Tumor <4 cm, confined to kidney
T1b: Tumor between 4 and 7 cm, confined to kidney
T2: Tumor >7 cm in greatest diameter, confined to kidney
T2a: Tumor >7 cm but ≤10 cm, confined to kidney
T2b: Tumor >10 cm, confined to kidney
T3: Tumor extends into major veins or perinephric tissues but not into ipsilateral adrenal gland or beyond Gerota fascia
T3a: Tumor grossly extends into the renal vein or its segmental branches, or tumor invades perirenal and/or renal sinus fat
T3b: Tumor grossly extends into the vena cava below the diaphragm
T3c: Tumor grossly extends into the vena cava above the diaphragm or invades the wall of the vena cava
T4: Tumor invades beyond Gerota fascia (including contiguous extension into the ipsilateral adrenal gland)
N: Regional lymph nodes
NX: Regional lymph nodes cannot be assessed
N0: No lymph node metastasis
N1: Metastasis in regional lymph nodes
M: Distant metastases
MX: Metastases cannot be assessed
MO: No distant metastases
M1: Distant metastases

Adapted from Edge et al. [120]

Table 13.2 Oncologic outcomes of open PN for T1 TCC (NR—not reported)

	Study	# of patients	Follow-up (months)	Local recurrence	Five-year disease-specific survival (%)
T1a	Crepel et al.	1622	24	NR	98.2
	Patard et al.	314	51	0.8%	97.8
	Antonelli et al.	176	59	0.6%	96.1
	Lee et al.	79	40	0	95.0
T1b	Crepel et al.	275	40	NR	93.8
	Patard et al.	65	51	3.6%	97.8
	Weight et al.	212	49	NR	93.0
	Antonelli et al.	52	54	1.9%	99.0
	Joniau et al.	67	40	4%	95.8
	Pahernik et al.	102	56	1.7%	

Adapted from Refs. [34–41]

T1a Tumors

A competing-risk population-based SEER analysis comparing oncologic outcomes after PN (n = 1622) versus RN (n = 5658) for T1aN0M0 was recently published. There was no difference in the 5-year cancer-specific mortality rate after adjusting for other causes of mortality (1.8% for PN vs. 2.5% for RN, p = 0.5) [34]. An international multi-institutional retrospective analysis of T1a also showed no difference in the rate of cancer-specific deaths (2.2% vs. 2.6%, p = 0.8) or local recurrence (0.8% vs. 0.6%, p = 0.6) after PN (n = 314) compared with RN (n = 499) [35]. Single-institution studies have published comparable 5-year disease-specific survival (95–96.1%) and local recurrence rates (0–0.9%) [36, 37].

T1b Tumors

A recent SEER population-based analysis of T1bN0M0 RCC compared matched PN (n = 275) and RN (n = 1100) groups. In regression models controlling for age, tumor size, and year of surgery, there was no difference in 5-year cancer-specific survival between PN and RN (91.4% vs. 95.3%, p = 0.2). Competing risk regression analysis also failed to demonstrate a difference in cancer-specific mortality [34]. A bi-institutional Mayo Clinic and Memorial Sloan Kettering study compared outcomes between RN (n = 286) and PN (n = 873) for T1b tumors. Type of surgery was not a significant factor in multivariate modeling of death from RCC (Hazard Ratio [HR] for RN vs. PN: 1.97, p = 0.079) [42]. A retrospective study from seven international centers had similar findings. In this study, the RN (n = 576) and PN (n = 65) groups had similar rates of cancer-specific death (9% vs. 6.2%, p = 0.6, respectively) and local recurrence (2.3% vs. 3.6%, p = 0.5, respectively). Type of surgery had no influence on survival in multivariable analysis (p = 0.8) [35]. Single-institution retrospective studies have published comparable local recurrence rates of 1.7%–4.0% and 5-year cancer-specific survival rates of 93.0–99.0% [36, 39–41].

>T1 Tumors

PN plays a vital role in treating select patients with >T1 RCC, such as those who would be rendered dialysis dependent after RN. The European Association of Urology recommends NSS for T2 RCC in selected patients [2]. In general, the available literature relies on pathologically diagnosed T2-3b and may not be unequivocally applicable to patients with clinically evident T2-3b disease prior to PN. The data from several studies reporting the oncologic outcomes of PN for T2-T3b RCC are reported in Table 13.3. A study from MD Anderson Cancer Center compared the oncologic efficacy of RN (n = 567) with PN

Table 13.3 Oncologic outcomes of open PN for >T1 RCC

Study	Number of patients per pathological stage	% elective	Follow-up (months)	Local recurrence	Disease-specific survival
Margulis et al.	T2–8	27%	62	0%	78%
	T3a–22				
	T3b–4				
Breau et al.	T2–32	42%	38	6%	83%
	T3a–28				
	T3b–9				
Karellas et al.	T2–34	86%	17	NR	89%
	T3a–0				
	T3b–0				

Adapted from Refs. [43–45]

(n = 34) for locally advanced RCC. The RN group had larger tumors with more advanced pathological stage. To control for the more advanced features in the RN group, multivariable Cox modeling was performed. In this analysis which included stage, grade, size, histology, and procedure type, PN versus RN was not an independent indicator of disease recurrence or RCC-specific mortality [43]. Breau et al. published a study comparing outcomes between RN ($n = 207$) and PN ($n = 69$) in populations matched for stage, tumor size, baseline renal function, age, and gender. There was no difference in the risk of cancer-specific survival (HR 0.80, $p = 0.5$) or overall survival (HR 1.11, $p = 0.6$) between the two groups [44].

The preceding data support a role for PN in select cases of advanced RCC. Unlike T1 RCC, however, the oncologic efficacy of PN remains uncertain due to the inherent selection biases in the aforementioned studies. **In general, PN should be utilized in locally advanced RCC only in cases that are favorable for NSS and/or in patients where RN would result in hemodialysis dependence.**

Preserving Renal Function: The Rationale Behind PN

The risks and benefits of treatment options for localized RCC extend beyond simply perioperative morbidity and cancer-specific outcomes. Understanding the influence of RN versus PN on postoperative CKD is central to this discussion, as advanced stages of CKD have been associated with increased mortality and morbidity [46]. Table 13.4 defines the stages of CKD per the National Kidney Foundation Disease Outcomes Quality Initiative CKD classification. The renal transplantation literature has been frequently cited as evidence to support the use of RN in patients with normal contralateral renal function, as kidney donors have similar risks of hypertension, renal dysfunction, and death compared with matched populations [47–49]. The donor nephrectomy and RCC populations are considerably different, however, as kidney donors tend to be young and lack medical comorbidities. On the contrary, 26% of patients with a renal mass and a normal contralateral kidney have preoperative Stage III–V CKD [12], while over 50% of patients with a renal mass in a solitary kidney have preexisting Stage III–V CKD [50, 51]. Pathological studies of nonneoplastic parenchymal tissue in nephrectomy specimens also show frequent evidence of underlying comorbidities. In a study of 110 specimens, only 38% had normal renal parenchyma, of which a majority exhibited pathologically evident vascular disease [52]. A greater decrement in renal function 6 months after surgery was demonstrated in patients with substantial pathological abnormalities compared to those with normal renal parenchyma [52]. The prevalence of preoperative CKD in RCC patients combined with the frequency of histologically evident renal parenchymal and vascular abnormalities in nonneoplastic tissue at

Table 13.4 National kidney foundation disease outcomes quality initiative CKD classification

Stage	Description	GFR (mL/min/1.73 m^2)
I	Kidney damage with normal or ↑ GFR	≥90
II	Kidney damage with mild ↓ GFR	60–89
III	Moderate ↓ GFR	30–59
IV	Severe ↓ GFR	15–29
V	Kidney failure	<15 (or dialysis)

Adapted from Ref. [53]

the time of nephrectomy indicates a potential for significant post-nephrectomy renal impairment.

In 2004, Go et al. published a landmark paper demonstrating a graded association between the degree of CKD and risk of cardiovascular events, hospitalization, and death [46]. This study included 1,120,295 adult patients in the Kaiser Permanente Renal Registry with a follow-up interval of 2.84 years. GFR was estimated using the Modification of Diet Renal Disease (MDRD) equation. Multivariable analysis, controlling for demographics and comorbidities, was performed to elucidate the relationship between CKD stage and adverse patient outcomes. A GFR >60 mL/min/1.73m^2 was used as the reference. As GFR decreased, the risk of death increased (HR 1.2, 1.8, 3.2, and 5.9 for GFR 45–59, 30–44, 15–29, and < 15 mL/min/1.73m^2, respectively). The adjusted HR for cardiovascular events and hospitalization also increased inversely with respect to GFR [46]. A study of 15,837 randomly selected patients from the Third National Health and Nutrition Examination Survey confirms the association between CKD and cardiovascular health. After adjustment in multivariable analysis, the presence of increasing numbers of cardiovascular risk factors was associated with a GFR <60 mL/min/1.73 m2 (odds ratios 1, 3.7, and 10.4 for 0, 1, and 2 risk factors, respectively, $p \leq 0.001$) [54].

In the early 2000s, investigators from both Memorial Sloan Kettering and Mayo Clinic reported a higher rate of renal failure (defined as serum creatinine >2.0 mg/dl) after RN compared to PN [32, 55]. Huang et al. published a retrospective cohort study from Memorial Sloan Kettering using the MDRD equation to estimate GFR in 662 patients with a single ≤4 cm renal tumor and normal contralateral renal function. They found that RN was associated with a lower 3-year postoperative probability of freedom from both GFR <60 mL/min/1.73m^2 (35% vs. 80%, $p < 0.0001$) and GFR <45 mL/min/1.73m^2 (64% vs. 95%, $p < 0.0001$) than PN. RN was an independent risk factor for the development of both GFR <60 mL/min/1.73m^2 (HR 3.82, $p < 0.0001$) and GFR <45 mL/min/1.73m^2 (HR 11.8, $p < 0.0001$) [12].

Several investigators have addressed whether enhanced renal preservation via NSS translates into improved overall survival and decreased risk of cardiovascular events compared to RN. Huang et al. performed an analysis of SEER-Medicare consisting of 2547 RN patients and 556 PN patients with T1a RCC. On multivariable analysis, RN was independently associated with an increased risk of cardiovascular events (HR 1.4, $p < 0.05$) and overall mortality (HR 1.38, $p < 0.001$). There was no association between RN and cardiovascular death or time to the first cardiovascular event [13]. In a study from the Mayo Clinic of ≤4 cm renal tumors, no difference was observed in overall survival when analyzing the entire cohort. In patients <65 years, however, RN was associated with an increased risk of overall mortality (relative risk 2.16, $p = 0.02$) after adjusting for comorbidities, preoperative creatinine, and year of surgery [56]. The trend toward improved overall survival with PN compared with RN has been studied in T1b renal tumors as well. Weight et al. performed a retrospective study of 212 PN and 298 RN patients with preoperative GFR > 60 mL/min/1.73m^2 and a normal contralateral kidney. New onset CKD was defined as postoperative GFR < 60 mL/min/1.73m^2. RN increased the odds of new onset CKD (odds ratio 3.4, $p < 0.001$) when controlling for gender, age, comorbidities, and preoperative renal function. Cancer-specific survival was equivalent between the two groups when adjusted for stage and grade. Multivariable models indicated that PN (HR 0.47, $p = 0.03$) and graded stratification of postoperative renal function ($p = 0.003$) independently predicted overall survival when controlling for pathological stage, age, and comorbidities [39].

Although the preceding evidence suggests that relative renal preservation by PN is associated with improved overall survival, several questions remain. Foremost, EORTC 30904 failed to show a survival benefit with PN [33]. Future studies will be required to elucidate the relative contributions of "surgically induced" renal failure and the continued effects of medical renal disease in postoperative patients. When planning surgery in RCC patients, urologists must consider the effects of surgical approach (RN vs. PN) on both oncologic control and renal function, given the deleterious effects of CKD on postoperative morbidity and mortality.

Underutilization of PN

Despite equivalent oncologic outcomes and the potential benefits of minimizing postoperative CKD risk, PN remains underutilized. Data from the Nationwide Inpatient Sample compiled from 2003 to 2008 demonstrates that RN consisted of 79.3% of renal surgeries while PN comprised the remaining 20.7% [57]. There was a trend toward increasing PN use over the study interval ($p < 0.001$) [57], and also the overall percentage of PN increased from a previous Nationwide Inpatient Sample study from 1988 to 2002 [58]. The Nationwide Inpatient Sample does not include information on tumor size, location, or histology. Given the downward stage migration of RCC, however, one would assume that a greater portion of detected renal masses would be amenable to NSS than the 20.7% frequency of PN reported in this sample. A retrospective study analyzing the NCDB stratified PN rates by clinical stage (cT1a, cT1b, and T2a), all of which they found to increase over time. They reported that the rate of PN for cT1a RCC tumors increased from 46.4% in 2004 to 76.8%, and for cT1b RCC tumors increased from 13.7% to 37.1% in 2013 [59]. Despite these trends, PN remains underutilized in these stages, where it is considered standard of care in most cases [1, 2].

Although not the only criterion impacting PN feasibility, tumor size is an important determinant in tumor complexity and is available in the SEER database. Dulabon et al. reported the use of PN in 18,330 patients from the SEER registry with ≤4 cm renal tumors from 1999 to 2006. A total of 6460 (35%) patients underwent PN, and the ratio of PN to RN increased every year ($p < 0.001$) with PN comprising 45% of renal surgeries in 2006. Additional analysis demonstrated noteworthy disparities in PN utilization in women, elderly, rural patients, patients with an earlier year of surgery, and patients with a larger tumor size [60].

Compared with population-based studies, tertiary care centers perform a higher percentage of PNs for T1 renal tumors. In a study of six European centers from 2004 to 2007, PN comprised 86.3% of renal surgeries for <2 cm tumors, 69.3% of renal surgeries for 2.1–4 cm tumors, and 35.3% of renal surgeries for 4.1–7 cm tumors [61]. Investigators from Memorial Sloan Kettering reported a similar trend with an increasing usage of PN from 2000 to 2007. In 2007, the frequency of PN was 89% for tumors ≤4 cm and 60% for tumors 4.1–7 cm [62]. Future endeavors aimed at understanding the underlying rationale for PN underutilization, and addressing these issues is paramount for widespread acceptance of PN throughout the urologic community.

Adoption of Minimally Invasive Techniques

Minimally invasive surgery has been increasingly common overall because of similar long-term outcomes with shorter recovery times in many surgeries. This scenario is the case for renal surgery, where traditionally open procedures are increasingly being replaced with laparoscopic or robotic-assisted partial or radical nephrectomies when feasible.

One cross-sectional study of renal surgery from state records in Maryland analyzed the trends in surgical approaches in renal surgery. Consistent with other literature [57–59], this study reported an increase in PN utilization for small renal tumors [63]. Despite the increase in PN overall, the proportion of laparoscopic RN also increased, whereas rates of laparoscopic PN remained low [63], likely related to the steep learning curve and technical difficulty of the procedure [64]. By contrast, the wider use of robotic technology for PN drastically increased over a very short time, from just 2% of all PNs in 2008 to 44% of PNs [64].

Despite the enthusiasm for minimally invasive techniques due to advantages such as shorter hospital stay, lower blood loss, and efforts at reducing warm ischemia time [65], the adoption of minimally invasive techniques may not have been uniformly beneficial, with recent studies positing a correlation between minimally invasive techniques and increased rates of positive surgical margins [59, 66, 67]. A separate study found that positive surgical margins after partial nephrectomy were associated with increased risk of recurrence in masses with high-risk features [68]. However, recent studies now demonstrate that in small renal tumors treated by OPN or LPN, positive margins are nearly equivalent.

It is clear that there is a role for both open and minimally invasive partial nephrectomy. Many studies emphasize the critical role of proper patient selection for OPN and LPN, with special reference to: tumor size, tumor complexity, prevention of ischemic injury, and preservation of as much functional parenchyma as possible (Chap. 12). In addition, the surgeon's skill set also significantly determines whether OPN or LPN is selected. In general, smaller lesions are managed by LPN and more complex lesions by OPN.

Objective Analysis of Tumor Complexity

In the 2017 AUA Renal Mass and Localized Renal Cancer Guideline, it states that for clinical T1 renal masses, nephron-sparing approaches should be prioritized whenever intervention is indicated [1]. Partial nephrectomy feasibility was not defined. Differences in opinion between surgeons regarding the feasibility of partial nephrectomy may contribute to the variability in the use of partial nephrectomy described above. An important characteristic that determines whether or not partial nephrectomy is feasible is the technical complexity of the tumor [68]. Traditionally, tumors were described with nonstandardized, subjective terms such as central, hilar, deep, superficial, exophytic, or endophytic. This descriptive approach was not quantifiable for research or comparative studies, making it impossible to compare series, techniques, or surgeons with rigor. Inability to quantify tumor complexity may contribute to the lack of uniformity in the assessment of partial nephrectomy feasibility and, consequently, may lead to variability in care of the small renal mass.

Starting in 2009, three systems were introduced that aimed to quantify the anatomic characteristics of renal masses in a reproducible way with meaningful clinical correlation: the RENAL nephrometry score, the Centrality Index (C-Index), and the PADUA classification [69–71]. The RENAL nephrometry scoring system was described by Uzzo in 2009 ([69], Table 13.5). Points are assigned to four morphometric tumor variables: diameter, exophytic versus endophytic properties, proximity to collecting system or renal sinus, and the tumor's location relative to the polar lines and axial midline (Fig. 13.1). Points are added together with total scores of 4–6, 7–9, and 10–12 corresponding to low, moderate, and high tumor complexity, respectively. A qualitative descriptor "h" is added after the nephrometry score if the lesion abuts the main renal artery or vein. A second descriptive term is added to describe the tumor's anterior (a) or posterior (p) location (or "x" if the tumor cannot be described as anterior or posterior).

The Preoperative Aspects and Dimensions Used for an Anatomical (PADUA) classification schema share many similarities with the RENAL nephrometry score [71]. Points are also assigned to anatomical features, and an "a" or "p" classifier is also used to denote anterior or posterior location, respectively (Table 13.6).

Table 13.5 RENAL nephrometry scoring system

Variable	1 point	2 points	3 points
Diameter (cm)	≤4	>4 and <7	≥7
Exophytic	≥50%	<50%	100% endophytic
Nearness to collecting system or renal sinus (mm)	≥7	>4 and <7	≤4
Anterior/posterior	Qualitative descriptor of "a," "p," or "x"; no points		
Location relative to polar lines	Above upper or below lower polar line	Crosses polar line	More than 50% across polar line, entirely between polar lines, or crosses axial midline

Kutikov and Uzzo [69]

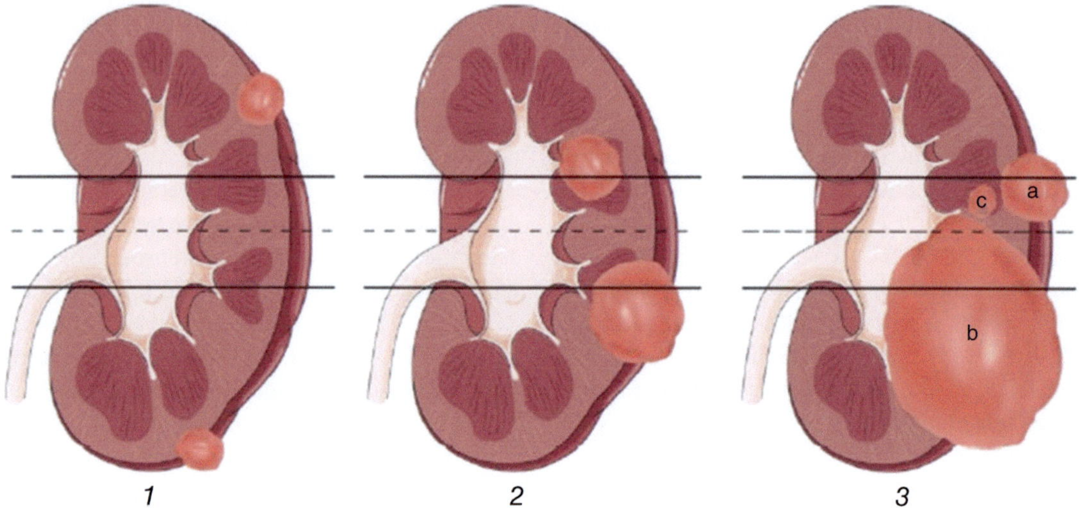

Fig. 13.1 L component of RENAL nephrometry score characterizes a tumor's location relative to the polar lines. A sagittal depiction of the kidney demonstrates the polar lines (solid) and renal axial midline (dashed), with the points (1, 2, or 3) that would be assigned to each tumor. The RENAL nephrometry score: a comprehensive standardized system for quantitating renal tumor size, location, and depth. (J Urol. 2009;182(3):844–53)

Table 13.6 PADUA classification scoring schema

Variable	1 point	2 points	3 points
Polar location	Polar	Interpolar	–
Exophytic	≥50%	<50%	100% endophytic
Renal rim	Lateral	Medial	–
Renal sinus	Uninvolved	Involved	–
Collecting system	Uninvolved	Displaced or invaded	–
Diameter (cm)	≤4	>4 and ≤ 7	>7

Adapted from Ref. [71]

The C-Index also aims to quantify the complexity of renal masses, but does so with a geometric approach [70]. The C-Index assesses the proximity of the tumor center to the kidney center and puts this value in context of the tumor size (Fig. 13.2). This schema makes use of the Pythagorean theorem in which the square of the hypotenuse (c) of a right-angle triangle is equal to sum of the squares of the other two sides (a and b) of the triangle (i.e., $a^2 + b^2 = c^2$). Using

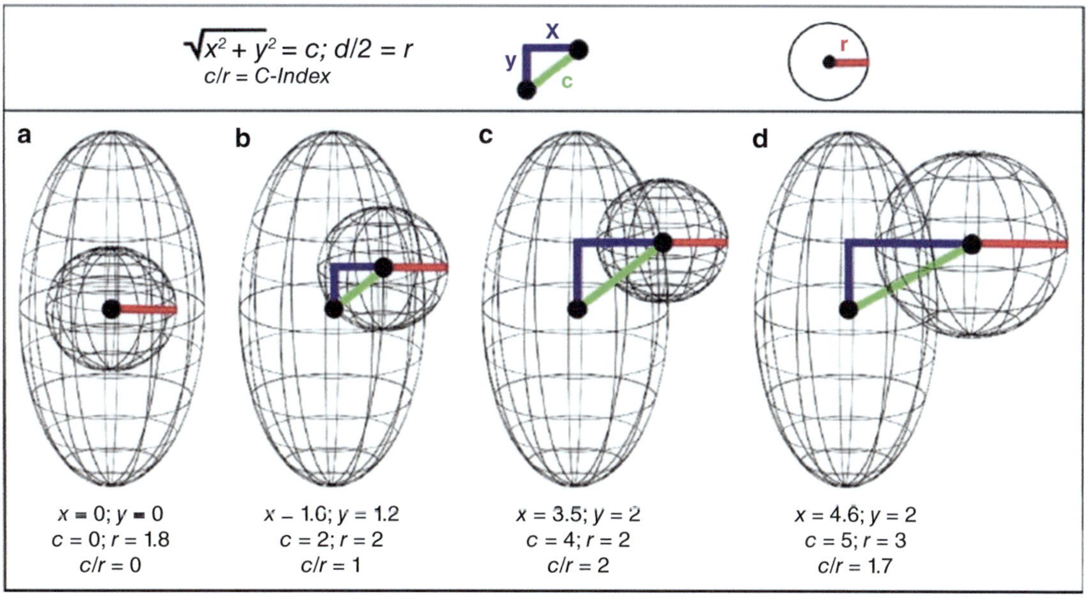

Fig. 13.2 C-Index method uses the Pythagorean theorem to measure the distance between the kidney center and tumor center, *c* (green line), which is the hypotenuse of a triangle formed by *x* and *y* (blue lines). Dividing *c* by *r* (red line) yields the C-Index kidney tumor location measurement using the C-Index method. (J Urol. 2010;183(5):1708–13)

axial imaging, the vertical distance from the kidney center to the level of the maximum tumor diameter is measured, as is the horizontal distance from the kidney center to the tumor center. The hypotenuse is then the distance from the kidney center to the tumor center (c). The tumor radius (*r*) is measured. The C-Index is calculated, where C-Index = *c*/*r*. A C-Index of 0 indicates that the tumor center is in the kidney center, while a C-Index of 1 indicates that the tumor periphery abuts the kidney center. The larger the C-Index, the farther the tumor center is from the kidney center.

There is retrospective evidence that these morphometric systems correlate with clinical markers of complexity, specifically a surgeon's choice of operation and approach, surgical technique including ischemia time and parenchymal preservation, as well as surgical outcomes and pathology. In a 2009 survey of members of the American Urologic Association, respondents were shown eight tumors with RENAL nephrometry scores ranging from 4 to 10 [68]. On multivariate analysis, each additional RENAL nephrometry score point increased the odds of a surgeon choosing to perform a radical nephrectomy instead of partial nephrectomy (OR 1.59, 95% CI 1.27–1.95). Respondents who were more likely to choose partial nephrectomy were high volume kidney surgeons (OR 1.57), high volume partial nephrectomy surgeons (OR 3.7), younger (OR 1.64), and in academic practice (1.80). The willingness of a surgeon to perform partial nephrectomy appears to be linked to tumor complexity, but the complexity threshold that triggers radical nephrectomy appears to vary among surgeons.

These findings are supported by retrospective data from clinical practice. In a single-institution retrospective review, Broughton et al. assessed 154 patients with clinical T1a renal tumors, of whom 120 (77.9%) had a planned partial nephrectomy [72]. Independent predictors of planned partial nephrectomy included tumor size, with each 1 cm decrease in diameter increasing the OR of partial nephrectomy 2.2-fold ($p = 0.011$). Tumor complexity was also an independent predictor, with each 1-point decrease in RENAL nephrometry score increasing the OR of partial nephrectomy 2.4-fold ($p < 0.001$). Similar retrospective studies have shown that increasing

RENAL nephrometry score is significantly associated with the use of radical instead of partial nephrectomy, and open instead of minimally invasive partial nephrectomy [73, 74].

The morphometric systems have also been found to correlate with technical aspects of partial nephrectomy including ischemia time and percentage of functional kidney volume preserved [75–78]. In a single-institution retrospective review, Simmons et al. calculated RENAL nephrometry score and C-Index for 237 partial nephrectomy patients and estimated the percentage of functional kidney volume that was preserved using postoperative imaging [78]. They noted that increasing tumor complexity was associated with parenchymal loss, with each 1 unit increase in RENAL nephrometry score correlating with a 5% decrease in functional volume preservation. Similarly, each 0.5-unit decrease in C-Index correlated with a 3% decrease in functional volume preservation.

Higher PADUA and RENAL nephrometry scores and lower C-Index have been associated with a higher risk of overall complications, including urine leak [71, 75, 76, 79, 80]. In addition, the morphometric systems may also be predictive of renal functional outcomes. For instance, the rate of ≥30% decrease in estimated GFR was significantly higher among patients with a C-Index ≤2.5 than those with C-Index >2.5 (70% vs. 32%, $p < 0.01$) [76].

It appears that quantitative scoring of tumor complexity by RENAL nephrometry score, PADUA classification, and C-Index may be a valuable addition to the clinical research armamentarium. The relative predictive abilities of the three systems remain unclear. Comparative research is needed, as are efforts to delineate the role of these systems in determining the feasibility of partial nephrectomy in moderate and highly complex lesions.

Preoperative Evaluation

A thorough preoperative evaluation is essential for patients undergoing open partial nephrectomy. The goals of the preoperative evaluation are clinical TNM staging, identifying and treating comorbid disease, selecting the proper patients for surgery, as well as reducing the risk of perioperative complications.

Cardiopulmonary Evaluation

Preoperative vigilance may identify patients at elevated risk of cardiopulmonary complications and allow for presurgical intervention. It has been recommended that cardiologists should evaluate and treat patients with unstable angina, decompensated heart failure, arrhythmias, substantial heart valve disease, and known or suspected coronary artery disease prior to noncardiac surgery [81]. A urologist should also inquire about cardiovascular symptoms and risk factors and refer for evaluation accordingly. Risk stratification tools such as the Revised Cardiac Risk Index may be helpful for preoperative risk stratification. The Revised Cardiac Risk Index is composed of six independent predictors of cardiac complications after major noncardiac surgery: high-risk surgical procedure (intraperitoneal, intrathoracic, suprainguinal vascular), ischemic heart disease, congestive heart failure, cerebrovascular disease, preoperative insulin use, and preoperative serum creatinine >2 mg/dL [82].

Predictors for pulmonary complications following non-cardiothoracic surgery include chronic obstructive pulmonary disease, age > 60 years, smoking, American Society of Anesthesiologists (ASA) Class ≥2, inability to perform activities of daily living, congestive heart failure, pulmonary hypertension, and low serum albumin [83, 84]. Patients without these risk factors may still be at risk for pulmonary complications due to surgical positioning and the surgical wound, since upper abdominal surgery and surgery that lasts >3 h are both independent predictors of pulmonary complications [84]. A pulmonary evaluation with chest x-ray, arterial blood gas, pulmonary function tests, and consultation by a pulmonologist may benefit some of these patients. Smokers should quit prior to surgery [83]. An anterior surgical approach may be preferable to a flank approach in patients with pulmonary risk factors.

Renal Evaluation

Assessment of renal function by urinalysis and serum creatinine is mandatory before partial nephrectomy, especially in light of the high rate of preexisting chronic kidney disease among patients with renal tumors [12]. Methods of estimating kidney function include serum creatinine, 24-h creatinine clearance, radionuclide imaging such as technetium-99 m diethylenetriaminepentaacetic acid, or estimating GFR using equations such as the Modification of Diet in Renal Disease (MDRD) equation [85]. Although serum creatinine and estimates of GFR based on serum creatinine such as the MDRD equation may not be as accurate as a 24 h urine collection or radionuclide imaging, they are commonly employed, relatively inexpensive, and typically adequate for clinical purposes.

Imaging

Adequate preoperative imaging is mandatory to identify locally advanced tumors or metastatic disease as well as to define regional anatomy and to characterize the renal vasculature. Renal angiography used to be commonly employed prior to partial nephrectomy, but it has been replaced by 3D CT angiography (CTA) at most centers. CTA is noninvasive and provides detailed anatomic images by incorporating arteriography, venography, excretory urography, and CT data into a single imaging modality. CTA can delineate renovascular anatomy including the subsegmental branches supplying the tumor, as well as renal tumor location, depth, and proximity to the collecting system [86]. In addition, preoperative imaging helps identify surgically relevant anatomic variants such as multiple renal arteries, retroaortic or circumaortic left renal vein, and duplex collecting system. Finally, Split Renal Function studies are of value in predicting new baseline eGFR (NBGFR) (Chap. 12).

Prophylaxis

Partial nephrectomy patients should have a preoperative urinalysis and culture to screen for bacteriuria. If a urinary tract infection or bacteriuria is discovered, antibiotics should be administered to sterilize the urine prior to surgery, especially in lesions in which collecting system entry is anticipated. The American Urologic Association recommends mechanical VTE prophylaxis (intermittent pneumatic compression devices or compression stockings) in all patients undergoing open surgery and consideration of pharmacologic VTE prophylaxis in patients with elevated risk for VTE [87, 88]. The use of pharmacologic VTE prophylaxis in partial nephrectomy is controversial [89].

Surgical Techniques

Broadly speaking, the steps of performing open partial nephrectomy are incision and surgical approach, isolation and control of the renal hilum, mobilization of the kidney while preserving the perinephric fat overlying the tumor, and tumor excision. This process is followed by renorrhaphy with hemostasis, collecting system repair if needed, and repair of the parenchymal defect.

Approach

Choosing a favorable surgical approach is the first step in a successful partial nephrectomy. The ideal approach provides excellent access to the kidney, renal vasculature, and tumor while minimizing wound-related morbidity. The position of the kidney relative to the ribs impacts the level of a flank incision and should be assessed on preoperative radiographic studies. Other factors to consider include the tumor location and size.

There are numerous surgical approaches to the kidney. For partial nephrectomy, the primary approaches are the supracostal flank, transcostal (classic) flank, and anterior subcostal incisions. Turner–Warwick described a rib-sparing extraperitoneal, extrapleural supracostal flank incision that is favored at some institutions [90]. For very large upper pole tumors, a thoracoabdominal approach can be useful. An 8-cm "mini-flank" supra 11th rib incision has been described as an effective alternative for radical or partial nephrectomy [91]. Other approaches to the kidney such as anterior midline, the dorsal lumbotomy, and subcostal flank incision are rarely, if ever, the most favorable approach for partial nephrectomy.

Vascular Control

After the surgical approach is complete and retraction is in place, controlling the renal pedicle is the initial priority with rare exceptions. The main renal artery and vein should be carefully dissected from surrounding structures. Vessel loops can be used to encircle the renal artery and vein without compromising blood flow. Establishing control of the renal vasculature gives the surgeon the ability to rapidly occlude the artery if necessary to stop unanticipated and uncontrolled bleeding.

Surgeons familiar with and experienced in the non-clamping technique rarely need to routinely encircle the renal vessels in OPN (JAL).

Kidney Mobilization

Having established vascular control, if necessary, one can proceed with mobilizing the remainder of the kidney. Gerota's fascia is opened. The ureter should be identified to reduce the risk of ureteral injury. It can be tagged with a vessel loop for identification. Great care should be taken to avoid injuring its blood supply. The kidney is mobilized within the perirenal fat, though the fat overlying the tumor should be left undisturbed in case there has been occult fat invasion. Mobilizing the kidney within the fat can be performed sharply or with cautery. It can be time-consuming and challenging in patients with prior kidney infections or other inflammatory processes that result in "sticky fat." Nevertheless, adequate mobilization of the kidney is an essential step in a high-quality, safe partial nephrectomy.

Vascular Clamping

During tumor excision and portions of renorrhaphy, the segmental artery supplying the tumor or the main renal artery is temporarily occluded with a vascular clamp. The purpose of clamping is to reduce intraoperative bleeding and improve visualization. Another proposed benefit is to ease access to intrarenal structures by reducing tissue turgor. Surgeons experienced in this technique may not need to clamp the segmental arteries, as they may be palpated or dissected intrarenally with a Frazier pediatric sucking device, exposed and ligated as each artery directly enters the tumor.

Traditionally, if the vasculature is clamped, mannitol is given intravenously 5–10 min before temporary renal arterial occlusion [92–94]. Recent research, including a randomized controlled trial, however, found that mannitol administration did not impact long-term renal function 6 months after partial nephrectomy [95, 96]. Anticoagulation to prevent intrarenal thrombosis is not necessary. The renal vein is not clamped, which may permit some oxygenation despite arterial occlusion [97–99]. In open partial nephrectomy, the kidney may be cooled immediately after clamping to protect against ischemic renal injury. The entire kidney is surrounded by ice slush for 10–15 min to obtain a core kidney temperature of approximately 20 °C, which permits as much as 3 h of ischemia time [94]. In cases where ischemia time is anticipated to be short, warm ischemia may be a reasonable option. Safe limits of warm ischemia have been proposed. Limits of 20 and 35 min have recently been advocated as safe [93, 100]. The clinical impact of ischemia time, if limited, remains unclear. The ischemia time itself may be a secondary variable with the quality and quantity of the preserved nephrons being the most important variable. Nonetheless, some data suggest that there is no safe limit of warm ischemia, with each additional minute increasing the risk of acute renal failure, chronic kidney disease, and end-stage renal disease [101]. Obviously in the nonischemic procedure, mannitol and ice slush are not necessary. This approach is favored by the senior author and used almost exclusively.

An open non-clamping technique has been described in detail [50, 102] to eliminate the potential impact of ischemia. The kidney is mobilized as described above. Similar to clamping partial nephrectomy, the hilar vessels are dissected out, and nonocclusive control is obtained with vessel loops in case vessel clamping is needed (Fig. 13.3). The perirenal fat overlying the tumor is left in situ (Fig. 13.4). Margins are marked out with the aid of intraoperative ultrasound. Again with increased surgical experience with this procedure, the pedicle dissection and vessel loops may not be necessary (JAL).

The renal capsule is opened either sharply with a tenotomy scissor or with a handheld needle pointed electrocautery. The renal parenchyma is opened with a tenotomy scissor circumferentially. Penfield dissectors are used to split the parenchyma, leaving a thin rim of grossly normal parenchyma on the tumor (Fig. 13.5). A Frazier pediatric suction device is used to keep the base of the nephrotomy free of blood. It also serves to locate cortical vessels which can be either coagulated if small or tied with 4-0 absorbable suture and divided (Fig. 13.6). At the base of the tumor, the specimen is gently lifted, and the remaining larger vessels can be clamped with a pediatric right-angle clamp, divided and ligated (Figs. 13.7 and 13.8, and Video 13.1). The specimen is inked to grossly evaluate resection margins. Frozen sections are routinely obtained. In the case of a positive margin, additional tissue can be resected and reanalyzed. Hemostasis and renorrhaphy proceed as described above. One advantage of non-clamping is that indigo carmine can be given intravenously to permit evaluation for openings in the collecting system. In cases of brisk hemorrhage, which is rare with experience, the surgeon can either clamp the renal vessels, apply manual compression adjacent to the cut renal paren-

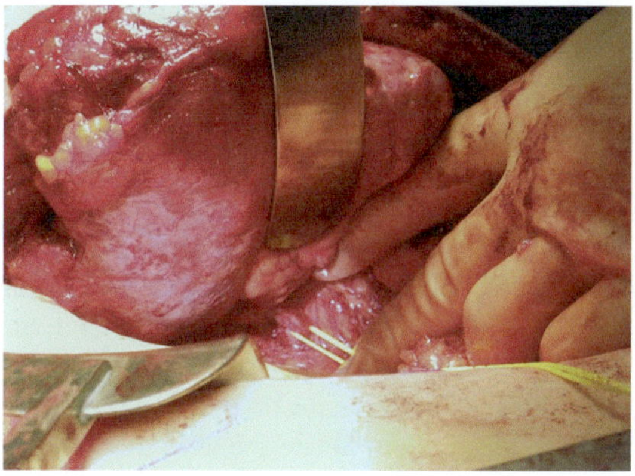

Fig. 13.3 Vascular control obtained if necessary to control bleeding

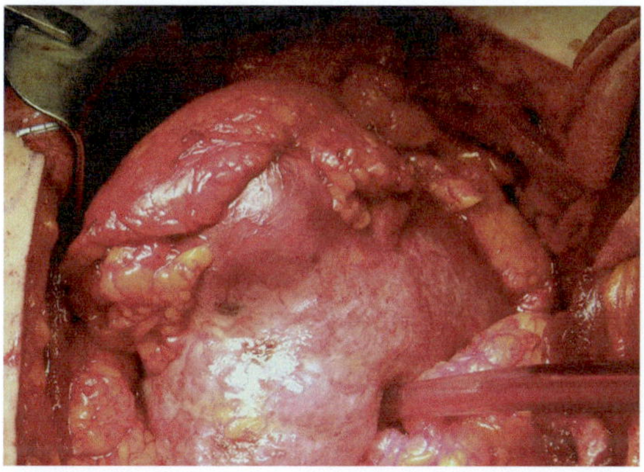

Fig. 13.4 Preservation of perinephric fat

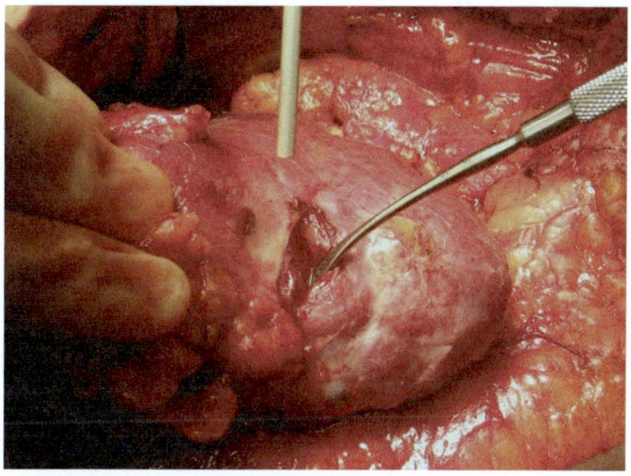

Fig. 13.5 Cleavage plane between tumor and normal parenchyma—note kidney totally perfused

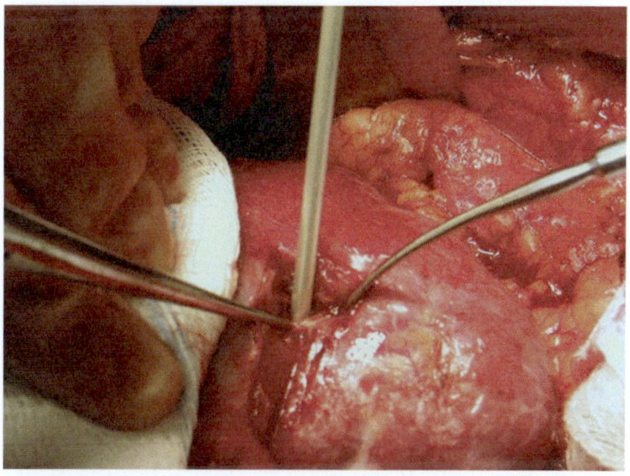

Fig. 13.6 Coagulation of small arteries at the corticomedullary junction—note kidney totally perfused

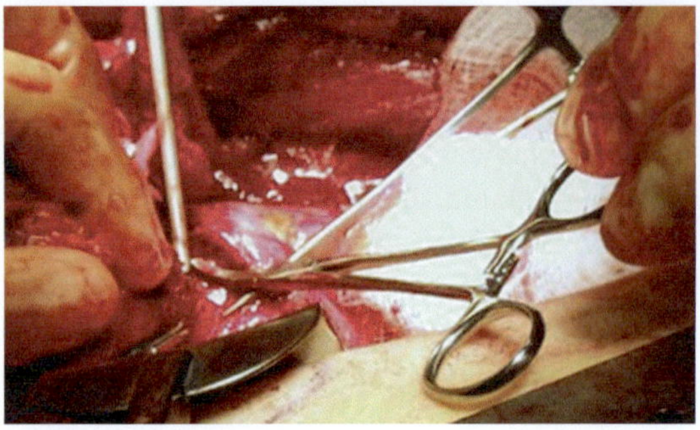

Fig. 13.7 Ligation of larger intrarenal arteries at the tumor base—kidney totally perfused

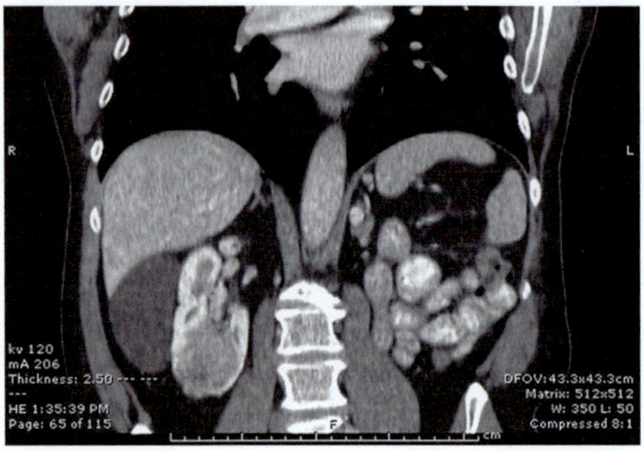

Fig. 13.8 Lower pole tumor—solitary kidney—Video of non-clamping, nonischemic, tissue-sparing partial nephrectomy is attached

chyma, or apply pressure with a Kittner dissector to control a bleeding vessel. The non-clamping technique allows excellent preservation of normal parenchyma, even with entirely endophytic tumors which can be approached through the hilum and sinus using Gil–Vernet's techniques and selective ligation of tertiary and quaternary arteries. Rarely does the senior surgeon (JAL) dissect the renal pedicle or put vessel loops around the segmental vessels, but exposes and ligates the intrarenal vessels directly as they enter the tumor itself.

With the passage of time and 30 years of experience with a very large series of non-clamping, nonischemic, tissue-sparing (enucleation) PNs, the senior author (JAL) rarely places vessel loops around the main renal pedicle or segmental arteries. Instead, the arcuate and interlobular vessels are identified within the renal parenchyma as they directly enter the tumor, as demonstrated in the illustrations above and the online video. When the collecting system is entered, stents are placed antegrade into the bladder. These modifications are routinely used and preferred by the senior author.

Excision of the Tumor

Once clamped and cooled, if utilized, the partial nephrectomy can proceed. There are various techniques of partial nephrectomy that can be employed, but all aim to fully excise the tumor with reliably negative margins and maximal preservation of functional parenchyma. There are a variety of partial nephrectomy techniques which include simple enucleation, polar nephrectomy, heminephrectomy and wedge resection, or resection of the tumor with a thin rim of normal parenchyma.

In enucleation, the tumor is separated from the surrounding normal parenchyma along a natural plane provided by the tumor pseudocapsule. No margin of normal parenchyma is taken. Most often, this technique is employed in patients with an inherited kidney cancer syndrome or multiple tumors [103]. Enucleation has traditionally been avoided in sporadic RCC due to concerns about local recurrence, as the tumor may extend for several millimeters through the pseudocapsule [104–107]. When enucleation is employed, it may be beneficial to ablate the resection margin to reduce the risk of recurrence [108]. Some surgeons believe that removing the tumor along with a margin of normal parenchyma is preferable to enucleation and provides lower rates of margin positivity. The senior surgeon (JAL) has evolved his PN technique over many years, and now prefers enucleation based on pathologic analysis of his margin positivity rate.

Polar nephrectomy can be employed for tumors that are limited to one pole of the kidney. Traditionally, this technique involved ligating and dividing the segmental apical or basilar artery supplying the upper or lower pole of the kidney, respectively. This selective vascular control results in a line on the kidney surface demarcating the ischemic pole from the rest of the kidney that remains perfused. The ischemic, tumor-bearing pole of the kidney is then excised along the line of ischemia. An alternative approach that we favor is to define the limits of resection by enucleation and not by the territory supplied by the segmental artery. This process permits preservation of the polar parenchyma that is uninvolved by the tumor. Large tumors that extensively involve the upper or lower portion of the kidney should be excised by heminephrectomy.

Centrally located tumors can prove particularly challenging given their intimate association with the renal hilum and collecting system. One option is to create an overlying radial or Y-shaped nephrotomy to expose the underlying tumor, which can then be excised by enucleation or with a thin rim of parenchyma. Alternatively, the tumor can be approached via the hilum using the intrarenal surgical techniques of Gil–Vernet. Small intrarenal venous branches can be ligated to improve exposure without compromising venous return. Segmental arteries supplying the tumor are divided. The tumor is excised, along with neighboring renal sinus fat if possible. Often, no normal adjacent tissue can be excised, and the tumor is essentially enucleated from the sinus.

Regardless of the surgical technique employed in partial nephrectomy, complete tumor excision should be confirmed in the operating room. Intraoperative ultrasound can be used to prospectively delineate resection margins and to identify additional occult tumors that are a potential source of ipsilateral recurrence [109, 110]. Frozen section is always employed to evaluate the margin status. The renal reconstruction is never begun until the margins are reported as pathologically negative. As long as the margin is negative, the size of the negative margin is not thought to be important [111].

Renorrhaphy

After excision of the tumor, the transected blood vessels on the renal surface are secured with figure-of-eight 4-0 Monocryl sutures. The argon laser can be used to achieve hemostasis on the renal cortex, but it should be used with caution as it may disrupt sutures or injure the collecting system. Openings in the collecting system should be carefully repaired with 4-0 Monocryl sutures. One can improve identification of collecting system defects by injecting methylene blue or indigo carmine either intravascularly or directly into the renal pelvis. Although it is rarely necessary, a ureteral stent can be placed in a retrograde fashion at the start of the procedure if significant repair of the intrarenal collecting system is anticipated. Alternatively, and more frequently, a stent can be placed antegrade over a wire through the opening in the collecting system.

Once suturing of vessels and the collecting system closure is complete, a bolster can be placed in the defect, though this is infrequently necessary if the cortical edges can be adequately opposed. The bolster can be composed of rolled Surgicel® or other absorbable hemostatic products. Floseal® (Baxter International Inc., Deerfield, IL, USA) or other hemostatic gels can also be used. The edges of the renal cortex are approximated, over the bolster, if one is used, with pledgeted interrupted 2-0 polyglactin sutures. These edges can be secured with knots or with a Weck clip (Pilling Weck Canada, L.P., Markham, ON, Canada) and a Lapra-Ty® clip (Ethicon Endo-Surgery, Cincinnati, OH, USA). Recently, we have used Evarrest Fibrin Sealant Patches (Ethicon) as an adjunct for hemostasis. The patches are composed of a combination of fibrinogen and thrombin in a cellulose matrix. The patches also eliminate the need for internal bolsters as the cellulose matrix provides excellent structural material which supports the renorrhaphy sutures used for parenchymal closure. If the renal artery is clamped, it can be preferably unclamped immediately after obtaining hemostasis or after the entire renorrhaphy is complete. A retroperitoneal drain should be placed, but can be omitted in small, superficial tumors in which the collecting system was not entered [112].

Addressing the Adverse Impact of Ischemia

Partial nephrectomy can be associated with a postoperative decline in renal function [97, 113, 114]. Numerous factors contribute to the decline in GFR after partial nephrectomy, including those that are not modifiable such as older age, female gender, larger tumor size, as well as solitary kidney and preexisting renal dysfunction [97, 113, 114]. Modifiable factors that contribute to decreased GFR include a reduction in functional renal parenchyma and ischemic injury [92, 101, 114–116]. Even when accounting for the percentage of functional renal parenchyma preserved after partial nephrectomy, renal ischemia is independently associated with postoperative renal dysfunction [116]. In a bi-institutional study of nephron-sparing surgery in solitary kidneys, warm and cold ischemia were associated with higher risk of acute ($p < 0.001$) and chronic ($p = 0.027$) renal failure, the need for temporary dialysis ($p = 0.028$), as well as urine leak ($p = 0.006$) when compared with partial nephrectomy without clamping [100].

To address the adverse impact of renal ischemia, several investigators have proposed performing partial nephrectomy with the kidney fully perfused and described above [50, 117–119]. In our experience, a partial nephrectomy series of 158 patients with solitary kidneys, when nadir GFR was compared during postoperative days 7–100, the non-clamping cohort was found to have a lower percentage decrease versus the clamping cohort (11.0% vs. 16.1%, $p = 0.08$) [50]. Additionally, when measured during postoperative days 101–365, there was a 27.7% decrease in GFR from preoperative GFR in the clamping group compared to 11.8% in the non-clamping group ($p = 0.01$). These data suggest a progressive renal insult after 100 days in the clamping group [50]. Despite this analysis, it remains unclear if zero ischemia has a clinically significant benefit over traditional short-duration warm ischemia.

A multivariate analysis of patients undergoing PN, which included tumor size, location, and focality as well as CKD risk factors, found that clamping was the only significant covariate. However, this study did not control for the percentage of functional parenchyma preserved [116]. Further analysis by the same authors suggests that ischemia is a secondary factor when accounting for the percentage of parenchyma that is preserved, which is a more important indicator [116]. There was no difference in median estimated blood loss, in their study, between the non-clamping and clamping groups (900 vs. 1000 mL, $p = 0.86$). The 5-year RCC-specific survival (excluding patients undergoing cytoreductive nephrectomy) was also similar between the non-clamping and clamping cohorts (79% vs. 75%, $p = 0.68$). Of note, while it is theorized that clamping may improve visualization, this process has not led to better surgical margins. In patients with two functioning renal units, margin-positive rates were similar between the clamping and non-clamping groups (6% vs. 4.7%) [117].

Future prospective studies are required to determine whether the volume of remaining renal parenchyma was adversely impacted by intraoperative renal ischemia (clamping vs. non-clamping) in the solitary kidney model. Axiomatically, preserving large volumes of renal tissue is important, but preserving renal parenchyma that has been injured by ischemia does little to enhance postoperative eGFR. This study would require clamping and unclamping cohorts in solitary kidneys (OPN and LPN) with accurate volumetric analysis, as ischemia and volume are the two most predictive parameters affecting postoperative renal function. The two-kidney model is woefully inadequate to determine the impact of ischemia and volume on postoperative renal function because of existing renal reserve in the normal contralateral kidney, which obscures the effects of ischemia and residual parenchymal volume on postoperative renal function.

References

1. Campbell S, Uzzo RG, Allaf ME, Bass EB, Cadeddu JA, Chang A, et al. Renal mass and localized renal cancer: AUA guideline. J Urol. 2017;198(3):520–9.
2. Ljungberg B, Bensalah K, Canfield S, Dabestani S, Hofmann F, Hora M, et al. EAU guidelines on renal cell carcinoma: 2014 update. Eur Urol. 2015;67(5):913–24.
3. Herr H. A history of partial nephrectomy for renal tumors. J Urol. 2005;173(3):705–8.
4. Herr HW. Surgical management of renal tumors: a historical perspective. Urol Clin North Am. 2008;35(4):543–9.

5. Bell E. A classification of renal tumors with observations on the frequency of the various types. J Urol. 1938;39:238.
6. Vermooten V. Indications for conservative surgery in certain renal tumors: a study based on the growth pattern of the cell carcinoma. J Urol. 1950;64(2):200–8.
7. Zinman L, Dowd JB. Partial nephrectomy in renal cell carcinoma. Surg Clin North Am. 1967;47(3):685–93.
8. Wickham JEA. Conservative renal surgery for adenocarcinoma. The place of bench surgery. Br J Urol. 1975;47(1):25–36.
9. Licht MR, Novick AC. Nephron sparing surgery for renal cell carcinoma. J Urol. 1993;149(1):1–7.
10. Herr HW. Partial nephrectomy for unilateral renal carcinoma and a normal contralateral kidney: 10-year follow-up. J Urol. 1999;161(1):33–5.
11. Fergany AFA, Hafez KSK, Novick ACA. Long-term results of nephron sparing surgery for localized renal cell carcinoma: 10-year followup. J Urol. 2000;163(2):442–5.
12. Huang WC, Levey AS, Serio AM, Snyder M, Vickers AJ, Raj GV, et al. Chronic kidney disease after nephrectomy in patients with renal cortical tumours: a retrospective cohort study. Lancet Oncol. 2006;7(9):735–40.
13. Huang WC, Elkin EB, Levey AS, Jang TL, Russo P. Partial nephrectomy versus radical nephrectomy in patients with small renal tumors—is there a difference in mortality and cardiovascular outcomes? J Urol. 2009;181(1):55–61. discussion 61–2
14. Ferlay J, Soerjomataram I, Dikshit R, Eser S, Mathers C, Rebelo M, et al. Cancer incidence and mortality worldwide: sources, methods and major patterns in GLOBOCAN. Int J Cancer. 2012;136(5):E359–86.
15. Siegel R, Miller K, Jemal A. Cancer statistics, 2018. CA Cancer J Clin. 2018;68(1):7–30.
16. Chow W-H, Dong LM, Devesa SS. Epidemiology and risk factors for kidney cancer. Nat Publ Group. 2010;7(5):13.
17. Storkel S, Eble JN, Adlakha K, Amin M, Blute ML, Bostwick DG, et al. Classification of renal cell carcinoma: Workgroup No. 1. Union Internationale Contre le Cancer (UICC) and the American Joint Committee on Cancer (AJCC). Cancer. 1997;80(5):987–9.
18. Chow W-H, Devesa SS. Contemporary epidemiology of renal cell cancer. Cancer J. 2008;14(5):288–301.
19. Curado MP, Edwards B, Shin HR, Storm H, Ferlay J, Heanue M, et al. Cancer incidence in five continents. Lyon: International Agency for Research on Cancer; 2007.
20. Hunt JD, van der Hel OL, McMillan GP, Boffetta P. Renal cell carcinoma in relation to cigarette smoking: meta-analysis of 24 studies. Int J Cancer. 2005;114(1):101–8.
21. Chow WH, Gridley G, Fraumeni JF, Järvholm B. Obesity, hypertension, and the risk of kidney cancer in men. N Engl J Med. 2000;343(18):1305–11.
22. Pischon T, Lahmann PH, Boeing H, Tjønneland A, Halkjaer J, Overvad K, et al. Body size and risk of renal cell carcinoma in the European Prospective Investigation into Cancer and Nutrition (EPIC). Int J Cancer. 2006;118(3):728–38.
23. Oh SW, Yoon YS, Shin S-A. Effects of excess weight on cancer incidences depending on cancer sites and histologic findings among men: Korea National Health Insurance Corporation Study. J Clin Oncol. 2005;23(21):4742–54.
24. Levi F, Ferlay J, Galeone C, Lucchini F, Negri E, Boyle P, et al. The changing pattern of kidney cancer incidence and mortality in Europe. BJU Int. 2008;101(8):949–58.
25. Kane CJ, Mallin K, Ritchey J, Cooperberg MR, Carroll PR. Renal cell cancer stage migration: analysis of the National Cancer Data Base. Cancer. 2008;113(1):78–83.
26. Cooperberg MR, Mallin K, Ritchey J, Villalta JD, Carroll PR, Kane CJ. Decreasing size at diagnosis of stage 1 renal cell carcinoma: analysis from the National Cancer Data Base, 1993 to 2004. J Urol. 2008;179(6):2131–5.
27. Frank I, Blute ML, Cheville JC, Lohse CM, Weaver AL, Zincke H. Solid renal tumors: an analysis of pathological features related to tumor size. J Urol. 2003;170(6 Pt 1):2217–20.
28. Remzi M, Ozsoy M, Klingler H-C, Susani M, Waldert M, Seitz C, et al. Are small renal tumors harmless? Analysis of histopathological features according to tumors 4 cm or less in diameter. J Urol. 2006;176(3):896–9.
29. Pahernik S, Ziegler S, Roos F, Melchior SW, Thüroff JW. Small renal tumors: correlation of clinical and pathological features with tumor size. J Urol. 2007;178(2):414–7. discussion 416–7
30. Nguyen MM, Gill IS. Effect of renal cancer size on the prevalence of metastasis at diagnosis and mortality. J Urol. 2009;181(3):8.
31. Thompson RH, Hill JR, Babayev Y, Cronin A, Kaag M, Kundu S, et al. Metastatic renal cell carcinoma risk according to tumor size. J Urol. 2009;182(1):41–5.
32. Lau WK, Blute ML, Weaver AL, Torres VE, Zincke H. Matched comparison of radical nephrectomy vs nephron-sparing surgery in patients with unilateral renal cell carcinoma and a normal contralateral kidney. Mayo Clin Proc. 2000;75(12):1236–42.
33. van Poppel H, Da Pozzo L, Albrecht W, Matveev V, Bono A, Borkowski A, et al. A prospective, randomised EORTC intergroup phase 3 study comparing the oncologic outcome of elective nephron-sparing surgery and radical nephrectomy for low-stage renal cell carcinoma. Eur Urol. 2011;59(4):543–52.
34. Crépel M, Jeldres C, Sun M, Lughezzani G, Isbarn H, Alasker A, et al. A population-based comparison of cancer-control rates between radical and partial nephrectomy for T1A renal cell carcinoma. Urology. 2010;76(4):883–8.

35. Patard J-J, Shvarts O, Lam JS, Pantuck AJ, Kim HL, Ficarra V, et al. Safety and efficacy of partial nephrectomy for all T1 tumors based on an international multicenter experience. J Urol. 2004;171(6 Pt 1):2181–5. quiz 2435
36. Antonelli A, Cozzoli A, Nicolai M, Zani D, Zanotelli T, Perucchini L, et al. Nephron-sparing surgery versus radical nephrectomy in the treatment of intracapsular renal cell carcinoma up to 7cm. Eur Urol. 2008;53(4):7.
37. Lee CT, Katz J, Shi W, Thaler HT, Reuter VE, Russo P. Surgical management of renal tumors 4 cm. or less in a contemporary cohort. J Urol. 2000;163(3):730–6.
38. Crépel M, Jeldres C, Perrotte P, Capitanio U, Isbarn H, Shariat SF, et al. Nephron-sparing surgery is equally effective to radical nephrectomy for T1BN0M0 renal cell carcinoma: a population-based assessment. Urology. 2010;75(2):271–5.
39. Weight CJ, Larson BT, Gao T, Campbell SC, Lane BR, Kaouk JH, et al. Elective partial nephrectomy in patients with clinical T1b renal tumors is associated with improved overall survival. Urology. 2010;76(3):631–7.
40. Joniau S, Vander Eeckt K, Srirangam SJ, Van Poppel H. Outcome of nephron-sparing surgery for T1b renal cell carcinoma. BJU Int. 2009;103(10):1344–8.
41. Pahernik S, Roos F, Röhrig B, Wiesner C, Thüroff JW. Elective nephron sparing surgery for renal cell carcinoma larger than 4 cm. J Urol. 2008;179(1):71–4. discussion 74
42. Thompson RH, Siddiqui S, Lohse CM, Leibovich BC, Russo P, Blute ML. Partial versus radical nephrectomy for 4 to 7 cm renal cortical tumors. J Urol. 2009;182(6):2601–6.
43. Margulis V, Tamboli P, Jacobsohn KM, Swanson DA, Wood CG. Oncological efficacy and safety of nephron-sparing surgery for selected patients with locally advanced renal cell carcinoma. BJU Int. 2007;100(6):1235–9.
44. Breau RH, Crispen PL, Jimenez RE, Lohse CM, Blute ML, Leibovich BC. Outcome of stage T2 or greater renal cell cancer treated with partial nephrectomy. J Urol. 2010;183(3):903–8.
45. Karellas ME, O'Brien MF, Jang TL, Bernstein M, Russo P. Partial nephrectomy for selected renal cortical tumours of ≥ 7 cm. BJU Int. 2010;106(10):1484–7.
46. Go AS, Chertow GM, Fan D, McCulloch CE, Hsu C-Y. Chronic kidney disease and the risks of death, cardiovascular events, and hospitalization. N Engl J Med. 2004;351(13):1296–305.
47. Ramcharan T, Matas AJ. Long-term (20–37 years) follow-up of living kidney donors. Am J Transplant. 2002;2(10):959–64.
48. Okamoto MM, Akioka KK, Nobori SS, Ushigome HH, Kozaki KK, Kaihara SS, et al. Short- and long-term donor outcomes after kidney donation: analysis of 601 cases over a 35-year period at Japanese single center. Transplantation. 2009;87(3):419–23.
49. Najarian JSJ, Chavers BMB, McHugh LEL, Matas AJA. 20 years or more of follow-up of living kidney donors. Lancet. 1992;340(8823):807–10.
50. Wszolek MF, Kenney PA, Lee Y, Libertino JA. Comparison of hilar clamping and non-hilar clamping partial nephrectomy for tumours involving a solitary kidney. BJU Int. 2011;107(12):1886–92.
51. La Rochelle J, Shuch B, Riggs S, Liang L-J, Saadat A, Kabbinavar F, et al. Functional and oncological outcomes of partial nephrectomy of solitary kidneys. J Urol. 2009;181(5):7.
52. Bijol V, Mendez GP, Hurwitz S, Rennke HG, Nosé V. Evaluation of the nonneoplastic pathology in tumor nephrectomy specimens: predicting the risk of progressive renal failure. Am J Surg Pathol. 2006;30(5):575–84.
53. Levey AS, Coresh J, Balk E, Kausz AT, Levin A, Steffes MW, et al. National Kidney Foundation practice guidelines for chronic kidney disease: evaluation, classification, and stratification. Ann Intern Med. 2003;139(2):137–47.
54. Foley RN, Wang C, Collins AJ. Cardiovascular risk factor profiles and kidney function stage in the US general population: the NHANES III study. Mayo Clin Proc. 2005;80(10):9.
55. McKiernan J, Simmons R, Katz J, Russo P. Natural history of chronic renal insufficiency after partial and radical nephrectomy. Urology. 2002;59(6):816–20.
56. Thompson RH, Boorjian SA, Lohse CM, Leibovich BC, Kwon ED, Cheville JC, et al. Radical nephrectomy for pT1a renal masses may be associated with decreased overall survival compared with partial nephrectomy. J Urol. 2008;179(2):468–71. discussion 472–3
57. Kim SP, Shah ND, Weight CJ, Thompson RH, Moriarty JP, Shippee ND, et al. Contemporary trends in nephrectomy for renal cell carcinoma in the United States: results from a population based cohort. J Urol. 2011;186(5):1779–85.
58. Hollenbeck BK, Taub DA, Miller DC, Dunn RL, Wei JT. National utilization trends of partial nephrectomy for renal cell carcinoma: a case of underutilization? Urology. 2006;67(2):254–9.
59. Fero K, Hamilton ZA, Bindayi A, Murphy JD, Derweesh IH. Utilization and quality outcomes of cT1a, cT1b and cT2a partial nephrectomy: analysis of the national cancer database. BJU Int. 2018;121:565–74.
60. Dulabon LM, Lowrance WT, Russo P, Huang WC. Trends in renal tumor surgery delivery within the United States. Cancer. 2010;116(10):2316–21.
61. Zini L, Patard JJ, Capitanio U, Mejean A, Villers A, de La Taille A, et al. The use of partial nephrectomy in European tertiary care centers. Eur J Surg Oncol. 2009;35(6):7.
62. Thompson RH, Kaag M, Vickers A, Kundu S, Bernstein M, Lowrance W, et al. Contemporary use of partial nephrectomy at a tertiary care center in the United States. J Urol. 2009;181(3):993–7.

63. Patel HD, Mullins JK, Pierorazio PM, Jayram G, Cohen JE, Matlaga BR, et al. Trends in renal surgery: robotic technology is associated with increased use of partial nephrectomy. J Urol. 2013;189(4):1229–35.
64. Link RE, Bhayani SB, Allaf ME, Varkarakis I, Inagaki T, Rogers C, et al. Exploring the learning curve, pathological outcomes and perioperative morbidity of laparoscopic partial nephrectomy performed for renal mass. J Urol. 2005;173(5):1690–4.
65. Gill IS, Kavoussi LR, Lane BR, Blute ML, Babineau D, Colombo JR, et al. Comparison of 1800 laparoscopic and open partial nephrectomies for single renal tumors. J Urol. 2007;178(1):41–6.
66. Tabayoyong W, Abouassaly R, Kiechle JE, Cherullo EE, Meropol NJ, Shah ND, et al. Variation in surgical margin status by surgical approach among patients undergoing partial nephrectomy for small renal masses. J Urol. 2015;194(6):1548–53.
67. Maurice MJ, Zhu H, Kim SP, Abouassaly R. Increased use of partial nephrectomy to treat high-risk disease. BJU Int. 2016;117(6B):E75–86.
68. Weight CJ, Crispen PL, Breau RH, Kim SP, Lohse CM, Boorjian SA, et al. Practice-setting and surgeon characteristics heavily influence the decision to perform partial nephrectomy among American Urologic Association surgeons. BJU Int. 2013;111(5):731–8. https://doi.org/10.1111/j.1464-410X.2012.11112.x/abstract.
69. Kutikov A, Uzzo RG. The R.E.N.A.L. nephrometry score: a comprehensive standardized system for quantitating renal tumor size, location and depth. J Urol. 2009;182(3):844–53.
70. Simmons MN, Ching CB, Samplaski MK, Park CH, Gill IS. Kidney tumor location measurement using the C index method. J Urol. 2010;183(5):1708–13.
71. Ficarra V, Novara G, Secco S, Macchi V, Porzionato A, De Caro R, et al. Preoperative aspects and dimensions used for an anatomical (PADUA) classification of renal tumours in patients who are candidates for nephron-sparing surgery. Eur Urol. 2009;56(5):786–93.
72. Broughton GJ, Clark PE, Barocas DA, Cookson MS, Smith JA, Herrell SD, et al. Tumour size, tumour complexity, and surgical approach are associated with nephrectomy type in small renal cortical tumours treated electively. BJU Int. 2012;109(11):1607–13. https://doi.org/10.1111/j.1464-410X.2011.10607.x/abstract.
73. Canter D, Kutikov A, Manley B, Egleston B, Simhan J, Smaldone M, et al. Utility of the R.E.N.A.L. nephrometry scoring system in objectifying treatment decision-making of the enhancing renal mass. Urology. 2011;78(5):1089–94. Available from: http://www.sciencedirect.com.ezproxyhost.library.tmc.edu/science/article/pii/S0090429511004353
74. Rosevear HM, Gellhaus PT, Lightfoot AJ, Kresowik TP, Joudi FN, Tracy CR. Utility of the RENAL nephrometry scoring system in the real world: predicting surgeon operative preference and complication risk. BJU Int. 2012;109(5):700–5. https://doi.org/10.1111/j.1464-410X.2011.10452.x/abstract.
75. Waldert M, Waalkes S, Klatte T, Kuczyk MA, Weibl P, Schüller G, et al. External validation of the preoperative anatomical classification for prediction of complications related to nephron-sparing surgery. World J Urol. 2010;28(4):531–5. Available from: http://www.springerlink.com.ezproxyhost.library.tmc.edu/content/712660p1144761q8/fulltext.pdf
76. Samplaski MK, Hernandez A, Gill IS, Simmons MN. C-index is associated with functional outcomes after laparoscopic partial nephrectomy. J Urol. 2010;184(6):2259–63.
77. Altunrende F, Laydner H, Hernandez AV, Autorino R, Khanna R, White MA, et al. Correlation of the RENAL nephrometry score with warm ischemia time after robotic partial nephrectomy. World J Urol. 2013;31(5):1165–9. Available from: http://www.springerlink.com.ezproxyhost.library.tmc.edu/content/7621231072217650/?MUD=MP
78. Simmons MN, Hillyer SP, Lee BH, Fergany AF, Kaouk J, Campbell SC. Nephrometry score is associated with volume loss and functional recovery after partial nephrectomy. J Urol. 2012;188(1):39–44.
79. Simhan J, Smaldone MC, Tsai KJ, Canter DJ, Li T, Kutikov A, et al. Objective measures of renal mass anatomic complexity predict rates of major complications following partial nephrectomy. Eur Urol. 2011;60(4):724–30.
80. Bruner B, Breau RH, Lohse CM, Leibovich BC, Blute ML. Renal nephrometry score is associated with urine leak after partial nephrectomy. BJU Int. 2011;108(1):67–72.
81. Fleisher LA, Beckman JA, Brown KA, Calkins H, Chaikof E, Fleischmann KE, et al. ACC/AHA 2007 guidelines on perioperative cardiovascular evaluation and care for noncardiac surgery: a report of the American College of Cardiology/American Heart Association Task Force on Practice Guidelines (Writing Committee to Revise the 2002 Guidelines on Perioperative Cardiovascular Evaluation for Noncardiac Surgery): developed in collaboration with the American Society of Echocardiography, American Society of Nuclear Cardiology, Heart Rhythm Society, Society of Cardiovascular Anesthesiologists, Society for Cardiovascular Angiography and Interventions, Society for Vascular Medicine and Biology, and Society for Vascular Surgery. Circulation. 2007;116(17):e418–99.
82. Lee TH, Marcantonio ER, Mangione CM, Thomas EJ, Polanczyk CA, Cook EF, et al. Derivation and prospective validation of a simple index for prediction of cardiac risk of major noncardiac surgery. Circulation. 1999;100(10):1043–9.
83. Bapoje SR, Whitaker JF, Schulz T, Chu ES, Albert RK. Preoperative evaluation of the patient with pulmonary disease. Chest. 2007;132(5):1637–45.
84. Qaseem A, Snow V, Fitterman N, Hornbake ER, Lawrence VA, Smetana GW, et al. Risk assessment for and strategies to reduce perioperative pulmonary

complications for patients undergoing noncardiothoracic surgery: a guideline from the American College of Physicians. Ann Intern Med. 2006;144(8):575–80.
85. Levey AS, Bosch JP, Lewis JB, Greene T, Rogers N, Roth D. A more accurate method to estimate glomerular filtration rate from serum creatinine: a new prediction equation. Modification of Diet in Renal Disease Study Group. Ann Intern Med. 1999;130(6):461–70.
86. Coll DM, Uzzo RG, Herts BR, Davros WJ, Wirth SL, Novick AC. 3-dimensional volume rendered computerized tomography for preoperative evaluation and intraoperative treatment of patients undergoing nephron sparing surgery. J Urol. 1999;161(4):1097–102.
87. Geerts WH, Bergqvist D, Pineo GF, Heit JA, Samama CM, Lassen MR, et al. Prevention of venous thromboembolism: American College of Chest Physicians Evidence-Based Clinical Practice Guidelines (8th Edition). Chest. 2008;133(6 Suppl):381S–453S.
88. Forrest JB, Clemens JQ, Finamore P, Leveillee R, Lippert M, Pisters L, et al. AUA Best Practice Statement for the prevention of deep vein thrombosis in patients undergoing urologic surgery. J Urol. 2009;181(3):1170–7.
89. Kenney PA, Wotkowicz C, Libertino JA. Contemporary open surgery of the kidney. In: Wein AJ, Kavoussi LR, Novick AC, Partin AW, Peters CA, editors. Campbell-Walsh urology. 10th ed. Philadelphia: Saunders; 2011. p. 1554–627.
90. Turner Warwick RT. The supracostal approach to the renal area. Br J Urol. 1965;37(6):671–2.
91. DiBlasio CJ, Snyder ME, Russo P. Mini-flank supra-11th rib incision for open partial or radical nephrectomy. BJU Int. 2006;97(1):149–56.
92. Simmons MN, Schreiber MJ, Gill IS. Surgical renal ischemia: a contemporary overview. J Urol. 2008;180(1):19–30.
93. Becker F, Van Poppel H, Hakenberg OW, Stief C, Gill I, Guazzoni G, et al. Assessing the impact of ischaemia time during partial nephrectomy. Eur Urol. 2009;56(4):625–34.
94. Novick AC. Renal hypothermia: in vivo and ex vivo. Urol Clin North Am. 1983;10(4):637–44.
95. Power NE, Maschino AC, Savage C, Silberstein JL, Thorner D, Tarin T, et al. Intraoperative mannitol use does not improve long-term renal function outcomes after minimally invasive partial nephrectomy. Urology. 2012;79(4):821–5.
96. Spaliviero M, Power NE, Murray KS, Sjoberg DD, Benfante NE, Bernstein ML, et al. Intravenous mannitol versus placebo during partial nephrectomy in patients with normal kidney function: a double-blind, clinically-integrated, randomized trial. Eur Urol. 2018;73(1):53–9.
97. Clark MA, Shikanov S, Raman JD, Smith B, Kaag M, Russo P, et al. Chronic kidney disease before and after partial nephrectomy. J Urol. 2011;185(1):43–8.
98. Gong EM, Zorn KC, Orvieto MA, Lucioni A, Msezane LP, Shalhav AL. Artery-only occlusion may provide superior renal preservation during laparoscopic partial nephrectomy. Urology. 2008;72(4):843–6.
99. Tracy CR, Terrell JD, Francis RP, Wehner EF, Smith J, Litorja M, et al. Characterization of renal ischemia using DLP hyperspectral imaging: a pilot study comparing artery-only occlusion versus artery and vein occlusion. J Endourol. 2010;24(3):321–5.
100. Thompson RH, Frank I, Lohse CM, Saad IR, Fergany A, Zincke H, et al. The impact of ischemia time during open nephron sparing surgery on solitary kidneys: a multi-institutional study. J Urol. 2007;177(2):471–6.
101. Thompson RH, Lane BR, Lohse CM, Leibovich BC, Fergany A, Frank I, et al. Every minute counts when the renal hilum is clamped during partial nephrectomy. Eur Urol. 2010;58(3):340–5.
102. Gill IS, Eisenberg MS, Aron M, Berger A, Ukimura O, Patil MB, et al. "Zero ischemia" partial nephrectomy: novel laparoscopic and robotic technique. Eur Urol. 2011;59(1):128–34.
103. Walther MM, Thompson N, Linehan W. Enucleation procedures in patients with multiple hereditary renal tumors. World J Urol. 1995;13(4):248–50.
104. Li QL, Guan HW, Zhang QP, Zhang LZ, Wang FP. Optimal margin in nephron-sparing surgery for renal cell carcinoma 4 cm or less. Eur Urol. 2003;44:448.
105. Blackley SK, Ladaga L, Woolfitt RA, Schellhammer PF. Ex situ study of the effectiveness of enucleation in patients with renal cell carcinoma. J Urol. 1988;140(1):6–10.
106. Marshall FF, Taxy JB, Fishman EK, Chang R. The feasibility of surgical enucleation for renal cell carcinoma. J Urol. 1986;135(2):231–4.
107. Rosenthal CL, Kraft R, Zingg EJ. Organ-preserving surgery in renal cell carcinoma: tumor enucleation versus partial kidney resection. Eur Urol. 1984;10(4):222–8.
108. Kutikov A, Vanarsdalen KN, Gershman B, Fossett LK, Guzzo TJ, Wein AJ, et al. Enucleation of renal cell carcinoma with ablation of the tumour base. BJU Int. 2008;102(6):688–91.
109. Assimos DG, Boyce H, Woodruff RD, Harrison LH, McCullough DL, Kroovand RL. Intraoperative renal ultrasonography: a useful adjunct to partial nephrectomy. J Urol. 1991;146(5):1218–20.
110. Campbell SC, Fichtner J, Novick AC, Steinbach F, Stöckle M, Klein EA, et al. Intraoperative evaluation of renal cell carcinoma: a prospective study of the role of ultrasonography and histopathological frozen sections. J Urol. 1996;155(4):1191–5.
111. Castilla EA, Liou LS, Abrahams NA, Fergany A, Rybicki LA, Myles J, et al. Prognostic importance of resection margin width after nephron-sparing surgery for renal cell carcinoma. Urology. 2002;60(6):993–7.
112. Godoy G, Katz DJ, Adamy A, Jamal JE, Bernstein M, Russo P. Routine drain placement after par-

tial nephrectomy is not always necessary. J Urol. 2011;186(2):411–6.

113. Lane BR, Babineau DC, Poggio ED, Weight CJ, Larson BT, Gill IS, et al. Factors predicting renal functional outcome after partial nephrectomy. J Urol. 2008;180(6):2363–8. discussion 2368–9
114. Lane BR, Russo P, Uzzo RG, Hernandez AV, Boorjian SA, Thompson RH, et al. Comparison of cold and warm ischemia during partial nephrectomy in 660 solitary kidneys reveals predominant role of nonmodifiable factors in determining ultimate renal function. J Urol. 2011;185(2):421–7.
115. Russo P. Partial nephrectomy for renal cancer (part II): the impact of renal ischaemia, patient preparation, surgical approaches, management of complications and utilization. BJU Int. 2010;105(11):1494–507.
116. Thompson RH, Lane BR, Lohse CM, Leibovich BC, Fergany A, Frank I, et al. Renal function after partial nephrectomy: effect of warm ischemia relative to quantity and quality of preserved kidney. Urology. 2012;79(2):356–60.
117. Smith GL, Kenney PA, Lee Y, Libertino JA. Non-clamped partial nephrectomy: techniques and surgical outcomes. BJU Int. 2011;107(7):1054–8.
118. Wszolek MF, Kenney PA, Libertino JA. Nonclamping partial nephrectomy: towards improved nephron sparing. Nat Rev Urol. 2011;8(9):523–7.
119. Rais-Bahrami S, George AK, Herati AS, Srinivasan AK, Richstone L, Kavoussi LR. Off-clamp versus complete hilar control laparoscopic partial nephrectomy: comparison by clinical stage. BJU Int. 2012;109(9):1376–81.
120. Edge SB, Byrd DR, Compton CC, Fritz AG, Greene FL, Trotti A, editors. AJCC cancer staging manual. 7th ed. Springer; 2009.

Minimally Invasive Partial Nephrectomy and Ablative Procedures for Small Renal Masses

14

Tony Luongo

Introduction

The surgical management of renal masses has evolved over the last century from removal of the entire kidney, to renal preservation surgery for necessity in the 1960s–1980s to performing partial nephrectomy (PN) for the majority of renal masses. The surgical management continued to evolve toward minimally invasive procedures, which include laparoscopic partial nephrectomy and thermal ablation of renal masses, especially for small renal masses (SRM) < 4 cm. This is relevant since the introduction and wide use of computed tomography (CT) and magnetic resonance imaging (MRI) in the twenty-first century has resulted in an increased incidence of these small renal masses (SRMs) [1]. As stated above, historically contrast-enhancing renal masses on cross-sectional imaging were treated with a radical nephrectomy. The treatment paradigm for renal masses has shifted toward nephron-sparing techniques, such as partial nephrectomy (PN) and ablative therapies, in response to the increased incidence of SRMs and has reduced the morbidity of a radical nephrectomy. PN provides comparable oncological outcomes for T1–T2 renal tumors while preserving the renal parenchyma and reducing the incidence of cardiovascular events [2–4]. The American Urological Association (AUA) currently recommends a PN for renal masses <4 cm [5]. Initial indications for minimally invasive partial nephrectomy (MIPN) were limited to SRMs, but improved technology, surgical skill set, and radiologic imaging has expanded indications to include more complex lesions [6]. Other nephron-sparing procedures are also available without compromising oncologic outcome [7, 8]. Improvements in technique and histological assessment have affected the surgical approach by way of a renal biopsy. In addition, technological advances in the form of augmented and virtual reality are beginning to enter the operating room and improve preoperative planning. In this chapter, we provide an update on the minimally invasive surgical techniques of laparoscopy and robotic-assisted laparoscopy, ablative techniques, as well as associated complications.

T. Luongo (✉)
Department of Urology, Tufts Medicine, Tufts University School of Medicine, Boston, MA, USA
e-mail: tluongo@tuftsmedicalcenter.org

Laparoscopic Partial Nephrectomy

Patient Selection (See Laparoscopic Partial Nephrectomy (LPN))

There are several factors (*see* Laparoscopic partial nephrectomy (LPN)) that should be taken into account when selecting a patient for minimally invasive partial nephrectomy (MIPN). These factors are similar when performed laparoscopic partial nephrectomy (LPN) as well as robot-assisted

J. A. Libertino, J. R. Gee (eds.), *Renal Cancer*, https://doi.org/10.1007/978-3-031-97599-8_14

laparoscopic partial nephrectomy (RALPN). Medical comorbidities such as cardiac and pulmonary disease can affect a patient's ability to tolerate pneumoperitoneum. Patients with severe chronic obstructive pulmonary disease are at risk for developing severe hypercarbia and acidosis [9]. The increased intraabdominal pressure induced by peritoneal insufflation is transmitted to the thoracic cavity, decreasing cardiac performance [10]. Obese patients present an additional challenge in that anatomic landmarks may be shifted, limited trocar movement, requiring longer instruments, and frequently requiring higher pneumoperitoneum [11]. There have been studies demonstrating a correlation between obesity and intraoperative blood loss. An overall difference in intraoperative time and transfusion rate has been demonstrated [12]. But, evidence suggests LPN can safely be performed in obese patients without increased morbidity [12–14]. Patient's surgical history is also important and should be carefully reviewed when determining the appropriate surgical approach and port placement. Some cases may require extensive lysis of adhesions, and may be at high risk for conversion to open procedure. A preoperative bowel preparation has historically been given to all patients to reduce the potential risk of infection, though this is increasingly being challenged with evidence showing no difference in infection risk or return of bowel function [15, 16]. The author does prescribe magnesium citrate bowel preparation preoperatively which improves intraoperative visualization.

Cross-sectional imaging should be carefully reviewed for identification of tumor location and proximity to the collecting system, number of vessels, and lymphadenopathy. The RENAL nephrometry score may be used to further classify renal lesion complexity and difficulty to resect [17].

Patient Positioning

Prior to positioning the patient, a time-in is performed confirming patient identity, team members, medication concern, and laterality of surgery. General endotracheal anesthesia is induced and then the patient is placed in the appropriate position. The positioning will depend on the access. For complex renal masses, particularly those that involve the collecting system, placement of an open-ended catheter into the ipsilateral ureter via cystoscopy can be done prior to positioning. Dilute methylene blue can then be injected in a retrograde fashion in order to identify entry into the collecting system and ensure adequate closure and prevention of urine leak. Bove et al., however, demonstrated no difference in urine leak with use of ureteral catheter versus no catheter [18].

In the transperitoneal approach, the patient is placed in a 45–60° modified flank position, as opposed to full flank position in the retroperitoneal approach with the ipsilateral side facing upward. The table is maximally flexed at the level of the iliac crest. Arms are then positioned on padded arm boards and secured in place in order to avoid brachial plexus injury. An axillary roll is typically used. The bottom lower extremity is bent 90° and the upper leg remains straight with pillows placed between the legs. All bony prominences are also carefully padded. The patient will be secured by a surgical bean bag positioner. Lower extremity sequential compression devices are utilized on all patients. The flank and shoulder are also supported, and the shoulders, hips, and lower extremities are secured with towels and tape in order to prevent movement with table rotation. The head is placed in a neutral position. Prior to prepping and draping the patient, laterality is again confirmed. The abdomen and flank are widely prepped and draped, allowing for potential conversion to open surgery.

Positioning of the patient is critical to the prevention of rhabdomyolysis and neuropathies, though despite careful attention to positioning, rhabdomyolysis has been reported [19, 20]. Following development of the pneumoperitoneum, trocars are placed. The trocar configuration, numbers and locations, depends on the approach and type of procedure. The following is a guide for trocar placement.

Access

Transperitoneal

As mentioned above, the patient is placed in a 45–60° modified flank position. A 12-mm incision is made at the ipsilateral border of the rectus muscle at a midpoint between the umbilicus and the anterior superior iliac spine. Intraperitoneal access can be obtained via Veress or Hassan (open) technique . Pneumoperitoneum is achieved to 15 mmHg [21]. Remaining trocars are placed under direct vision. Depending on the laterality of the tumor, a 12-mm subcostal port is placed on the contralateral side for the surgeon's hand. The camera port is also placed using a 12-mm trocar, medial and caudal to the subcostal trocar. A 12-mm trocar is placed for the assistant along the anterior axillary line. On the right side, if the surgeon decides to a liver retractor, a 5-mm subxiphoid trocar is inserted (Fig. 14.1).

Retroperitoneal

The patient is placed in full flank position (90°), a 12-mm incision is made in the posterior axillary line between the iliac crest and the tip of the 12th rib, and a working space is created using blunt dissection between the kidney and psoas muscle.

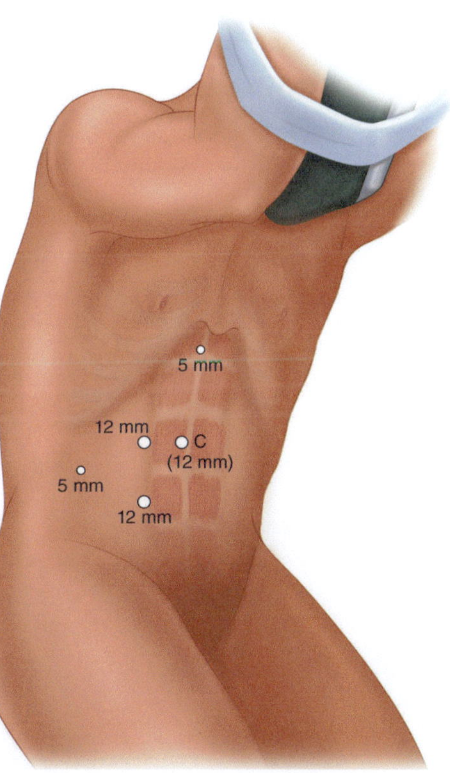

Fig. 14.1 Transperitoneal laparoscopic partial nephrectomy. (Original work submitted by the authors.) Key: C—camera port

This creates a tract from the skin through the muscle into the retroperitoneal space. A balloon dilator is introduced in this space and expanded to displace the peritoneum and retroperitoneal fat to create the working space; a blunt tip trocar is then inserted through the incision with cuff expanded and cinched up to the abdominal wall to prevent air leakage. The alternative is to use a visual obturator with 0° lens to enter the retroperitoneal space. Using blunt dissection with the laparoscope and insufflation, the working space is created. Once the working space is established, the rest of the trocars can be placed. A 5-mm port is placed at the tip of the 12th rib, a 12-mm port along the axillary line at the level of the umbilicus, and a 12-mm port in the midaxillary line just superior to the umbilicus [22] (Fig. 14.2). The retroperitoneal access is technically more challenging due to reduced working space, but best suited for posterior tumors and for patients with "hostile" abdomen due to prior abdominal surgeries to avoid the risk of bowel injury . Transperitoneal and retroperitoneal approaches have been shown to have similar outcomes, including blood loss, complications, and postoperative creatinine [23].

Hand-Assisted

Hand-assisted LPN allows for hand-facilitated dissection, suturing, and hemostasis, while maintaining the cosmesis of minimally invasive surgery. When the surgeon's dominant hand is contralateral to the tumor side, a midline periumbilical working port is made for the nondominant hand [24]. However, in ipsilateral cases, when the surgeon's dominant hand is the same side of the tumor, the hand incision is made in the ipsilateral lower quadrant for the dominant hand. In order to preserve pneumoperitoneum, the incision made is based upon the size of the surgeon's hand. There are multiple hand ports available which include the Omniport, LapDisc, and GelPort. The author prefers the use of the GelPort Laparoscopic System (Applied Medical, Rancho Santa Margarita, CA) to prevent loss of pneumoperitoneum. Two or three additional ports may be placed depending upon tumor location and surgeon preference. An example of trocar placement

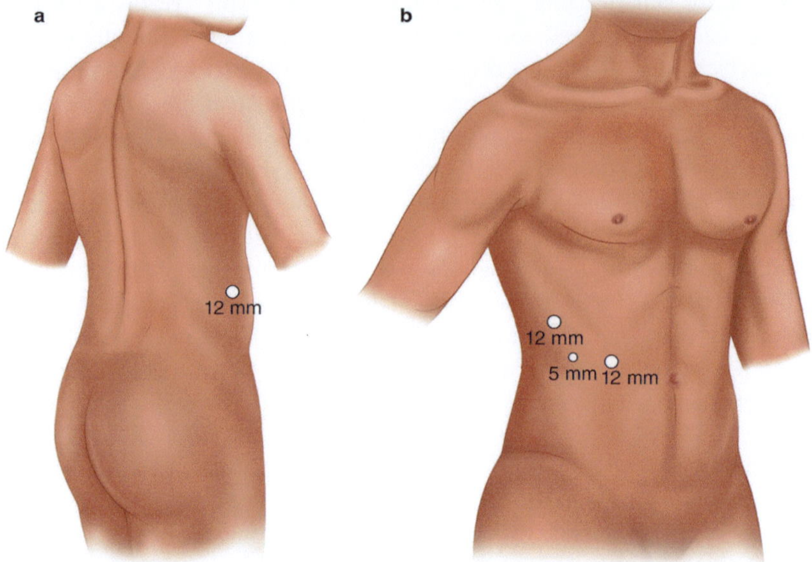

Fig. 14.2 (a, b) Retroperitoneal laparoscopic partial nephrectomy. (Original work submitted by the authors)

for a right-sided case is as follows: a 12-mm camera trocar is placed lateral to the rectus above the umbilicus. After using a 30-degree lens to ensure successful initial port placement, an additional 12-mm trocar is placed in the subxiphoid area, right midaxillary line, and right anterior axillary line above the level of the umbilicus. The hand port is placed in the right lower quadrant in a transverse fashion as described above (Fig. 14.3).

Procedure

The partial nephrectomy procedure involves six fundamental steps which include colon mobilization, ureter/gonadal vein identification, renal hilum dissection, exposure of renal mass, hilar clamping, resection of renal mass, and renorrhaphy (closure of the renal defect with or without closure of collecting system).

Once access is obtained, the first step in the transperitoneal approach is medial mobilization of the colon (ascending or descending). For right-sided tumors, the hepatic flexure is mobilized and the duodenum is Kocherized. The gonadal vessels and ureter are identified, and the ureter is retracted laterally while keeping the gonadal vein medial adjacent to the inferior vena cava. On the left, the

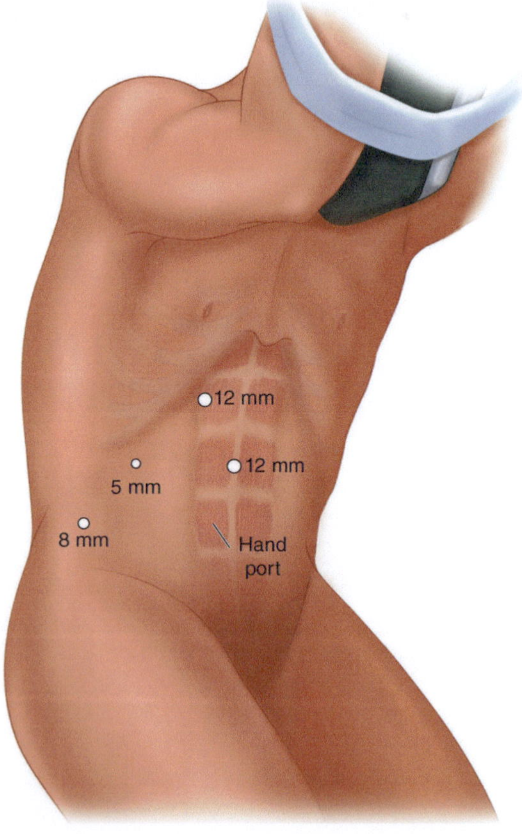

Fig. 14.3 Hand-assisted laparoscopic partial nephrectomy (right). (Original work submitted by the authors)

splenorenal, splenocolic, and splenophrenic ligaments are released, and the spleen and pancreas tail are mobilized medially. The gonadal vessels and ureter are identified and retracted laterally. Prudent dissection of the ureter is critical to preventing devascularization. The renal hilum is dissected with care taken to identify accessory vessels. There was a 96% correlation rate between 3-D magnetic resonance angiogram and intraoperative findings [25]. Once the hilar vessels are adequately exposed, Gerota's fascia is dissected and the tumor identified, preserving a portion over the tumor for T3 staging. This portion of Gerota's fascia may also serve as a handle during tumor excision. The 2017 American Urologic Association update on renal mass and localized renal cancer recommend adrenalectomy if preoperative imaging suggest metastasis or direct invasion into the adrenal gland [26]. Otherwise, the adrenal gland is separated from the upper pole. Patients with clinically regional lymphadenopathy should undergo lymph node dissection for staging purposes [26], as there is no survival benefit of lymph node dissection in patients with stage 1 renal cell carcinoma and no clinically concerning lymph nodes [27]. Despite the controversy, some still advocate for lymph node dissection for patients with large T1b tumors in order to detect and cure micrometastasis [28, 29].

Hilar Clamping

There are various devices utilized for hilar clamping: a Satinsky clamp for en bloc clamping, or bulldog clamps for selective clamping. Clamping technique varies by surgeon preference. Artery-only clamping has been described, with reported findings of similar blood loss [30]. Gong et al. [30] found that clamping the artery and vein resulted in increased postoperative creatinine compared to artery-only clamping in a case-controlled study, though there was no significant difference in the development of renal insufficiency in patients with normal preoperative renal function.

In attempts to minimize cellular oxidative damage during renal ischemia, renal hypothermia and administration of intravenous diuretics have been employed. There are various methods for inducing renal hypothermia, including perfusing renal arteries with cold crystalloid, infusion of retrograde transurethral saline, and intraperitoneal ice slush [31–33]. Mannitol and/or Lasix may be given prior to clamping, though recent studies suggest there may not be benefit to use of intraoperative diuretics. In a double-blind, randomized clinical trial, Spaliveiro et al. [34] found that in patients with normal renal function, there is difference in postoperative eGFR of patients who received mannitol.

Typically, the tumor excision and renorrhaphy are done while the hilum is clamped. A safe renal warm ischemia time is felt to be 30 min. But, there are studies suggesting that 90 min may be reasonably safe. Other studies suggest every minute of warm ischemia counts toward worse renal damage [35, 36]. Some surgeons have adopted various modifications of the surgical technique to reduce shorter ischemia times, including early unclamping, before the completion of the renorrhaphy [37]. The clamps are removed immediately after the initial central running suture is placed and prior to placement of mattress or bolster sutures [35]. In a series of 100 patients comparing early unclamping to the standard clamping technique, similar intraoperative blood loss was seen. Also, compared with the average clamping times for open partial nephrectomy at 20 min [38], the average clamp time in the early unclamping group was 6 min shorter.

Nonclamping, nonischemic partial nephrectomy was originally described by Libertino (Chap. 12). Performance of LPN without the use of a clamp, particularly in select tumors such as small, exophytic lesions, has been described. In a retrospective comparison of clamping and off-clamping techniques in 26 patients, Guillonneau et al. [39] described an off-clamping technique with the use of ultrasonic shears and bipolar electrocautery for hemostasis of the tumor bed. Similar complication rates were reported, and all patients had negative margins. Conversely, Rais-Bahrami et al. [40] found in their series of 126 patients that the off-clamp group had significantly more blood loss but had similar rates of transfusions compared to the clamped group. A meta-analysis of 10 studies that assessed off-clamp and on-clamp partial nephrectomies revealed that off-clamp compared to on clamp surgery had a higher blood transfusion rate, but lower overall postoperative complication and positive margin rate, and better preservation of renal function [41]. Also, at 6 months follow-up, the off-clamp group had significantly less changed postoperative creatinine [40].

Selective clamping involves the microdissection of tumor-specific arterial branches, thus eliminating global ischemia. This has the advantage compared to standard clamping of achieving a relatively bloodless field for tumor resection while not compromising blood flow to the whole kidney. This can be facilitated with the use of intraoperative use of ultrasound and fluorescence imaging [42, 43] Gill et al. [44] described this technique with the use of preoperative three-dimensional (3D) CT imaging and intraoperative color Doppler ultrasonography. Retrospective studies that have compared selective clamping to hilar clamping revealed selective clamping to be associated with improved postoperative renal function, similar perioperative complication rates and length of hospital stay, but longer operative times and transfusion rates [45,46].

Tumor Resection

Once the kidney is fully mobilized, the tumor is identified. An intraoperative ultrasound may be used to determine the size, depth, and location of a tumor, particularly endophytic or centrally located tumors. The tumor is circumferentially demarcated using electrocautery. This demarcation is incised with cold scissors, and using a grasper on the other arm providing countertraction the renal tumor is completely excised. The resection of the tumor can be performed in the standard partial nephrectomy approach with a rim of normal parenchymal tissue or no rim of normal parenchyma (i.e., enucleation). Comparisons between standard resection and enucleation have shown similar surgical margin rates and perioperative outcomes [47–49]. Also, the two techniques show comparable progression-free and cancer-specific survivals in the two groups after a 10-year follow-up [49]. Tumor enucleation should be considered in patients with chronic renal impairment, multifocal/bilateral tumors to maximize renal preservation. With respect to the significance of positive surgical margin status, there appears to be minimal metastatic or recurrence risk associated with positive surgical margin [50], though long-term data are lacking. Frozen section and random tissue sampling from the tumor bed remain controversial [51–53]; however, it may play a role in cases of suspected remaining tumor, as data suggest that gross inspection provides an accurate margin assessment [53].

Reconstruction of the Collecting System

Tumors abutting or invading the collecting system often require entry into the collecting system. Methylene blue may be injected in a retrograde fashion through an open-ended ureteral catheter. If the kidney is perfused, intravenous indigo carmine may also be used. The collecting system can be closed with 2-0 Vicryl or a 3-0 unidirectional barbed suture with a Lapra-Ty (Ethicon Endo-Surgery, Cincinnati, OH, USA) at the end. Methylene blue is again injected to confirm a watertight closure. Bylund et al. [54] described an alternative closure technique using a fibrin glue absorbable gelatin sponge sutured in place without formal collecting system reconstruction and reported a urine leak rate of 2/104 patients.

Hemostasis of the Tumor Bed

Hemostasis of the resected bed of the kidney is one of the most crucial steps of a partial nephrectomy procedure since delayed bleeding is the most common postoperative complication requiring a secondary intervention [38]. Suture renorrhaphy is the most reliable technique to achieve hemostasis of the partial nephrectomy bed. This involves a central running suture, typically a barbed suture, such as 3.0 Quill or V-lock, to oversew any bleeding vessels. Closure of the defect is then performed typically with Braided suture, 0 or 2-0 Vicryl sutures with a Weck Hem-o-lok clip (Teleflex Medical, Kenosha, WI) on one end, using four to six sutures placed in a mattress fashion. The other end of the sutures are then secured with a Weck Hem-o-lok clip and a Lapra-Ty. This eliminates the need for knot tying. Hemostatic agents or a bolster may also be utilized [55], with bolsters aiding particularly with cases in which apposition of the sides of the renal bed are not possible. But there are no studies that have demonstrated a clear benefit of any of these hemostatic agents.

Closure

Ensuing the confirmation of hemostasis, Gerota's fascia is re-approximated, and the specimen is removed. Resumption of pneumoperitoneum allows reconfirmation of hemostasis. A Blake or Jackson-Pratt drain is then delivered through the most lateral port site. Under direct visualization, all remaining trocars are removed, and local anesthesia is injected into the port sites. The fascia is then closed with 0 Vicryl. A Carter-Thomason device may then be used to close the remaining 12-mm trocar sites. Monocryl (Ethicon, Somerville, NJ, USA) is used to seal the skin and adhesives may be applied.

Robotic-Assisted Laparoscopic Partial Nephrectomy (RALPN)

Multi-Port Robotic-Assisted Laparoscopic Partial Nephrectomy (MP RALPN)

RALPN improves depth perception by use of 3D visualization of the surgical field, provides greater degree of motion via articulating instruments, enhancing precision and dexterity, elimination of tremor, and ergonomics. Aboumarzouk et al. [56] performed a systematic review comparing LPN and RALPN, finding similar outcomes including conversion rates, operative time, intraoperative blood loss, duration of hospital stay, positive margins, and complications. The robotic group demonstrated shorter warm ischemia time. Recent studies demonstrate similar findings [57, 58]. Robotic surgery on the kidney can be performed transperitoneal or retroperitoneal via multiple or single-site port(s).

Patient Positioning

The positioning of the patient is similar to the transperitoneal laparoscopic approach at a modified 45–60° flank position [58]. However, the patient's posterior is placed near to the edge closer to the robot rather than being centered on the table to improve the reach of the robotic arms. For retroperitoneal access, the patient is in full flank position with the umbilicus at the break of the table, and the table maximally flexed to maximize operative space [58]. Lower extremity positioning and securing the patient are similar to the laparoscopic approach described in the section above.

Access

In general, for robotic-assisted laparoscopic procedures, four robotic ports are utilized with one to two assistant ports arranged between the robotic trocar and the camera trocar . The trocar configuration depends on the robotic system platform utilized. There should be sufficient distance between the trocars, with at least 7.5 to 8 cm distance between trocars and camera in order to ensure adequate instrument working room. First, a 12-mm para-umbilical incision is made through which the 30°-down laparoscope is placed. For the da Vinci Xi robotic system, four 8-mm robotic ports are arranged and appropriately spaced along the paramedian line. Finally, a 5 mm laparoscopic port is placed in the midline cephalad to the camera port (robotic right arm for renal tumors on the right side). The robot is docked nearly perpendicular to the table. Figure 14.4 illustrates the port placements for transperitoneal robotic access for the da Vinci Xi.

Counter retraction may be provided by the fourth arm with a prograsper during bowel takedown and hilar dissection. The fourth arm may also assist in kidney and tumor dissection.

Retroperitoneal access with an incision made at the tip of the 12th rib through the external oblique fascia. After careful dissection through the internal oblique muscle fibers, an incision is made through the internal oblique fascia and a space is created. Porreca et al. describe blind creation of a space using a finger and a glove connected to a nasogastric tube for inflation thereafter [59]. While retroperitoneal access may be more technically challenging with the potential for disorientation due to unfamiliar landmarks and limited working space, it does offer the advantages of direct access to the renal hilum, the order of vessel identification changed with the renal artery being encountered before the renal vein [59–61]. The lack of bowel manipulation allows for earlier return of bowel function and reduced risk of ileus, which in turn minimizes the length of stay, as well as significantly reduces the risk of potential bowel injury [60].

Figure 14.5 demonstrates an example of retroperitoneal robotic access.

Procedure

The techniques described for transperitoneal and retroperitoneal laparoscopic partial nephrectomy can be used in a similar fashion for the da Vinci (Intuitive Surgical, Sunnyvale, CA, USA) robotic surgical system. Technically challenging steps, such as closure of the collecting system, may be performed more easily with the robot due to the use of articulating arms. The bedside assistant is responsible for suctioning, delivery of sutures, placement of clips, and possibly placement of the hilar clamp (Fig. 14.5).

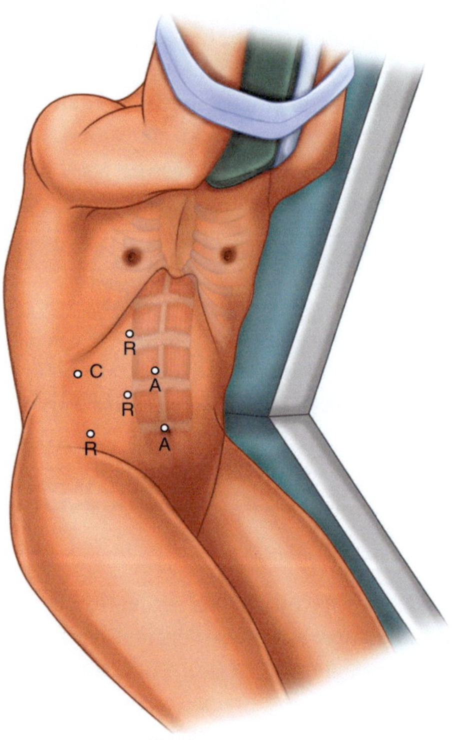

Fig. 14.4 Transperitoneal robotic-assisted laparoscopic partial nephrectomy for da Vinci Xi. (Original work submitted by the authors.) Key: L—liver, R—robot port, A—assistance port, C—camera port

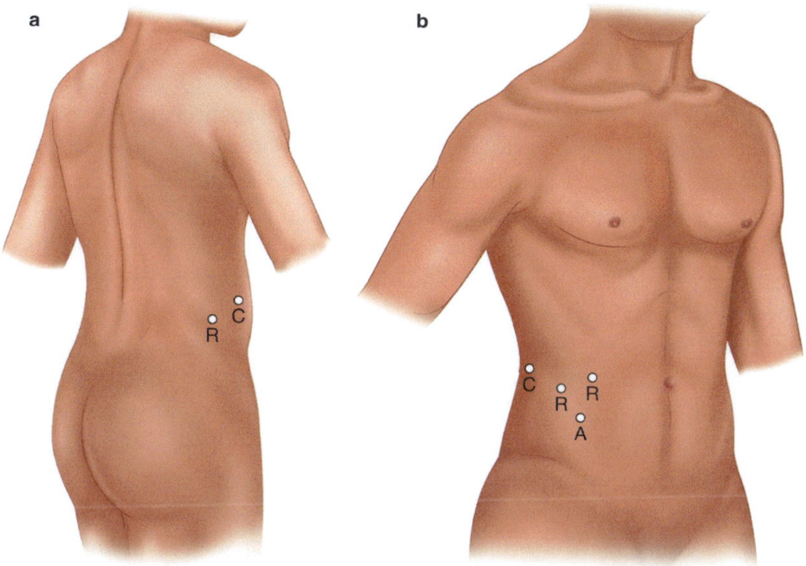

Fig. 14.5 (**a**, **b**) Retroperitoneal robotic-assisted laparoscopic partial nephrectomy. (Original work submitted by the authors.) Key: R—robot port, A—assistance port, C—camera port

Single-Port Robotic-Assisted Laparoscopic Partial Nephrectomy (SP RALPN)

SP RAPN is emerging as another effective minimally invasive approach for the treatment of SRM. Studies comparing SP RALPN to standard MP RALPN suggest similar peri- and postoperative outcomes compared to MP RALPN. It may also offer additional benefits such as lower opioid use and improved cosmetic results. This approach may facilitate the expansion of the role of retroperitoneal kidney surgery. This can translate into faster postoperative recovery, which could ultimately lead to the implementation of outpatient surgery. SP RAPN has been mainly used for low to intermediate complexity tumors, but increased experience will likely extend its indications to more complex renal tumors. Further research is needed to confirm its early promising results and better define the role of SP RAPN.

Complications of Minimally Invasive Partial Nephrectomy

Complication rates have been reported higher in partial nephrectomy compared to total nephrectomy. Surgical approach may also correlate with complications. Previously reported complication rates for LPN and RALPN ranged from 11% to 36% and from 8.5% to 35.3%, respectively. Cacciamani et al. [57] performed a meta-analysis reviewing 20,282 cases of open, LPN, and RALPN from 2000 to 2016, and found overall postoperative complication rates of 23.4% for LPN, and 19.2% for RALPN. Another meta-analysis of 2240 partial nephrectomies, although the risk of complications was similar between robotic and laparoscopic approaches, robotic partial nephrectomy was associated with a nearly 50% lower risk of conversion to open surgery [62]. There are several patient factors such as obesity and prior abdominal surgery that are associated with a higher complication risk [63]. Tumor-related factors such as size and location of tumor, and infection (pyelonephritis) correlate with higher complication rate [64, 65]; surgeon-related factors, particularly surgical experience. Studies have shown that many of the complications occur during the first 20 cases and a learning curve of at least 20 laparoscopic cases [66, 67]. It is important to emphasize that when complications occur, early recognition and intervention, if needed, can often minimize their morbid consequences.

Intraoperative Complications

Vascular Injury

Renal hilum injuries can result in significant morbidity and mortality if not managed in a timely fashion. Hemostatic agents such as Surgiflo (Ethicon, Somerville, NJ, USA) or Floseal (Baxter, Deerfield, IL, USA), or direct pressure with Surgicel (Ethicon, Somerville, NJ, USA) may be sufficient to treat small venous bleeding. Adequate hemostasis is confirmed by decreasing pneumoperitoneum. Larger venous injuries may be oversewn with nonabsorbable suture such as 4-0 Prolene (Ethicon, Somerville, NJ, USA); however, significant injury may require total nephrectomy. Fortunately, major vascular injuries during laparoscopic surgery are rare [68]. It can occur at any point of the procedure. The life-threatening vascular complications occur during the access stage of the procedure, which includes insertion of Veress needle or the first trocar, or during the dissection of the renal hilum. Direct injury to the aorta, IVC, renal artery, or vein as well as their branches can result and lead to significant bleeding. Vascular injuries to the renal hilum usually occur when structures, in particular vascular structures, are not completely identified during dissection [69]. These vascular injuries can be corrected with the use of cautery, surgical clips, or suturing depending on the location, size, and severity of the injury . It is important to have a full understanding of the **anatomic orientation, identification of vascular structures, and** complete **surgical dissection to prevent vascular complications.**

Injury to Intra-abdominal Organs

Bowel injury may occur in a traumatic fashion, such as during access, or thermal with the use of electrocautery. Minor thermal injury may be managed with simple imbrication, whereas major thermal injury may require bowel resection and re-anastomosis. In rare cases, diversion is indicated. Postoperative identification of bowel injury often requires surgical exploration. Clinical presentations of bowel injury include peritonitis, nausea, vomiting, signs, and symptoms of sepsis. Excessive bowel manipulation may also increase the risk of postoperative ileus. Early adhesion formation may also cause small bowel obstruction.

Prior surgical history requires special consideration given the resulting intra-abdominal adhesions and increased possibility of bowel injury during access and insufflation, trocar placement, and/or surgical dissection. Strategies to minimize bowel injuries is to gain access, and place Veress needle and initial trocar away from previous scars and surgical fields, consider open trocar placement, or retroperitoneal approach.

Pancreatic and splenic injuries typically occur during left-sided procedures [70]. Injury to the pancreatic tail is most common. Most commonly, pancreatic injury is identified during the postoperative period with increased, often milky-appearing drain output. Confirmation is by obtaining drain fluid and serum amylase and lipase. Management includes elemental diet or total parenteral nutrition, nasogastric tube placement, somatostatin to suppress pancreatic exocrine function, and percutaneous drainage. Minor splenic injuries are typically managed conservatively with hemostatic agents and/or tamponade. Rarely, splenectomy is performed in cases of significant splenic laceration.

Diaphragmatic injury is rare in laparoscopic renal surgery, occurring in 0.4% of cases [71]. Intraoperatively, clinical signs of pleural entry may include changes in respiratory requirements or simply billowing of the diaphragm. Repair can be performed intraoperatively using laparoscopy. If there is a clinical concern for diaphragmatic injury and no defect is visualized, an upright chest X-ray may be obtained postoperatively in the recovery area. However, routine postoperative chest X-rays are not required [72].

Postoperative Complications

Hemorrhage

Pseudoaneurysm (PA) and arteriovenous fistula (AVF) are rare, but potentially fatal causes of postoperative hemorrhage. However, delayed hemorrhage is the most common complication requiring secondary procedure after LPN [38]. In a systematic review by Jain et al., the mean presentation occurred 14.9 days after surgery, and 87.3% presented with gross hematuria [73]. Other symptoms patients may have include flank pain and potentially ecchymosis, particularly in cases with significant retroperitoneal hematoma formation. Patients' diagnosis may be made with CT angiogram; however, in some cases depending on severity, the patient may be taken directly by Interventional Radiology for angiography and angioembolization [74]. Selective angioembolization is the preferred method of treatment of PA and AVF; however, in some cases, complete renal embolization and even re-exploration and potentially completion nephrectomy are performed.

Urine Leak

Urine leakage is a potential complication of any renal surgery in which the pelvicalyceal system is violated. Postoperative urine leak following laparoscopic and robotic partial nephrectomy is not common. The reported rate range from 1% to 10% [75, 76]. Factors associated with urinary leak include large tumor size, hilar location, pelvicalyceal repair, prolonged operative, and warm ischemia time.

Larger or more endophytic tumors may require intentional entry into the collecting system. As a result, great care is taken to ensure that during repair, the collecting system is adequately closed. The use of methylene blue assists with closure, as mentioned above. However, despite prudent efforts, a urine leak may occur. Zorn et al. demonstrated that collecting system entry alone does not correlate with increased risk of leakage of urine [77]. A drain placed intraoperatively aids in the diagnosis of both hemorrhage and urine leak. Clinic symptoms include abdominal or flank pain, ileus, increased serous-appearing drain output, and rising serum creatinine. Urine leak may be confirmed by checking a drain fluid creatinine, which would reveal an elevated value when compared to serum. Most cases of urinary leak require no intervention other than percutaneous drainage. If conservative management fails, additional interventions may be needed with ureteral stent, drain, and foley catheter for bladder decompression. Occasionally, a percutaneous nephrostomy tube is required, and rarely a second surgery for closure is indicated. Antibiotics may be indicated if there is concern for infection with fevers or leukocytosis.

Postoperative Management

In the immediate postoperative period, patients are continued on intravenous fluids and started on a clear liquid diet. Postoperative day 1, patients are transitioned to a regular diet and intravenous fluids are stopped once the patient has had adequate oral intake. Pain control is managed with intermittent intravenous and oral analgesics, and antibiotics are continued for 24 h. Laboratory data are checked postoperatively and postoperative day 1. For deep vein thrombosis (DVT) prophylaxis, sequential compression devices are worn at all times, subcutaneous heparin is administered, and early ambulation is encouraged. Our institution utilizes the Caprini Score for determination of postoperative DVT risk. Patients with elevated risk of DVT are transitioned to enoxaparin, depending on renal function and risk of bleeding, which is determined by intraoperative blood loss.

A drain is placed for monitoring of bleeding or urine leak, and if drain output is elevated, the fluid is checked for creatinine. The Foley catheter is typically removed postoperative day 1 and the drain is removed prior to discharge from the hospital, on average postoperative day 2 at our institution. Given minimal intraoperative bowel manipulation, full return of bowel function is not required for diet advancement or discharge. In a 90-patient series presented by Shah and Abaza, a clinical pathway was proposed in which 94% patients were discharged on postoperative day 1, with a 5% readmission rate [78]. Minimal data exist regarding perioperative antiplatelet use. In a retrospective review of 430 consecutive cases, Leavitt et al. found no significant difference in major postoperative complications or intraoperative blood loss in patients for whom aspirin was continued when performing laparoscopic partial nephrectomy [79]. Generally, antiplatelet agents are safely resumed within 7–10 days.

Thermal Ablative Treatments for Small Renal Masses

Minimally invasive thermal ablative (TA) therapies for renal tumors have typically been performed percutaneously with real-time imaging guidance in an interventional radiology suite. Renal ablation offers several advantages such as the procedures are technically less challenging than a partial nephrectomy as there is no need for hilar clamping, collecting system reconstruction, renorrhaphy, or adjacent organ dissection. In addition, it has less blood loss, shorter length of procedure, and fewer complications [80]. Ablative therapy is typically limited to clinical cT1a (<3 cm) tumors and patients with increased surgical risks [5]. The American Urological Association recommends a tissue diagnosis prior to treatment as the ablative process destroys the tissue and prevents a definitive diagnosis [5]. Cryoablation (CA), radiofrequency ablation (RFA), and microwave therapy are the energy delivery systems that are currently being used.

Cryoablation causes cellular damage from both the freezing temperatures induced by ice ball formation from rapid expansion of high-pressure argon gas and subsequent reperfusion injury during thawing. The freezing temperature is delivered by cryoprobes. The number and spacing of the probes are determined by the probe-specific ablative shape and size, and size of the tumor. The probes are placed in parallel to each other in a manner that ensures an overlap freezing effect of each probe. The probes are advanced just beyond the edge of the tumor. The treatment effect (i.e., ice ball formation) is monitored with real-time imaging (ultrasound) and the ice ball should extend up to 1 cm beyond the tumor margin.

Radiofrequency Ablation (RFA) utilizes alternating current transmitted to cells via electrodes. The energy causes agitation, resulting in tissue heating to temperatures over 60–100 °C. At these high temperatures, irreversible cell damage and necrosis occur. The RFA probe is introduced into the tumor, and the tines are deployed to a diameter that ensures ablation of the tumor and up to 1-cm margin of normal renal tissue. There is no current imaging technique that adequately monitors the progress of RFA treatment effect intraoperatively, and most of the treatment is based on direct temperature measurement.

The choice of approach—open, laparoscopic, or percutaneous—depends on tumor location and its proximity to the bowel, adjacent organs, and the great vessels; body habitus; and prior abdominal surgery. Complication rates and oncologic outcomes between percutaneous and laparoscopic approaches appear to be equivalent [81–83]. In patients with recurrent disease, ablative therapy did not preclude radical nephrectomy [84, 85]. Thermal ablation can be used to treat most small renal masses, particularly in patients who are poor surgical candidates due to significant comorbidities, solitary kidney, and hereditary renal cell carcinoma.

A number of studies and systematic reviews have compared MIPN (LPN or RALPN) to TA [86–92]. These studies have demonstrated similar oncological outcomes (local recurrence-free and metastatic-free survival) between partial nephrectomy (PN) and TA, but a superior metastasis-free survival for PN when compared to RFA. Of note, the overall survival favors PN, but these studies have a high selection bias—PN patients tend to be younger and healthier. Thompson et al. presented 1424 cT1a patients that underwent PN (n = 1057), RFA (n = 180), and CA (n = 187) with a median follow-up of 5.2, 3.6, and 1.9 years, respectively [93]. The PN recurrence-free survival and metastasis-free survival was comparable to CA (98% vs 98%, and 99% vs 100%, respectively), but a superior metastasis-free survival was noted for PN compared to RFA (99% vs 93%, respectively). Similarly, patients with cT1b (n = 379) managed with PN (n = 326) and CA (n = 53) had comparable oncological outcomes. A recent review by Pierorazio et al. identified an inferior 1-year recurrence-free survival for patients undergoing

TA compared to PN; however, a secondary TA procedure eliminates this difference [88]. The perioperative side effect profile appears more favorable for TA compared to PN, but the renal function outcomes for either procedure are similar [88, 92, 93]. Moreover, RFA and CA appear to share similar oncological, perioperative, and functional outcomes, but further data are required to delineate differences between the two techniques. Thoughtful consideration is necessary when comparing MIPN and ablative therapies as the indications for each vary and the patient populations are often significantly different with the MIPN population being younger and healthier [56]. At the present time, minimally invasive ablative procedures require further validation prior to widespread utilization.

Microwave therapy is a newer thermal ablative treatment modality but some still regard it as investigational. It is beginning to gain ground as it has been shown in a few studies to be safe and as effective as PN, but further data are required [6, 7]. An international group has reported their experience with extracorporeal and laparoscopic approach, demonstrating its feasibility and safety [94, 95]. Further trials with optimized device settings and longer-term follow-up are needed to demonstrate the oncologic safety and efficacy of these novel techniques.

Future Directions

In line with the principle of "no surgery is the best surgery," renal mass biopsy (RMB) is beginning to gain ground. It has been documented that nearly a quarter of renal masses removed are benign [8]. When considering the rigorous cancer guidelines set forth for other organ systems, the lack of a definitive tissue diagnosis prior to surgical management remains unique to renal masses. Technological and histological advancements provide a high diagnostic accuracy with acceptable morbidity for RMB, and the procedure itself does not preclude surgical therapy [96]. With these improvements and advances, it is possible that the future of renal cancer will be guided by renal mass biopsies.

We are also likely to see improvement in imaging for renal masses, such as the development of molecular imaging for renal cancer. Radiolabeled 89Zr-DFO-girentuximab (TLX250-CDx) is a highly specific monoclonal antibody for CAIX, an enzyme highly expressed in clear cell renal carcinoma (ccRCC), and can differentiate between ccRCC and other renal lesions [97]. This partly addresses the unmet need for accurate noninvasive techniques to guide patient management. Currently, cross-sectional imaging cannot reliably differentiate benign and malignant renal masses, and biopsy, which is invasive, is subject to sampling errors. The ZIRCON study has evaluated the performance of TLX250-CDx PET/CT for detection of ccRCC in adult patients with indeterminate renal masses (IDRM). The primary end points were the sensitivity and specificity of TLX250-CDx PET/CT imaging in detecting ccRCC in patients with IDRM . A total of 284 renal mass cases were included in primary analysis. The average sensitivity and specificity among three blinded, independent reviewers revealed an impressive 86% [80%, 90%] and 87% [79%, 92%], respectively [97].

The improvement in surgical technology, particularly robotic surgery. The upgrade in the Intuitive Surgical da Vinci multiport surgical system in March 2024 with the FDA clearance for the fifth-generation robotic system, da Vinci 5. Da Vinci 5 design and engineering will improve accuracy and precision with new surgeon controllers and powerful vibration and tremor controls, next-generation 3D display and image processing, and first-of-its-kind force-sensing technology for surgeons to feel subtle forces exerted on tissue during surgery. Da Vinci 5 has innovative features that are designed to help increase surgeon autonomy and streamline surgeon and care team workflow.

Also the development and, hopefully, approval of new robotic surgical platforms. This would include multiport platforms such as Medtronic's HUGO, Johnson & Johnson's Ottava, Asensus' Senhance Surgical System, CMS Surgical's Versius Surgical Robot, and single-port platforms such as Titan Medical's Enos Surgical System and Vicarious Surgical's robotic system.

High-intensity focused ultrasound (HIFU) is being studied and evaluated as a thermal ablative treatment modality for small renal masses. This may represent a safer ablative option compared to existing options. The feasibility, safety, and oncologic efficacy needs to be established.

Another noteworthy development is the use of advanced imaging technology in the form of augmented (AR) and virtual reality (VR). AR is the overlay of virtual images onto the real world, whereas VR is the simulation of the real world. AR has already entered the clinical field and has been used intraoperatively to improve surgical outcomes, particularly negative margins in a PN and the preservation of normal ischemia by guiding selective arterial clamping [2, 3]. Moreover, VR has the potential to further improve surgical outcomes by creating an accurate and detailed mental map of the surgical anatomy prior to surgery. Wake et al. illustrated that experienced surgeons, after reviewing a CT scan, fail to identify the correct location of a renal tumor on a 3D reconstructed kidney [4]. Interestingly, studies on VR from the University of California, Irvine, investigated the use of a VR head-mounted display along with hand-motion tracking for preoperative planning for a PN. Their use of VR technology allows the surgeons to peer inside and interact with patient-specific 3D-VR models. Experienced surgeons indicated that the review of the VR model provides superior anatomical understanding compared to CT alone. Additionally, the VR experience improved surgical confidence for the planned PN and altered the operative approach on numerous occasions [98]. Although AR and VR technologies are promising, further studies are required to evaluate their clinical impact and address the time constraints that come with creating these advanced images.

Conclusion

Minimally invasive nephron-sparing techniques have proven similar oncologic outcomes while reducing morbidity and improving outcomes [38]. While LPN remains the gold standard nephron-sparing approach for SRMs, RALPN has emerged as a safe, effective, and widely used technique among many surgeons who otherwise may not be proficient with laparoscopy. Current literature suggests that RALP has equivalent and potentially superior outcomes when compared to LPN and OPN.

References

1. Chen DY, Uzzo RG. Evaluation and management of the renal mass. Med Clin North Am. 2011;95(1):179–89.
2. Detmer FJ, Hettig J, Schindele D, Schostak M, Hansen C. Virtual and augmented reality systems for renal interventions: a systematic review. IEEE Rev Biomed Eng. 2017;10:78–94.
3. Rassweiler J, Rassweiler MC, Muller M, Kenngott H, Meinzer HP, Teber D. Surgical navigation in urology: European perspective. Curr Opin Urol. 2014;24(1):81–97.
4. Wake N, Bjurlin M, Wysock J, Chandarana H, Huang W. MP63-13 "pin the tumor on the kidney": an evaluation of how surgeons translate CT and MRI data to 3d models. J Urol. 2018;199(4):e845–6.
5. Campbell S, Uzzo RG, Allaf ME, et al. Renal mass and localized renal cancer: AUA guideline. J Urol. 2017;198(3):520–9.
6. Cornelis FH, Marcelin C, Bernhard JC. Microwave ablation of renal tumors: a narrative review of technical considerations and clinical results. Diagn Interv Imaging. 2017;98(4):287–97.
7. Zhou W, Arellano RS. Thermal ablation of T1c renal cell carcinoma: a comparative assessment of technical performance, procedural outcome, and safety of microwave ablation, radiofrequency ablation, and cryoablation. J Vasc Interv Radiol. 2018;29(7):943–51.
8. Millet I, Doyon FC, Hoa D, et al. Characterization of small solid renal lesions: can benign and malignant tumors be differentiated with CT? AJR Am J Roentgenol. 2011;197(4):887–96.
9. Whelan RL, Fleshman JW, Fowler DL. The SAGES manual of perioperative care in minimally invasive surgery. Chapter 35 Pulmonary implications of CO2 pneumoperitoneum in minimally invasive surgery. New York: Springer; 2005. p. 360–5.
10. Harris SN, Ballantyne GH, Luther MA, Perrino AC. Alterations of cardiovascular performance during laparoscopic colectomy: a combined hemodynamic and echocardiographic analysis. Anesth Analg. 1996;83(3):482–7.
11. Guh DP, Zhang W, Bansback N, Amarsi Z, Birmingham CL, Anis AH. The incidence of comorbidities related to obesity and overweight: a

systematic review and meta-analysis. BMC Public Health. 2009;9(1):88.
12. Eaton SH, Thirumavalaven N, Katz MH, Babayan RK, Wang DS. Effect of body mass index on perioperative outcomes for laparoscopic partial nephrectomy. J Endourol. 2011;25(9):1447–50.
13. Fugita OEH, Chan DY, Roberts WW, Kavoussi LR, Jarrett TW. Laparoscopic radical nephrectomy in obese patients: outcomes and technical considerations. Urology. 2004;63(2):247–52.
14. Doublet J, Belair G. Retroperitoneal laparoscopic nephrectomy is safe and effective in obese patients: a comparative study of 55 procedures. Urology. 2000;56(1):63–6.
15. Chi AC, McGuire BB, Nadler RB. Modern guidelines for bowel preparation and antimicrobial prophylaxis for open and laparoscopic urologic surgery. Urol Clin North Am. 2015;42(4):429–40.
16. Deng S, Dong Q, Wang J, Zhang P. The role of mechanical bowel preparation before ileal urinary diversion: a systematic review and meta-analysis. Urol Int. 2014;92(3):339–48.
17. Kutikov A, Uzzo RG. The R.E.N.A.L. nephrometry score: a comprehensive standardized system for quantitating renal tumor size, location and depth. J Urol. 2009;182(3):844–53. American Urological Association.
18. Bove P, Bhayani SB, Rha K-H, Allaf ME, Jarrett TW, Kavoussi LR. Necessity of ureteral catheter during laparoscopic partial nephrectomy. J Urol. 2004;172(2):458–60.
19. Glassman DT, Merriam WG, Trabulsi EJ, Byrne D, Gomella L. Rhabdomyolysis after laparoscopic nephrectomy. JSLS. 2007;11(4):432–7.
20. Reisiger KE, Landman J, Kibel A, Clayman RV. Laparoscopic renal surgery and the risk of rhabdomyolysis: diagnosis and treatment. Urology. 2005;66(5):29–35.
21. Szabó I, László A. Veres needle: in memoriam of the 100th birthday anniversary of Dr János Veres, the inventor. Am J Obstet Gynecol. 2004;191:352–3.
22. Gill IS, Delworth MG, Munch LC. Laparoscopic retroperitoneal partial nephrectomy. J Urol. 1994;152(5 Pt 1):1539–42.
23. Ng C, Gill IS, Ramani AP, Steinberg A, Spaliviero M, Abreu SC, et al. Transperitoneal versus retroperitoneal laparoscopic partial nephrectomy: patient selection and perioperative outcomes. J Urol. 2005;174(3):846–9.
24. Kavoussi LR, Schwartz MJ, Gill IS. Laparoscopic surgery of the kidney. In: Campbell walsh urology. 10th ed. Philadelphia: Elsevier Inc; 2012. p. 1628–69. e7: chap 55.
25. Wang DS, Stolpen AH, Bird VG, Ishigami K, Rayhill SC, Winfield HN. Correlation of preoperative three-dimensional magnetic resonance angiography with intraoperative findings in laparoscopic renal surgery. J Endourol. 2005;19(2):193–9. 2005;19(2):193–9.
26. Renal Mass and localized renal cancer: AUA Guideline. American Urological Association Research and Education. 2017. http://www.auanet.org/content/guidelines-and-quality-care/clinical-guidelines/main-reports/renalmass09.pdf
27. Blom JHM, van Poppel H, Maréchal JM, Jacqmin D, Schröder FH, de Prijck L, et al. Radical nephrectomy with and without lymph-node dissection: final results of European Organization for Research and Treatment of Cancer (EORTC) randomized phase 3 trial 30881. Eur Urol. 2009;55(1):28–34.
28. Capitanio U, Jeldres C, Patard J-J, Perrotte P, Zini L, de La Taille A, et al. Stage-specific effect of nodal metastases on survival in patients with non-metastatic renal cell carcinoma. BJU Int. 2009;103(1):33–7.
29. van Poppel H. Lymph node dissection is not obsolete in clinically node-negative renal cell carcinoma patients. Eur Urol. 2011;59(1):24–5. European Association of Urology.
30. Gong EM, Zorn KC, Orvieto MA, Lucioni A, Msezane LP, Shalhav AL. Artery-only occlusion may provide superior renal preservation during laparoscopic partial nephrectomy. Urology. 2008;72(4):843–6.
31. Marley CS, Siegrist T, Kurta J, O'Brien F, Bernstein M, Solomon S, et al. Cold intravascular organ perfusion for renal hypothermia during laparoscopic partial nephrectomy. J Endourol. 2011;185(6):2191–5. American 8Urological Association Education and Research, Inc.
32. Landman J, Venkatesh R, Lee D, Vanlangendonck R, Morissey K, Andriole GL, et al. Renal hypothermia achieved by retrograde endoscopic cold saline perfusion: technique and initial clinical application. Urology. 2003;61(5):1023–5.
33. Gill IS, Abreu SC, Desai MM, Steinberg AP, Ramani AP, Ng C, et al. Laparoscopic Ice slush renal hypothermia for partial nephrectomy: the initial experience. J Urol. 2003;170(1):52–6.
34. Spaliveiro M, Power NE, Sjoberg DD, Benfante NE, Berstein ML, Wren J, Russo P, Colemen JA. Intravenous mannitol versus placebo during partial nephrectomy in patients with normal kidney function: a double blind, clinically-integrated, randomized trial. Eur Urol. 2018;73(1):53–9.
35. Orvieto MA, Tolhurst SR, Chuang MS, et. al.: Defining maximal renal tolerance to warm ischemia in porcine laparoscopic and open surgery model. Urology 2005; 66: pp. 1111-1115.
36. Thompson RH, Lane BR, Lohse CM, et. al.: Every minute counts when the renal hilum is clamped during partial nephrectomy. Eur Urol 2010; 58: pp. 340-345.
37. Nguyen MM, Gill IS. Halving ischemia time during laparoscopic partial nephrectomy. J Urol. 2008;179(2):627–32.
38. Gill IS, Kavoussi LR, Lane BR, Blute ML, Babineau D, Colombo JR Jr, et al. Comparison of 1,800 lapa-

roscopic and open partial nephrectomies for single renal tumors. J Urol. 2007;178(1):41–6.
39. Guillonneau B, Bermúdez H, Gholami S, Fettouh El H, Gupta R, Adorno Rosa J, et al. Laparoscopic partial nephrectomy for renal tumor: single center experience comparing clamping and no clamping techniques of the renal vasculature. J Urol. 2003;169(2):483–6.
40. Rais-Bahrami S, George AK, Herati AS, Srinivasan AK, Richstone L, Kavoussi LR. Off-clamp versus complete hilar control laparoscopic partial nephrectomy: comparison by clinical stage. BJU Int. 2012;109(9):1376–81.
41. Liu W, Li Y, Chen M, et. al.: Off-clamp versus complete hilar control partial nephrectomy for renal cell carcinoma: a systematic review and meta-analysis. J Endourol 2014; 28: pp. 567-576.
42. Borofsky MS, Gill IS, Hemal AK, et. al.: Near-infrared fluorescence imaging to facilitate super-selective arterial clamping during zero-ischaemia robotic partial nephrectomy. BJU Int 2013; 111: pp. 604-610.
43. Rao AR, Gray R, Mayer E, et. al.: Occlusion angiography using intraoperative contrast-enhanced ultrasound scan (CEUS): a novel technique demonstrating segmental renal blood supply to assist zero-ischaemia robot-assisted partial nephrectomy. Eur Urol 2013; 63: pp. 913-919.
44. Gill IS, Patil MB, de Castro Abreu AL, Ng C, Cai J, Berger A, et al. Zero ischemia anatomical partial nephrectomy: a novel approach. J Urol. 2012;187(3):807–15. Elsevier Inc.
45. Desai MM, de Castro Abreu AL, Leslie S, et. al.: Robotic partial nephrectomy with superselective versus main artery clamping: a retrospective comparison. Eur Urol 2014; 66: pp. 713-719.
46. Cacciamani GE, Medina LG, Gill TS, Mendelsohn A, Husain F, Bhardwaj L, Artibani W, Sotelo R, Gill IS. Impact of renal hilar control on outcomes of robotic partial nephrectomy: systematic review and cumulative meta-analysis. Eur Urol Focus. 2018; https://doi.org/10.1016/j.euf.2018.01.012.
47. Sutherland SE, Resnick MI, Maclennan GT, Goldman HB. Does the size of the surgical margin in partial nephrectomy for renal cell cancer really matter? J Urol. 2002;167(1):61–4.
48. Marszalek M, Carini M, Chlosta P, Jeschke K, Kirkali Z, Knüchel R, et al. Positive surgical margins after nephron-sparing surgery. Eur Urol. 2012;61(4):757–63.
49. Minervini A, Ficarra V, Rocco F, Antonelli A, Bertini R et al. Simple Enucleation is Equivalent to Traditional Partial Nephrectomy for Renal Cell Carcinoma: Results of a Nonrandomized, Retrospective, Comparative Study. J Urol. 2011;185(5):1604-10.
50. Bensalah K, Pantuck AJ, Rioux-Leclercq N, Thuret R, Montorsi F, Karakiewicz PI, et al. Positive surgical margin appears to have negligible impact on survival of renal cell carcinomas treated by nephron-sparing surgery. Eur Urol. 2010;57(3):466–73.
51. Kubinski DJ, Clark PE, Assimos DG, Hall MC. Utility of frozen section analysis of resection margins during partial nephrectomy. Urology. 2004;64(1):31–4.
52. Duvdevani M, Laufer M, Kastin A, Mor Y, Nadu A, Hanani J, et al. Is frozen section analysis in nephron sparing surgery necessary? A clinicopathological study of 301 cases. J Urol. 2005;173(2):385–7.
53. Timsit M-O, Bazin J-P, Thiounn N, Fontaine E, Chrétien Y, Dufour B, et al. Prospective study of safety margins in partial nephrectomy: intraoperative assessment and contribution of frozen section analysis. Urology. 2006;67(5):923–6.
54. Bylund JR, Clark CJ, Crispen PL, LaGrange CA, Strup SE. Hand-assisted laparoscopic partial nephrectomy without formal collecting system closure: perioperative outcomes in 104 consecutive patients. J Endourol. 2011;25(12):1853–7.
55. Tsivian A, Tsivian M, Benjamin S, Sidi AA. Simplified hemostatic technique during laparoscopic partial nephrectomy. Int Braz J Urol. 2012;38(1):84–8.
56. Aboumarzouk OM, Stein RJ, Eyraud R, Haber G-P, Chlosta PL, Somani BK, et al. Robotic versus laparoscopic partial nephrectomy: a systematic review and meta-analysis. Eur Urol. 2012;62(6):1023–33.
57. Cacciamani GE, Medina LG, Gill T, Abreu A, Sotelo R, Artibani W, Gill IS. Impact of surgical factors on robotic partial nephrectomy outcomes: comprehensive systemic review and meta-analysis. J Urol. 2018;200(2):258–74.
58. Kaul S, Laungani R, Sarle R, Stricker H, Peabody J, Littleton R, et al. Da Vinci-assisted robotic partial nephrectomy: technique and results at a mean of 15 months of follow-up. Eur Urol. 2007;51(1):186–92.
59. Porreca A, D'Agostino D, Dente D, Dandea M, Salvaggio A, Cappa E, Zuccala A, Del Rosso A, Chessa F, Romagnoli D, Mengoni F, Borghesi M, Sciavina R. Retroperitoneal approach for robotic-assisted partial nephrectomy: technique and early outcomes. Int Braz J Urol. 2018;44(1):63–8.
60. Pavan N, Derweesh I, Hampton LJ, White WM, Porter J, Challacombe BJ, Dasgupta P, Bertolo R, Kaouk J, Mirone V, Porpiglia F, Autorino R. Retroperitoneal robotic partial nephrectomy: systemic review and cumulative analysis of comparative outcomes. J Endourol. 2018;32(7):591–6.
61. Marconi L, Challacombe B. Robotic partial nephrectomy for posterior renal tumors: retro or transperitoneal approach? Eur Urol Focus. 2018;4:632. https://doi.org/10.1016/j.euf.2018.08.003
62. Choi JE, You JH, Kim DK, et. al.: Comparison of perioperative outcomes between robotic and laparoscopic partial nephrectomy: a systematic review and meta-analysis. Eur Urol 2015; 67: pp. 891-901.
63. Zaid HB, Parker WP, Lohse CM, et. al.: Patient factors associated with 30-day complications after

partial nephrectomy: a contemporary update. Urol Oncol 2017; 35: pp. 153 e151-153 e156.
64. Simhan J, Smaldone MC, Tsai KJ, et. al.: Objective measures of renal mass anatomic complexity predict rates of major complications following partial nephrectomy. Eur Urol 2011; 60: pp. 724-730.
65. Rassweiler J, Fornara P, Weber M, et. al.: Laparoscopic nephrectomy: the experience of the laparoscopy working group of the German Urologic Association. J Urol 1998; 160: pp. 18-21.
66. Fahlenkamp D, Rassweiler J, Fornara P, et. al.: Complications of laparoscopic procedures in urology: experience with 2,407 procedures at 4 German centers. J Urol 1999; 162: pp. 765-770. discussion 770–761
67. Keeley FX, Tolley DA: A review of our first 100 cases of laparoscopic nephrectomy: defining risk factors for complications. Br J Urol 1998; 82: pp. 615-618.
68. Simforoosh N, Basiri A, Ziaee SA, et. al.: Major vascular injury in laparoscopic urology. JSLS 2014; 18:
69. Meraney AM, Samee AA, Gill IS: Vascular and bowel complications during retroperitoneal laparoscopic surgery. J Urol 2002; 168: pp. 1941-1944.
70. Varkarakis IM, Allaf ME, Bhayani SB, Inagaki T, Su LM, Kavoussi LR, et al. Pancreatic injuries during laparoscopic urologic surgery. Urology. 2004;64(6):1089–93.
71. Aron M, Colombo JR Jr, Turna B, Stein RJ, Haber G-P, Gill IS. Diaphragmatic repair and/or reconstruction during upper abdominal urological laparoscopy. J Urol. 2007;178(6):2444–50.
72. Simon SD, Castle EP, Ferrigini RG, Andrews PE. Routine postoperative chest x-ray following laparoscopic nephrectomy. JSLS. 2005;9(1):205–7.
73. Jain S, Nyirenda T, Yates J, Munver R. Incidence of renal artery pseudoaneurysm following open and minimally invasive partial nephrectomy: a systematic review and comparative analysis. J Urol. 2013;189(5):1643–8.
74. Uberoi J, Badwan KH, Wang DS. Renal-artery pseudoaneurysm after laparoscopic partial nephrectomy. J Endourol. 2007;21(3):330–3.
75. Meeks JJ, Zhao LC, Navai N, et. al.: Risk factors and management of urine leaks after partial nephrectomy. J Urol 2008; 180: pp. 2375-2378.
76. Potretzke AM, Knight BA, Zargar H, et. al.: Urinary fistula after robot-assisted partial nephrectomy: a multicentre analysis of 1 791 patients. BJU Int 2016; 117: pp. 131-137.
77. Zorn KC, Gong EM, Orvieto MA, Gofrit ON, Mikhail AA, Shalhav AL. Impact of collecting-system repair during laparoscopic partial nephrectomy. J Endourol. 2007;21(3):315–20
78. Shah K, Abaza R. Clinical pathway for discharge on postoperative day one after robotic partial nephrectomy. [moderated poster] In: American Urological Association annual meeting. Washington, DC; 2011 May 14–19; May 30.
79. Leavitt DA, Keheila M, Siev M, Shah PH, Moreira DM, George AK, et al. Outcomes of laparoscopic partial nephrectomy in patients continuing aspirin therapy. J Urol. 2016;195(4 Pt 1):859–64.
80. Long JA, Bernhard JC, Bigot P, et. al.: Partial nephrectomy versus ablative therapy for the treatment of renal tumors in an imperative setting. the; C. French association of Urology Cancerology World J Urol 2017; 35: pp. 649-656.
81. Lian H, Guo H, Zhang G, Yang R, Gan W, Li X, et al. Single-center comparison of complications in laparoscopic and percutaneous radiofrequency ablation with ultrasound guidance for renal tumors. Urology. 2012;80(1):119–25. Elsevier Inc.
82. Long CJ, Kutikov A, Canter DJ, Egleston BL, Chen DYT, Viterbo R, et al. Percutaneous vs surgical cryoablation of the small renal mass: is efficacy compromised? BJU Int. 2010;107(9):1376–80.
83. Goyal J, Verma P, Sidana A, Georgiades CS, Rodriguez R. Single-center comparative oncologic outcomes of surgical and percutaneous cryoablation for treatment of renal tumors. J Endourol. 2012;26(11):1413–9.
84. Tracy CR, Raman JD, Donnally C, Trimmer CK, Cadeddu JA. Durable oncologic outcomes after radiofrequency ablation. Cancer. 2010;116(13):3135–42.
85. Aron M, Kamoi K, Remer E, Berger A, Desai M, Gill I. Laparoscopic renal cryoablation: 8-year, single surgeon outcomes. J Urol. 2010;183(3):889–95. Elsevier Inc.
86. Caputo PA, Zargar H, Ramirez D, et al. Cryoablation versus partial nephrectomy for clinical T1b renal tumors: a matched group comparative analysis. Eur Urol. 2017;71(1):111–7.
87. Patel HD, Pierorazio PM, Johnson MH, et al. Renal functional outcomes after surgery, ablation, and active surveillance of localized renal tumors: a systematic review and meta-analysis. Clin J Am Soc Nephrol. 2017;12(7):1057–69.
88. Pierorazio PM, Johnson MH, Patel HD, et al. Management of renal masses and localized renal cancer: systematic review and meta-analysis. J Urol. 2016;196(4):989–99.
89. Desai MM, Aron M, Gill IS. Laparoscopic partial nephrectomy versus laparoscopic cryoablation for the small renal tumor. Urology. 2005;66(5):23–8.
90. O'Malley RL, Berger AD, Kanofsky JA, Phillips CK, Stifelman M, Taneja SS. A matched-cohort comparison of laparoscopic cryoablation and laparoscopic partial nephrectomy for treating renal masses. BJU Int. 2007;99(2):395–8.
91. Haramis G, Graversen JA, Mues AC, Korets R, Rosales JC, Okhunov Z, et al. Retrospective comparison of laparoscopic partial nephrectomy versus laparoscopic renal cryoablation for small. J Laparoendosc Surg. 2012;22(2):152–7.
92. Guillotreau J, Haber G-P, Autorino R, Miocinovic R, Hillyer S, Hernandez A, et al. Robotic partial nephrectomy versus laparoscopic cryoablation for the small renal mass. Eur Urol. 2012;61(5):899–904.

93. Thompson RH, Atwell T, Schmit G, et al. Comparison of partial nephrectomy and percutaneous ablation for cT1 renal masses. Eur Urol. 2015;67(2):252–9.
94. Ritchie RW, Leslie TA, Turner GDH, Roberts ISD, D'Urso L, Collura D, et al. Laparoscopic high-intensity focused ultrasound for renal tumours: a proof of concept study. BJU Int. 2010;107(8):1290–6.
95. Ritchie RW, Leslie T, Phillips R, Wu F, Illing R, Haar Ter G, et al. Extracorporeal high intensity focused ultrasound for renal tumours: a 3-year follow-up. BJU Int. 2010;106(7):1004–9.
96. Marconi L, Dabestani S, Lam TB, et al. Systematic review and meta-analysis of diagnostic accuracy of percutaneous renal tumour biopsy. Eur Urol. 2016;69(4):660–73.
97. Shuch BM, Pantuck AJ, Bernhard JC, Morris MA, Master VA, Scott AM, Van Praet C et al. Results from phase 3 study of 89Zr-DFO-girentuximab for PET/CT imaging of clear cell renal cell carcinoma (ZIRCON). 2023 ASCO Genitourinary Cancers Symposium LBA602.
98. Parkhomenko E, Safiullah S, Owyong M, et al. MP26–06 initial experience with renal virtual reality models as educational and preoperative planning tools for partial nephrectomy. J Urol. 2018;199(4, Supplement):e337–8.

Surgery for Renal Cell Carcinoma with Thrombus Extension into the Vena Cava

15

John A. Libertino, Chad Wotkowicz, and Jason R. Gee

Introduction

Since the second edition of this textbook, new, important observations regarding the management of renal cell carcinoma involving the venous system have emerged and will be incorporated into this revised chapter.

Renal cell carcinoma (RCC) has a propensity, within the natural course of progression, to infiltrate into the venous system of the affected renal unit with rates of extension varying between 4% and 10% [1]. Within this subgroup, an additional 1% of patients may have thrombus extending into the right atrium or ventricle [2, 13, 14, 29].

The increased utilization of imaging studies will no doubt lead to a decrease in these numbers in the future; however, the gold standard of RCC treatment will remain surgical intervention as first described by Robson in 1969 [3]. For RCC with tumor thrombus extending into the vena cava, radical nephrectomy, tumor thrombectomy, and retroperitoneal lymph node dissection remains the mainstay treatment for these complex tumors. Occasionally, IVC resection and reconstruction are necessary as well.

Although the radiographic appearance of these renal masses and associated tumor thrombus can be alarming, their removal can be performed in a safe and effective fashion by following the surgical tenets to be discussed in this chapter. In addition to discussing the management of these tumors, we will also present the first author's (JAL) personal outcome data from 359 patients treated with venous tumor thrombi, 347 patients with RCC, and the remainder with adrenal cortical carcinoma, angiomyolipoma, and leiomyosarcoma of the renal vein or IVC. Despite the tremendous improvements in cancer therapeutics, the basic tenets of surgical oncology have been constant in our algorithm for managing these complicated cases (13, 14, 17, 18, 27, 28, 29).

Staging

Staging of RCC, or any other tumor, is an important adjunct in the management of patients' clinical situations and further allows for future outcomes studies to be critically compared.

Supplementary Information The online version contains supplementary material available at https://doi.org/10.1007/978-3-031-97599-8_15.

J. A. Libertino (✉)
Professor of Urology, Tufts University School of Medicine, Department of Urology Tufts University Medical Center, Boston, MA, USA

C. Wotkowicz
Midcoast Hospital, Brunswick, ME, USA
e-mail: chad.wotkowicz@Lahey.org

J. R. Gee
Associate Professor of Urology, Tufts University School of Medicine, Department of Urology, Tufts University Medical Center, Boston, MA, USA

Department of Urology, MGH Cancer Center, Emerson Hospital, Concord, MA, USA

J. A. Libertino, J. R. Gee (eds.), *Renal Cancer*, https://doi.org/10.1007/978-3-031-97599-8_15

2010 AJCC TNM clinical staging system for renal cell carcinoma Tumor status.

- TX: The primary tumor cannot be evaluated.
- T0: There is no evidence of a primary tumor in the kidney(s).
- T1: The tumor is found only in the kidney and is 7 centimeters (cm) or smaller in size at its largest area.
- T1a: The tumor is found only in the kidney and is 4 cm or smaller in size at its largest area.
- T1b: The tumor is found only in the kidney and is between 4 and 7 cm at its largest area.
- T2: The tumor is found only in the kidney and is larger than 7 cm in size at its largest area.
- T2a: The tumor is only in the kidney and is more than 7 cm but 10 cm or less at its largest area.
- T2b: The tumor is only in the kidney and is more than 10 cm at its largest area.
- T3: The tumor has grown into major veins or perinephric tissue (connective, fatty tissue around the kidneys). It has not grown into the adrenal gland (gland on top of each kidney that produces hormones and adrenaline to help control heart rate, blood pressure, and other body functions) on the same side of the body as the tumor, and it has not spread beyond Gerota's fascia (an envelope of tissue that surrounds the kidney).
- T3a: The tumor has spread to the large vein leading out of the kidney, called the renal vein, or the muscles of the vein, or it has spread to the fat surrounding the kidney and/or the fat inside the kidney. The tumor has not grown beyond Gerota's fascia.
- T3b: The tumor has grown into the large vein leading out of the heart, called the vena cava, below the muscle known as the diaphragm under the lungs that helps breathing.
- T3c: The tumor has spread to the vena cava above the diaphragm or the walls of the vena cava.
- T4: The tumor has spread to areas beyond Gerota's fascia and extends into the adrenal gland on the same side of the body as the tumor.

Nodal status. The "N" in the TNM staging system stands for lymph nodes. Lymph nodes near the kidneys are called regional lymph nodes. Lymph nodes in other parts of the body are called distant lymph nodes.

- NX: The regional lymph nodes cannot be evaluated.
- N0: The cancer has not spread to the regional lymph nodes.
- N1: The cancer has spread to regional lymph nodes. Distant metastasis.

The "M" in the TNM system indicates whether the cancer has spread to other parts of the body. Common areas where kidney cancer may spread include the bones, liver, lungs, brain, and distant lymph nodes.

- M0: The disease has not metastasized.
- M1: The cancer has spread to other parts of the body beyond the kidney area.

Used with the permission of the American Joint Committee on Cancer (AJCC), Chicago, Illinois. The original source for this material is the AJCC Cancer Staging Manual, Seventh Edition (2010) published by Springer Science and Business Media LLC, http://www.springer.com.

Our personal experience utilizing the AJCC TNM System is outlined in Fig. 15.1.

However, another important adjunct in the management of RCC invading the vena cava is an alternative, Mayo Staging System, which provides an important classification and helpful anatomical landmarks for planning the surgical removal of the IVC tumor thrombus. Our personal experience utilizing the Mayo classification is outlined in Fig. 15.2.

In this system: renal vein thrombus <2 cm into the IVC is staged as a level 1, infrahepatic thrombus is staged as a level II thrombus (below hepatic veins), and supra-hepatic IVC thrombus (above the hepatic veins) but below the diaphragm is staged as level III and an IVC tumor thrombus extending above the diaphragm is staged as level IV. The senior author's (JAL) experience with a

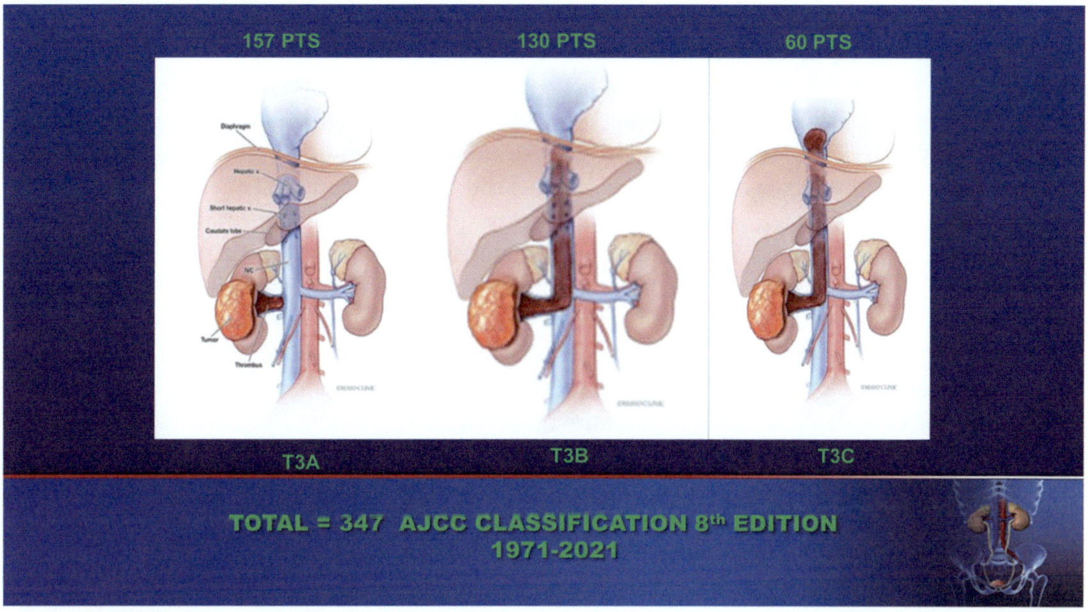

Fig. 15.1 AJCC RCC staging system and our experience

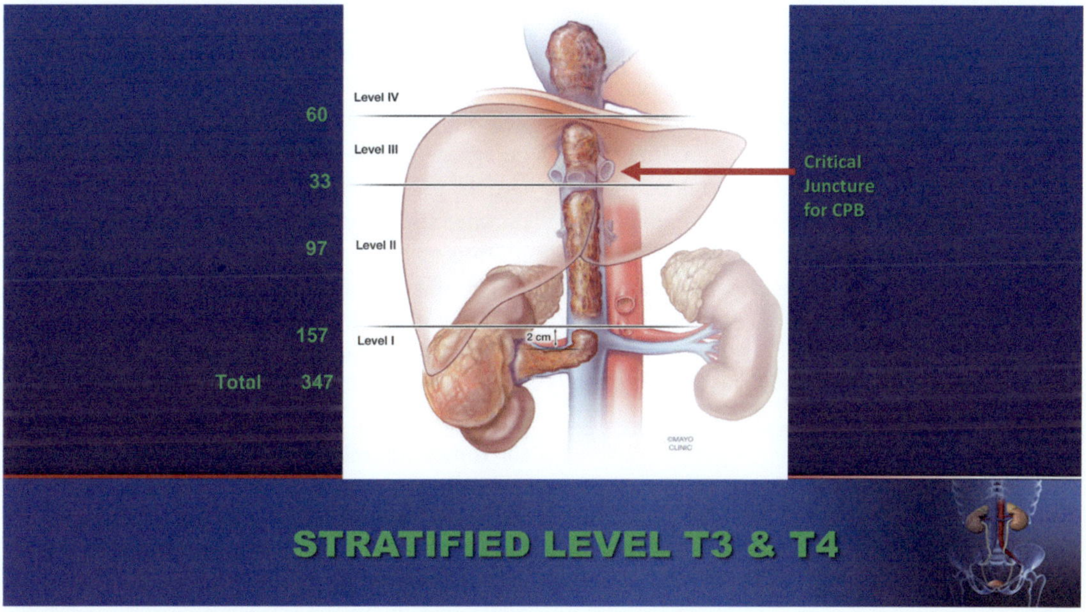

Fig. 15.2 Neves, Zincke-Mayo alternative staging system and our experience

total of 347 RCC patients stratified by level I–IV is outlined in Fig. 15.2 (36).

Like most malignancies, the outcomes are improved significantly if there is no invasion of the surrounding structures and absence of lymph node metastasis. Studies suggest 5-year survival rates of between 40% and 68% following radical nephrectomy with tumor thrombectomy [4, 5]. The level of tumor extent has been shown in some studies to correlate with survival, and at our institution we have published our results indicating improved survival for patients with renal vein involvement versus involvement of the IVC suggesting the need for revision of the previous TNM system, which occurred in the latest revision of the AJCC TNM system [6]. Different institutions have devised a variety of categories based on thrombus extension, and for the purposes of this chapter, we will use the Neves Zincke-Mayo system as illustrated above (fig. 15.2) (36). The operative approach for the most part can be based on the level of tumor thrombus extension: renal vein, infrahepatic IVC, suprahepatic venous IVC, and intracardiac. Although a host of authors have proposed a variety of classification systems, the primary outcome in most cases will depend on the biology of the tumor, the surgical experience, and confidence of the surgeon and his team. In our institution, the team consists of a urologist with vascular training and experience, an interventional cardiologist, a cardiothoracic surgeon, and a cardiac anesthesiologist to optimize perioperative outcomes.

Renal cell carcinoma has long been called the internist's tumor because of the myriad of symptoms this particular malignancy can present with (Chart 15.1) [7]. More concerning are the symptoms that tumor thrombi can produce (Chart 15.2). It is also worth noting that surgeons need to become familiar with the venous anatomy of the kidney and retroperitoneum which can often vary based on collateral drainage associated with venous tumor thrombus (Fig. 15.3).

Chart 15.1 Clinical manifestations of renal cell carcinoma

Renal cell carcinoma—Paraneoplastic manifestations
Stauffer syndrome—Elevated liver function tests with fever and hepatic necrosis
Neuromyopathy
Neuromyopathy
Polycythemia—Increased erythropoietin production
Hypertension—Increased renin production
Elevated erythrocyte sedimentation rates
Anemia of chronic disease
Cachexia and weight loss
Fever of unknown origin
Elevated alkaline phosphatase
Hypercalcemia—Increased parathyroid-related hormone/osteolytic bone mets

Imaging

Imaging is a critical step in the management of RCC with IVC thrombus for evaluating the cranial and caudal extent, volume of tumor thrombus, and potential of caval wall invasion, thus providing the information necessary to determine the best surgical approach for a given patient. This becomes very important for larger tumors and higher levels of IVC tumor thrombus (level III & IV). Currently, MRI is the gold standard that has proven to be the most effective in detecting IVC tumor thrombus with a 100% sensitivity (32). MRI images should be recent and completed no longer than 30 days prior to scheduled surgery, as these lesions may grow and change rapidly.

The radiologic presentation and diagnostic evaluation of RCC and tumor thrombus have been described elsewhere in this textbook and will not be discussed in detail in this section. However, some of the more common imaging studies preferred by our group include 3D-CTA reconstructions and MRI with dedicated venous phases (Fig. 15.4). MRV can delineate between bland and tumor thrombus which assists greatly in surgical planning and often dictates the need to start pre surgical anticoagulation to limit the risk of clot embolus. MRI has replaced traditional cavagrams which are no longer done routinely but are performed rarely to evaluate potential caval wall invasion (Fig. 15.5).

Additionally, we employ TEE preoperatively for tumor thrombus localization and intraoperatively for routine real-time imaging of the tumor thrombus. We utilize coronary angiography if

Chart 15.2 Renal cell carcinoma thrombus: signs and symptoms of venous extension

Renal cell carcinoma thrombus signs and symptoms
Caput medusae
Pulmonary embolism
Budd–Chiari syndrome (hepatomegaly, abdominal pain, and ascites)
Varicocele
Bilateral lower extremity edema
Proteinuria

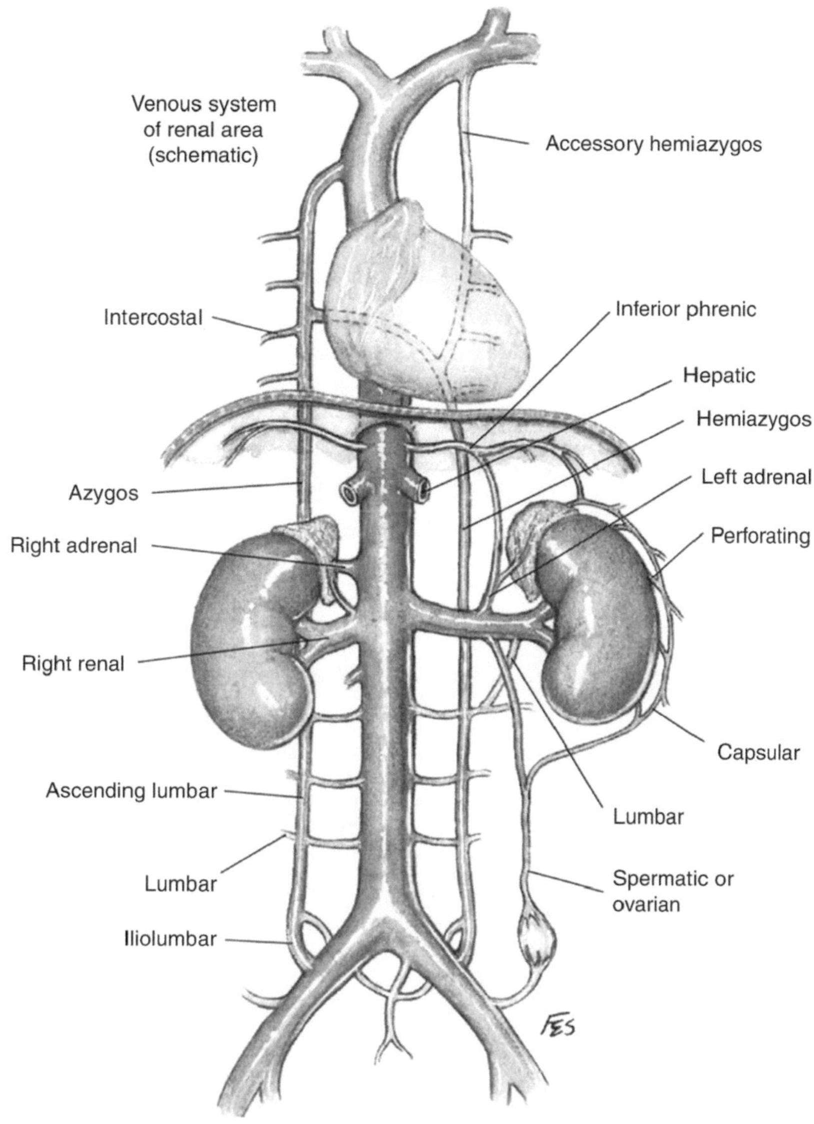

Fig. 15.3 Relevant venous anatomy of the kidney and retroperitoneum

indicated by stress echocardiogram results or a history of angina, to assess the potential for cardiac revascularization which we have occasionally performed concomitantly.

The primary goal of preoperative imaging is to determine the level of the tumor thrombus and to evaluate for metastatic disease. Zini and colleagues have suggested that preoperative measurements of renal vein and IVC diameters with associated tumor thrombus can correlate with rates of ostial wall invasion [8]. The presence of metastatic disease does not necessarily preclude an aggressive approach as data has been accumulating to suggest that solitary metastasectomy and cytoreductive procedures improved survival rates [9].

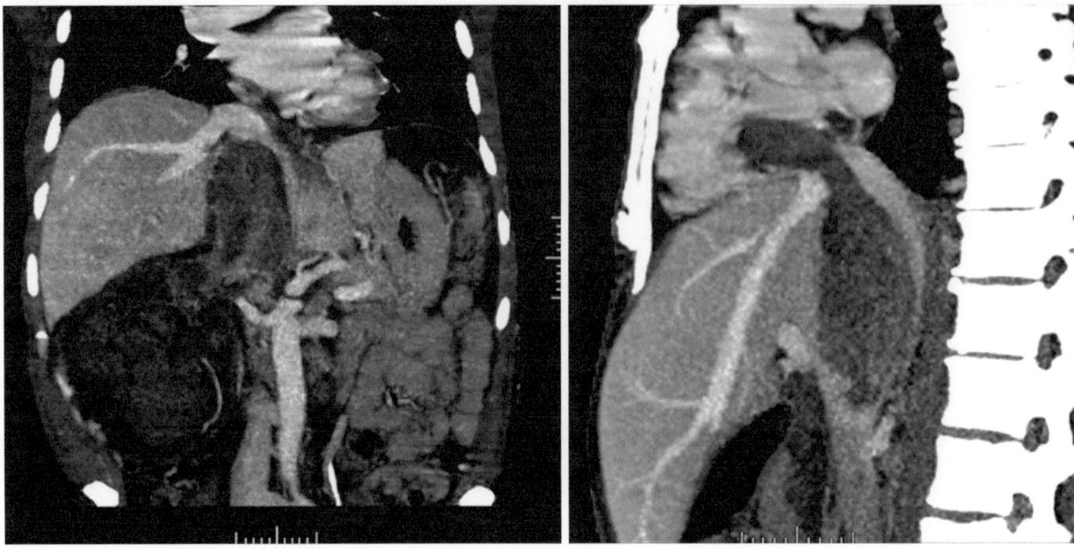

Fig. 15.4 Imaging reconstructions demonstrate extension of a large right renal cell carcinoma with tumor extension into the right atrium

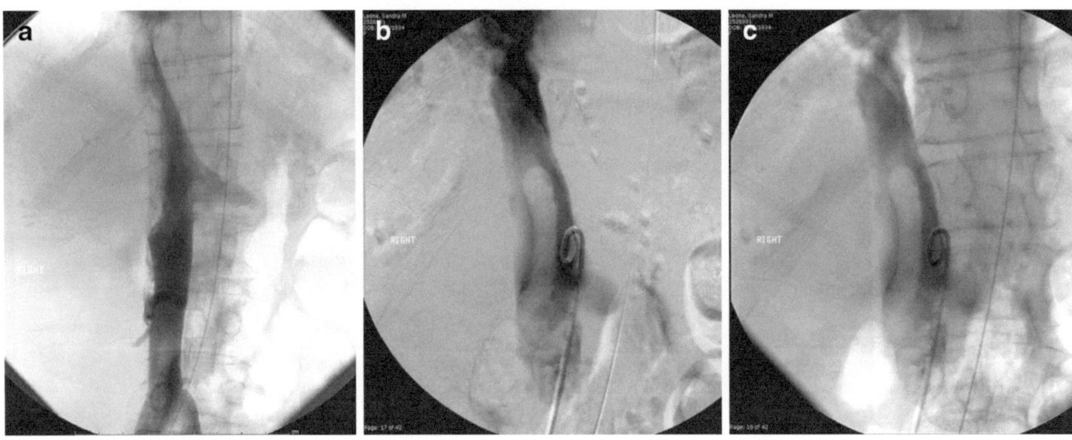

Fig. 15.5 Cavagram series demonstrating thrombus within the inferior vena cava. MRI may be used in conjunction to differentiate tumor wall invasion from bland thrombus

Preoperative Renal Embolization

Although somewhat controversial, we have found preoperative renal artery angio infarction to be very beneficial in dealing with large renal cell carcinomas with tumor thrombus. We prefer to perform our embolization 2–4 weeks prior to planned surgery (Fig. 15.6). The primary purpose of this technique is to provide some insurance against excessive blood loss via extensive venous collaterals which undergo thrombosis after renal artery occlusion, and to facilitate ligation of the renal vein prior to controlling or ligating the renal artery, which is a major intraoperative benefit. It allows the surgeon to approach the IVC tumor thrombus without having to control the renal artery. **Not having to manipulate the pedicle, especially the renal vein & IVC for vascular control of the renal artery, reduces the risk of tumor embolization, and allows one the ability to deal with the venous system directly. This is the major intraoperative benefit of renal**

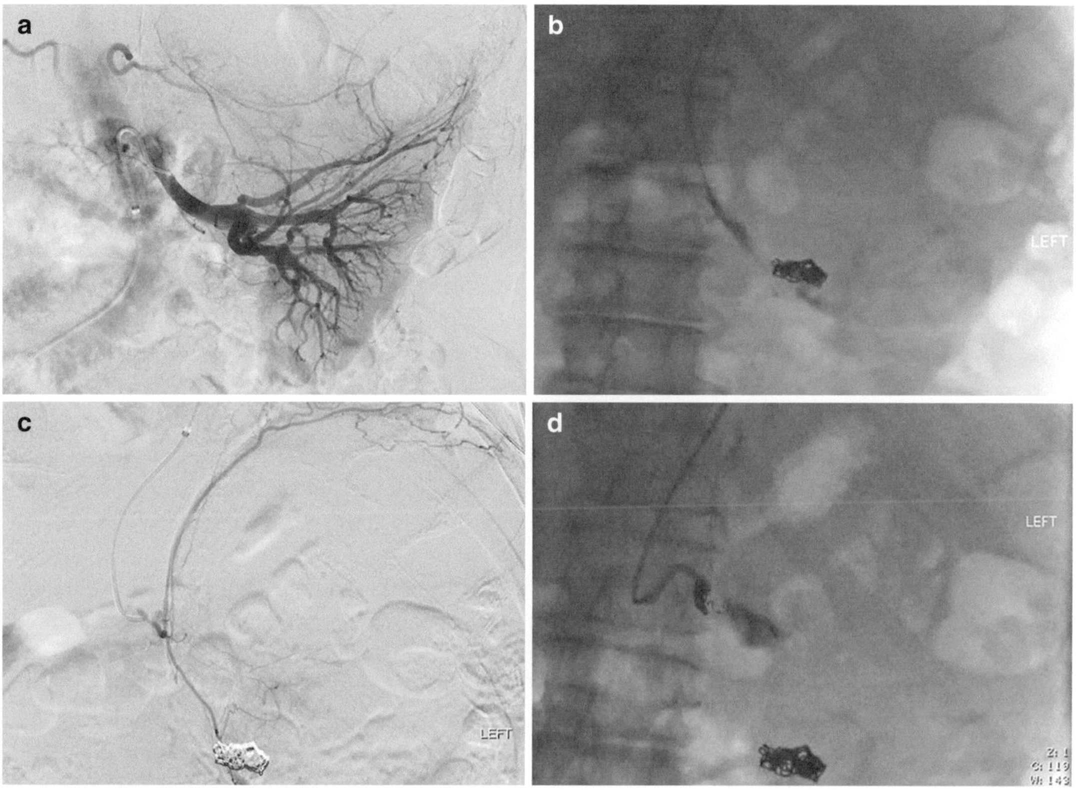

Fig. 15.6 (**a**) Left aortogram demonstrating hypovascular left renal mass. (**b**) Left brachial artery was accessed for embolization of left renal artery using purified ethanol followed by platinum coils. (**c**) Inferior phrenic artery was cannulated and demonstrated tumor vascularity. Embolization performed with purified ethanol and coils. (**d**) Successful embolization of inferior phrenic artery with diminished flow to left kidney

artery embolization, more so than reduction of intraoperative blood loss.

In some instances, the embolization can also result in tumor shrinkage and thrombus regression. The natural response to embolization often creates a moderate degree of edema (tissue hypoxia and necrosis) which can actually enhance dissection around the renal pedicle, especially in patients with extensive hilar adenopathy. This same process can induce tumor necrosis that activates natural killer cells [10, 11]. Embolization success can often be determined intraoperatively by assessing the fullness of the venous system via renal vein palpation. Postinfarction syndrome (5% of patients) is often characterized by flank pain, fevers, chills, malaise, hematuria, transient hypertension, and hyponatremia [12]. In our experience, younger, healthier patients tend to present with more severe symptoms which may require a brief hospitalization for analgesics and monitoring; however, all symptoms are eventually self-limiting.

Placement of an IVC filter is ineffective and has in our experience very problematic. We have had patients referred for surgery after filter placement where the filter was incorporated into the thrombus, or the filter tip actually penetrating the wall of the IVC. Removal of the filter damages the IVC making subsequent reconstruction much more difficult and occasionally requiring pericardial, vein, or synthetic grafting reconstruction.

We tailor our surgical approach to the specific needs of each patient according to the Cephalad level of the tumor thrombus, size and location of the tumor, regional lymphadenopathy, and unusual vascular anatomy. **The critical surgical decision is based on the upper limit of the tumor thrombus, and whether it is above or**

below the hepatic veins. Tumor thrombus below the hepatic veins (Level I & II) do not usually require CPB, but tumor thrombus extending above the hepatic veins (Level III & IV) are best performed with DHCA and CPB, in our experience. Later in this chapter, we will introduce the new, original concept of **endovascular downstaging** as a potential method for eliminating the need for DHCA and CPB in patients with tumor thrombi above the hepatic veins.

Surgical Techniques

Renal Vein Tumor Thrombus Level I

Right renal tumors with renal vein thrombus into the IVC can be managed with an approach similar to a radical nephrectomy; however, we do advocate, in large right renal tumors, a thoracoabdominal incision with generous exposure to provide insurance against blood loss (Fig. 15.7). After exposure is obtained, the kidney and renal pedicle are exposed as well as the inferior vena cava (IVC). As mentioned previously, the renal artery is palpated to assure that a successful embolization has been completed. The tumor thrombus can usually be palpated and in some instances milked out of the IVC to provide room for placement of two Debakey vascular clamps at the confluence of the renal vein and IVC. A scalpel is used at the level of the IVC to circumscribe

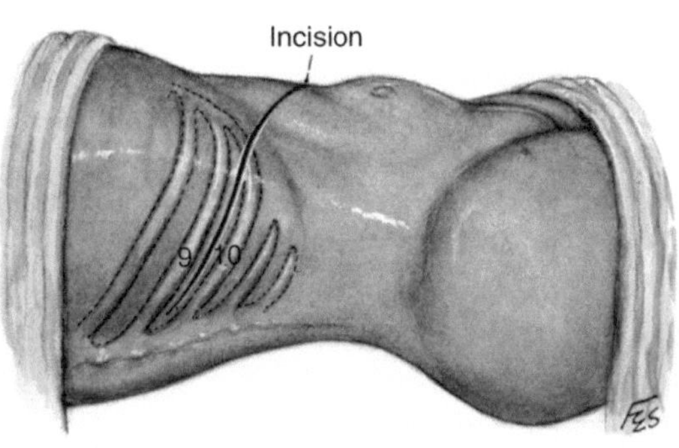

Fig. 15.7 Thoracoabdominal incision for renal vein tumor thrombus. Curve-linear supratenth incision extending to the midline

the renal vein ostium, and the vascular clamp nearest the renal vein is removed leaving a cuff of IVC above the second clamp in place to facilitate reconstruction of the IVC with 4–0 polypropylene suture in a running fashion (Figs. 15.8, 15.9, 15.10, and 15.11).

Infrahepatic Tumor Thrombus Level II

As discussed earlier, preoperative imaging is crucial to establish the cranial and caudal extension of the thrombus and rule out the need for cardiopulmonary bypass (CPB). The anesthesiologist should perform transesophageal echocardiography prior to the start of the case. We have published our approach to these tumors multiple times over the past 20 years and still approach most of these thrombi with a chevron or thoracoabdominal incision in the majority of cases [13, 14]. Right upper pole masses can be mobilized more easily with a thoracoabdominal incision. With left-sided tumors, posing some difficulty because of the length of the renal vein and associated collaterals that tend to develop, these patients will also undergo renal angio infarction prior to resection. We usually approach left-sided tumors through a chevron incision. It should be mentioned that these cases can be prolonged and the initial placement of Bookwalter retractors must be done with caution to prevent excessive pressure on the bowel and most importantly the liver. A liver hematoma can occur during the case and become somewhat troublesome to deal with at the end of the procedure. The caudate lobe will need to be exposed and retracted, often exposing the porta hepatis. Perforating minor hepatic veins can be sacrificed with impunity to improve mobility of the caudate lobe and IVC. Simple lacerations to the liver can be treated with argon laser or electrocautery, with larger defects requiring Surgicel or Gel Foam bolsters.

Unlike cases involving cardiopulmonary bypass and IVC thrombus, the portion of the IVC with the thrombus should be approached with a "no-touch technique," as much as possible, until the Rummel tourniquet has been placed cephalad and caudal to the thrombus with an additional

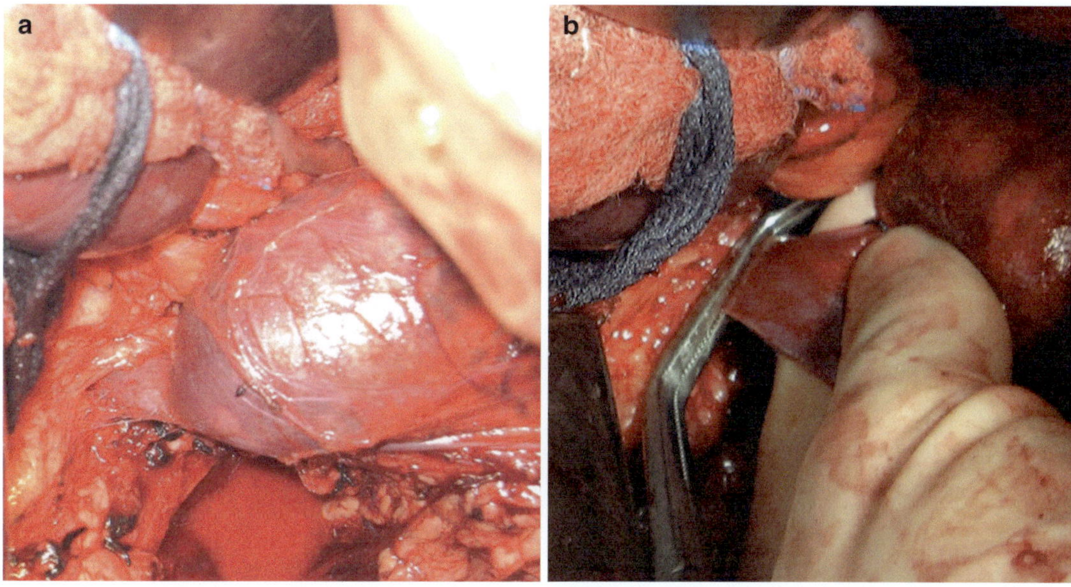

Fig. 15.8 Large renal vein thrombus is milked back to expose the confluence of the RV/IVC for placement of the Debakey vascular clamp

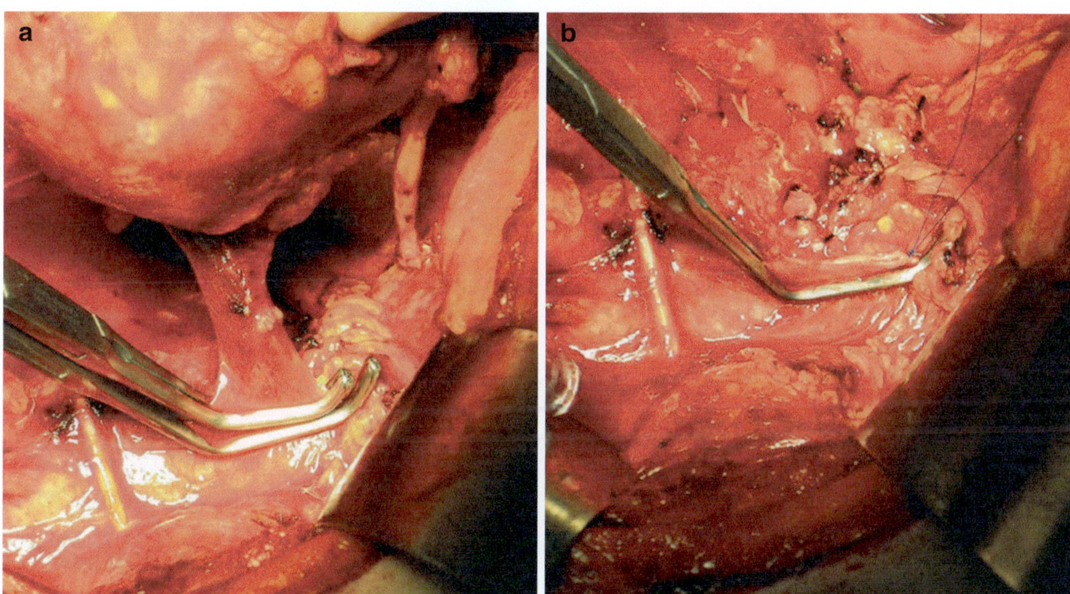

Fig. 15.9 A second Debakey clamp is placed taking caution not to limit the circumference of the IVC following caval reconstruction

tourniquet on the contralateral renal vein (Fig. 15.12). Inadvertent injuries to the IVC will occur if one performs enough resections, and these injuries are best dealt with utilizing gentle pressure proximally and distally. We advocate utilizing sponge sticks for pressure and then Allis clamps to reapproximate the defect before oversewing with 4–0 Prolene sutures; followed by placement of an Evarrest fibrin sealant patch over the defect if necessary. Likewise, inadvertent

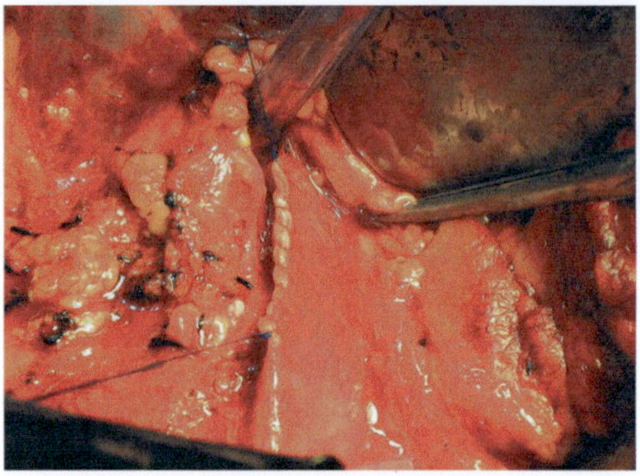

Fig. 15.10 Closed cavotomy with running 4–0 polypropylene (Prolene)

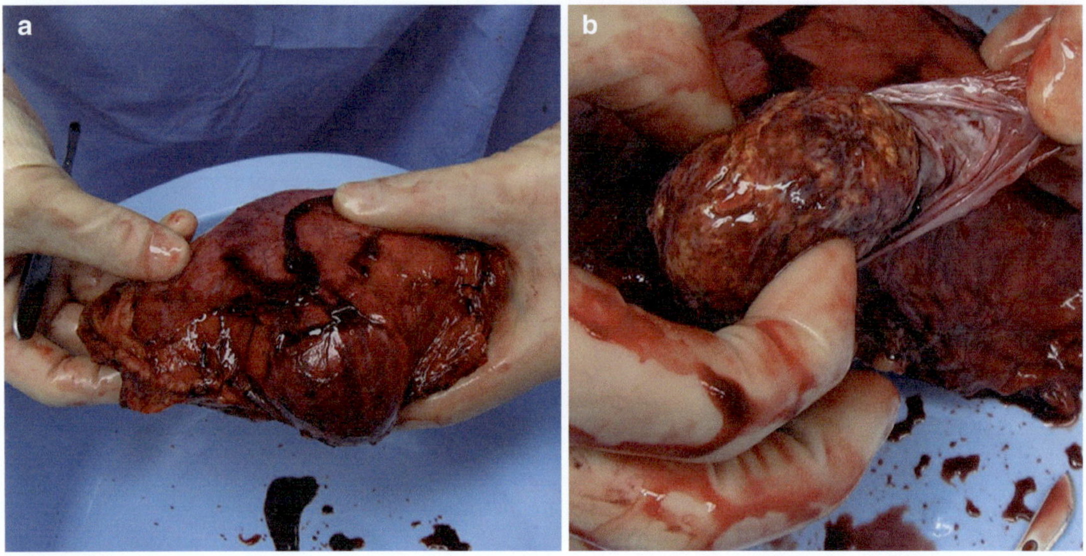

Fig. 15.11 Kidney specimen with thrombus in the renal vein

damage to the aorta is best approached with gentle pressure and closure with Prolene figure-of-eight pledgeted sutures then placement of Evarrest fibrin sealant patch, Surgicel or Gelfoam, over the repair. A common sense approach when dealing with injuries of large vessels is to avoid making more than one opening at a time.

In many instances, preoperative imaging will detect significant lumbar veins that deserve respect during dissection. Once these major venous tributaries are isolated, the surgeon can then address the ipsilateral renal artery. Although our colleagues in radiology have certainly perfected the embolization technique, we still palpate the renal artery to rule out incomplete embolization. If any question exists, one can utilize intraoperative Doppler. If there is still concern about the completeness of the renal angio infarction, we strongly advocate isolation, ligation, and division of the renal artery before tumor thrombectomy with large Hem-o-Lok clips-or Suture ligation.

Tumor thrombectomy should only be started after the arterial supply has been addressed with ligation and division or successful embolization. Before making the cavotomy, we like to take a moment to reassess all our tourniquets and have the attention of the operating room staff in case of unexpected blood loss. Once the tourniquets are tightened, we start with, a simple anterior longitu-

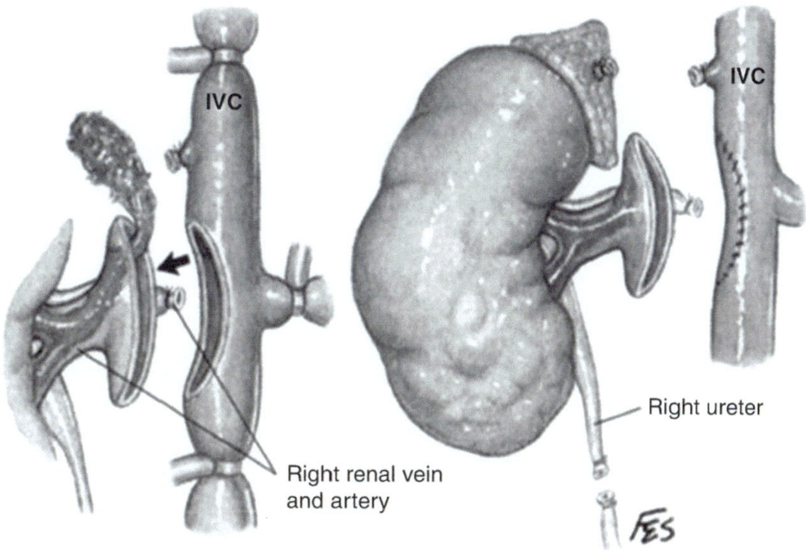

Fig. 15.12 Removal of infrahepatic tumor thrombus with a cuff of renal vein demonstrating placement of the Rummel tourniquets. Occasionally, large lumbar veins will need to be dissected and treated as well

dinal cavotomy with Potts scissors over the thrombus (Figs. 15.13, 15.14, 15.15, 15.16, 15.17, 15.18, and 15.19). Once there is adequate exposure, a small vascular endarterectomy spatula or narrow 1/8-in malleable ribbon is used to free the thrombus from the caval wall. Significant back bleeding following cavotomy is almost always due to a missed posterior lumbar vein. An Allis clamp can serve as a tag while placing figure-of-eight stitches, in some cases; however, if the vein retracts, one must be prepared to place large figure-of-eight sutures into the musculature below the lumbar vein.

After the tumor thrombus has been cleared, the caval wall should be inspected for any evidence of invasion. Although the infrarenal and suprarenal IVC may need to be partially resected in some cases, we do advocate primary repair with PTFE grafts or a pericardial patch. Prior to completing the primary caval closure, the Rummel tourniquets are released sequentially starting at the infrarenal position to purge the system and minimize embolism risk. A running 4–0 polypropylene (Prolene) is our suture of choice. The inferior vena cava can be approximated primarily as long as the circumference is maintained at above 50% of its original size. Suture line bleeding can be managed with placement of Surgicel or fibrin sealant patch over the incision. After the cavotomy is closed, we then proceed with a standard radical nephrectomy.

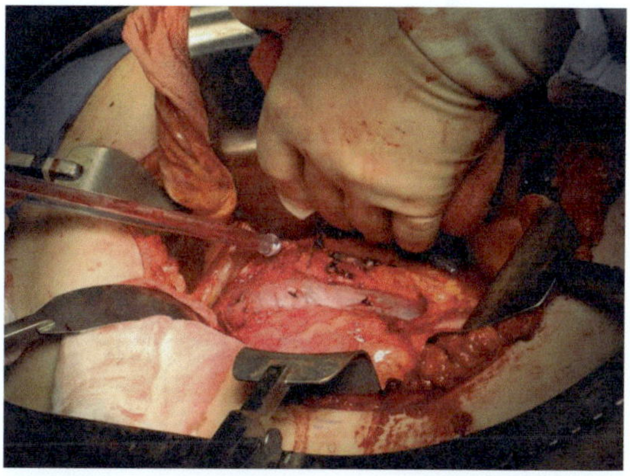

Fig. 15.13 Left renal cell carcinoma with tumor thrombus above the renal vein confluence. Patient had a previous caval filter placed precluding atraumatic placement of Debakey clamps

Retrohepatic, Supradiaphragmatic, and Atrial Tumor Thrombus Level III & IV

Our experience with deep hypothermic cardiac arrest (DHCA) with cardiopulmonary bypass (CPB) is one of the earliest and largest experiences in the literature and remains our gold standard for resection of tumors at or above the major hepatic veins or within the right atrium (Level III & IV) [13, 14, 17, 18]. In addition to describing our technique, we would also like to highlight other surgical techniques

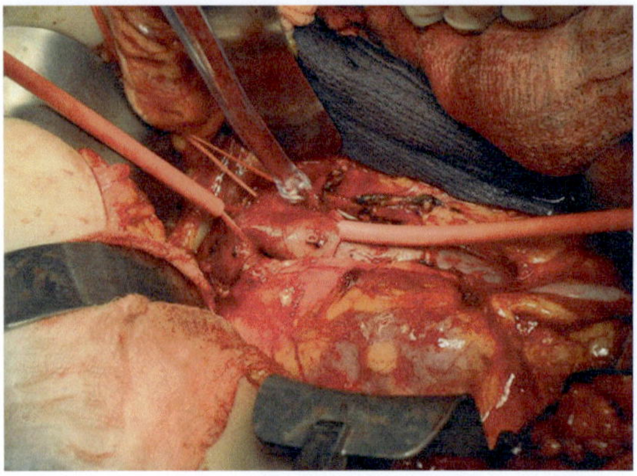

Fig. 15.14 Smaller *red* vessel loop in the background isolating the retrocaval right renal artery. The caudal Rummel tourniquet is around the inferior vena cava above the previous filter. The cephalad Rummel tourniquet encompasses the suprarenal IVC and contralateral right renal vein

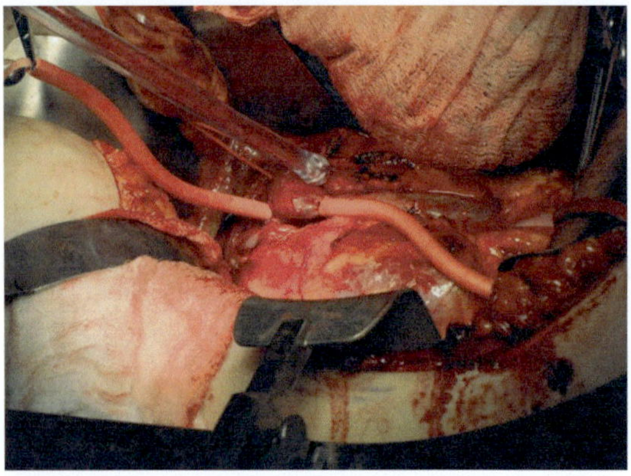

Fig. 15.15 Rummel tourniquets are cinched in place in preparation for anterior longitudinal cavotomy

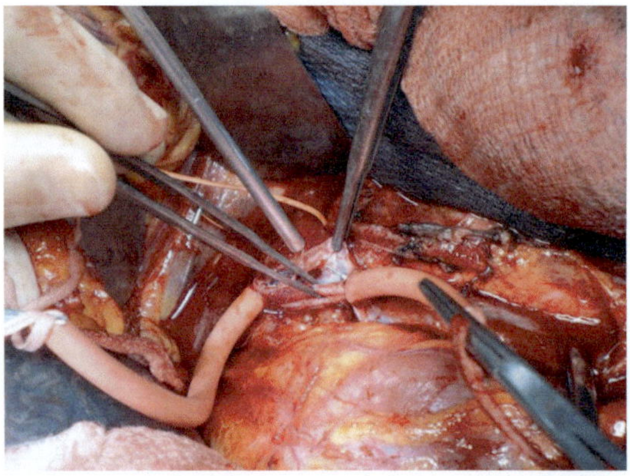

Fig. 15.16 Cavatomy demonstrates IVC filter penetrating the wall of the IVC

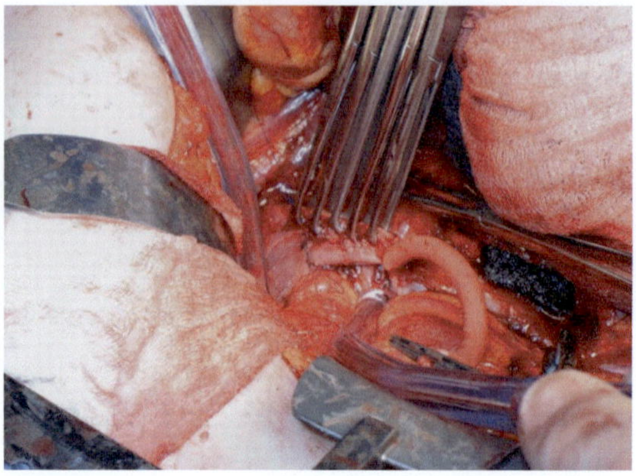

Fig. 15.17 After removal of thrombus and ligation of the left renal vein, Allis clamps are utilized to reapproximate IVC prior to reconstruction

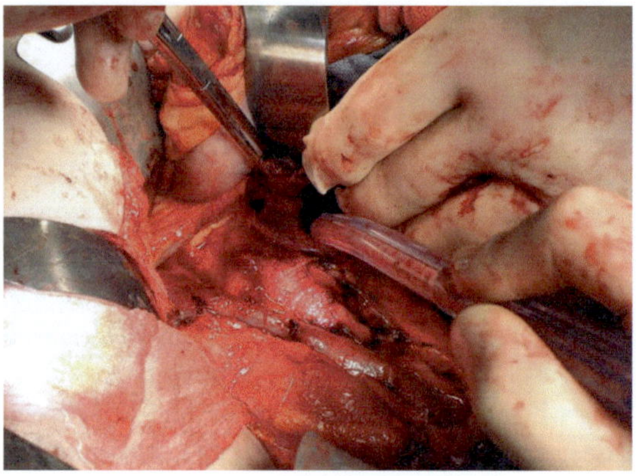

Fig. 15.18 Left renal vein and cuff IVC with tumor thrombus noted in the lumen. Cavatomy has been closed with running 4–0 Prolene suture

utilized by us and our contemporary colleagues in managing these complex cases via an intra-abdominal approach focusing on maximizing mobilization of the right lobe of the liver.

Venovenous Bypass (Caval–Atrial Shunt)

Our colleagues at other institutions have reported their utilization of venovenous bypass for caval tumor thrombectomy in patients not able to tolerate the loss of cardiac output (hypotension), and whose tumor thrombus is believed to be nonadherent, and fails to extend into the right atrium

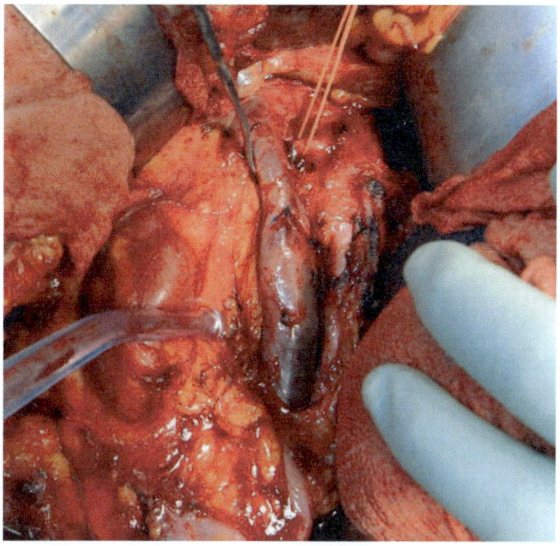

Fig. 15.19 Closed IVC cavotomy after removal of tumor thrombus and impacted IVC filter

[15]. The vena cava is mobilized and controlled at the infrarenal level, below both renal veins and the intrapericardial portion. With adequate control, a 20-F venous cannula may be placed in the IVC caudal to the tumor thrombus. An 8–14 F cannula is then inserted into the right brachial vein or right atrium for venous return. The cannulas are connected to an electromagnetic centrifugal pump, and a bypass is initiated to maintain the flow to the right side of the heart. Hepatic venous bleeding can be quite bothersome with this technique and may be addressed with a Pringle maneuver for a total of 45 min. Likewise, the major hepatic veins can also be cross clamped if necessary. Additional bleeding is sure to arise from the lumbar/azygos systems and can be difficult to control; however, it may be a necessary risk to take in those patients unable to tolerate cross clamping of the caval system. We do not recommend VVBP as there is usually too much back bleeding into the IVC. In addition if the wall of the IVC is invaded by a tumor, it may be technically difficult to replace it while the patient is on VVBP. This approach also precludes visual endoscopic visualization of the wall of the IVC, which is occasionally required to be certain that all adherent tumor thrombus has been removed.

Liver Mobilization

We have used liver mobilization for retrohepatic exposure of the IVC for tumor thrombectomy since the late 1970s. We initially reported our technique and the results of completely mobilizing the liver by dividing the triangular and coronary ligaments to facilitate exposure of the retrohepatic IVC in the mid-1980s [13, 14, 32]. After complete mobilization, the liver is attached to the IVC solely by the hepatic veins. We have utilized this technique successfully in many patients with retrohepatic tumors extending to the level of the hepatic veins or the intrapericardial IVC. We are delighted that our colleagues at other major institutions have published equivalent results utilizing similar liver mobilization techniques that expose the retrohepatic IVC, allowing access to the IVC at the level of the hepatic veins or just above. In 2007, Ciancio and colleagues at the University of Miami have utilized a technique, similar to the one we originally described, dividing the ligaments (falciform, triangular, superior coronary, and ligamentum teres) and utilizing the Pringle maneuver via the foramen of Winslow [16] (Figs. 15.20 and 15.21). Again, following these steps, the major hepatics are the only structures in continuity with the IVC. Tumor thrombus can be gently milked below the hepatics in some instances without the need for bypass, unless there appears to be invasion of the hepatic venous system, the thrombus extends into the atrium, or there is concern that the thrombus has invaded the supradiaphragmatic wall of the IVC. The essential maneuver in this approach is to displace the tumor thrombus below the hepatic veins to avoid liver congestion.

Russo and colleagues at MSKCC have published their experience with off-bypass techniques for the removal of tumor thrombus in 78 patients between 1989 and 2009. These authors also utilized venovenous bypass and liver mobilization techniques as previously described to remove suprarenal tumor thrombus, concluding that retrohepatic ($n = 7$) and suprahepatic ($n = 3$) tumor thrombus could be removed without the need for bypass.

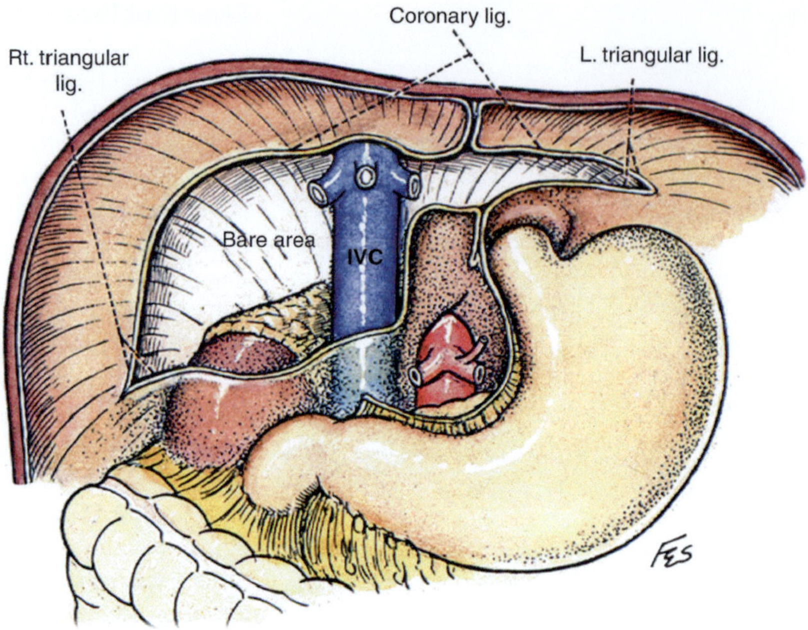

Fig. 15.20 Anterior schematic of the infrahepatic IVC demonstrating the relationship between the major hepatic veins and the diaphragm

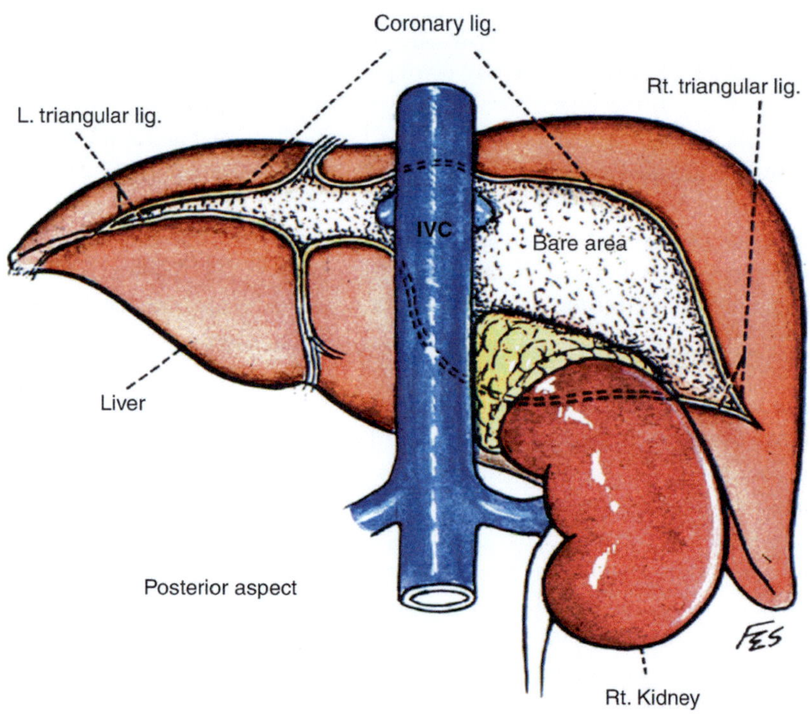

Fig. 15.21 Posterior view of the IVC

Traditional Cardiopulmonary Bypass (Median Sternotomy)

At our institution [17], we utilize a chevron incision to evaluate for any metastatic disease that may have been undetected by preoperative imaging. A Kocher maneuver is performed to expose the IVC and interaortocaval region. The retrohepatic IVC is exposed with a Langenbeck maneuver (liver mobilization cephalad and to the left by division of the right triangular and coronary ligaments) (Fig. 15.22). The kidney is mobi-

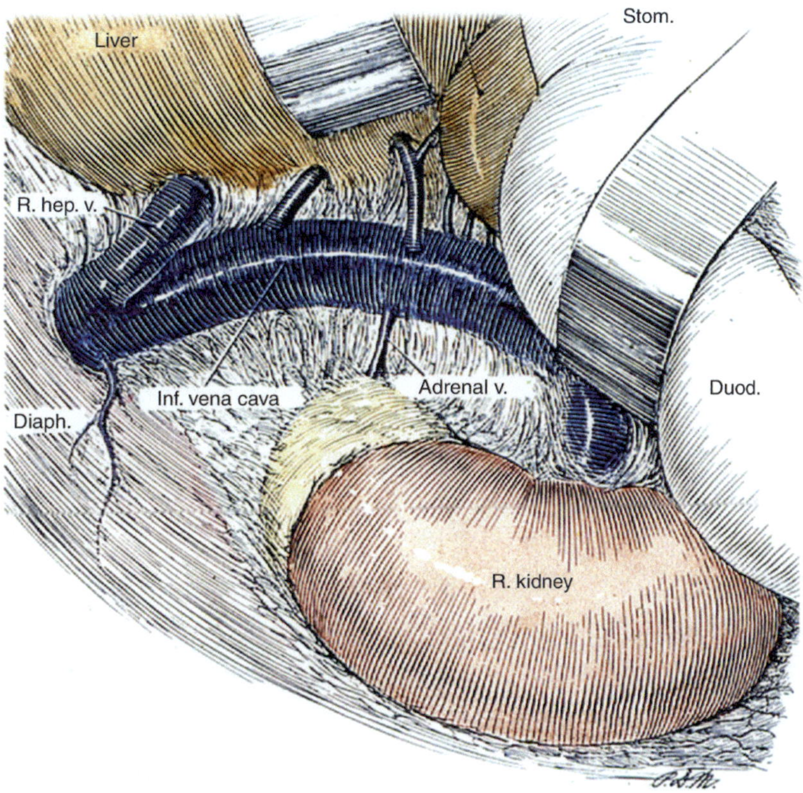

Fig. 15.22 Langenbeck

lized with the exception of the renal vein and tumor thrombus paying close attention to hemostasis (Figs. 15.23 and 15.24). The renal artery is divided with a pair of Hem-O-Lok clips and a 0-silk suture, leaving the renal vein as the sole attachment [17]. Any significant bleeding will be exposed and difficult to control following systemic heparinization for cardiopulmonary bypass. After the kidney has been mobilized, the entire inferior vena cava is exposed to the level of the diaphragm and distal to the common iliac bifurcation. The contralateral renal vein is also exposed to avoid damage during the cavotomy. Utilizing this approach mandates complete mobilization of the IVC in order to secure complete hemostasis, and avoid bleeding from anticoagulation necessary to initiate cardiopulmonary bypass. **A major, undesirable consequence of this approach is that the complete mobilization of the IVC exposes the patient to a greater risk of a pulmonary embolism rather than the minimal access approach to be discussed in the next section**.

At this point in the procedure, patients are placed on systemic heparin and traditional bypass initiated with cannulation of the ascending aorta providing arterial return and venous drainage by means of the superior vena cava and right common femoral vein. Thiopental and methylprednisolone are administered as the core temperature is cooled to 18–20 C and the head and abdomen are packed with ice. Approximately 95% of the blood volume is removed providing an essentially bloodless operating field for at least 40 min before neurological sequelae can develop. Retrograde cerebral perfusion or utilization of trickle flow rates between 5 and 10 ml/kg per minute can exceed this length of time.

Next, the right atrium is opened and distal control obtained, and any atrial thrombus may be removed to prevent any embolic events during the cavotomy and removal of the infradiaphragmatic tumor thrombus (Fig. 15.25). After distal control is obtained, anterior cavotomy is made from the renal vein ostium to the level of the minor hepatic veins above the caudate lobe of the liver. The thrombus is

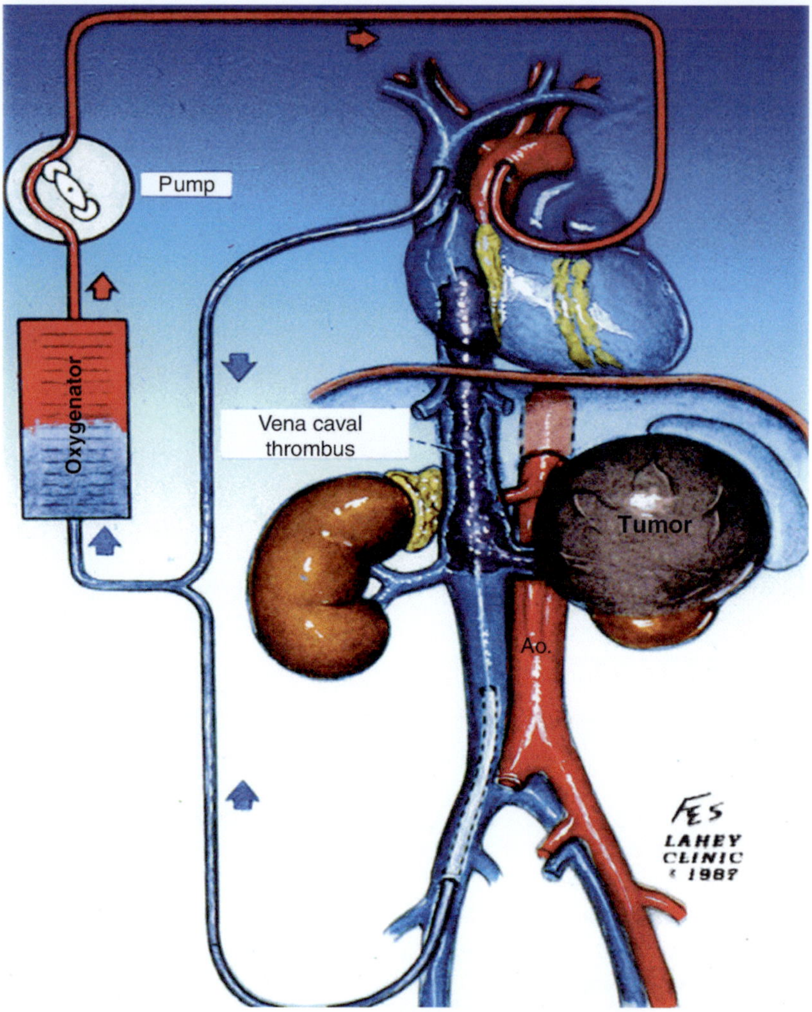

Fig. 15.23 Traditional cardiopulmonary bypass

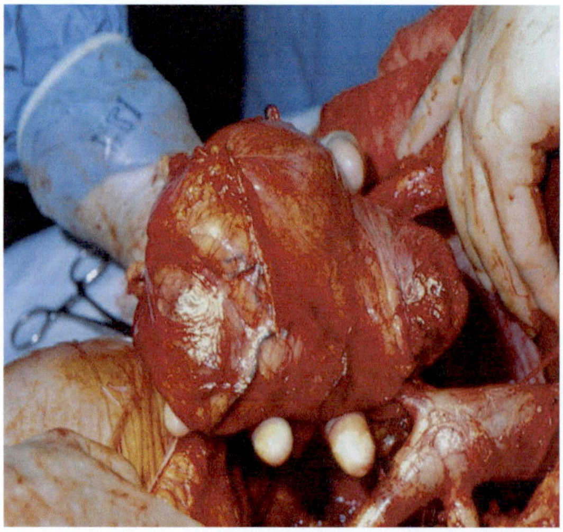

Fig. 15.24 Complete mobilization of the affected kidney with traditional cardiopulmonary bypass

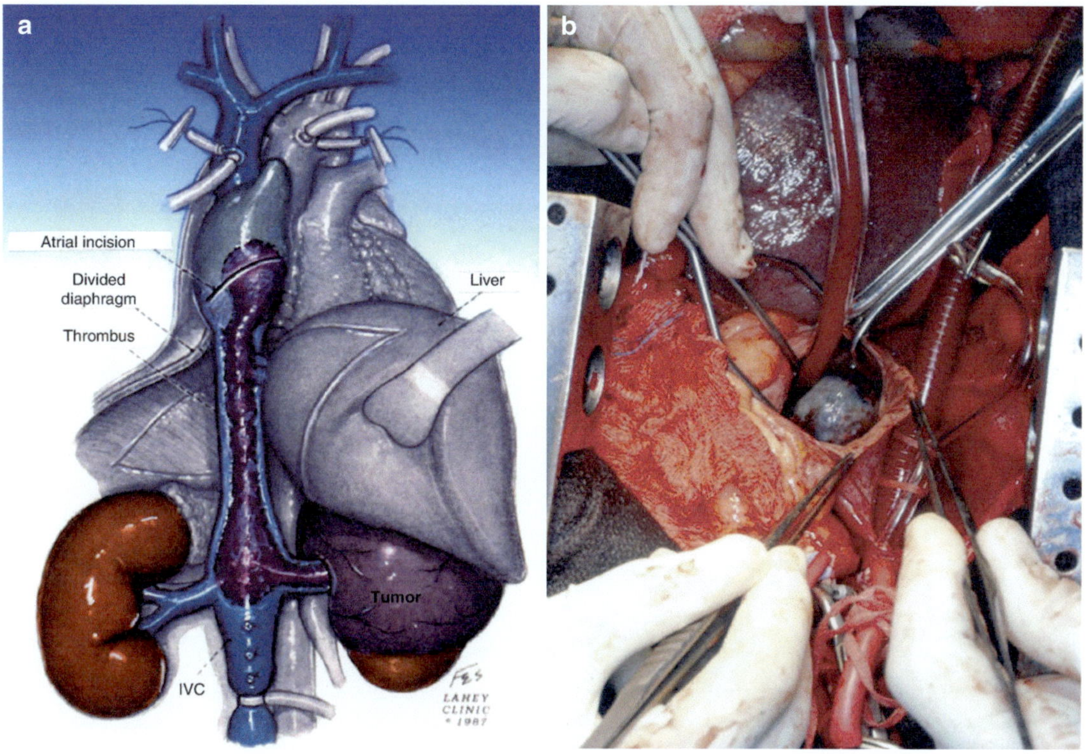

Fig. 15.25 Right atriotomy demonstrating tumor thrombus in the right atrium

removed with the patient in Trendelenburg's position and using positive pressure respirations. Ideally, the thrombus and the kidney are removed as one unit. Venacavascopy can be performed via the right atriotomy or the cavotomy from below to assure complete removal of the thrombus. The cavotomy is closed with a running 4–0 Prolene suture (Figs. 15.26, 15.27, 15.28, and 15.29). **This standard approach with median sternotomy has been completely replaced, in our practice, by the minimal access approach discussed in the next section.** If there is a need for coronary revascularization, this traditional median sternotomy approach should still be employed.

Cardiopulmonary Bypass (Minimally Access Approach)

First described at our institution in 1998 for RCC and IVC tumor management [18], and since then we have adopted this technique in all patients requiring cardiopulmonary bypass in an effort to reduce intraoperative embolism to shorten the length of surgery and improve postoperative outcomes (decreased mechanical ventilation support and transfusion rates).

Surface anatomy is important in planning the minimal access approach. The surgeon must outline the right third to fourth ribs whose cartilage must be divided in order to obtain direct access to the right atrium, which is required for the atriotomy and cardiac tumor extraction (Fig. 15.29).

Following a chevron incision, the IVC is exposed only along its anterior surface **without mobilization of the IVC or the kidney as performed in the standard procedure**, thus reducing the possibility of a fatal pulmonary embolism. At this point, the CT surgeon begins with a 3-cm infraclavicular incision to mobilize and isolate the right subclavian artery. A right 3-cm vertical parasternal incision is made over ribs 3–4, and the respective cartilage is divided. Occasionally, the right internal thoracic artery may require liga-

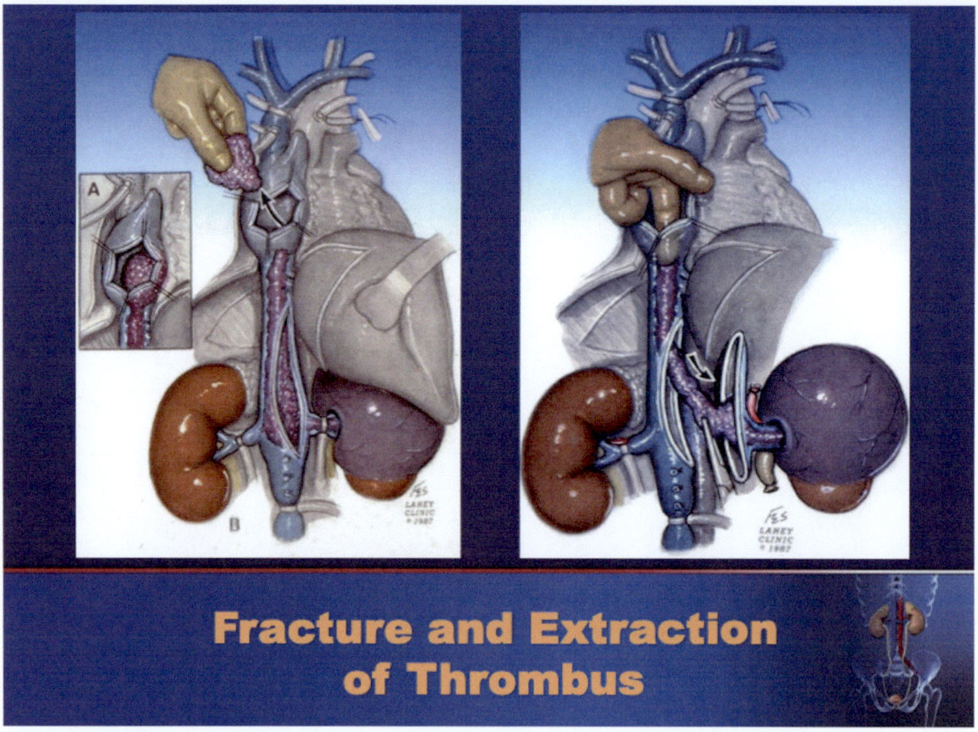

Fig. 15.26 Fracture of thrombus and extraction

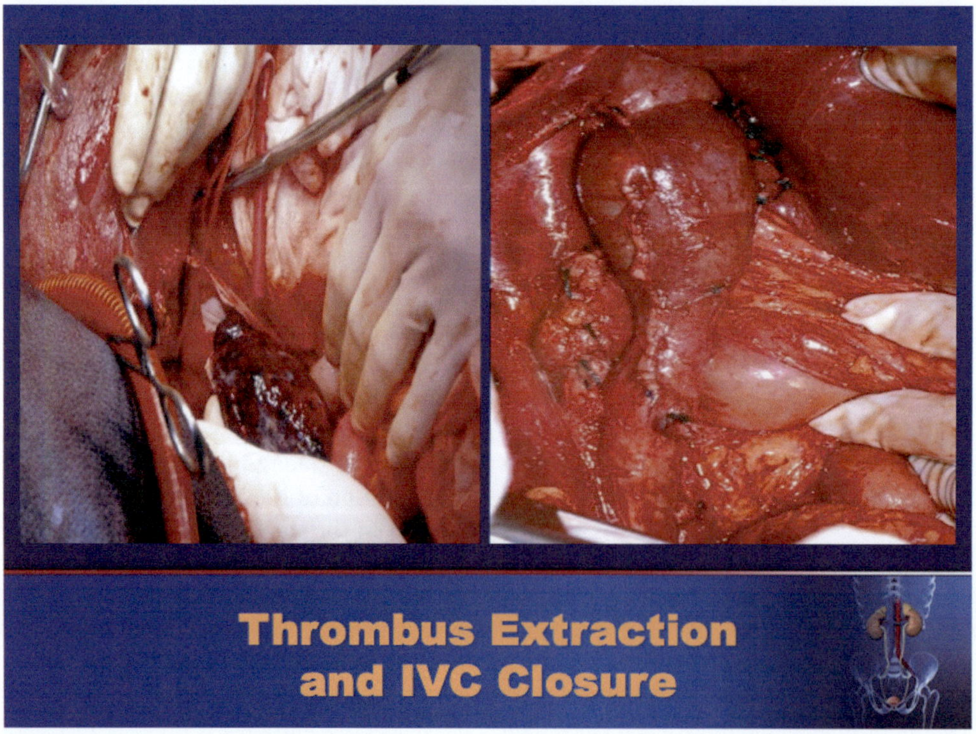

Fig. 15.27 Thrombus extraction and IVC closure

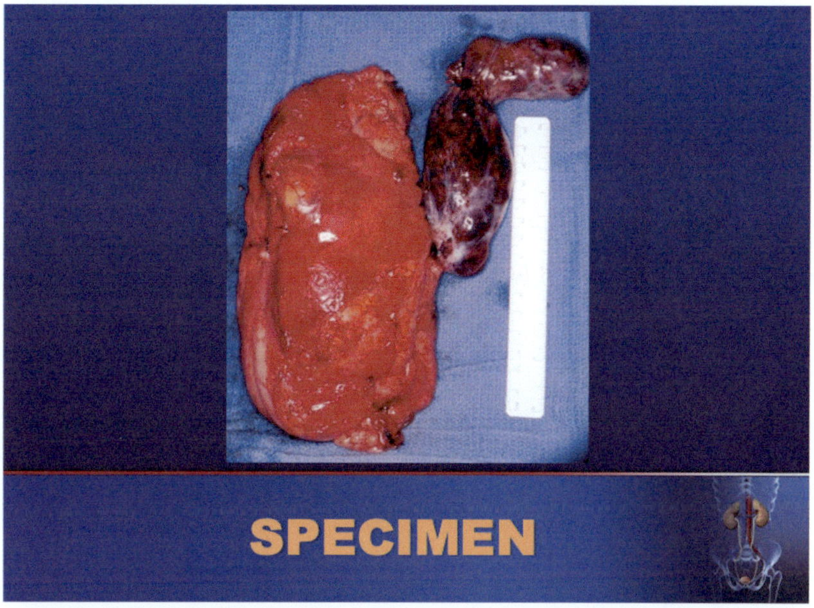

Fig. 15.28 Surgical specimen

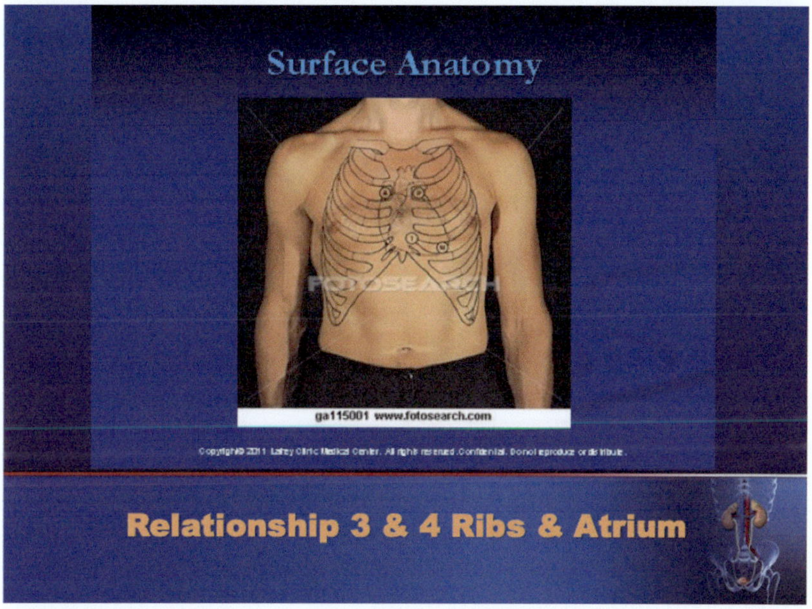

Fig. 15.29 Relationship with 3rd & fourth ribs and atrium

tion. A pericardial incision is made, and stay sutures are placed in the right atrium in anticipation for a formal atriotomy. An 8-mm synthetic graft is anastomosed to the previously exposed right subclavian artery as systemic heparinization is instituted. A two-staged venous cannula is inserted into the right atrium and directed into the superior vena cava tor venous return. Cardiopulmonary bypass and deep hypothermic circulatory arrest (DHCA) are initiated as discussed earlier (Fig. 15.30). After appropriate cooling, a formal atriotomy is made and the tumor thrombus is extracted from the heart. Now, complete exposure of the anterior surface of the IVC is achieved, again paying attention to potential bleeding that will resurface during rewarming of the heparinized patient. A cavotomy is performed and the tumor thrombus removed as

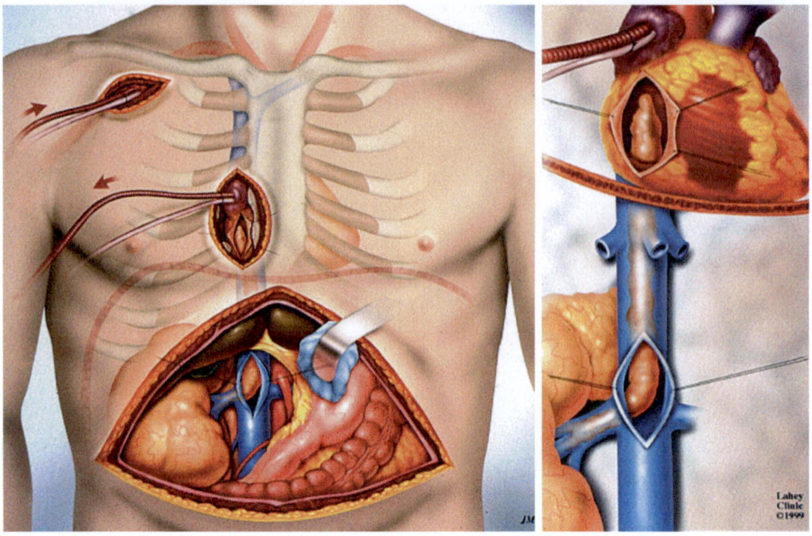

Fig. 15.30 Minimally invasive cardiopulmonary bypass for removal of a large right renal mass with tumor thrombus extending to the right atrium. Schematic demonstrates right subclavian artery graft and right atrial venous cannulation (Video 15.1)

described in the previous section. Radical nephrectomy is performed, after the IVC is closed, and at the same time the patient is being rewarmed, and while protamine sulfate, fresh frozen plasma, platelets, and desmopressin are administered in order to offset coagulopathies.

This approach obviates the need for extensive mobilization of the IVC reducing the risk of embolism, and reduces operating time in that the nephrectomy is carried out at the same time as the patient is being weaned off CPB and rewarmed following DHCA and CPB.

Comparative Effectiveness of Median Sternotomy (MS) Versus Minimal Access (MA) Cardiopulmonary Bypass and Circulatory Arrest for Resection of Renal Cell Carcinoma with Inferior Vena Caval and Cardiac Extension

We recently published our outcomes of cardiopulmonary bypass using the traditional median sternotomy (MS) vs minimal access (MA) surgery for patients with RCC above the level of the hepatic veins [27, 28]. From 1986 to 2012, 70 radical nephrectomies with concomitant inferior vena cava (IVC) thrombectomies (Level III & IV) were performed at our institution using median sternotomy ($n = 23$ patients) and minimal access technique ($n = 47$ patients). Preoperative patient characteristics, pathologic data, organ-specific postoperative complications and follow-up data were compared between these groups. Estimates of overall and recurrence-free survival were constructed using Kaplan–Meier curves and compared using log-rank testing.

There were no significant differences with respect to patient demographics or preoperative comorbid conditions between the minimal access (MA) and median sternotomy (MS) groups. The MA group showed a significant reduction ($P < 0.05$) in the duration of postoperative mechanical ventilation, length of ICU and hospital stay, decreased operative time, and the number of blood transfusions compared to MS patients. Overall and organ-system-specific complications demonstrated a decreased incidence of wound infection (37.9% v. 12.5%, $P = 0.0135$) and sepsis (14.3% v. 0%, $P = 0.0137$) in patients undergoing the MA approach. Perioperative mortality was significantly reduced in the MA group (30.4% v. 8.5% $P = 0.0179$). Recurrence-free survival in the MS group was 0.59 years and 1.2 years in the MA group ($P = 0.06$).

For all of the above reasons, since our original description of the MA technique in 1998, we have not performed the traditional median sternotomy approach and clearly prefer the

minimal access approach for cardiopulmonary bypass (CPB) and deep hypothermic circulatory arrest (DHCA) during the resection of RCC with extensive tumor thrombus, because it provides similar oncologic control with decreased duration of mechanical ventilation, length of stay, and infection-related complications. **We believe that our findings suggest that MA techniques provide significant advantages over MS and suggest its use to our surgical colleagues elsewhere as a safe and effective replacement of the MS approach.** These observations were confirmed in 2018 by Hua and colleagues in a multi institutional study in China (33).

Occluded Vasculature Management

In certain situations, there may be extensive tumor thrombus involving the contralateral renal vein, hepatic veins, or common iliac veins. In some situations, the thrombus may be of a bland vascular nature, secondary to venous stagnation, and is often easiest removed with gentle flushing. For adherent clot, we recommend using an endarterectomy spatula and Fogarty balloon catheters for removal. In theory, one could also utilize endoscopy techniques with stone basket retrieval systems although we have yet to personally need to perform this procedure. Bland thrombus is occasionally more difficult to remove from the venous system because of its gelatinous nature and adherence.

Caval Wall Resection and Caval Interruption

Regardless of the level of the tumor thrombus, one must inspect the caval wall for suspected invasion and perform a partial or complete resection. Studies suggest that invasion may be present in up to 23% of cases with the majority occurring at the renal vein ostium [13, 14, 19]. Caval reconstruction can be performed with synthetic patches (polytetrafluoroethylene) or biological substitutes (autologous saphenous vein or pericardial patches). During a right radical nephrectomy, if the IVC cannot be patched or replaced IT can be ligated or resected, provided the left renal vein is sacrificed distal to the gonadal, lumbar, and adrenal tributaries. Left renal masses with associated thrombus can undergo suprarenal IVC ligation only following procedures that allow right venous outflow (autotransplantation or saphenous interposition vein graft to the splenic, portal, or inferior mesenteric vein).

Minimally Invasive Techniques and Tumor Thrombectomy

Renal cell carcinoma with tumor thrombi limited to the renal vein can be treated with pure laparoscopic approaches in many instances, if room is available to place Hem-O-Lok clips without compromising the vena cava or risking a thrombotic event [20]. Laparoscopy has been utilized in the past with hand-assist for removal of IVC tumor thrombus, utilizing intraoperative ultrasound to identify the extent of the tumor thrombus [21]. Hand-assist provides a tactile advantage over pure laparoscopy that is crucial in some cases to confirm ultrasound estimates of tumor thrombus and assist in placing clamps involving the inferior vena cava. The Ohio State University group has published their results utilizing the da Vinci robot to treat five patients with tumor involving the inferior vena cava [22]. While Gill and other reports in the literature have explored the possibility of robotic radical nephrectomy and IVC thrombectomy and reconstruction, in my opinion, the risks outweigh the benefits of this approach. In addition, in my experience, the very large size of most of these renal tumors obviates the benefits of the minimally invasive approach for this clinical problem, as they will require a large incision for removal of the renal tumor. Finally, the potential complication of air embolism and the limited number of skilled minimally invasive surgeons capable of performing RCC and TT for level III & IV limits its general use.

Endovascular Downstaging: A New Approach, Combination of Interventional Radiologic Tumor Extraction and Surgery

A 53-year-old male, with a right renal cell cancer and IVC thrombus at the cavoatrial junction, unfortunately developed a pulmonary embolism, requiring catheter-directed thrombolysis therapy 2 weeks before being referred to us for surgery (fig. 15.31). Following our evaluation, the cardiothoracic surgeons were concerned about the possibility of a massive cytokine release from recently infarcted lung tissue resulting in death that might occur after cardiopulmonary bypass and circulatory arrest. The tumor was angio infarcted and the patient heparinized, in an effort to delay the needed surgery for 3 months. In spite of angio infarction, the patient began having severe gross hematuria requiring transfusions. He was reevaluated with cardiac ultrasound, and it was discovered that the IVC thrombus had grown into the right ventricle, in a very brief period of time (fig. 15.32).

This critical situation demanded a creative, novel approach. In conjunction with our interventional cardiologist, we were able to place the patient on an extracorporeal oxygen membrane (ECMO) device, whereupon the interventional cardiologist extracted the tumor thrombus from the right ventricle down to the level of the renal vein (figs. 15.33, 15.34). We were subsequently able to do a radical nephrectomy and IVC thrombectomy without the need of cardiopulmonary bypass and circulatory arrest, thus avoiding the expected massive cytokine storm. The patient did extremely well, and he is alive with disease 8 years following this new approach [29]. A link to the video of this procedure is listed below.

Endovascular downstaging combines the interventional cardiologists initial removal of tumor thrombus above the hepatic veins or diaphragm (level III & IV) with subsequent radical nephrectomy and IVC thrombectomy. The goal is to remove the tumor thrombus to a level below the level of the hepatic veins, making subsequent surgery easier and to eliminate the need for DHCA and CPB for level III and IV stage tumors. **This approach creates a new paradigm for the management of suprahepatic and supra diaphragmatic (level III & IV) tumors in properly selected patients**.

We recently reviewed our small series of four patients with Level 3 and Level 4 IVC tumor thrombus who underwent endovascular downstaging as an alternative to cardiopulmonary bypass and circulatory arrest.

The technique consists of the following: Placement of a transesophageal echocardiogram device for continuous monitoring during the procedure, the right internal jugular or femoral vein is accessed percutaneously, and an occlusive balloon catheter is inserted into the main pulmonary artery to prevent pulmonary embolism. Subsequently, an AngioVac system (Angiodynamics) is inserted into the vena cava or the heart as deter-

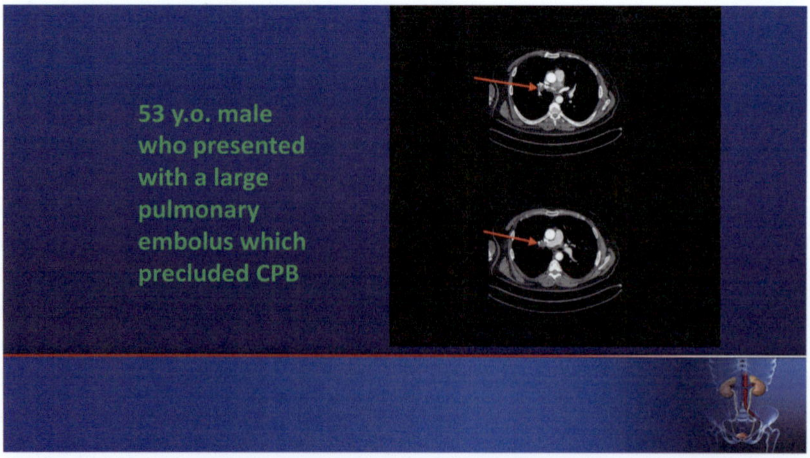

Fig. 15.31 Massive pulmonary embolism

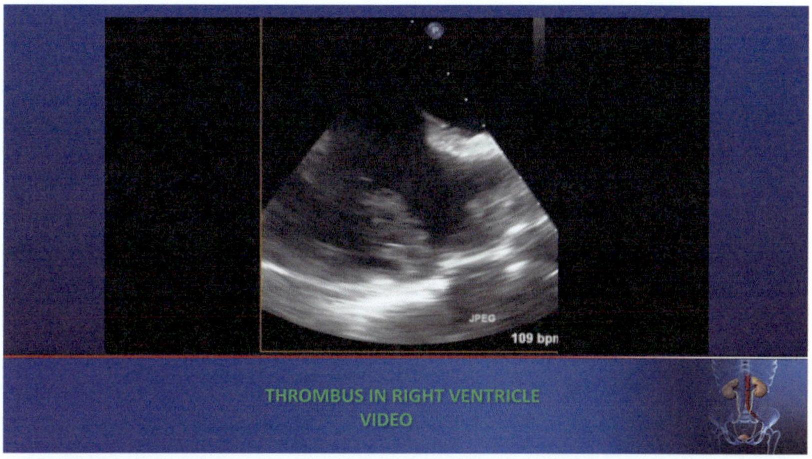

Fig. 15.32 Thrombus in the right ventricle abutting the pulmonary valve (Video 12)

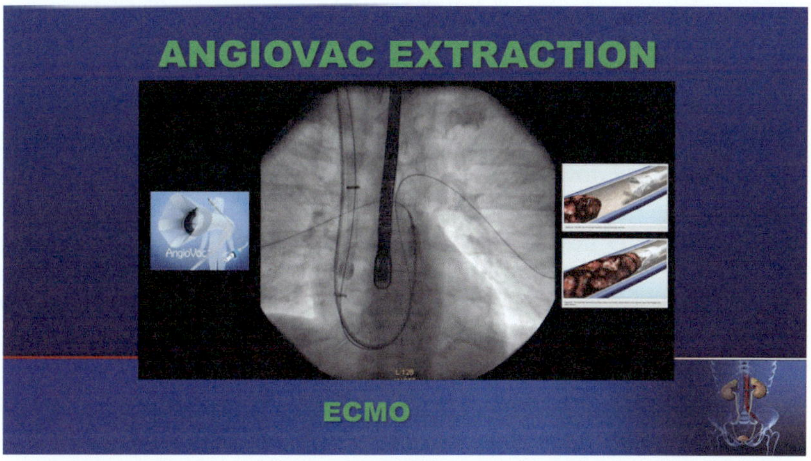

Fig. 15.33 Illustration of AngiVac procedure (Video 15.3)

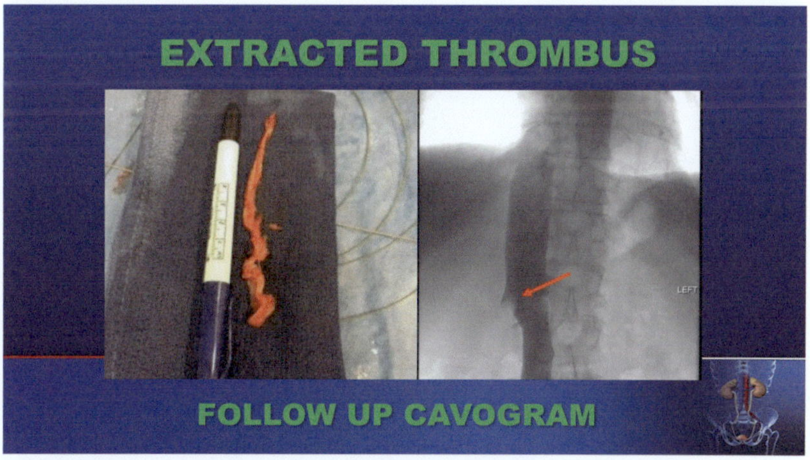

Fig. 15.34 Extracted tumor thrombus and post extraction cavogram (Video 15.3)

mined by the level of the tumor thrombus. In the initial case described above, the tumor thrombus extended into the right ventricle and ECMO was added to that procedure. In three other cases the tumor thrombus was evacuated to a level below the hepatic veins without ECMO. At a subsequent surgical procedure, resection of the remaining tumor thrombus and radical nephrectomy are accomplished (figs. 15.35, 15.36, 15.37).

We have compared the results achieved in these four patients with our own personal experience of 347 cases of venous invasion, 93 patients with tumors above the hepatic veins (Level III and IV), 70 of whom had undergone cardiopulmonary bypass and circulatory arrest. Because endovascular downstaging made the remaining infrahepatic vein IVC thrombectomy technically less difficult, it also eliminated cardiopulmonary bypass and circulatory arrest (thereby eliminating all of the potential complications); we found that **endovascular downstaging resulted in less complex surgery, shorter operating times, less blood loss, shorter hospital lengths of stay, and fewer surgical complications, thus resulting in less surgical morbidity and mortality and improved patient outcomes.**

We appreciate the complexity of managing RCC with IVC tumor thrombus. In a report from the Mayo Clinic, a large series of patients were reviewed from 1970 to2000 (34). Complications occurred in 15% of nephrectomies undergoing concomitant IVC thrombectomy. This study reported an increased rate of both major and minor complications proportional to the level of the tumor thrombus. For IVC tumor thrombus levels I to IV, adverse event rates were noted as 18%, 20%, 26%, and 47%, respectively. A 26% complication rate for level III and a 47% complication rate for level IV tumor thrombi is formidable, especially in the hands of this very experienced and respected surgical team. Among their most frequent complications were hemorrhage (3.0%), pulmonary embolism (2.7%), wound infection (2.6%), acute renal failure (1.8%), ileus (5.3%), and the need for additional surgery (3.6%).

Endovascular downstaging is a new, original concept we believe worthy of consideration, which reduces the surgical risk and surgical morbidity and mortality of these complex level III & level IV procedures, by lowering the level of the tumor thrombus, making the subsequent radical nephrectomy and inferior vena caval tumor thrombectomy easier and safer by eliminating DHCA and CPB.

In addition, it allows this life-saving surgery to be carried out in medical centers where cardiothoracic surgery is not available or when cardiopulmonary bypass is medically contraindicated.

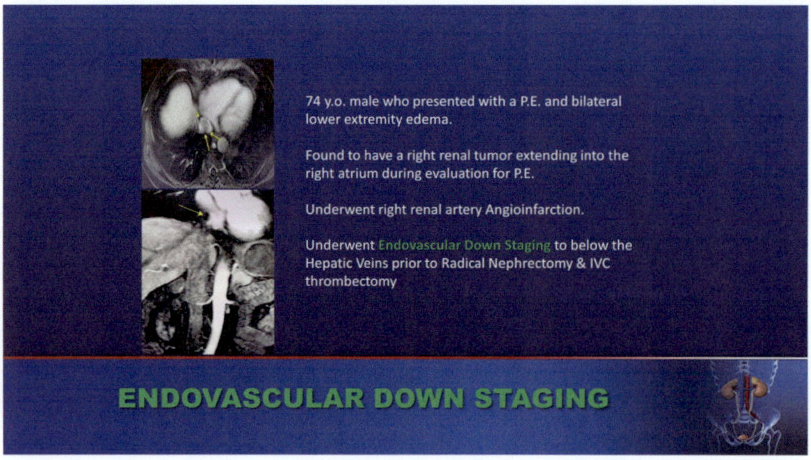

Fig. 15.35 A 74 y.o. patient with a level IV who underwent endovascular downstaging prior to radical nephrectomy and tumor thrombectomy of the remaining tumor below the hepatic veins

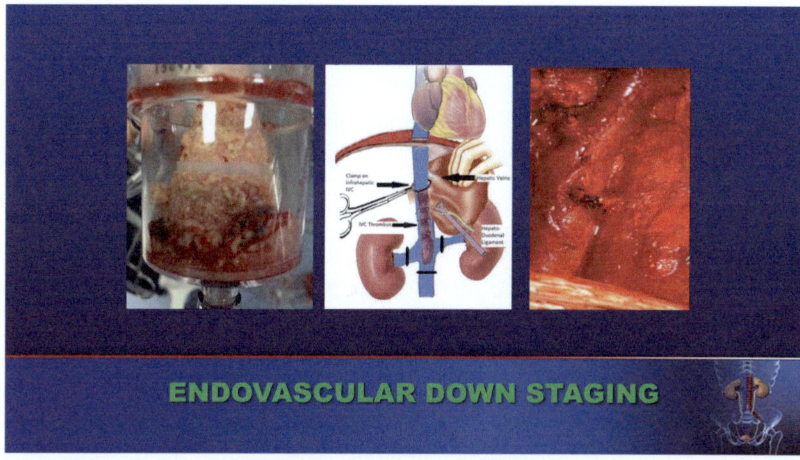

Fig. 15.36 Tumor aspirate collected by the AngioVac device, surgical approach for the remaining tumor thrombus and IVC closure

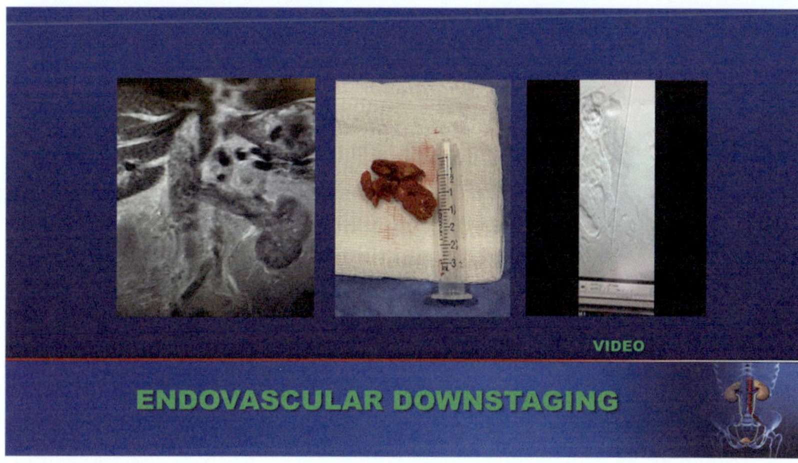

Fig. 15.37 A 84 y.o. female with a left renal tumor extending above the hepatic veins, who underwent endovascular downstaging and subsequent radical nephrectomy (Video 15.4)

Partial Nephrectomy and Tumor Thrombus

Radical nephrectomy (RN) with/without thrombus excision (ThE) is the undisputed standard treatment for kidney cancer (KC) with renal and/or caval thrombus (Th). However, partial nephrectomy (PN) ± ThE may be considered in rare cases when imperative indications exist.

The International RCC-IVC tumor thrombus consortium, founded in 2007, retrospectively reviewed our database of 3000 patients undergoing surgery for RCC with tumor thrombus at 23 institutions between 1971 and 2014. Primary outcomes analyzed were overall (OS) and cancer-specific survival (CSS), renal function variation after surgery, and complications. Secondary outcomes were predictors of OS and CSS for imperative partial nephrectomy cases (IPN). To reduce bias, the IPN group was matched with the RN using a propensity score algorithm on the basis of age, gender, tumor size, TNM, and histology.

Forty-two patients, reported by Giancarlo Marra and associates, underwent imperative partial nephrectomy and tumor thrombectomy. All thrombi were ≥ level I; five patients experienced Clavien ≥3 complications with two complication-related deaths. At 27.3 (IQR = 7.1–47.7) months OS and CSS were 54.8% and 78.6%, whereas at 9.7 (IQR = 1.4–43.7) months, eGFR change was −17.3 ± 27.0 mL/min. On univariate analysis tumor size, preoperative eGFR, transfusions, hospital stay, high serum creatinine, operating time (OT), complications, lymphadenectomy, and metastases related to an increased risk of death. After matching (n = 38 per arm), no significant differences were present except for tumor necrosis (IPN 39.5%; 15.8%; $P = 0.01$), thrombus level ($P = 0.02$), so too for OT ($P = 0.27$), perioperative transfusions ($P = 0.74$), and complications ($P = 0.35$). Five-year OS and CSS for imperative partial nephrectomy (IPN were 57.9% and 73.7%, respectively, with no significant differences with RN (OS 63.2 $P = 0.611$; CSS 68.4 $P > 0.99$). After 14.9 months, creatinine and eGFR changes were (+0.4 ± 0.6 mg/dL and − 23.2 ± 37.3 ml/min; $P = 0.2879$). It would appear that in unusual, highly selected cases due to imperative indications, partial nephrectomy and tumor extraction may be an alternative to radical nephrectomy, and tumor extraction for RCC with tumor thrombus, yielding noninferior oncological outcomes, functional outcomes, and complications. Further studies are needed to determine the role of partial nephrectomy and thrombus extraction (PN ± ThE) for RCC patients with a tumor thrombus [30].

At our institution, we have an extensive experience utilizing partial nephrectomy to preserve renal function, and have done several partial nephrectomies with renal vein involvement with good results; however, we would only advocate this approach with tumor thrombus in patients with imperative indications for partial nephrectomy, or with tumor involving the major branches of the renal vein with a patent main renal vein, or in a patient with a solitary kidney. However, the work of the International consortium, as well as Kim and colleagues, who described two surgical cases with solitary kidneys and tumor thrombus in the renal vein, that were spared hemodialysis and remained disease-free at 9 and 24 months, respectively, is noteworthy [23]. We applaud these outcomes; however, we recommend that surgeons undertaking this approach be familiar with extracorporeal bench surgery and renal autotransplantation.

Neoadjuvant Chemotherapy and Tumor Thrombus

As discussed earlier, on rare occasions, thrombus in the renal vein or IVC has dramatically decreased in size with the neoadjuvant use of improved chemotherapeutic agents and has resulted in downgrading in some instances. The hypervascular nature of these tumors makes them ideal targets for vascular endothelial growth factor (VEGF) inhibitors. A report from Takeda and colleagues discusses a case in which Sorafenib was used pre surgically resulting in a 43% regression in the size of the tumor thrombus, which retracted into the renal vein from the vena cava allowing nephrectomy to proceed [24]. Rini and colleagues recently published supportive phase II trial data in patients with renal vein or IVC extension with tumor shrinkage after neoadjuvant Sunitinib for locally advanced renal cell carcinoma [25]. Data from current investigational studies will help determine the appropriate timing of nephrectomy. The role of adjuvant chemotherapy and immunotherapy will be discussed in greater detail in other chapters in this textbook.

Tumor Thrombectomy and Metastectomy

Metastatic RCC has been shown in some patients to disappear following removal of the affected kidney, a concept known as the Lazarus effect. At our institution, we advocate removal of accessible pulmonary metastatic disease when possible. In most instances a pulmonary metastasectomy, first described by Barney and Churchill, for anterior lower lobe lesions is concomitantly performed with nephrectomy utilizing endovascular staplers and Doyen clamps [26]. We remain optimistic that nonpulmonary metastatic sites may become amenable to resection as we continue to see great strides in molecular-targeted chemotherapeutic agents. Our colleagues at the European Organization for Research and Treatment of Cancer are randomizing patients with metastatic disease to neoadjuvant Sunitinib, followed by nephrectomy and vice versa.

Personal Experience

The senior surgeon (JAL) of our group has treated 347 patients with renal cell carcinoma and renal vein or caval tumor thrombus. Tumor thrombus level of extension and survival outcomes data are illustrated in Figs. 15.38, 15.39, 15.40, 15.41, and 15.42. Our patient population includes a 2/3 male predominance with an average age of 62. Our complication and survival rates are well within the average of our contemporary colleagues at other major centers. One of our major contributions to managing these complex cases has been the implementation of a minimally invasive approach for cardiopulmonary bypass resulting in decreased blood loss, length of mechanical ventilation, analgesic requirements, duration of surgery, and hospital stay [28].

Another area of involvement in which we have personally participated in is the IRCC-IVC Tumor Thrombus Consortium. Dr. Juan I. Martinez-Salamanca and Dr. John A. Libertino formed the International IRCC-IVC Thrombus Consortium in 2007. The consortium now maintains a database for over 3000 patients, from 23 institutions around the globe, suffering from this condition. It is a very valuable resource for studying patients with RCC & IVC tumor thrombus.

International Renal Cell Carcinoma: Venous Thrombus Consortium (IRCC-VTC)

Many lessons have been learned as a result of the collaborative efforts of this international consortium and are best summarized in a recent publication from the consortium [31]. On the basis of the analysis of a clinical, surgical, and pathologic data set from the largest cohort of patients with RCC and venous involvement to date, several issues concerning prognostic factors, operative procedures, and surgical outcomes in this setting have been addressed.

Lessons learned from the consortium include the recognition of tumor thrombus anatomic level as an independent survival predictive factor, the confirmation of radical surgery as the mainstay of treatment for these patients even in the metastatic setting, the identification of papillary histological subtypes as a magnifier of oncologic risk when compared to other pathological subtypes, and the description of a direct relationship between the

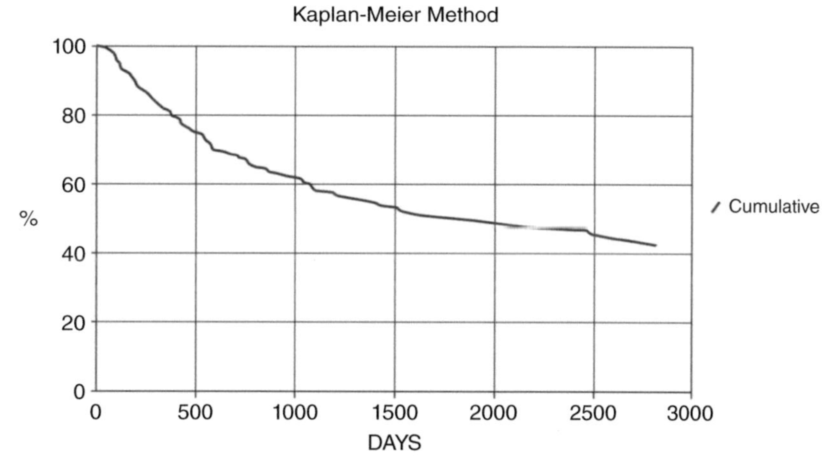

Fig. 15.38 Overall disease-specific survival ($n = 300$): median—18 months, mean—44 months

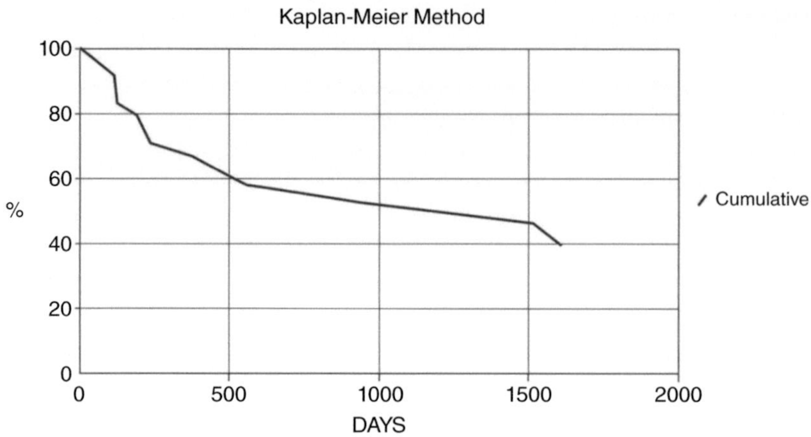

Fig. 15.39 Overall disease-specific survival—atrium ($n = 31$)

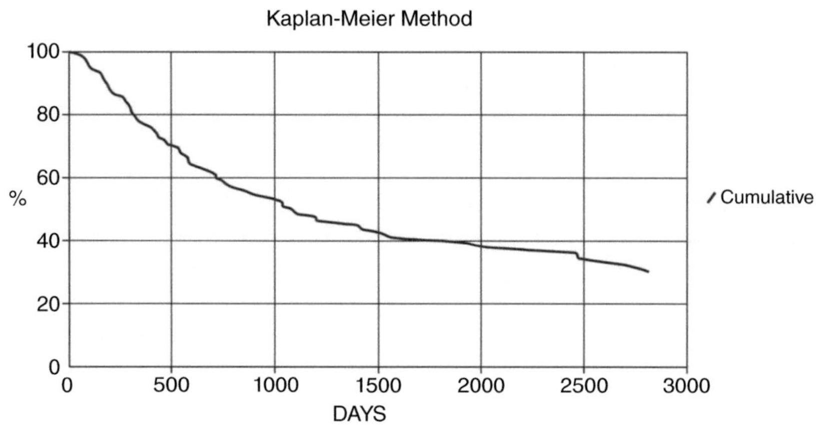

Fig. 15.40 Overall disease-specific survival—vena cava ($n = 146$)

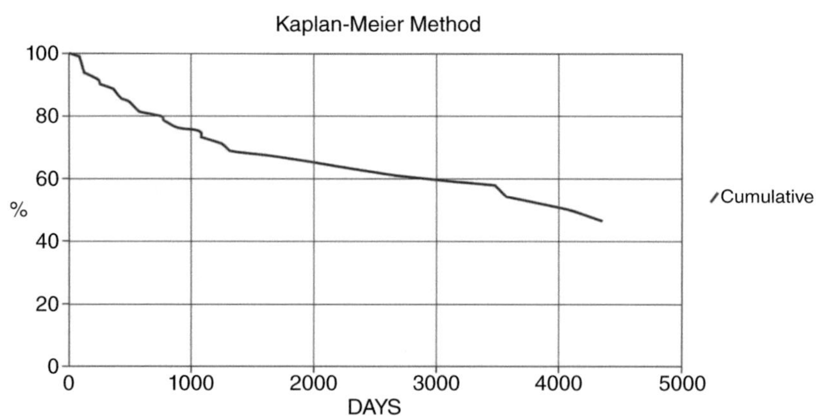

Fig. 15.41 Overall disease-specific survival—renal vein ($n = 123$)

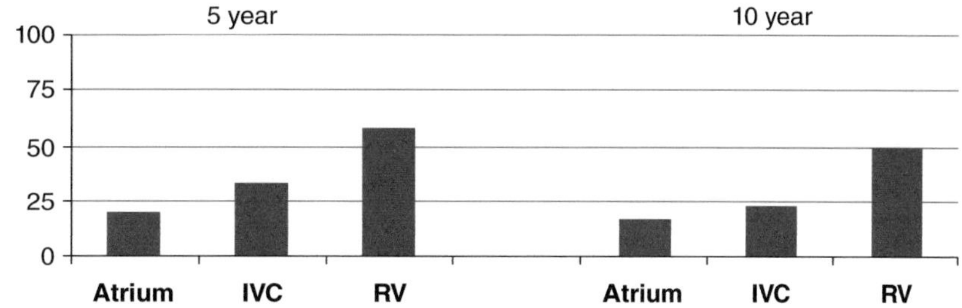

Fig. 15.42 Cancer-specific survival

tumor thrombus level and severity of complications, making this a strong predictor of perioperative complications in patients with RCC and tumor thrombus. The multinational, important work of this consortium must continue to unravel the complexities of managing patients with RCC and Venous extension.

References

1. Marshall VF, Middleton RG, Holswade GR, Goldsmith EI. Surgery for renal cell carcinoma in the vena cava. J Urol. 1970;103:414–20.
2. Scheft P, Novick AC, Strafton RA, Stewart BH. Surgery for renal cell carcinoma extending into the vena cava. J Urol. 1978;120:28–31.
3. Robson CJ, Churchill BM, Anderson W. The results of radical nephrectomy for renal cell carcinoma. J Urol. 1969;101:297–301.
4. Glaser A, Novick AC. Long-term follow-up after surgical treatment for renal cell carcinoma extending into the right atrium. J Urol. 1996;155:448–50.
5. Zisman A, Wieder JA, Pantuck AJ. Renal cell carcinoma with tumor thrombus extension: biology, role of nephrectomy and response to immunotherapy. J Urol. 2003;169:909 16.
6. Moinzadeh A, Libertino J. Prognostic significance of tumor thrombus level in patients with renal cell carcinoma and venous thrombus extension. Is all T3b the same? J Urol. 2004;171:598–601.
7. Kim HL, Belledegrun AS, Freitas DG. Paraneoplastic signs and symptoms of renal cell carcinoma: implications for prognosis. J Urol. 2003;170:1742–6.
8. Zini L, Destriuex-Garnier L, Leroy X. Renal vein ostium invasion of renal cell carcinoma with an inferior vena cava thrombus: prediction by renal and vena caval vein diameters and prognostic significance. J Urol. 2008;179(2):450–4.
9. Lam JS, et al. Evolving principles of surgical management and prognostic factors for outcome in renal cell carcinoma. J Clin Oncol. 2006;24:5565–75.
10. Nakano H, et al. Treatment of renal cancer patients by transcatheter embolization and its effects on lymphocyte proliferative responses. J Urol. 1983;130:24–7.
11. Bakke A, et al. Augmentation of natural killer cell activity after arterial embolization of renal carcinomas. Cancer Res. 1982;42:3880–3.
12. Schwartz MJ, et al. Renal artery embolization: clinical indications and experience from over 100 cases. BJU Int. 2006;99:881–6.
13. Libertino JA, Zinman L, Watkins E Jr. Long-term results of resection of renal cell cancer with extension into inferior vena cava. J Urol. 1987;137(1):21–4.
14. Swierzewski DJ, Swierzewski MJ, Libertino JA. Radical nephrectomy in patients with renal cell carcinoma with venous, vena caval and atrial extension. Am J Surg. 1994;168(2):205–9.
15. Kaag MG, Toyen C, Cronins RP. Radical nephrectomy with vena caval thrombectomy: a contemporary experience. BJU Int. 2010;107:1386–93.
16. Cianco G, Vaidya A, Savoie M. Management of renal cell carcinoma with tumor thrombus in the renal and inferior vena cava: the University of Miami experience in using liver transplantation techniques. Eur Urol. 2007;51(4):988–94.
17. Shahian DM, Libertino JA, Zinman LN, et al. Resection of cavoatrial renal cell carcinoma employing circulatory arrest. Arch Surg. 1990;125:727–31. Discussion 731–2
18. Fitzgerald JM, Tripathy U, Svensson LG, Libertino JA. Radical nephrectomy with vena caval thrombectomy using a minimal access approach for cardiopulmonary bypass. J Urol. 1998;159(4):1292–3.
19. Rabbani F, Hakimian P, Reuter V. Renal vain or inferior vena caval extension in patients with renal cortical tumors: impact of tumor histology. J Urol. 2004;172(3):1057–61.
20. Kapoor A, Nguan C, Al-Ahaiji T. Laparoscopic management of advanced renal cell carcinoma with level I renal vein thrombus. Urology. 2006;68(3):514–7.
21. Varkarakis I, Bhayani S, Allaf M. Laparoscopic-assisted nephrectomy with inferior vena cava tumor thrombectomy: preliminary results. Urology. 2004;64(5):925–9.
22. Abaza R. Initial series of robotic radical nephrectomy with vena caval tumor thrombectomy. Eur Urol. 2011;59:652–6.
23. Kim EH, Jain S, Bm B, Figneshau RS. Partial nephrectomy in two patients with known T3a tumours involving the renal vain. BJU Int. 2012;109(9):1345–8.
24. Takeda H, Nakano Y, Kashiwgi Y, Yoshino Y, Gotoh M. Downsizing a thrombus of advanced renal cell car-

cinoma in a presurgical setting with sorafenib. Urol Int. 2012;88:235–7.
25. Rini BI, Garcia J, Elson P, Wood L. The effect of sunitinib on primary renal cell carcinoma and facilitation of subsequent surgery. BJU Int. 2012;1987:1548–54.
26. Barney J, Churchill E. Adenocarcinoma of the kidney with metastases to the lung: cured nephrectomy and lobectomy. J Urol. 1939;42:269–76.
27. Wotkowicz C, Libertino JA, Sorcini A, Mourtzinos A. Management of renal cell carcinoma with vena cava and atrial thrombus: minimal access vs median sternotomy with circulatory arrest. BJU Int. 2006;98:289–97.
28. Faust W, D'Agostino R, Libertino J. Comparative effectiveness of median sternotomy vs minimal access cardiopulmonary bypass and circulatory arrest for resection of RCC with IVC extension. JCT. 2016;7(10):752–61.
29. Palmer D, Humpfrey J, Fredrick A, Piemonte T, Libertino J. Endovascular removal of intracardiac thrombus prior to radical nephrectomy and IVC thrombectomy. Urology. 2016;96:85–6.
30. Marra G, Bratttoli M, Gontero P, Libertino JA. Is imperative partial nephrectomy feasible for kidney cancer with venous thrombus involvement? Outcomes of 42 cases and matched pair analysis with a large radical nephrectomy cohort. Urol Oncol. 2018;36(7):339.e1–8.
31. Salamanca JI, Linares E, et al. Lessons learned from the International Renal Cell-Venous Thrombus Consortium (RCC-VTC). Curr Urol Rep. 2014;15:404.
32. Libertino, J.A. Renal cell carcinoma with extension into the vena cava. Chapter in Rob & Smith's operative surgery. McDougal, W.S. (Ed.), Fourth Edition Butterworth London, 1986.

Role of Lymphadenectomy in Renal Cell Cancer

16

Jacqueline Bultiauw, Mattias van Hattem, Maarten Albersen, Hendrik Van Poppel, and Eduard Roussel

Summary

Surgical extirpation of regional lymph nodes in the treatment of renal cell carcinoma (RCC) is still accepted as the most accurate staging procedure for the detection of lymphatic spread. However, the therapeutic benefit remains controversial. The renal lymphatic drainage is unpredictable, and the optimal extent of lymph node dissection (LND) is a matter of debate. Small lymph node metastases cannot be reliably visualized by the currently available imaging techniques. The prospective, randomized European Organization for Research and Treatment of Cancer trial (EORTC) 30881 showed that performing LND in patients with T1-T2 clinically node-negative (cN0) RCC offers limited staging information and no benefit in terms of decreasing disease recurrence or improving survival in patients undergoing radical nephrectomy. Several retrospective studies have suggested that high-risk patients with advanced or metastatic disease should undergo LND because of the important staging role of LND and because some of them might benefit from a therapeutic effect, however more recent studies contest a therapeutic benefit of LND, suggesting only a staging role of LND in the contemporary surgical management of RCC. In this chapter, the available evidence is summarized, and the implications for clinical practice of lymph node staging in RCC are discussed.

Introduction

After William S. Halsted demonstrated the efficacy of extensive surgical extirpation of regional lymph nodes (lymphadenectomy or lymph node dissection (LND)) for breast cancer in 1894, radical excision and regional LND gradually evolved as the standard of care for most carcinomas. Although LND has become an integral part of management for most other genitourinary malignancies, this has to date not been standardized in the management of renal cell carcinoma (RCC). Indeed, no data have clearly demonstrated which patients should undergo LND in the treatment of RCC, and which can be spared this adjunct surgical procedure. Despite decades of evaluation—since Robson and colleagues first reported increased survival in a small cohort of patients who underwent LND in 1969 [1]—the therapeutic benefit of LND in the management of RCC remains controversial. The increasing use of routine cross-sectional imaging techniques has resulted in the earlier diagnosis of incidental renal masses. Contemporary series suggest that the incidence of isolated lymph node metastases (pN+) in clinically localized disease is small (1–%) [2–6].

J. Bultiauw · M. van Hattem · M. Albersen (✉) ·
H. Van Poppel · E. Roussel
Department of Urology, University Hospitals Leuven, Leuven, Belgium
e-mail: jacqueline.bultiauw@student.kuleuven.be; maarten.albersen@uzleuven.be; hendrik.vanpoppel@kuleuven.be; eduard.roussel@uzleuven.be

J. A. Libertino, J. R. Gee (eds.), *Renal Cancer*, https://doi.org/10.1007/978-3-031-97599-8_16

The five-year overall survival (OS) in these patients with lymph node invasion is poor and ranges from 15% to 30% [3, 4, 7–9]. The anatomic localization of metastases is unpredictable due to the relatively heterogeneous metastatic spread of RCC through both hematogenous and lymphatic routes [10]. The absence of a therapeutic benefit of LND in patients with resectable, clinically node-negative localized renal tumors undergoing radical nephrectomy (RN), as reported in the phase III, prospective randomized European Organization for Research and Treatment of Cancer (EORTC) trial number 30881 [2] has created controversy regarding the usefulness and extent of LND, formerly considered mandatory surgery [1]. Moreover, patients in contemporary cohorts are more likely to undergo partial nephrectomy (PN) rather than RN and are less likely to undergo concomitant LND [11–13].

In a recent systematic review and meta-analysis, Bhindi et al. concluded that LND in RCC does not show a clear survival benefit in existing studies, despite biological reasoning for its potential [9]. In nonmetastatic RCC, removing all disease sites, including lymph nodes, may be curative. In metastatic RCC, reducing nodal disease could improve systemic therapy response and reduce immunological suppression. However, lymph node involvement often signals hidden systemic disease, even in nonmetastatic cases. Retroperitoneal lymphatic drainage, with connections to major veins, may explain RCC's blood-based spread. Furthermore, lymph node involvement in RCC is a poor prognostic factor, associated with a more aggressive disease course.

In this chapter, we assess the role of LND at the time of nephrectomy in patients with renal tumors. The main controversy is whether the role of LND is limited to a staging procedure or whether LND may prevent local recurrence and improve OS.

Anatomy of Regional Lymph Nodes

Historically, RCC has been associated with early hematogenous dissemination rather than a predictable lymphatic spread [10, 14–16]. The patterns of renal lymphatic drainage were initially described by Parker in 1935 [17], during anatomical studies of the posterior lymphatic channels of the abdomen. He found that the pathways of retroperitoneal drainage could be quite variable. Assouad et al. [16] confirmed the unpredictable anatomy of the renal lymphatic drainage. The most frequent lymphatic landing sites are paracaval and retrocaval nodes (right kidney), para-aortic and preaortic nodes (left kidney), and interaortocaval nodes (both right and left kidneys). Figure 16.1 shows a

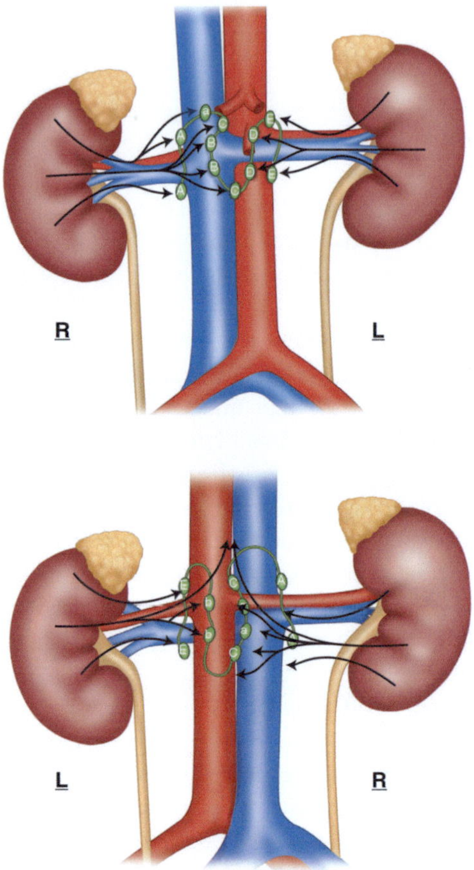

	Anterior Efferent Lymphatic Vessels	Posterior Efferent Lymphatic Vessels
Right Kidney	A. Paracaval B. Precaval C. Interaortocaval a. Retrocaval	A. Paracaval a. Retrocaval C. Interaortocaval - Thoracic duct
Left Kidney	D. Preaortic E. Para-aortic	D. Para-aortic b. Retroaortic - Thoracic duct

Fig. 16.1 Diagram illustrating the lymphatic vessels of the kidneys. The top image shows the anterior view, with labeled lymph nodes and vessels connecting the kidneys to the central lymphatic system. The bottom image displays the posterior view, highlighting similar structures

summary of the anatomical review of the lymphatic drainage of the kidney. However, in one-third of the patients, renal lymphatics have been found draining directly, without passing through any lymph nodes, into the thoracic duct [16]. Brouwer and colleagues confirmed this direct lymphatic drainage into the thoracic duct for the first time in vivo in humans [18]. They reported on four patients where early lymphatic drainage was visualized along the course of the thoracic duct using lymphoscintigraphy and single photon emission computed tomography (SPECT/CT). In one patient, this was observed without any retroperitoneal lymph node interposition. Saitoh, in an autopsy study of 1828 cases of renal cancer, observed extremely wide variation in the anatomic localization of lymph node metastases from RCC. There was a low incidence of metastases to the ipsilateral adrenal and renal hilar lymph nodes in nephrectomy cases [14]. In another autopsy study, analyzing 554 patients with renal cancer, Johnsen and Hellsten [19] found lymph node metastases in 80 patients (14%), of which 75 had additional distant metastases. Exclusively paracaval or para-aortic positive lymph nodes were noted in only five patients (0.9%). Therefore, the therapeutic benefit of extensive retroperitoneal LND in association with RN is likely to be low. However, more limited LND may be useful, mainly as a staging procedure to inform disease prognosis [19]. The predilection of RCC for early hematogenous dissemination without lymph node infiltration has been shown in several other studies [16, 18, 20, 21]. Vasselli et al. reported an incidence of 53% of distant metastasis without lymph node invasion (LNI) [15]. In a more recent study, of 797 patients with metastatic RCC treated with cytoreductive nephrectomy and LND, 57% were found to have no lymph node metastases [22]. This hematogenous dissemination was confirmed by Capitanio et al. in 2016 [20]. A later study by Kuusk et al. in 2018 observed lymphatic drainage to be outside the locoregional retroperitoneal templates in 35% and one in five patients had supradiaphragmatic sentinel nodes [21].

Scope of Lymph Node Dissection and Oncological Outcomes

Currently, there is no consensus on the anatomic extent of LND for RCC management [23]. Most of the studies available report only the presence or the absence of a nonstandardized, surgeon-related LND.

The limits of the extended LND (eLND) during RN for RCC have changed over the years. In 1969, Robson and colleagues [1] included an eLND and demonstrated a 22.7% incidence of positive lymph nodes. They supported the removal of the para-aortic and paracaval lymph nodes from the bifurcation of the aorta to the crus of the diaphragm as an essential element of RN. They suggested that the improved survival was due in part to this retroperitoneal LND. It is reasonable that a template for LND should be based on the primary lymphatic drainage of the kidney and the location of metastatic disease observed in surgical series [24].

Templates proposed for eLND for tumors on the right kidney included the hilar, para-, pre-, retro-, and interaortocaval lymph nodes, whereas for left-sided tumors, inclusion of the hilar para-, pre-, and retro-aortic, and interaortocaval lymph nodes was recommended [25]. Figure 16.2 shows an eLND after removal of the specimen (Fig. 16.2a) and the specimen with RN and "en bloc" LND (Fig. 16.2b). Crispin et al. [24] proposed a standard surgical template for LND based on the locations of lymph node involvement. Of the 169 high-risk RCC patients who underwent LND in conjunction with nephrectomy, 64 patients (38%) had lymph node metastases. Of these 64 patients, 29 (45%) had no metastases in the perihilar lymph nodes, demonstrating the poor staging ability of a hilar-only node dissection. The authors recommend that when performing an LND, the paracaval and interaortocaval lymph nodes are removed in patients with right-sided tumors and the para-aortic and interaortocaval lymph nodes are removed from the crus of the diaphragm to the common iliac artery.

Although there are no formal rules regarding the extent and boundaries of LND at the time of

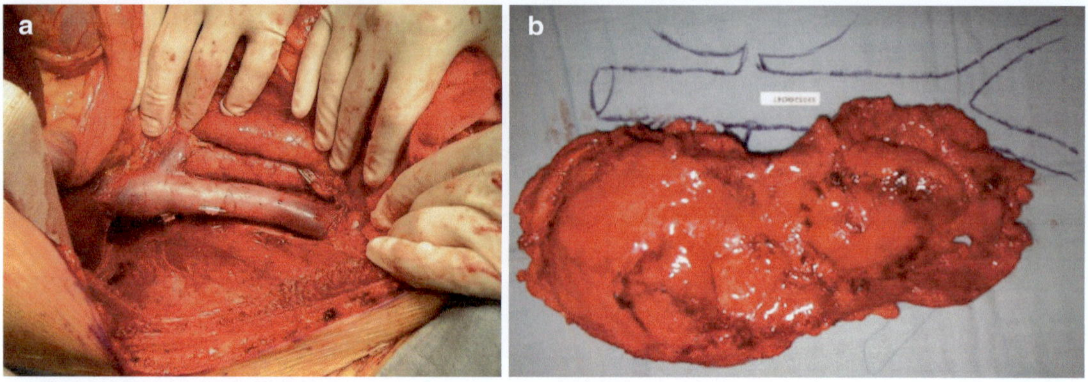

Fig. 16.2 (**a**) Extended lymph node dissection, view after removal of the specimen. (**b**) Specimen with radical nephrectomy and "en bloc" lymph node dissection

RN, the staging accuracy of LND can be improved if the template for LND is extended compared to limited node sampling [26–30]. Herrlinger et al. retrospectively compared outcomes of 320 patients who underwent eLND with data of 191 patients who underwent only "facultative" LND (removal of no or only a few nodes for staging purposes) to evaluate whether the extent of LND had any significant effect on survival outcomes [26]. They concluded that eLND improves the prognosis of RCC patients without any additional morbidity and suggest that eLND is superior compared to facultative LND. Terrone et al. [27] and Joslyn et al. [29] found a positive correlation between the increasing number of nodes examined and the number of positive lymph nodes (LNs) detected. According to Terrone et al., at least 13 nodes should be excised to provide adequate staging. They reviewed the reports of 725 patients with RCC submitted for RN [27]. When ≥13 lymph nodes were removed, the rate of pN+ increased from 10.2% to 20.8% ($P < 0.001$). Schafhauser et al. found a similar cutoff of 14 lymph nodes [28]. Capitanio et al. reported that, when clinically indicated, staging LND in RCC should be extended [30]. According to Capitanio et al., extended lymph node dissection (LND) is clinically indicated when unfavorable clinical or pathological features are evident, either at diagnosis or during surgery. These scenarios include suspected nodal metastases identified through preoperative imaging, advanced pathological features such as higher tumor stages (e.g., pT3–4), larger tumor sizes, high Fuhrman grades, presence of lymphovascular invasion, or the presence of aggressive histological traits like coagulative tumor necrosis or sarcomatoid differentiation. This study suggests that the removal of 15 lymph nodes is the minimum threshold for deeming a staging LND adequate. Moreover, they stated that the greatest accuracy in staging the disease is achieved when about 20 LNs are removed. Their study, however, did not report on the impact on survival of (extended) LND.

The required number of lymph nodes examined to provide optimal nodal staging is not well defined by the American Joint Committee on Cancer (AJCC) staging manual, while the European Association of Urology (EAU) recommends that at least 15 LNs should be removed to obtain adequate staging information [31].

Disagreement continues about the ideal limits of LND. Whitson et al. (2011) analyzed the Surveillance, Epidemiology, and End Results (SEER) database and found that increasing the number of lymph nodes removed significantly improved disease-specific survival in lymph node-positive, nonmetastatic RCC patients [32]. Increasing lymph node yield by ten nodes was associated with a 10% absolute increase in 5-year cancer-specific survival (CSS) in this subset of patients; however, the study has notable limitations, including potential misclassification in the node-negative group due to low lymph node yields, lack of critical data in the SEER database (e.g., performance status, comorbidities, lymphadenectomy templates, and adjuvant therapy), and the absence of clinical node status, which raises methodological concerns and limits the generalizability of results based on pathological node status [2, 32]. More recently, Capitanio et al. reported improved CSS with a greater extent of LND among patients with pT2, pT3c-pT4 tumors, or tumors with sarcomatoid features [5]. Conversely, Gershman et al. recently reported no association of the extent of LND with oncologic outcomes [6]. In another study based on the SEER database (2004–2014), Dong et al. found that in lymph node-negative clear cell RCC (ccRCC) patients, removing three or more lymph nodes significantly improved OS. Patients who had three or more nodes removed had a 5-year OS of 93%, compared to 83% for those with fewer than three [33]. In a population of patients with nonmetastatic pT2–3Nany RCC from the SEER database (2001–2013), those who underwent RN with or without LND were studied [35]. In this cohort, a higher number of removed nodes were associated with improved cancer-specific mortality, including pT2 and subgroups, although this was not the case for patients with clear cell histology. According to their findings, the number of positive nodes is associated with higher cancer-specific mortality in pT3 patients. Consequently, LND and its extent appear to provide little therapeutic benefit for pT2–3NanyM0 patients, apart from their prognostic significance.

A study by Tachibana et al. included 45 non-metastatic RCC patients with 1 or 2 positive lymph nodes, comparing outcomes of limited LND and template retroperitoneal lymph node dissection (RPLND) [34]. Median lymph nodes removed were significantly higher in the RPLND group (18 vs. 4). Patients undergoing RPLND had better median OS (27.39 vs. 17.07 months) and a higher 5-year OS rate (60.3% vs. 39.3%). These results highlight improved survival with more extensive lymph node removal. The differences in CSS and recurrence-free survival (RFS) did not reach statistical significance. Nevertheless, there was a trend toward improved CSS and RFS in the template RPLND group. Recurrence analysis revealed that six patients in the limited LND group developed retroperitoneal lymph node recurrences in the ipsilateral node packet, suggesting that template RPLND might have provided additional benefit. For left-sided tumors, a template RPLND involved the removal of para-aortic nodes, with dissection boundaries extending from the crus of the diaphragm superiorly, the left ureter laterally, the aorta medially, and the common iliac artery inferiorly. For right-sided tumors, paracaval and inter-aortocaval nodes were removed, with the dissection boundaries defined by the crus of the diaphragm superiorly, the right ureter laterally, the aorta medially, and the right common iliac artery inferiorly. The choice to perform a template RPLND was left at the surgeon's discretion. This decision was guided by factors including suspected nodal disease on preoperative imaging, detection of abnormal nodes during surgery, the aggressive nature of the primary tumor, and the patient's overall health and ability to withstand a more extensive procedure. The study by Rosiello et al. highlighted the crucial role of eLND in patients with clinically node-positive (cN1) renal cell carcinoma (RCC) [35]. It was observed that 50% of cN1 patients had pathologically confirmed lymph node metastases upon performing eLND. Identifying pathological node-positive (pN1) patients could not only allow for more precise follow-up strategies but could potentially guide the use of adjuvant therapies in the future [36]. Additionally, the study revealed that among cN1 patients, only 24% had pathologically confirmed lymph node metastases within the anatomically suspicious area identified on preoperative imaging. In contrast, 18% of patients exhibited metastases both within and outside this anatomical field, and 8% showed metastases exclusively outside the field. These results suggest that limiting LND to the suspicious anatomical area would fail to properly stage more than 50% of pathological node-positive (pN1) patients. Patients with LNs measuring 4 cm or more had a substantially higher risk (ranging from 20% to over 70%) of harboring pN1 disease outside the suspicious anatomical field. Their analyses showed that the occurrence of lymph node metastases varies based on the preoperative nodal stage observed on CT scans. Specifically, in patients with cN1 disease, 50% had confirmed pN1 status, whereas only 6.5% of those with cN0 disease at preoperative imaging were pN1.

Nevertheless, selection bias in these reports cannot be excluded and any recommendation regarding the optimal extent of LND in RCC treatment is based on a low level of evidence.

Morbidity of LND

Several studies evaluated the perioperative morbidity of LND [2, 7, 37–39], none of these studies reported an increased perioperative morbidity for LND. However, unmeasured confounding may impact the observed results since none provided adjusted effect estimates. The prospective, randomized EORTC 30881 trial reported an overall complication rate of 22% and 26% for surgery without or with LND respectively [2]. The most common complications associated with the surgical treatment of RCC are lymphocele, chylous ascites, bleeding from lumbar or major vessels, and damage to adjacent organs. However, it is difficult to determine a direct correlation between these surgical complications with the LND procedure. Compared to nephrectomy alone, nephrectomy associated with LND did not significantly increase morbidity. Only a slightly higher risk of bleeding was observed among those undergoing LND. LND remains a highly complex procedure and should be performed by well-trained surgeons. A recent study by Gershman et al. [39] reported that LND at the time of RN was associated with an overall complication rate of 9% and a 4% rate for Clavien-Dindo grade ≥3 complications. In this study, LND was not associated with 30-day complications or prolonged hospitalization. Likewise, in another recent study (a secondary analysis of the ASSURE trial investigating the use of adjuvant sunitinib or sorafenib in localized RCC), there was no difference in complication rates between patients who did and did not undergo LND [38].

With the increased use of minimally invasive techniques, there has been some concern about the limited use of LND and about difficulties in performing an adequate laparoscopic LND that may negatively impact treatment outcomes. However, a report by Chapman et al. [37] showed that laparoscopic LND in clinically node-negative patients undergoing nephrectomy for RCC is feasible and safe and may improve staging accuracy. A mean of 12.1 nodes were recovered using an eLND. The overall risk of intraoperative and postoperative complications was similar between the group undergoing laparoscopic RN with LND and the group without LND.

In the study conducted by Tachibana et al. [34], a total of 45 patients with one or two isolated lymph nodes underwent radical nephrectomy with curative intent for locally advanced renal cell carcinoma. Among these patients, 23 received limited LND, while 22 underwent template RPLND. The operative techniques were distributed as follows: Laparoscopic (3 limited, 0 extended), Robotic (4 limited, 2 extended), and Open (16 limited, 20 extended). Within the template RPLND cohort, only one patient had a bilateral dissection, with the remainder undergoing ipsilateral procedures. The minimally invasive laparoscopic approach was more frequently used in the limited LND dissection group. No statistically significant differences were observed in operative time, estimated blood loss, perioperative mortality, or length of stay. However, the limited LND group exhibited a higher incidence of Clavien grade 3 or greater complications. Notably, grade 4 complications included severe events such as respiratory failure, pneumothorax, fascial dehiscence, and the need for hemodialysis. Additionally, two patients experienced postoperative mortality, with the majority of serious complications, classified as Clavien grade 4 or 5, occurring in those who had undergone inferior vena cava (IVC) thrombectomy within the limited LND group. Importantly, based on the findings, they observed no significant differences in surgical outcomes between the template RPLND and limited LND groups, indicating that incorporating a templated RPLND into nephrectomy is both feasible and safe.

Imaging for the Detection of Lymph Node Invasion

Currently, imaging techniques are unable to accurately identify patients with micrometastases in normal-sized lymph nodes who could benefit from LND [40, 41]. Therefore, the absence of any evident lymph node metastasis with modern imaging technology should not formally rule out a regional LND. Figure 16.3a, b shows an LND for CT-scan suspicious nodes, in conjunction with PN. In the detection of microscopic LNI, CT scans can give both false-positive and false-negative images [20, 42]. Studer et al. reviewed CT scans of 163 patients with RCC to evaluate the predictive value for the diagnosis of regional lymph node metastases. False-negative CT scans were found in five patients: two had metastatic nodes in the renal hilus, and three had micrometastases in nodes <1 cm. In 43 CT scans, enlarged lymph nodes with a diameter of 1–2.2 cm (median 1.4 cm) were observed. Only 18 of the 43 patients (42%) had lymph node metastases. In 58%, the enlarged lymph nodes showed only inflammatory changes and/or follicular hyperplasia (false positivity). This finding was significantly more frequent in patients with renal vein invasion and tumor necrosis [42]. Demir et al. [43] report that current imaging techniques have a false-negative rate of approximately 10%, suggesting that micrometastases may be more common than detected. They also note that while lymph nodes larger than 2 cm in the abdomen or retroperitoneal area are often indicative of malignancy on computed tomography, pathological confirmation is crucial. Reactive lymph nodes frequently cause false-positive results. A study by Studer et al. [42] found that only 42% of patients were accurately diagnosed. Capitanio et al. [20] performed a systematic analysis of 2954 patients who underwent RN or PN for RCC. Preoperative axial CT scans revealed 424 patients showing at least one enlarged lymph node, i.e., cN1 disease. Of those, LNI (i.e., pN1 disease) was pathologically confirmed in only 122 patients (28.8%). However, a recent study by Connolly et al. [44] suggested a sufficient accuracy of modern CT scan predicting metastasis within regional lymph nodes. They reported sensitivity, specificity, positive and negative predictive values of 82, 71, 56, and 90% respectively. Despite these findings, the overall consensus remains that currently it is not possible to preoperatively differentiate LNI from enlarged inflammatory nodes by using the existing imaging techniques [20, 23, 45]. These studies support the need for eLND in patients where accurate staging is important.

In a study from Muttin et al. [46], they mention that several series have evaluated the likelihood of metastatic nodal disease based on radiologic lymph node size greater than 1 cm. Furthermore, in a previous report of the same group, LNI was pathologically confirmed in less than 30% of patients with clinical suspicion of LNI. Consequently, several predictive models were developed to predict pathologically positive lymph nodes, thus reducing false-positive or false-negative results. Gershman et al. demonstrated that only the maximum lymph node short diameter at imaging had excellent predictive performance on pN1 disease [47]. The area under the receiver operating characteristic curve (AUC) of this predictor was 0.84. In this series, the observed percentage of lymph node metastases

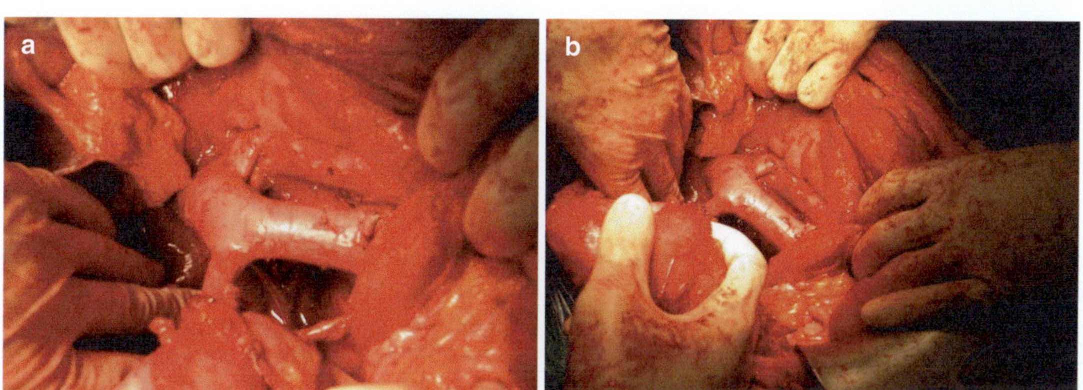

Fig. 16.3 (**a**) Lymph node dissection for CT-scan suspicous nodes, in conjunction with partial nephrectomy. (**b**) Lymph node dissection for CT-scan suspicious nodes, in conjunction with partial nephrectomy

was 20, 29, and 90% for lymph nodes 7, 10, and 30 mm in short-axis size, respectively. Considering the cT stage, the observed percentage of lymph node metastases was 1, 33, and 38% for cT1–2, cT3a, and cT3b–4, respectively. A multivariable model consists of maximum LN short-axis diameter and radiographic perinephric/sinus fat invasion. This model predicted pN1 disease with an AUC of 0.85.

Muttin et al. found that inflammatory lymphadenopathies were associated with unfavorable clinical and pathological characteristics, as well as a 2.4-fold increased cancer-specific mortality in univariable analyses. However, after adjusting for potential confounders, the presence of inflammatory lymphadenopathies did not significantly impact CSM and did not achieve independent predictor status for survival [46].

Radadia et al. [48] reported a sensitivity of 67% and a specificity of 95% in clinical staging for detecting pathological lymph node positivity (pLN) in patients undergoing lymph node dissection (LND), with a negative predictive value (NPV) of 94% for cLN-negative patients and a positive predictive value (PPV) of 74% for cLN-positive patients. These findings, consistent with Conolly et al. [44], support a strong association between clinical (cN) and pathological (pN) nodal statuses when assessed via CT imaging. However, the methodology for determining cLN status within the national cancer database (US) remains unclear, as this database does not specify the imaging modality employed by physicians. This limitation complicates the interpretation of cLN staging accuracy, potentially affecting the generalizability of these findings [48]. While clinically positive lymph nodes (cLN) significantly increase the likelihood of LND being performed, cT stage was the strongest predictor for LND among cLN-negative patients. In both cLN-positive and cLN-negative cohorts, the likelihood of undergoing LND rose with increasing cT stage, aligning with the clinical rationale that patients with more advanced tumors may benefit from LND due to an elevated risk of microscopic nodal disease. This highlights the importance of precise cLN staging and improved imaging for effective RCC management. Gershman et al. identified that predictors of pathological node-positive (pN1) disease in RCC include larger retroperitoneal lymph nodes and signs of perinephric or sinus fat invasion observed on CT imaging [47]. Babaian et al. looked at other preoperative clinical factors that can predict positive pLN via a nomogram, including lactate dehydrogenase, cLN status, local symptoms, and performance status [49].

The use of positron emission tomography (PET)/CT imaging for detecting lymph node metastases in RCC has been explored to a limited extent, and its current application remains constrained [35]. While novel tracers such as radiolabeled girentuximab and [18F]-FDG have demonstrated potential for characterizing renal masses and detecting nodal or distant metastases, PET/CT is primarily used in research settings [50]. Despite its promising specificity and sensitivity in some studies, the high false-positive rate and increased radiation exposure limit its practicality for routine RCC staging. Current guidelines do not recommend its use for RCC staging based on available evidence, further emphasizing the reliance on conventional imaging methods as the standard for assessing nodal involvement [35].

Prevalence of Lymph Node Metastasis

The incidence of lymph node metastasis has decreased over time, most likely due to increased tumor detection resulting in surgery being performed in earlier disease stages [51]. The early study of Robson et al. (1969) and the later published EORTC 30881 study of Blom et al. (2009) reported an incidence of positive lymph nodes of 22.7% and 4%, respectively [1, 2].

In most historical series, the incidence of positive lymph nodes among patients undergoing RN and LND ranges from 23% to 35% [1, 52]. In contemporary series, smaller asymptomatic lesions are diagnosed with rising frequency, and the prevalence of LNI has decreased significantly [13]. Nowadays, the incidence of pN+ in a low-risk population of clinically node and metastasis negative (cN0M0) patients ranges from 1% to 5% [2–4, 45].

Higher clinical stage and higher pathological tumor grade are associated with higher rates of positive nodes. Giuliani et al. reported 13.2% and 36.1% positive nodes in stage pT1–2 and pT3–4, respectively [53]. Pantuck et al. observed 5.2% and 23.4% positive nodes for T1–2 and T3–4, respectively. They reported nodal metastasis in 32% of Fuhrman grade 1–2 tumors and in 68% of grade 3–4 tumors [7]. Sun et al. and Capitanio et al. reported similar findings of increasing prevalence of LNI with increasing tumor stage and grade [4, 5]. In another study, Capitanio et al. reported that the percentage of LNI remained stable over time for locally advanced disease, 12% against 12% in 1988–1996 and 2008–2014, respectively [13]. Blute et al. noted on a multivariate analysis that the risk of dying from RCC was 7.87-fold higher with LNI at nephrectomy than without [3]. Tilki et al. confirmed this worse CSS for LNI at nephrectomy in a cohort of patients with RCC and tumor thrombus. They showed a significantly worse 5-year CSS for pN1 patients compared to pN0- and pNx patients, 22.6%, 68.3%, and 62.5% respectively [54]. Finally, Pantuck et al. reported that patients who did not undergo LND were three times more likely to die than those who did undergo LND. Recurrence rates were similar regardless of the extent of LND [7].

Farber et al. [53] suggest that LND may be overused, particularly in patients with lower-stage RCC. They refer to an earlier study indicating that lymph node metastasis rates range from 13% to 21% across all RCC stages, with higher stages showing a greater incidence. For instance, Capitanio et al. analyzed 3507 patients and found that only 1.1% of those with stage T1 disease and 2.3% of those with stage T2 disease had positive lymph nodes. In contrast, Farber et al.'s analysis showed that 5% of stage T1 patients and 23% of stage T2 patients underwent LND.

Predicting Lymph Node Involvement

Several series indicate that lymph node metastasis is one of the most significant prognostic factors for survival in patients with RCC [1, 7, 8, 29, 54, 55]. The great challenge is to accurately identify those patients who would most benefit from LND.

Protocols and Nomograms

Different clinical predictive tools have been proposed in RCC to identify those patients at risk of harboring LNI. Blute et al. retrospectively reviewed an institutional cohort of 1652 patients from the Mayo Clinic surgically treated for clinically nonmetastatic (M0) ccRCC (68/1652 or 4.1% were pN+). They developed an intraoperative risk factor protocol to predict the probability of regional LNI based on metastatic risk. On multivariate analysis, the primary tumor pathological features of nuclear grade (Fuhrman 3 or 4), tumor size ≥10 cm, pathological stage pT3 or pT4, sarcomatoid differentiation, and the presence of coagulative tumor necrosis can be used to predict patients at the greatest risk for regional LNI at RN [3]. If two or more of these five features are present in the primary tumor, there is a 15-fold higher incidence of N+. Moreover, the same authors recently validated their results in an updated series of 169 patients who received LND in conjunction with nephrectomy for high-risk RCC. Lymph node metastases were identified in 64 (38%) patients. When two or more of the five primary tumor pathological features were identified during surgery, patients were considered high risk for nodal metastasis and LND was performed at the time of nephrectomy [24]. The challenge with applying this protocol is that its utility is limited in routine clinical practice, as frozen section analysis to assess risk features is not available at all institutions [40]. Hutterer et al. [56] developed a preoperative nomogram based on patient age, symptom classification, and tumor size to predict the probability of LNI. On multivariate analysis, only tumor size and symptom classification were independent predictors of nodal metastases. External validation demonstrated 78.4% accuracy [56]. However, the nomogram was based on only hilar node dissection, which does not represent the exclusive landing zone for RCC. This may result in significant underestimation of the exact number of pN+ patients. Another limitation of the study is that the clinical node status of these patients was not reported.

Capitanio et al. developed a preoperative nomogram, to estimate the risk of LN involvement and/or LN progression during follow-up, based on clinical TNM stage and tumor size [57]. This predictive model had a discrimination of 86.9%. External validation of the nomogram is needed to confirm these findings. Babaian et al. [49] also developed a nomogram based on ECOG performance status, cN stage, lactate dehydrogenase, and local symptoms to estimate the probability of LN involvement with an 89% discrimination after internal validation. In this study, patients with distant metastasis were excluded. Recently Gershman et al. [47] developed two predictive models based on maximum LN short-axis diameter and presence of radiographic perinephric/sinus fat invasion. These radiographic features outperformed, in their models, traditional clinical variables—as used in the abovementioned protocols and nomograms [3, 24, 49, 56, 57]—in predicting pN1 risk [47].

Bhindi et al. [9] examined a total of ten studies and developed multivariable models to predict the likelihood of pN1 disease, including three nomograms, three risk scores, and four multivariable regression models. The most frequently used predictors in these models were tumor stage, tumor size, and radiographic lymphadenopathy (cN1), which were consistently associated with an increased risk of lymph node metastasis. Muttin et al. [46] found that patients with cN1pN0 RCC exhibited greater morbidity and systemic disease at diagnosis than those with cN0pN0, suggesting a preference for hematogenous dissemination over lymphatic invasion. Lymph node enlargement was primarily due to inflammation and fibrosis. While inflammatory lymphadenopathies correlated with larger tumors and adverse pathological features, they were not independent predictors of worse CSM. Pathologically confirmed LNI remains a critical predictor of survival in RCC. Furthermore, a radiological suspicion of nodal metastases should not be considered a poor prognostic factor until nodal involvement is confirmed by final pathology. The study by Golijanin et al. [58] investigated the relationship between clinicopathologic features and OS in patients using both univariable and multivariable analyses. The researchers identified patients aged 18–89 years who underwent radical or partial nephrectomy with LND for pN1M0 RCC between 2006 and 2013 from the National Cancer Database. Key findings revealed that factors such as older age, rural residence, larger tumor size, higher pT stage, positive surgical margins, an increased number of positive lymph nodes, and nonclear cell histologic subtype were significantly associated with higher mortality. Additionally, in patients treated between 2010 and 2013, histologic tumor necrosis, sarcomatoid differentiation, and adrenal gland invasion were linked to poorer outcomes. Based on these prognostic factors, a risk score was developed, showing that five-year OS rates decreased as risk scores increased, offering a practical tool to facilitate postoperative prognostication and selection of patients for consideration of adjuvant therapy [2, 58].

Rosiello et al. [35] reported that, in multivariable analyses adjusting for clinical tumor size and the number of LNs removed, an increase in the diameter of suspicious LNs on preoperative imaging was independently associated with an elevated risk of finding positive LNs outside the suspicious anatomical region.

Intraoperative Lymph Node Assessment

In the EORTC study 30881, 84 patients had palpably enlarged lymph nodes at nephrectomy. In only 14 of these 84 patients (17%), the palpably enlarged lymph nodes were positive for RCC metastases at the time of surgery. That means that in many patients, the enlargement of the nodes was not due to metastasis [2]. Intraoperative frozen section has been assessed to guide the decision to perform a full LND. In a recent study, 114 patients with RCC underwent frozen section examination of retroperitoneal enlarged lymph nodes and concurrent regional LND. The final histopathologic results indicated that only 36 patients (31.6%) had nodal metastases at

LND. The frozen section examination revealed positive findings in 32 patients and negative findings in four patients [59]. The study by Rosiello et al. [35] highlighted the limitations of conventional imaging techniques such as CT and MRI, which are often inadequate in detecting metastases in normal-sized or shaped LNs, which likely contribute to the low detection rates of pathologic lymph nodes. Fewer than 20% of the visibly enlarged lymph nodes during surgery were confirmed as positive upon histopathological examination. Therefore, intraoperative imaging technologies, such as radio-guided surgery using intravenously administered tracers, could improve the accuracy of staging during surgery. This approach may enhance the identification of occult metastatic LNs, allowing for more precise surgical management and potentially better outcomes for patients.

Sentinel Lymph Nodes

Sentinel node biopsy is widely used for nodal staging of melanoma and breast cancer.

Intraoperative sentinel lymph node mapping in the kidney was first described in a live porcine model by Bernie et al. in 2003 [60]. Since then, several other groups successfully applied sentinel lymph node mapping techniques to study lymphatic drainage in RCC [18, 61–63]. Bex et al. were the first to explore the sentinel node technique for RCC in humans [61, 62]. They prospectively evaluated the feasibility of intratumoral injection of radiolabeled technetium-99 m (^{99m}Tc) nano colloid under ultrasound guidance, followed by lymphoscintigraphy and hybrid SPECT/CT to image and sample the draining lymph nodes in eight patients with clinical T1-T2N0M0 RCC. Surgery with sampling was performed the following day using a gamma probe and a portable mini gamma camera. Lymphatic mapping was successful in identifying lymphatic drainage in 75% (6 of 8) of patients with visualization of one or more nodes [61]. In a study performed by the same group, of 20 patients with pT1–2pN0cM0 RCC, visualization of at least one sentinel node in 14/20 (60%) patients was reported [62]. Most of the nodes were within the template as described by Crispen et al. [24]. A Swedish group evaluated the feasibility of performing SN detection in patients with T1b-T3b RCC by preoperative injection of radiolabeled ^{99m}Tc nano colloid and preoperative lymphoscintigraphy followed by SPEC/CT. They reported SN detection in 10/11 patients with a total of 32 SN identified [63]. Recently, Kuusk et al. conducted a phase II, prospective single-arm study investigating the distribution of sentinel nodes from renal tumors on SPECT/CT in 68 patients. They observed lymphatic drainage outside the locoregional retroperitoneal templates in 14 patients (35%). Further, they reported a nonvisualization of SN on preoperative imaging in more than a third of patients [21]. The different authors all conclude that sentinel lymph node sampling is feasible and safe, and its use may improve the insight into renal lymphatic drainage. Further studies are needed to demonstrate if identification of lymphatic landing sites may have diagnostic and/or therapeutic significance [21, 61–63].

Future Options

New approaches, such as PET with fluorine-18 fluorodeoxyglucose (FDG) or detecting labeled antibodies against carbonic anhydrase IX (CAIX) [64], have been proposed to improve preoperative staging of RCC patients. However, future studies are needed to confirm these promising findings [23, 45]. Clinical studies have demonstrated the exceptional effectiveness of cG250 PET (girentuximab PET) in accurately targeting and diagnosing both localized and metastatic clear cell renal cell carcinoma (ccRCC). The advancement of similar imaging modalities is expected to be crucial for the precise detection of lymph node metastases in the future [65]. Notably, advancements in molecular imaging, particularly with radiolabeled girentuximab ([^{89}Zr] Zr-girentuximab), have shown significant potential, as highlighted in the ZIRCON study [66]. This phase 3 trial reported that [^{89}Zr] Zr-girentuximab PET/CT achieved high sensitivity (85.5%) and specificity (87.0%) for detecting ccRCC, including small lesions. These findings represent a notable improvement over conventional imaging methods, underscoring the reliability of [^{89}Zr]Zr-girentuximab as a noninvasive and accurate diagnostic tool. This advancement could drive the adoption of PET/CT for RCC staging in clinical practice in the near future.

Molecular and Genomic Biomarkers

Kroeger et al. [67] demonstrated that low levels of carbonic anhydrase IX and elevated expression of epithelial vascular endothelial growth factor 2 protein were linked to increased rates of lymph node involvement. Additionally, the loss of chromosome 3p was associated with a reduced risk of lymph node metastasis. Abbas et al. [68] found that intratumoral expression of programmed death ligand 1 (PD-L1) in RCC was associated with more advanced disease at diagnosis, including both lymph node and distant metastasis, and was linked to significantly reduced overall survival. Chen et al.'s systematic review identified high expression of metastasis-associated lung adenocarcinoma transcript 1 (MALAT1) as a potential biomarker for early detection of lymph node metastasis in RCC. Furthermore, elevated MALAT1 levels were linked to poor survival outcomes, significantly reducing overall survival in patients [69]. Pu et al.'s meta-analysis found that surviving expression was strongly linked to higher tumor grade, advanced tumor stage, and lymph node metastasis, but showed no association with age, sex, or distant metastasis [70]. The identification and validation of accurate biomarkers through clinical trials will hopefully equip clinicians with the necessary tools to identify patients who are likely to benefit from lymph node dissection (LND), ultimately enhancing outcomes for those with RCC.

When to Perform an LND?

Localized Disease (cT1abN0M0)

Prospective data on LND in the treatment of RCC is limited to the EORTC 30881 study, which randomized 732 patients with clinically node-negative RCC to either RN plus eLND or RN alone [2]. The study found that adding LND to RN did not improve survival outcomes. This lack of benefit was primarily due to the low incidence of unexpected lymph node metastases (4.0%) detected by LND. In patients with low-stage (T1-T2) RCC and cN0 lymph nodes, LND provided no benefit in reducing disease recurrence or improving survival (level 1 evidence). The EORTC 30881 trial remains the only prospective, randomized clinical trial assessing the impact of LND with a high level of evidence to date. However, it focused exclusively on patients with pT1–3 disease and no clinically detectable lymph nodes, potentially missing a subset of patients who could have benefited from LND. An older study presented by Pantuck et al. [7] retrospectively studied 900 patients who underwent nephrectomy for RCC. LND did not show a survival benefit in patients without enlarged lymph nodes at diagnosis. They reported that in the setting of patients with clinically localized, clinically node-negative RCC (cT1–2N0M0), LND would only be "useful" for staging and not for a proposed therapeutic benefit. Pantuck et al. conducted two studies on lymph node dissection (LND) in RCC patients. In one retrospective study of 900 patients, they found that LND did not provide a survival benefit for those without enlarged lymph nodes at diagnosis. They concluded that in patients with clinically localized, node-negative RCC (cT1–2N0M0), LND is primarily useful for staging rather than therapeutic purposes. At diagnosis, 59% of RCC patients (n = 535) had no evidence of regional lymph nodes or distant metastasis (N0M0), 14% (n = 129) had evidence of regional lymph node involvement (N+), and 26% (n = 236) had evidence of distant metastasis only (N0M1). Of the patients with N0M0 disease, 238 underwent LND, but no survival benefit was observed compared to those who had nephrectomy alone. However, in patients with node-positive (N+) disease, LND was associated with a significant survival advantage, extending median survival by about 5 months [7]. Currently, the EAU guidelines state that in patients with localized disease and clinically negative (cN0) lymph nodes, LND is not recommended (level 1 evidence) [31]. Demir et al. [43] categorized 181 patients into four groups based on their diagnostic stages: Group 1 (T1–3N0M0), Group 2 (T1–3NXM0), Group 3 (T1–3N1M0), and Group 4 (T1–4N0/XM1). Their analysis showed no statistically significant difference between Groups 1 and 2. The median survival for the Nx group, which did not undergo lymph node dissection, was 89 months—worse than the N0 group but better than the N1 group. These findings indicate that the Nx group is a heterogeneous cohort, comprising both N0 and N1 patients, and lymph node dissection can help achieve a more accurate risk stratification for these individuals.

Localized Disease: Larger Tumors (cT2abN0M0)

Capitanio et al. [5] reported an independent protective effect on survival for LND and its extent in patients with pT2a-pT2b RCC (Hazard ratio (HR) 0.91) and large tumors (tumor size >10 cm). Conversely, Feuerstein et al. [71] did not find a difference in recurrence-free survival in patients with ≥7-cm tumors, whether they underwent LND. The authors suggest, however, a role for LND to acquire important staging information. As mentioned above, Blute et al. and Crispen et al. presented data indicating that patients with larger tumor masses may benefit from LND, at least for staging purposes, due to the higher risk of LNI [3, 24]. Recently, Dell'Oglio et al. [45] reported that patients with RCC larger than 7 cm (cT2a or higher) might still benefit from LND because of a nonnegligible risk of LNI and/or LN progression. However, as well as Blute et al., Crispen et al. and Dell'Oglio et al. did not evaluate the impact of LND on survival [3, 24, 45].

Locally Advanced Disease (cT3-T4N0M0)

The value of LND in patients with locally advanced disease (cT3–4N0M0) has not been adequately assessed in a prospective randomized study. The EORTC trial has been criticized because most of the patients included in it were at low risk of developing lymph node metastases, suggesting that the study cannot conclude that the outcome in both arms is equivalent for all tumor stages [5, 23, 41, 72]. However, Bekema et al. [72] presented a subanalysis of the prospective EORTC trial focusing on cT3 tumors. They showed a not statistically significant improved survival at 5 years for the RN + LND group compared with the no-LND group. This not statistically significant result might reflect the results from the EORTC trial which could not evaluate the impact of LND in this subgroup [23]. Older retrospective studies by Herrlinger et al. and Schafhauser et al. reported improved five- and ten-year survival rates for patients who underwent RN + eLND compared to patients who underwent RN + LND or simple RN [26, 28]. However, in both studies, selection biases cannot be excluded. Blute et al. and Crispen et al. showed that patients with high stage (pT3-pT4) were twice as likely to have regional LNI compared with low-stage RCC [3, 24]. Tilki et al. [54] studied the effect of LND on oncological outcome in a specific subset of 1978 patients with RCC and tumor thrombus in the absence of metastatic diseases, using data from the International Renal Cell Carcinoma–Venous Thrombus Consortium (IRCC-VTC). They showed that the number of positive nodes harvested during LND and LN density was a strong prognostic indicator of CSS. The rate of pN1 patients among clinically node-negative patients was relatively high (9.6%), since the removal of positive nodal disease appears to provide a survival benefit, the authors conclude that LND may be warranted in this patient population. In the setting of patients with locally advanced, clinically node-negative RCC (cT3–4 N0M0), LND has a staging as well as a possible therapeutic benefit. Routine LND should at least be offered to these very high-risk patients. This aligns with the conclusion of Tachibana et al., who stated that since more extensive surgery may not necessarily increase morbidity in these cases, it should be considered for healthy patients with locally advanced RCC. This approach allows for the potential of improved outcomes without imposing significant additional risks on patients who are otherwise in good health [34]. In a study by Zhuang et al. [73] on patients with localized high-risk RCC—specifically nonmetastatic patients exhibiting two or more high-risk factors such as Fuhrman grade 3–4, tumor diameter ≥10 cm, pathological stage T3–T4, sarcomatoid features, or coagulative tumor necrosis—LND was associated with improved survival outcomes. Patients who underwent LND had a significantly longer average survival time of 43.10 months compared to 40.52 months for those who did not undergo LND. Additionally, patients with lymph node metastasis (N1) experienced a shorter survival of 31.50 months, whereas those without metastasis (N0) had a survival of 46.75 months. The study also found that survival decreased significantly with an increasing number of positive lymph nodes: 46.79 months for patients with no positive nodes, 32.30 months for those with 1–4 positive nodes, and 26.90 months for those with ≥5 positive nodes. These findings underscore the prognostic significance of lymph node status and indicate that LND may enhance survival outcomes in high-risk RCC patients. On the other hand, according to Kokorovic et al. [74], there was no correlation between the performance of LND and OS, RFS, or CSS in patients with nonmetastatic RCC treated with RN at varying probability thresholds of pN1 disease, which ranged from 5% to 40%. Additionally, a higher count of removed lymph nodes did not show any association with improved OS or CSS.

Clinical Node-Positive (cT1–4, N + M0) RCC

Several older retrospective reports have suggested a role of LND in the presence of clinically positive lymph nodes and no distant metastases [26, 75–78]. Already in 1980, Peters and Brown demonstrated an improved survival associated with LND, with an increase in the five-year survival from 25.8% to 43.5% [75]. Similar findings, of a survival benefit attributed to LND, were reported by Herrlinger et al. [26], Giberti et al. [76], and Canfield et al. [77]. Another retrospective analysis of pooled data of 171 RCC patients with positive nodal metastases and absence of distant metastases showed a 10- to 15-year CSS of approximately 30%, suggesting that LND of positive nodal metastases in patients undergoing RN for RCC may be beneficial for some patients [78]. However, these historical series comprise small cohorts, and biases such as selection bias must be considered. Among contemporary studies, the Mayo Clinic reported on a large RN cohort: 1797 patients of whom 606 underwent an LND. Here, no survival benefit was associated with LND at RN [6, 79]. Recently, the same group presented an extended RN cohort of 2722 patients, of whom 1215 underwent LND. Overall, 171 patients (6.3%) had pN1 disease. Median follow-up was 9.6 years [6]. This analysis confirmed their previous findings that LND is not associated with improved oncological outcomes among patients at high risk who undergo RN for M0 RCC. This included patients with radiographic lymphadenopathy across increasing probability thresholds of pN1 disease. However, a methodological issue was reported by Porter since 153 high-risk patients were excluded from the propensity matching analysis because there were no suitable matches in the non-LND group [80]. A recent secondary analysis of the ASSURE (ECOG-ACRIN 2805) adjuvant trial by Ristau et al. reported no improvement in survival, for adjuvant therapy relative to placebo, in patients with pN+ who underwent LND [31, 38, 81]. Gershman et al. [8] report a poor prognosis for isolated pN1 disease with a five-year probability of metastasis-free survival of only 16%. Nevertheless, they state that a subset of patients experience durable long-term survival to 10 years after surgical resection of isolated lymphatic metastases, suggesting a potential therapeutic role of LND for a small subset of patients. Current EAU guidelines state that in patients with localized disease and clinically enlarged lymph nodes, use of LND can provide staging information and thus is always justified (level 3 evidence) [31, 81].

Regional Lymph Node Recurrence

Therapeutically, LND might help reduce the incidence of local recurrences. Kwon et al. followed 1503 patients who had undergone nephrectomy for RCC and found that 2.4% (36/1503) had a local recurrence with the most common site being regional lymph nodes (30/36) [82]. A recent series of the Mayo Clinic examined the outcomes of 15 patients who underwent salvage retroperitoneal LND for isolated lymph node recurrence after RN. Median time from nephrectomy to resection was 10.3 months (3–159). Approximately two-thirds (66.7%) of patients progressed after salvage retroperitoneal LND at a median of 6 months [3–27] after RN. Median progression-free survival (9.1 months) was comparable to that of patients who had lymph node-positive RCC (8.7 months) at the time of RN. The authors concluded that a proportion of patients with isolated lymph node recurrence would benefit from salvage surgery [83]. More recently, a multiinstitutional study by Russell et al. reported the largest cohort of patients ($n = 50$) after surgical resection of isolated retroperitoneal lymph node recurrence of RCC after nephrectomy and no evidence of distal metastases [84]. These reports indicate the potential benefit of resection of isolated nodal recurrence in highly selected patients. Furthermore, they highlight the potential for undertreatment that may occur when LND is not incorporated into the initial resection for some patients. Figure 16.4 shows salvage LND for recurrence after RN (Fig. 16.4a) and a view after removal of lymph node recurrence (Fig. 16.4b).

Distant Metastasis and Cytoreduction (cTanyNanyM1)

The value of LND in patients with metastatic disease during cytoreductive nephrectomy has been assessed by several older and recent retrospective studies in the era of immunotherapy [7, 15, 22, 55, 85, 86]. These studies have shown conflicting results. Older studies have suggested a potential role for LND in patients in the metastatic RCC setting. Vasselli et al. [15] evaluated the presence of lymphadenopathy (radiographic cN+) in 154 patients with metastatic RCC undergoing cytoreductive nephrectomy prior to treatment with interleukin-2 (Il-2). No significant difference in survival was observed between patients with preoperative positive lymph nodes who had a complete regional LND and those with preoperative negative lymph nodes, suggesting a possible benefit of LND. No significant differences in response rate for IL-2 were detected with respect to the absence or presence of lymphadenopathy. Similarly, Pantuck et al. [7] reported a significant survival advantage (approximately 5 months) in 112 node-positive patients who underwent LND at the time of cytoreductive nephrectomy prior to immunotherapy, compared with 17 node-positive patients who did not undergo LND.

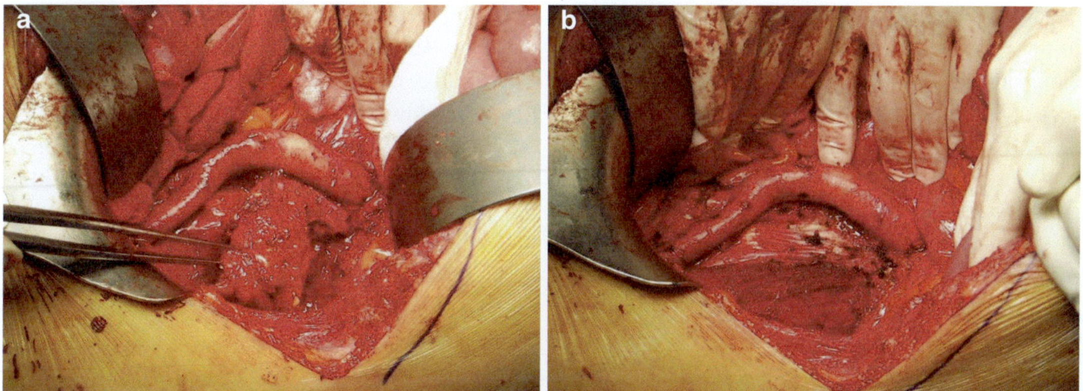

Fig. 16.4 (**a**) Salvage LND for recurrence after radical nephrectomy. (**b**) After removal of lymph node recurrence

Contemporary studies have not demonstrated a survival benefit between patients with metastases at diagnosis who did or did not undergo LND. Capitanio et al. [5] observed that in a cohort of 1938 patients (M0 and M+), there is no effect of LND and its extent in the group of M+ patients; they state that an effect of LND may be expected in a proportion of those patients, e.g., when the patient shows a bulky mass or a tumor with sarcomatoid features. Feuerstein et al. [85] reported that on a cohort of 256 patients who underwent cytoreductive nephrectomy, there is no significant difference in five-year survival between patients who did and did not undergo LND, 21% against 31% respectively. The five-year overall survival was 27% and 9% for negative and positive nodal status, respectively. Similarly, Gershman et al. [86] presented data using propensity score techniques, on 305 patients undergoing cytoreductive nephrectomy, not supporting an oncological benefit of LND. Chipollini et al. [87] found that in patients with metastatic RCC undergoing cytoreductive nephrectomy with LND, the number of positive lymph nodes was associated with short-term survival. They observed that patients with pN+ status had a median CSS of 11.3 months compared to 24.2 months for those with pN− status, emphasizing the prognostic significance of nodal involvement. The proportion of positive lymph nodes was identified as an independent risk factor, reflecting aggressive tumor biology and providing valuable insights for high-risk patients with RCC. Additionally, Chipollini et al. [87] posited that the aggressive phenotypes observed in their study facilitated early lymphatic spread alongside hematogenous dissemination, underscoring the importance of LND for staging purposes. However, they noted that nonstandardized LND did not demonstrate therapeutic advantages, with its utility limited to prognostic insights. They highlighted the necessity for prospective studies employing standardized templates to more effectively evaluate the therapeutic benefits of LND. Furthermore, nodal involvement may indicate a poor response to systemic therapies, suggesting that complete removal of regional nodal disease could have potential advantages in carefully selected cases. According to Chipollini et al. [84], the introduction of new systemic therapies will enhance the ability to better stratify patients, allowing for more targeted and personalized treatment approaches. This includes identifying those who may benefit from aggressive surgical interventions while providing additional prognostic information to improve predictions of disease survival. Population studies using data from the Surveillance, Epidemiology, and End Results (SEER) registry indicate that patients undergoing CN with concurrent LND have worse disease-specific survival compared to those who undergo CN alone [88]. The presence of a positive lymph node reduced median CSS from 22 months to 9 months, with additional positive nodes further decreasing survival. Another SEER study found that nodal disease negatively impacted CSS and OS by 68% and 69%, respectively, with each additional positive node contributing to a decline of 5.1% and 5.6% [89]. Additionally, a study from the Mayo Clinic showed that patients with pN+ disease exhibited more aggressive characteristics in their primary tumors, supporting these findings [90]. Notwithstanding the discordance concerning the therapeutic benefit of LND in metastatic RCC, all authors report presence of lymphatic involvement as an independent worse predictor of survival in patients with distant metastases [5, 7, 22, 53, 82, 84]. Indicating that LND may still serve as an important tool for staging purposes.

In summary, in patients with T1-T2N0 RCC and an absence of unfavorable characteristics, regional LND offers limited staging information and no benefit in terms of decreasing disease recurrence or improving survival (level 1 evidence). However, it cannot be concluded that LND is of no benefit in clinically node-negative patients. Removal of LNs containing microscopic metastases may be beneficial to some patients [8, 9, 40]. In high-risk patients (cT3-T4N0M0 or cTanyN+M0), discordance exists with some of the retrospective nonrandomized studies suggesting a possible benefit of regional LND on CSS. In the setting of patients with clinical node-positive RCC (cTanyN+M0), LND has a staging as well as a possible therapeutic benefit. Demir et al.

concluded that their findings demonstrated significant differences in disease-free survival and OS between T1–3N0M0 and T1–3N1M0 patients, suggesting that these groups should not be classified under the same staging category. It would be more appropriate to classify node-positive patients as stage 4 in a staging system where pT3N0 patients are designated as stage 3 [43]. If RN or PN is planned, enlarged lymph nodes either at imaging or palpation during surgery should be resected when technically feasible (level 3 evidence). A systematic review and meta-analysis by Bhindi et al. reported that the existing literature does not support a survival benefit with LND in either M0 or M1 RCC [9]. However, a small subset of patients with isolated nodal metastases experience long-term survival after surgical resection. They conclude that LND may play an important staging role in the contemporary management of RCC.

Conclusion and Future Research

The role of LND in the management of RCC continues to be an area of active investigation and debate. For patients with localized RCC (cT1–2N0M0) without lymphadenopathy, the risk of lymph node involvement is low, and LND can safely be omitted based on high-level evidence. In higher risk RCC, while historical studies have suggested a survival benefit from LND, contemporary research has failed to consistently demonstrate a therapeutic advantage. However, LND retains value for its staging role, as pN1 status has consistently been associated with worse survival outcomes in both M0 and M1 RCC. Thus, it is prudent to reserve LND for carefully selected patients at high risk for nodal metastasis.

Standardization of LND templates and techniques is critical to improve consistency in outcomes and guide future research pathology. Prospective, well-designed, multiinstitutional, randomized clinical trials are urgently needed to clarify the prognostic and therapeutic benefits of LND, particularly in high-risk cohorts. Future research should focus on improving imaging modalities, which could improve the detection of occult nodal metastases. Additionally, advancements in tumor molecular profiling, preoperative biopsies, and biomarkers could help identify patients at higher risk of lymphatic spread, facilitating personalized treatment strategies.

Due to the aggressive behavior of nodal metastases, some researchers propose redefining RCC with lymph node involvement as Stage IV disease. Such a reclassification could profoundly impact postoperative monitoring, facilitate earlier detection of recurrence, and refine the selection of patients for adjuvant treatments or enrolment in clinical trials. Ultimately, the integration of standardized LND techniques with modern systemic therapies, advanced imaging technologies, and tumor molecular profiling is likely to provide a more evidence-based approach to the management of RCC. These advancements hold the promise of enhancing prognostic accuracy, improving patient stratification, and optimizing survival outcomes in this challenging disease.

References

1. Robson CJ, Churchill BM, Anderson W. The results of radical nephrectomy for renal cell carcinoma. J Urol [Internet]. 1969;101(3):297–301. https://doi.org/10.1016/s0022-5347(17)62331-0.
2. Blom JHM, van Poppel H, Maréchal JM, Jacqmin D, Schröder FH, de Prijck L, et al. Radical nephrectomy with and without lymph-node dissection: final results of European Organization for Research and Treatment of Cancer (EORTC) randomized phase 3 trial 30881. Eur Urol [Internet]. 2009;55(1):28–34. https://doi.org/10.1016/j.eururo.2008.09.052.
3. Blute ML, Leibovich BC, Cheville JC, Lohse CM, Zincke H. A protocol for performing extended lymph node dissection using primary tumour pathological features for patients treated with radical nephrectomy for clear cell renal cell carcinoma. J Urol [Internet]. 2004;172(2):465–9. https://doi.org/10.1097/01.ju.0000129815.91927.85.
4. Sun M, Bianchi M, Hansen J, Abdollah F, Trinh QD, Lughezzani G, et al. Nodal involvement at nephrectomy is associated with worse survival: a stage-for-stage and grade-for-grade analysis. Int J Urol [Internet]. 2013;20(4):372–80. https://doi.org/10.1111/j.1442-2042.2012.03170.x.
5. Capitanio U, Suardi N, Matloob R, Roscigno M, Abdollah F, Trapani D. Extent of lymph node dissection at nephrectomy affects cancer-specific survival

and metastatic progression in specific sub-categories of patients with renal cell carcinoma (RCC). BJU Int. 2014;114(2):210–5.
6. Gershman B, Thompson RH, Moreira DM, Boorjian SA, Tollefson MK, Lohse CM, et al. Radical nephrectomy with or without lymph node dissection for nonmetastatic renal cell carcinoma: a propensity score-based analysis. Eur Urol [Internet]. 2016;71(4):560–7. https://doi.org/10.1016/j.eururo.2016.09.019.
7. Pantuck A, Zisman A, Dorey F, Chao D, Han KR, Said J, et al. Renal cell carcinoma with retroperitoneal lymph nodes: role of lymph node dissection. J Urol. 2003;169:2076–83.
8. Gershman B, Moreira DM, Thompson RH, Boorjian SA, Lohse CM, Costello BA, et al. Renal cell carcinoma with isolated lymph node involvement: long-term natural history and predictors of oncologic outcomes following surgical resection. Eur Urol [Internet]. 2017;72(2):300–6. https://doi.org/10.1016/j.eururo.2016.12.027.
9. Bhindi B, Wallis CJD, Boorjian SA, Thompson RH, Farrell A, Kim SP, et al. The role of lymph node dissection in the management of renal cell carcinoma: a systematic review and meta-analysis. BJU International. Blackwell Publishing Ltd. 2018;121:684–98.
10. Karmali RJ, Suami H, Wood CG, Karam JA. Lymphatic drainage in renal cell carcinoma: back to the basics. BJU International. Blackwell Publishing Ltd. 2014;114:806–17.
11. Russo P, Jang TL, Pettus JA, Huang WC, Eggener SE, O'Brien MF, et al. Survival rates after resection for localized kidney cancer: 1989 to 2004. Cancer [Internet]. 2008;113(1):84–96. https://doi.org/10.1002/cncr.23520.
12. Kates M, Lavery HJ, Brajtbord J, Samadi D, Palese MA. Decreasing rates of lymph node dissection during radical nephrectomy for renal cell carcinoma. Ann Surg Oncol [Internet]. 2012;19(8):2693–9. https://doi.org/10.1245/s10434-012-2330-6.
13. Capitanio U, Stewart GD, Larcher A, Ouzaid I, Akdogan B, Roscigno M, et al. European temporal trends in the use of lymph node dissection in patients with renal cancer. Eur J Surg Oncol. 2017;43(11):2184–92.
14. Saitoh H, Nakayama M, Nakamura K, Satoh T. Distant metastasis of renal adenocarcinoma in nephrectomised cases. J Urol [Internet]. 1982;127(6):1092–5. https://doi.org/10.1016/s0022-5347(17)54243-3.
15. Vasselli JR, Yang JC, Linehan WM, White DE, Rosenberg SA, Walther MM. Lack of retroperitoneal lymphadenopathy predicts survival of patients with metastatic renal cell carcinoma. J Urol [Internet]. 2001;166(1):68–72. https://doi.org/10.1016/s0022-5347(05)66078-8.
16. Assouad J, Riquet M, Foucault C, Hidden G, Delmas V. Renal lymphatic drainage and thoracic duct connections: implications for cancer spread. Lymphology [Internet]. 2006;39(1):26–32. Available from: https://www.ncbi.nlm.nih.gov/pubmed/16724507
17. Parker AE. Studies on the main posterior lymph channels of the abdomen and their connections with the lymphatics of the Genito-urinary system. Am J Anatomy [Internet]. 1935;56(3):409–43. https://doi.org/10.1002/aja.1000560305.
18. Brouwer OR, Noe A, Olmos RAV, Bex A. Lymphatic drainage from renal cell carcinoma along the thoracic duct visualized with SPECT/CT. Lymphat Res Biol [Internet]. 2013;11(4):233–8. https://doi.org/10.1089/lrb.2013.0017.
19. Johnsen JA, Hellsten S. Lymphatogenous spread of renal cell carcinoma: an autopsy study. J Urol [Internet]. 1997;157(2):450–3. Available from: https://www.ncbi.nlm.nih.gov/pubmed/8996329
20. Capitanio U, Deho' F, Dell'Oglio P, Larcher A, Capogrosso P, Nini A, et al. Lymphadenopathies in patients with renal cell carcinoma: clinical and pathological predictors of pathologically confirmed lymph node invasion. World J Urol [Internet]. 2015;34(8):1139–45. https://doi.org/10.1007/s00345-015-1747-5.
21. Kuusk T, De Bruijn R, Brouwer OR, De Jong J, Donswijk M, Grivas N, et al. Lymphatic drainage from renal tumors in vivo: a prospective sentinel node study using SPECT/CT imaging. J Urol [Internet]. 2017;199(6):1426–32. https://doi.org/10.1016/j.juro.2017.11.112.
22. Lughezzani G, Capitanio U, Jeldres C, Isbarn H, Shariat SF, Arjane P, et al. Prognostic significance of lymph node invasion in patients with metastatic renal cell carcinoma: a population-based perspective. Cancer [Internet]. 2009;115(24):5680–7. https://doi.org/10.1002/cncr.24682.
23. Capitanio U, Leibovich BC. The rationale and the role of lymph node dissection in renal cell carcinoma. World J Urol [Internet]. 2016;35(4):497–506. https://doi.org/10.1007/s00345-016-1886-3.
24. Crispen PL, Breau RH, Allmer C, Lohse CM, Cheville JC, Leibovich BC, et al. Lymph node dissection at the time of radical nephrectomy for high-risk clear cell renal cell carcinoma: indications and recommendations for surgical templates. Eur Urol [Internet]. 2010;59(1):18–23. https://doi.org/10.1016/j.eururo.2010.08.042.
25. Wood DP Jr. Role of lymphadenectomy in renal cell carcinoma. Urol Clin North Am [Internet]. 1991;18(3):421–6. Available from: https://www.ncbi.nlm.nih.gov/pubmed/1877102
26. Herrlinger A, Schrott KM, Schott G, Sigel A. What are the benefits of extended dissection of the regional renal lymph nodes in the therapy of renal cell carcinoma. J Urol [Internet]. 1991;146(5):1224–7. https://doi.org/10.1016/s0022-5347(17)38052-7.
27. Terrone C, Guercio S, De Luca S, Poggio M, Castelli E, Scoffone C, et al. The number of lymph nodes examined and staging accuracy in renal cell carcinoma. BJU Int [Internet]. 2003;91(1):37–40. https://doi.org/10.1046/j.1464-410x.2003.04017.x.
28. Schafhauser W, Ebert A, Brod J, Petsch S, Schrott KM. Lymph node involvement in renal cell carcinoma

and survival chance by systematic lymphadenectomy. Anticancer Res [Internet]. 1999;19(2C):1573–8. Available from: https://www.ncbi.nlm.nih.gov/pubmed/10365148
29. Joslyn SA, Sirintrapun SJ, Konety BR. Impact of lymphadenectomy and nodal burden in renal cell carcinoma: retrospective analysis of the National Surveillance, Epidemiology, and End Results database. Urology [Internet]. 2005;65(4):675–80. https://doi.org/10.1016/j.urology.2004.10.068.
30. Capitanio U, Suardi N, Matloob R, Abdollah F, Castiglione F, Briganti A, et al. Staging lymphadenectomy in renal cell carcinoma must be extended: a sensitivity curve analysis. BJU Int [Internet]. 2012;111(3):412–8. https://doi.org/10.1111/j.1464-410X.2012.11313.x.
31. Ljungberg B, Bensalah K, Canfield S, Dabestani S, Hofmann F, Hora M, et al. EAU guidelines on renal cell carcinoma: 2014 update. Eur Urol [Internet]. 2015;67(5):913–24. https://doi.org/10.1016/j.eururo.2015.01.005.
32. Whitson J, Harris C, Reese A, Meng M. Lymphadenectomy improves survival of patients with renal cell carcinoma and nodal metastases. J Urol. 2011;185:1615–20.
33. Dong F, Xu L, Peng X, Xu T, Shen Y, Gao F, et al. Pathologically examining a minimum of three lymph nodes could better determine node negativity in patients with non-metastatic chromophobe renal cell carcinoma. Jpn J Clin Oncol. 2018;48(10):942–9.
34. Tachibana I, Vasquez R, Mahmoud M, Kern SQ, Patel RS, King J, et al. Can Retroperitoneal Lymph Node Dissection (RPLND) be feasibly performed to prolong survival in Renal Cell Carcinoma (RCC) with limited lymph node involvement? An analysis of recurrence patterns. Urol Oncol: Seminars and Original Investigations. 2022;40(11):495.e11–7.
35. Rosiello G, Scilipoti P, Larcher A, Fallara G, Colandrea G, Basile G, et al. Neglected lymph nodal metastases in patients with renal cancer: when to extend the anatomical template of lymph node dissection during nephrectomy. World J Urol. 2023;41(6):1573–9.
36. Choueiri TK, Tomczak P, Park SH, Venugopal B, Ferguson T, Chang YH, et al. Adjuvant Pembrolizumab after nephrectomy in renal-cell carcinoma. N Engl J Med. 2021;385(8):683–94.
37. Chapman TN, Sharma S, Zhang S, Wong MK, Kim HL. Laparoscopic lymph node dissection in clinically node-negative patients undergoing laparoscopic nephrectomy for renal carcinoma. Urology [Internet]. 2008;71(2):287–91. https://doi.org/10.1016/j.urology.2007.08.057.
38. Ristau BT, Manola J, Haas NB, Heng DYC, Messing EM, Wood CG, et al. Retroperitoneal lymphadenectomy for high risk, nonmetastatic renal cell carcinoma: an analysis of the ASSURE (ECOG-ACRIN 2805). Adjuvant Trial J Urol [Internet]. 2017;199(1):53–9. https://doi.org/10.1016/j.juro.2017.07.042.
39. Gershman B, Moreira DM, Thompson RH, Boorjian SA, Lohse CM, Costello BA, et al. Perioperative morbidity of lymph node dissection for renal cell carcinoma: a propensity score–based analysis. Eur Urol. 2018;73(3):469–75.
40. Van Poppel H. Lymph node dissection is not obsolete in clinically node-negative renal cell carcinoma patients. Eur Urol [Internet]. 2010;59(1):24–5. https://doi.org/10.1016/j.eururo.2010.09.033.
41. Studer UE, Birkhäuser FD. Lymphadenectomy combined with radical nephrectomy: to do or not to do? Eur Urol [Internet]. 2008;55(1):35–7. https://doi.org/10.1016/j.eururo.2008.09.056.
42. Studer UE, Scherz S, Scheidegger J, Kraft R, Sonntag R, Ackermann D, et al. Enlargement of regional lymph nodes in renal cell carcinoma is often not due to metastases. J Urol [Internet]. 1990;144(2 Pt 1):243–5. https://doi.org/10.1016/s0022-5347(17)39422-3.
43. Demir T, Aliyev A, Beşiroğlu M, Araz M, Köstek O, Sakin A, et al. Is lymph node dissection necessary for staging while undergoing nephrectomy in patients with renal cell carcinoma? Curr Probl Cancer. 2021;45(1):100619.
44. Connolly SS, Raja A, Stunell H, Parashar D, Upponi S, Warren AY, et al. Diagnostic accuracy of preoperative computed tomography used alone to detect lymph-node involvement at radical nephrectomy. Scand J Urol [Internet]. 2015;49(2):142–8. Available from: http://europepmc.org/abstract/MED/25623950
45. Dell'Oglio P, Larcher A, Muttin F, Di Trapani E, Trevisani F, Ripa F, et al. Lymph node dissection should not be dismissed in case of localized renal cell carcinoma in the presence of larger diseases. Urol Oncol: Seminars and Original Investigations. 2017;35:35.
46. Muttin F, Pecoraro A, Larcher A, Dell'Oglio P, Nini A, Cianflone F, et al. Predictive and prognostic effect of inflammatory lymphadenopathies in renal cell carcinoma. World J Urol. 2019;37(4):701–8.
47. Gershman B, Takahashi N, Moreira DM, Thompson RH, Boorjian SA, Lohse CM, et al. Radiographic size of retroperitoneal lymph nodes predicts pathological nodal involvement for patients with renal cell carcinoma: development of a risk prediction model. BJU Int [Internet]. 2016;118(5):742–9. https://doi.org/10.1111/bju.13424.
48. Radadia KD, Rivera-Núñez Z, Kim S, Farber NJ, Sterling J, Falkiewicz M, et al. Accuracy of clinical nodal staging and factors associated with receipt of lymph node dissection at the time of surgery for nonmetastatic renal cell carcinoma. Urol Oncol: Seminars and Original Investigations. 2019;37(9):577.e17–25.
49. Babaian K, Kim D, Kenney P, Wood C, Sanchez C, Fang J, et al. Preoperative predictors of pathologic lymph node metastasis in patients with renal cell carcinoma undergoing RPLND. J Urol. 2014;193:1101.
50. Roussel E, Capitanio U, Kutikov A, Oosterwijk E, Pedrosa I, Rowe SP, et al. Novel imaging methods for renal mass characterization: a collaborative review. Eur Urol. Elsevier B.V. 2022;81:476–88.

51. Capitanio U, Becker F, Blute ML, Mulders P, Patard JJ, Russo P, et al. Lymph node dissection in renal cell carcinoma. Eur Urol. 2011;60:1212–20.
52. Skinner DG, Vermillion CD, Colvin RB. The surgical management of renal cell carcinoma. J Urol [Internet]. 1972;107(5):705–10. https://doi.org/10.1016/s0022-5347(17)61121-2.
53. Giuliani L, Giberti C, Martorana G, Rovida S. Radical extensive surgery for renal cell carcinoma: long-term results and prognostic factors. J Urol [Internet]. 1990;143(3):468–73.; discussion 473–4. https://doi.org/10.1016/s0022-5347(17)39992-5.
54. Tilki D, Chandrasekar T, Capitanio U, Ciancio G, Daneshmand S, Gontero P, et al. Impact of lymph node dissection at the time of radical nephrectomy with tumor thrombectomy on oncological outcomes: results from the International Renal Cell Carcinoma-Venous Thrombus Consortium (IRCC-VTC). Urol Oncol [Internet]. 2017;36(2):79.e11–7. https://doi.org/10.1016/j.urolonc.2017.10.008.
55. Pantuck AJ, Zisman A, Dorey F, Chao DH, Han KR, Said J, et al. Renal cell carcinoma with retroperitoneal lymph nodes. Impact on survival and benefits of immunotherapy. Cancer [Internet]. 2003;97(12):2995–3002. https://doi.org/10.1002/cncr.11422.
56. Hutterer GC, Patard JJ, Perrotte P, Ionescu C, de La Taille A, Salomon L, et al. Patients with renal cell carcinoma nodal metastases can be accurately identified: external validation of a new nomogram. Int J Cancer [Internet]. 2007;121(11):2556–61. https://doi.org/10.1002/ijc.23010.
57. Capitanio U, Abdollah F, Matloob R, Suardi N, Castiglione F, Di Trapani E, et al. When to perform lymph node dissection in patients with renal cell carcinoma: a novel approach to the preoperative assessment of risk of lymph node invasion at surgery and of lymph node progression during follow-up. BJU Int [Internet]. 2013;112(2):E59–66. https://doi.org/10.1111/bju.12125.
58. Golijanin B, Pereira J, Mueller-Leonhard C, Golijanin D, Amin A, Mega A, et al. The natural history of renal cell carcinoma with isolated lymph node metastases following surgical resection from 2006 to 2013. Urol Oncol: Seminars and Original Investigations. 2019;37(12):932–40.
59. Ming X, Ningshu L, Hanzhong L, Zhongming H, Tonghua L. Value of frozen section analysis of enlarged lymph nodes during radical nephrectomy for renal cell carcinoma. Urology [Internet]. 2009;74(2):364–8. https://doi.org/10.1016/j.urology.2008.12.075.
60. Bernie JE, Zupkas P, Monga M. Intraoperative mapping of renal lymphatic drainage: technique and application in a porcine model. J Endourol [Internet]. 2003;17(4):235–7. https://doi.org/10.1089/089277903765444375.
61. Bex A, Vermeeren L, de Windt G, Prevoo W, Horenblas S, Olmos RAV. Feasibility of sentinel node detection in renal cell carcinoma: a pilot study. Eur J Nucl Med Mol Imaging [Internet]. 2010;37(6):1117–23. https://doi.org/10.1007/s00259-009-1359-7.
62. Bex A, Vermeeren L, Meinhardt W, Prevoo W, Horenblas S, Valdés Olmos RA. Intraoperative sentinel node identification and sampling in clinically node-negative renal cell carcinoma: initial experience in 20 patients. World J Urol [Internet]. 2010;29(6):793–9. https://doi.org/10.1007/s00345-010-0615-6.
63. Sherif AM, Eriksson E, Thörn M, Vasko J, Riklund K, Ohberg L, et al. Sentinel node detection in renal cell carcinoma. A feasibility study for detection of tumour-draining lymph nodes. BJU Int [Internet]. 2011;109(8):1134–9. https://doi.org/10.1111/j.1464-410X.2011.10444.x.
64. Divgi CR, Uzzo RG, Gatsonis C, Bartz R, Treutner S, Yu JQ, et al. Positron emission tomography/computed tomography identification of clear cell renal cell carcinoma: results from the REDECT trial. J Clin Oncol [Internet]. 2012;31(2):187–94. https://doi.org/10.1200/JCO.2011.41.2445.
65. Oosterwijk-Wakka J, Boerman O, Mulders P, Oosterwijk E. Application of monoclonal antibody G250 recognizing carbonic anhydrase IX in renal cell carcinoma. Int J Mol Sci. 2013;14:11402–23.
66. Shuch B, Pantuck AJ, Bernhard JC, Morris MA, Master V, Scott AM, et al. [89Zr]Zr-girentuximab for PET–CT imaging of clear-cell renal cell carcinoma: a prospective, open-label, multicentre, phase 3 trial. Lancet Oncol. 202;
67. Kroeger N, Seligson D, Klatte T, Rampersaud E, Birkhäuser F, Rao N, et al. Clinical, molecular, and genetic correlates of lymphatic spread in clear cell renal cell carcinoma. Eur Urol. 2012;61:888–95.
68. Abbas M, Steffens S, Bellut M, Eggers H, Anika G, Becker J, et al. Intratumoral expression of programmed death ligand 1 (PD-L1) in patients with clear cell renal cell carcinoma (ccRCC). Med Oncol. 2016;33
69. Chen J, Chen Y, Gu L, Li X, Gao Y, Lyu X, et al. LncRNAs act as prognostic and diagnostic biomarkers in renal cell carcinoma: a systematic review and meta-analysis. Oncotarget. 2015;7:7.
70. Pu Z, Guangzhen W, Xie H, Wang G, Hao H. Clinicalpathological and prognostic significance of survivin expression in renal cell carcinoma: a meta-analysis. Oncotarget. 2017;8:8.
71. Feuerstein MA, Kent M, Bazzi WM, Bernstein M, Russo P. Analysis of lymph node dissection in patients with ≥7-cm renal tumors. World J Urol [Internet]. 2014;32(6):1531–6. https://doi.org/10.1007/s00345-013-1233-x.
72. Bekema HJ, MacLennan S, Imamura M, Lam TBL, Stewart F, Scott N, et al. Systematic review of adrenalectomy and lymph node dissection in locally advanced renal cell carcinoma. Eur Urol [Internet]. 2013;64(5):799–810. https://doi.org/10.1016/j.eururo.2013.04.033.
73. Zhuang W, Chen J, Li Y, Liu W. Valuation of lymph node dissection in localized high-risk renal cell

cancer using X-tile software. Int Urol Nephrol. 2020;52(2):253–62.
74. Kokorovic A, Breau RH, Kapoor A, Finelli A, So AI, Lavallee LT, et al. Lymph node dissection during radical nephrectomy: a Canadian multi-institutional analysis. Urol Oncol: Seminars and Original Investigations. 2021;39(6):371.e17–25.
75. Peters PC, Brown GL. The role of lymphadenectomy in the management of renal cell carcinoma. Urol Clin North Am [Internet]. 1980;7(3):705–9. Available from: https://www.ncbi.nlm.nih.gov/pubmed/7456182
76. Giberti C, Oneto F, Martorana G, Rovida S, Carmignani G. Radical nephrectomy for renal cell carcinoma: long-term results and prognostic factors on a series of 328 cases. Eur Urol [Internet]. 1997;31(1):40–8. https://doi.org/10.1159/000474416.
77. Canfield SE, Kamat AM, Sánchez-Ortiz RF, Detry M, Swanson DA, Wood CG. Renal cell carcinoma with nodal metastases in the absence of distant metastatic disease (clinical stage TxN1-2M0): the impact of aggressive surgical resection on patient outcome. J Urol [Internet]. 2006;175(3 Pt 1):864–9. https://doi.org/10.1016/S0022-5347(05)00334-4.
78. Karakiewicz PI, Trinh QD, Bhojani N, Bensalah K, Salomon L, de la Taille A, et al. Renal cell carcinoma with nodal metastases in the absence of distant metastatic disease: prognostic indicators of disease-specific survival. Eur Urol [Internet]. 2006;51(6):1616–24. https://doi.org/10.1016/j.eururo.2006.12.015.
79. Gershman B, Thompson RH, Boorjian SA, Larcher A, Capitanio U, Montorsi F, et al. Radical nephrectomy with or without lymph node dissection for high risk nonmetastatic renal cell carcinoma: a multi-institutional analysis. J Urol [Internet]. 2018;199(5):1143–8. https://doi.org/10.1016/j.juro.2017.11.114.
80. Porter JR. The role of lymphadenectomy for renal cell carcinoma: are we any closer to an answer? Eur Urol [Internet]. 2017;71(4):568–9. Available from: https://www.sciencedirect.com/science/article/pii/S0302283816307424
81. Renal Cell Carcinoma EAU Guidelines on. 2018.
82. Kwon T, Song C, Hong JH, Kim CS, Ahn H. Reassessment of renal cell carcinoma lymph node staging: analysis of patterns of progression. Urology [Internet]. 2011;77(2):373–8. https://doi.org/10.1016/j.urology.2010.06.015.
83. Boorjian SA, Crispen PL, Lohse CM, Leibovich BC, Blute ML. Surgical resection of isolated retroperitoneal lymph node recurrence of renal cell carcinoma following nephrectomy. J Urol [Internet]. 2008;180(1):99–103.; discussion 103. https://doi.org/10.1016/j.juro.2008.03.025.
84. Russell C, Lue K, Fisher J, Kassouf W, Schwaab T, Sexton W, et al. Oncologic control associated with surgical resection of isolated retroperitoneal lymph node recurrence from renal cell carcinoma. BJU Int. 2015;117
85. Feuerstein MA, Kent M, Bernstein M, Russo P. Lymph node dissection during cytoreductive nephrectomy: a retrospective analysis. Int J Urol [Internet]. 2014;21(9):874–9. https://doi.org/10.1111/iju.12457.
86. Gershman B, Thompson RH, Moreira DM, Boorjian SA, Lohse CM, Costello BA, et al. Lymph node dissection is not associated with improved survival among patients undergoing cytoreductive nephrectomy for metastatic renal cell carcinoma: a propensity score based analysis. J Urol [Internet]. 2016;197(3 Pt 1):574–9. https://doi.org/10.1016/j.juro.2016.09.074.
87. Chipollini J, Abel EJ, Peyton CC, Boulware DC, Karam JA, Margulis V, et al. Pathologic predictors of survival during lymph node dissection for metastatic renal-cell carcinoma: results from a multicenter collaboration. Clin Genitourin Cancer. 2018;16(2):e443–50.
88. Patel H, Gorin M, Gupta N, Kates M, Johnson M, Pierorazio P, et al. Mortality trends and the impact of lymphadenectomy on survival for renal cell carcinoma patients with distant metastasis. Can Urol Assoc J. 2016;10:389–95.
89. Trinh QD, Sukumar S, Schmitges J, Bianchi M, Sun M, Shariat S, et al. Effect of nodal metastases on cancer-specific mortality after Cytoreductive nephrectomy. Ann Surg Oncol. 2012;20:2096
90. Gershman B, Thompson R, Moreira D, Boorjian S, Lohse C, Costello B, et al. Lymph node dissection is not associated with improved survival among patients undergoing Cytoreductive nephrectomy for metastatic renal cell carcinoma: a propensity-score based analysis. J Urol. 2016;197:574.

Role of Surgery in Locally Recurrent and Metastatic Renal Cancer

17

Katiana Vazquez-Rivera, Marc Ganz, and A. Ari Hakimi

Kidney Cancer and Recurrence

It is estimated that there will be about 81,610 new cases of kidney cancer diagnosed in the United States in 2024 (52,380 in men and 29,230 in women). About 14,390 people will die from this disease [1]. While the vast majority of the patients present with localized renal cell carcinoma (RCC), up to 30% of individuals diagnosed with RCC exhibit synchronous metastases at the time of diagnosis, and 30% experience a recurrence following the complete resection of the primary tumor [2]. Current management options for localized RCC includes radical nephrectomy (RN), partial nephrectomy (PN) when surgically feasible, thermal ablation (TA), and active surveillance (AS). While RN or PN are currently the gold standard for treating localized RCC, these procedures are not without limitations. Recurrence rates remain significant at 7%, 26%, and 39% for T1, T2, and T3 staged diseases, respectively [3, 4]. Risk factors include locally advanced or node-positive disease and adverse histopathologic features [5–7]. Adjuvant therapy can also play a role in the management of localized RCC with an increased risk of recurrence after surgery.

The surgical resection of isolated local recurrence of RCC following radical or partial nephrectomy warrants consideration, as it has been associated with achieving long-term cancer-free status in 30% to 40% of patients [8–11]. However, it is imperative for surgeons to remain cognizant of the heightened surgical morbidity and potential long-term compromise to renal function inherent in this approach [12–14]. Fortunately, the array of tools at surgeons' disposal grows annually. As the treatment paradigm for advanced and metastatic RCC undergoes a transformation with the advent of targeted systemic agents, clinicians are increasingly integrating these therapies into both neoadjuvant and adjuvant contexts for recurrent disease [15, 16].

Management of metastatic renal cell carcinoma (mRCC) has undergone rapid evolution over the past two decades, marked by the emergence of targeted therapies and immune checkpoint inhibitors as the new benchmark in care [17]. With the addition of increasingly effective systemic treatments, there has been growing scrutiny regarding the role of surgical therapy in the management of mRCC, although several studies have indicated potential benefits in appropriately selected patients [18–21].

K. Vazquez-Rivera
Department of Urology, Maimonides Health, Brooklyn, NY, USA
e-mail: kvazquez@maimo.org

M. Ganz
Department of Urology, SUNY Downstate Health Sciences University, Brooklyn, NY, USA

A. A. Hakimi (✉)
Department of Surgery, Urology Service, Memorial Sloan Kettering Cancer Center, New York, NY, USA
e-mail: hakimia@mskcc.org

J. A. Libertino, J. R. Gee (eds.), *Renal Cancer*, https://doi.org/10.1007/978-3-031-97599-8_17

The multicenter, randomized, double-blind, placebo-controlled, phase 3 KEYNOTE-564 trial demonstrated a significant improvement in disease-free survival with adjuvant pembrolizumab compared to placebo following surgery [22]. Subgroup analyses within the study further highlighted the benefit in patients classified as M1 with no evidence of disease (NED). Pembrolizumab also showed superior distant metastasis-free survival compared to placebo [22]. As one of the first trials to establish the efficacy of immune checkpoint inhibitors in the adjuvant setting for RCC, this study potentially sets a new standard of care for patients with high-risk RCC post-nephrectomy or metastasectomy.

Recurrence After RN

Kidney cancer is typically diagnosed at a localized stage and generally carries a favorable prognosis, with an approximately 93% 5-year survival rate [23]. Since the early twenty-first century, partial nephrectomy has increasingly supplanted radical nephrectomy, particularly in the treatment of organ-confined disease. Nonetheless, radical nephrectomy remains the preferred treatment for larger and/or locally advanced renal tumors. The location and risk of local recurrence depend on the primary treatment. In the absence of distant metastatic disease, local retroperitoneal recurrence (RPR) following RN occurs in up to 3% of cases, with a poor prognosis and a 5-year cancer specific survival (CSS) of 27% to 52%, posing a significant management challenge [24–26]. Tumors can still recur in the soft tissue of the ipsilateral renal fossa, ipsilateral adrenal gland, renal vein stump or adjacent inferior vena cava (IVC), ipsilateral retroperitoneal lymph node tissue, and psoas muscle, with or without evidence of other metastatic sites [27]. Risk factors include locally advanced or node-positive disease, positive surgical margins, and adverse histopathologic features. It is noteworthy that patients may also harbor micrometastatic disease undetected at the time of extirpative surgery [5–7, 28].

One of the most challenging aspects of this phenomenon is the absence of an established standardized treatment protocol and the lack of large-scale evidence supporting any specific management approach. Open surgical excision of locoregional recurrence following radical nephrectomy appears to be an effective treatment option and is typically performed with curative intent. Long-term survival has been achieved in a significant proportion of patients, indicating that aggressive surgical resection can be a prudent approach. Although laparoscopic approaches have been described [29, 30], an open surgical approach allows for wide and radical excision, potentially facilitating the resection of adjacent organs such as the spleen, colon, or pancreas when necessary.

The diagnosis and surgical evaluation of RPR can be further complicated by the presence of an inferior vena cava tumor thrombus, which may extend into the right atrium. This situation often requires the involvement of additional surgical teams, such as vascular surgery for potential vena caval reconstruction or grafting, and cardiac surgery for the utilization of cardiac bypass when the tumor reaches the heart. Margulis et al. identified prognostic features for cancer-specific survival (CSS) at RPR extirpation that can be used to help appropriately select patients for surgery. On multivariate analysis, the following were adverse risk factors associated with an increased risk of cancer-specific death after resection for recurrent RCC: a positive surgical margin following RPR resection ($p = 0.04$), the size of the recurrent tumor ($p = 0.004$), and the presence of sarcomatoid features in the RPR ($p = 0.04$) [9]. Meanwhile, on a multivariate analysis, Thomas et al. identified pathological nodal stage at original nephrectomy (HR: 4.08; 95%CI, 1.89–8.83; $p < 0.001$) and maximum diameter of RPR mass (HR: 1.21; 95%CI, 1.12–2.32; $p < 0.001$) as independent risk factors for cancer-specific death after RPR surgery. Additionally, 14.7% of patients in their series experienced grade 3 or higher complications, underscoring the importance of conducting this complex surgery in specialized referral centers [24]. Despite these technical difficulties, surgical resection can be effective and is recommended for selected patients [31–34]. Treatment paradigms are evolving to embrace a multidisciplinary approach that integrates both medical and surgical interventions. With the advent of targeted therapies for advanced and metastatic RCC, reliance on surgery alone is no longer necessary. Clinicians are now employing these therapies in both neoadjuvant and adjuvant settings, achieving promising results. Thus, the improved outcomes observed in recent series of patients with RPR likely reflect the transformative impact of the targeted systemic therapy era on the management of locally advanced and metastatic disease [15].

The largest reported series of patients with RPR was conducted at MD Anderson by Thomas et al. [24], involving 102 cases of isolated local recurrence with a 32-month median follow-up. They found a 3-year and 5-year CSS of 71% and 52%, respectively. Notable findings from this study include that 45.1% of patients received neoadjuvant therapy, while 47.1% received adjuvant systemic therapy, such as immunotherapy or targeted therapy; additionally, 41.2% remained free of disease (NED) after RPR surgery without any further therapies. The authors identified pathological nodal stages at time of RN and size of RPR as adverse prognostic indicators. When they compared CSS in patients that received immunotherapy versus targeted therapy in the salvage setting, they found a significant survival benefit in those receiving targeted therapy. It is worth emphasizing that in this study, none of the patients had detectable distant metastases at the time of RPR surgery and all cases were performed at a single institution. This is in contrast with a multi-institutional French cohort reported by Paparel et al., encompassing over 12 centers with 72 patients (26-month median follow-up). They reported a 1, 3, and 5-year CSS of 74%, 55%, and 46%, respectively [35]. In univariate analysis only, they noted that time to recurrence and surgical intervention remained independent predictive factors for cancer-specific mortality. However, in this study, 30% of patients had concomitant distant metastases at the time of RPR.

Another recent retrospective multi-institutional study by Huang et al. compared the oncological outcomes of patients with RPR treated either with RPR surgery or targeted therapy alone. The study included 243 patients, with 182 undergoing surgical resection of RPR and 61 receiving targeted therapy alone. The median CSS was 99 months in the surgery group and 42 months in those treated with targeted therapy alone. For patients treated with RPR surgery, 1, 3, and 5-year recurrence free survival (RFS) rates after surgery were 75%, 42%, and 27%, and 1, 3, and 5-year CSS rates were 93%, 76%, and 69%, respectively. In contrast to patients treated with targeted therapy alone, 1, 3, and 5-year CSS rates were 83%, 51%, and 27%, respectively [14]. This study reinforces the role of aggressive surgical resection for local control and potential improvement in CSS of RCC patients after prior RN.

The improved outcomes observed in recent studies of patients with RPR likely reflect the significant impact of the targeted systemic therapy era on the management of locally advanced and metastatic disease. The KEYNOTE-564 study (median follow-up 57.2 months), the first positive phase III study of an adjuvant immunotherapy in RCC, demonstrated that adjuvant pembrolizumab post-nephrectomy had an improvement in disease-free survival (DFS) versus placebo (estimated DFS at 24 months, 77.3% vs. 68.1%) [36]. Overall survival (OS) for the pembrolizumab group was 91.2% at 48 months compared to 86.0% in the placebo group. These findings provide patients more treatment options with the goal of obtaining better outcomes and extended survival.

In selected patients who do not have distant metastatic disease, performing an aggressive surgical resection of RPR following RN is a viable option. This approach has acceptable complication rates and can potentially cure over 40% of patients. Additional research is necessary to explore the potential benefits and effects of targeted neoadjuvant therapy for this group of patients.

Recurrence After PN

Partial nephrectomy is currently the standard treatment for small renal masses (clinical T1a) when there is a normal contralateral kidney, assuming the mass is suitable for this procedure

[37–40]. Furthermore, PN is being extended to include tumors of any size, provided that optimal oncologic control can be achieved [37, 39, 40]. Incomplete tumor resection and risk of residual disease represented by positive surgical margin (PSM) could occur after PN, regardless of the approach. Consequently, a small percentage of patients (1–5% [41–45]) will develop ipsilateral recurrent disease following PN, and the main risk factors are advanced T stage or high tumor grade. Most local recurrences in this context are likely due to undetected microscopic multifocal RCC, often discovered distant from the previous tumor site. Although recent data suggest that positive surgical margins, especially in patients with high-grade or high-stage disease, may indicate a worse prognosis for recurrence-free and metastases-free survival [46, 47], the overall impact on oncologic outcomes remains less clear.

The literature shows no consensus on whether there is a statistical correlation between surgical margins and recurrence rates or specific survival. At one end of the spectrum, Petros et al. demonstrated a strong association between positive surgical margins (PSM) and disease progression following partial nephrectomy (PN). In their study at a large single-institution center, they reviewed 2297 cases of PN and observed a PSM rate of 1.48%. They found that PSM impacted the 5-year survival probability for OS (0.99 for negative surgical margins (NSM) vs. 0.97 for PSM), local RFS (0.98 vs. 0.77), and metastases-free survival (MFS) [48]. Similarly, Khalifeh et al. reported significantly lower 3-year disease-free survival rates of 47% and 3-year metastasis-free survival rates of 63% in PSM compared to their NSM counterparts [46].

At the opposite end of the spectrum, Yossepovich et al. investigated 1344 patients undergoing PN over more than three decades at Memorial Sloan Kettering and the Mayo Clinic, observing a PSM rate of 5.5%. They found no significant differences in local or metastatic recurrence rates between patients with PSM and those with NSM [49]. Similarly, in the French study by Morrone et al., 2922 patients who underwent robotic-assisted partial nephrectomy (RAPN) were reviewed. Among these, 136 patients (6.3%) had a PSM, with a median follow-up period of 19 months. The study reported a total of 160 (7.4%) recurrences, comprising 88 local recurrences and 72 metastases. Specifically, 9 recurrences (6.6%) occurred in the PSM group, while 151 recurrences (7.4%) were observed in the NSM group. This study found no significant effects on RFS, MFS, or OS [50]. These findings are further corroborated by Bensalah et al., who conducted a multi-institutional cohort study comparing 111 patients with PSM to a matched cohort of 664 patients with NSM. They found no significant differences in RFS, CSS, or OS between the two groups [51].

In general, experts recommend watchful waiting rather than salvage nephrectomy in the setting of a positive surgical margin until visible disease develops [42]. This recommendation is partly due to the challenges associated with re-do surgery, which include obliterated and scarred surgical planes, altered anatomy, surgical landmarks replaced with fibrosis, extensive abdominal adhesions, and the presence of multiple previously placed surgical clips. These technical difficulties greatly increase the risk of complications and the PSM rate in salvage PN compared to the initial surgery [52–54]. Nevertheless, there are several advantages to repeat partial nephrectomy. For patients where repeat nephron-sparing surgery (NSS) could prevent the need for dialysis, it should be considered whenever possible due to the high cardiovascular morbidity and mortality associated with dialysis. Additionally, NSS can have a positive economic impact by avoiding the substantial costs associated with end-stage renal disease and its ongoing care expenses. We must also consider that performing a completion nephrectomy after prior NSS leaves the patient with a solitary kidney, which remains at risk for metachronous, contralateral disease.

Historically, salvage open partial nephrectomy has been well established and provides acceptable oncologic outcomes. In the early 2000s, Magera et al. and colleagues from the Mayo Clinic evaluated intraoperative and postoperative outcomes through a paired analysis. Their study reported that repeat nephron-sparing surgery (NSS) is a safe procedure, with complication rates comparable to those of the initial surgery [55]. More recent series from the group at the National Cancer Institute (NCI) reported experiencing more of the anticipated complications with re-do surgery, citing a 19.6% major complication rate and significant renal functional decline. Nevertheless, they reported acceptable oncologic outcomes, with a 95% MFS at 57 months for salvage PN in a solitary kidney [12].

In another recent study, the MD Anderson group analyzed 44 patients with local tumor bed recurrence (or ipsilateral recurrence [IR]) following PN and compared them with 163 control patients who underwent PN without recurrence [41]. They defined local tumor bed recurrence strictly as the detection of a new enhancing lesion specifically in the surgical defect or in the same region as the initial partial nephrectomy site. The patients with tumor bed recurrence were more likely to have bilateral disease at presentation and a solitary kidney. These patients underwent more complex operations, characterized by longer operative times, higher estimated blood loss (EBL), and extended ischemia time. They were also more likely to have pT3 disease and PSMs, with a rate of 15.6%. Among the patients with IR, 55% underwent salvage surgery, while the remainder received alternate therapies (e.g., ablation, systemic therapy). No significant difference in OS was noted, with a 5-year OS of 77.5% (+/− 6.5%) in the IR group vs. 83.2% (+/− 3.4%) in the control group ($p = 0.22$). However, the IR group experienced significantly worse 5-year CSS, with rates of 86.4% (+/− 5.5%) compared to 99% (+/− 1%) in the control group ($p < 0.001$). Although PSMs have not been shown to affect overall survival in initial PN cases, they have been associated with poor prognosis following salvage PN for local tumor recurrence [14].

Robotic surgery offers significant advantages for patients and clinicians when making surgical decisions. It can reduce intraoperative and postoperative complications while providing less surgical incisional pain, shorter hospital stays, and faster recovery times. This approach was first reported in the salvage setting by Autorino et al. in 2013 and Watson et al. in 2016, where they found similar surgical outcomes after repeat and initial robotic-assisted PN [13, 56]. Most recently, using a prospectively maintained multi-institutional database, Okhawere et al. reviewed 36 patients who underwent salvage robotic-assisted partial nephrectomy (sRPN) from 2012 to 2020. There were three intraoperative complications ($p = 1.000$) and two major postoperative complications ($p = 1.000$) with a rate of conversion to open surgery of 0%. Regarding oncologic outcomes, the PSM rate was 8%, and the recurrence rate was 3% at median follow-up of 7 months [54].

In the current era, robot-assisted laparoscopy has emerged as the predominant approach for minimally invasive surgery (MIS) in the treatment of renal malignancies [57]. However, concerns have been raised within the urologic community due to atypical tumor recurrences (ATR), particularly following robotic surgeries. These recurrences, including those occurring at port sites, have sparked apprehension as they deviate from expected recurrence patterns and challenge the perceived safety of MIS techniques in oncologic control. Russo et al. conducted a study at Memorial Sloan Kettering Cancer Center (MSKCC) involving 58 patients with localized renal cell carcinoma (RCC) who underwent minimally invasive surgery (MIS), either partial or radical nephrectomy, and later developed atypical tumor recurrence (ATR) [58]. The recurrences primarily manifested as perinephric or nephrectomy bed tumor implants in 48% of cases ($n = 28$). Additionally, 29% of patients exhibited intraperitoneal and port-site metastases. A noteworthy finding from this study was the disparity in recurrence timing between high-grade and low-grade tumors, with high-grade tumors recurring significantly sooner (median of 7 months) compared to low-grade tumors (median of 31 months) [58].

In contrast, the large, randomized ASSURE trial demonstrated no significant differences in oncologic outcomes—such as overall survival, cancer-specific survival, or local recurrence patterns—between open and minimally invasive surgery (MIS) approaches [59]. Building on this, Lee et al. utilized the ASSURE trial cohort to propose a novel classification system for local recurrence following surgery, categorizing recurrences into four types: Type I, involving a single recurrence in the remnant kidney or ipsilateral renal fossa; Type II, featuring a single recurrence in the ipsilateral vasculature, adrenal gland, or a lymph node; Type III, indicating a single recurrence in other intra-abdominal soft tissues or organs; and Type IV, encompassing any combination of Types I–III or multiple recurrences within a single type [59]. The worldwide adoption of a standardized definition and classification for local recurrence, such as this one, could facilitate validation and foster discussions on specific treatment strategies for distinct recurrence patterns.

Patients who present with tumor recurrence after an initial partial nephrectomy are generally older and have more significant comorbidities than at the time of their initial surgery. Given the high surgical risk associated with re-do surgery, coupled with these additional health risks, there is certainly a subset of patients for whom targeted therapy may be more appropriate than undergoing major surgery. Tumor ablation for local recurrence may also offer a less invasive treatment alternative. While this treatment modality is beyond the scope of this chapter, it is important to mention it as another option for patients for whom surgery is too risky.

Local Recurrence Following Primary Ablative Therapy

The daily utilization of advanced imaging techniques by clinicians to assess patients' complaints has significantly increased the rate of diagnosis of incidental renal masses, particularly small, low-stage renal masses [60]. In recent years, thermal ablation (TA) has gained widespread acceptance as a management option for small renal masses, particularly for patients with multiple comorbidities who are considered poor candidates for surgery [61]. Consequently, since 2017, both the American Urological Association (AUA) and European Association of Urology (EAU) guidelines have recommended ablative techniques as a valid alternative to surgery for pT1a renal masses (<4 cm), except for those located at the hilum or in proximity to the proximal ureter [39, 62]. Studies have demonstrated that PN and TA offer comparable metastasis-free survival rates. Additionally, TA has been shown to have a favorable morbidity profile when compared to extirpative surgery, including lower transfusion rates, shorter hospital stays, and reduced conversion rates to RN [63]. However, the long-term efficacy of TA is not as well established as the other surgical modalities, and local recurrences tend to be more frequent after TA than after surgery [44, 64]. Proposed management of a failed ablative procedure include active surveillance, tissue biopsy, salvage ablation, and salvage surgery. Considering that most patients who undergo primary TA were initially deemed poor candidates for surgery, repeat TA (rTA) is frequently advocated as a viable option for addressing residual or locally recurrent renal cell carcinoma (RCC). Approximately 66% to 73% of patients who undergo initial ablative treatment and then experience local tumor recurrence are estimated to undergo repeated ablation [65]. However, patients who are unsuitable for rTA due to large or complex recurrences, or those who are viable candidates for surgery, may opt for salvage surgery.

The rates of local recurrence can vary based on the initial treatment modality chosen—whether cryosurgery or radiofrequency ablation—and on tumor-related risk factors such as stage and histologic subtype. In general, local recurrence rates following TA are higher compared to those after surgery, with TA having a recurrence rate of 2–10% versus 1–2% for surgical excision [66–68]. Diagnosing local recurrence after TA can be challenging due to the evolving fibrosis within the tumor bed, which can make it difficult to distinguish from residual tumor. Typically, central or nodular enhancement within the tumor bed on extended follow-up imaging is considered indicative of local recurrence. It is important to highlight that persistent contrast enhancement can be detected up to 9 months after the cryoablation, although this does not necessarily indicate malignancy [69]. The AUA Guidelines recommend performing a post-ablative biopsy in cases of new enhancement, progressive increase in the size of the ablated tumor, new nodularity in or around the treated zone, failure of the ablated tumor to regress over time, or the appearance of satellite or port site lesions [70].

The majority of local recurrences can be addressed through repeat ablation, although a subset of patients with progressive disease may eventually necessitate conventional surgical intervention. These cases include instances of rapid tumor growth following primary treatment or tumors situated in unfavorable locations, such as the collecting system or renal hilum. Salvage renal surgery following ablation is technically demanding and complicated by severe fibrosis surrounding the previously ablated lesion, which distorts normal anatomical planes and makes dissections particularly challenging. The choice between PN and RN depends on several factors, including the type of lesion, the patient's overall health, and, crucially, the surgeon's experience and expertise. This issue was underscored in a study by Nguyen et al., in which half of the patients initially scheduled for partial nephrectomy had to be converted to radical nephrectomy due to extensive scarring and fibrosis [71]. Karam et al. subsequently evaluated the feasibility, safety, and pathological, radiological, and functional outcomes of salvage surgery following ablation. The majority of surgeries were performed using an open approach, with only one laparoscopic and one robotic-assisted procedure. No deaths were observed after a median follow-up period of 26.5 months. While surgery was feasible in all but one attempted case, they reported a high rate of perioperative complications and noted postoperative complications in nine patients, four of which were Clavien grade III [72]. Abarzua-Cabezas et al. reported their experience with 13 patients, where 10 underwent salvage partial nephrectomy (sPN) and 3 underwent salvage radical nephrectomy (sRN). They observed no major intraoperative complications or injuries to adjacent organs. They concluded that, despite being a challenging procedure, salvage surgery is both feasible and capable of achieving adequate oncologic outcomes [73].

Treating post-ablation local recurrence with salvage surgery is technically challenging and may result in a radical nephrectomy for patients who were initially candidates for partial nephrectomy. This approach carries a significantly higher morbidity compared to primary kidney surgery. Therefore, it is crucial to accurately select suitable candidates for ablation at the initial diagnosis and confirm local recurrence before considering salvage surgery. Current studies suggest that, in properly selected patients, surgical salvage for post-ablation local recurrence, including partial nephrectomy, is feasible, though demanding. Further investigations are required to evaluate the long-term efficacy of salvage techniques, with particular focus on the outcomes of robotic surgery.

Renal Cell Carcinoma Metastasectomy

Despite the success of surgical interventions for localized renal cell carcinoma, 20 to 30% of patients will eventually develop asynchronous metastatic disease or local recurrence after treatment [39, 74]. Moreover, even with the advent of novel immune-oncologic (IO) therapies and vascular endothelial growth factor (VEGF)-targeted combination therapies for metastatic renal cell carcinoma (mRCC), the complete response rate for medical treatment remains modest, ranging between 3% and 16%, as evidenced by phase III randomized studies [75–77]. However, in carefully selected patients, surgical resection of metastatic disease, when technically feasible, offers a potentially curative treatment option. Although only a limited number of studies have explored the role of surgical metastasectomy in mRCC, and no Level 1 evidence exists to demonstrate its superiority over systemic therapy, retrospective and observational studies have shown promising results. These studies report a 5-year survival rate approaching 50% following metastasectomy for mRCC [78–80].

Approximately 61% of patients with metastatic renal cell carcinoma (mRCC) develop solitary metastatic lesions, while 39% present with multifocal metastatic disease [81]. This multifocal disease often includes concurrent bone and brain metastases in addition to metastases at other sites. The prognosis of RCC patients is significantly influenced by the site of metastasis [81]. The National Comprehensive Cancer Network (NCCN) guidelines indicate that patients with oligometastatic recurrences after nephrectomy may be eligible for metastasectomy in certain cases, including metastases in the lung, bone, and brain [82]. In contrast, the European Association of Urology (EAU) suggests metastasectomy as a viable local treatment option for most mRCC sites, except for brain and bone metastases [39].

Zaid et al. conducted a systematic review, revealing that complete metastasectomy in patients with mRCC resulted in reduced overall mortality rates [83]. Nevertheless, patients with mRCC constitute a diverse population based on the number and locations of metastases, the duration between localized and metastatic RCC, the stage of the primary tumor, and individual patient attributes. While some advocate for metastasectomy in patients with solitary or multiple metastases [83], others suggest that the best candidates are those with solitary or oligometastatic lesions [84].

The lung is the most common site for metastasis in RCC, representing 43.6% of kidney cancer metastases [85]. Lung metastases from RCC (LM-RCC) are often observed as either solitary or multiple pulmonary nodules. In certain clinical settings, solitary nodules can be mistaken for primary lung carcinoma [86]. Research has demonstrated that aggressive surgical removal of LM-RCC provides potential survival benefits, with reported 5-year survival rates ranging from 18% to 75% [87]. Complete resection has been demonstrated to be a significant predictor of favorable prognosis, positively impacting survival by delaying the need for immunotherapy or targeted therapy, and potentially facilitating a complete response following these treatments [88, 89]. Nevertheless, certain risk factors are consistently associated with poorer outcomes in this group: pulmonary nodules larger than 3 cm, involvement of hilar or mediastinal lymph nodes, reduced pulmonary reserve, prolonged disease-free interval between definitive therapy and the onset of pulmonary metastases, and incomplete metastasectomy [90–93].

Meimarakis and colleagues [94] developed a prognostic tool known as the Munich score, which is designed to assist in long-term outcome prediction after pulmonary metastasectomy. They identified key risk factors post-surgery, including pleural invasion, the presence of synchronous metastases, primary tumor nodal status (pN), metastases smaller than 3 cm, and involvement of hilar or mediastinal lymph nodes. According to this score, patients classified as Munich I (complete metastasectomy with no risk factors) had a median survival of 90.1 months, those in Munich II (complete metastasectomy with one or more risk factors) had a median survival of 31.4 months, and Munich III (incomplete metastasectomy) had a median survival of 14.2 months.

In the case of RCC, the bone is the primary site for hematogenous spread of tumor cells [95] and is the second most common site of metastasis after the lungs. Bone metastases are observed in approximately 20% to 35% of patients with metastatic RCC (mRCC), and the 5-year survival rate for these patients is less than 11% [96]. The lesions are predominantly osteolytic, resulting in significant skeletal destruction, accompanied by subsequent pain, pathological fractures, hypercalcemia, and nerve compression. Consequently, the primary treatment objectives for these patients are to alleviate pain and prevent or delay skeletal-related events (SREs) [97].

The treatment of brain metastases poses significant challenges, as success rates in this patient group have been notably lower. Brain metastases occur in approximately 17% of patients with metastatic RCC, where the median overall survival (OS) is reported as 10.7 months, and the 5-year survival rate is only 12% [98]. Clinical trials with systemic therapies such as sunitinib and nivolumab have demonstrated limited efficacy in treating intracranial metastases in patients with renal cell carcinoma (RCC) [99]. However, retrospective analyses have shown promising outcomes with other tyrosine kinase inhibitors, notably cabozantinib, which has yielded encouraging responses in this patient population [100]. Radiotherapy (RT), with or without surgical resection, continues to serve as the primary approach for managing brain metastases. Surgical resection is typically reserved for patients with a limited number of intracranial metastases (generally up to five) and favorable performance status, where the benefit of removing lesions can be maximized.

In a study by Ikushima et al. [101], patients receiving local therapy for brain metastases demonstrated varying survival outcomes based on treatment modality. Median survival was 25.6 months for those treated with fractionated stereotactic radiotherapy, 18.7 months for patients undergoing surgical resection followed by conventional radiotherapy, and 4.3 months for those treated with conventional radiotherapy alone. Similarly, Ippen et al. [102] compared different therapeutic approaches, showing a median survival of 21.9 months in patients treated with stereotactic radiosurgery combined with surgical resection, 13.9 months for stereotactic radiosurgery alone, and 5.9 months for whole-brain radiotherapy. More recent findings from Ma et al. further explored the outcomes of radiotherapy for brain metastases in RCC at Memorial Sloan Kettering Cancer Center (MSKCC) [103]. In this cohort, 91 patients with RCC brain metastases underwent stereotactic radiosurgery (SRS) to 212 lesions, with a median follow-up of 38.3 months for surviving patients. Median intracranial progression-free survival and overall survival were 7.8 months and 21 months, respectively, with durable local control of 83% at 12 months post-SRS [103]. These studies collectively highlight the paucity of data regarding the local treatment of brain metastases in RCC, emphasizing the importance of multimodal strategies and the need for further research to optimize management approaches.

The concept of metastasectomy for cases involving multiple sites, beyond a single site or organ, has been gaining attention. Retrospective studies, many of which were conducted before the advent of targeted therapies, suggest that resection of metastatic disease at multiple locations may be linked to improved cancer-specific survival (CSS) [78, 79]. In a single-institution study by Kavolius et al. [78], the authors reported a 5-year overall survival (OS) rate of 44% for patients who underwent complete metastasectomy, compared to just 11% for those who did not receive resection or systemic therapy. However, the study also found that patients with multiple metastatic sites had a significantly lower 5-year OS compared to those with only a single site resected (29% vs. 54%, $P < 0.001$) [78].

Alt et al. [79] presented findings from another single-institution study, reporting a 5-year cancer-specific survival (CSS) rate of 49.4% for patients who underwent complete metastasectomy at multiple sites, compared to just 13.9% for those who did not achieve complete resection ($P < 0.001$). This survival benefit was maintained even for patients with three or more metastases when complete resection was achieved [79]. When controlling for factors such as the number of lesions, location, timing of metastases, and ECOG performance status, patients who underwent complete resection of all metastatic disease exhibited a threefold decrease in the risk of cancer-specific death (HR 2.91; 95% CI, 2.17–3.90; $P < 0.001$). In a separate study, Naito et al. [104] analyzed 556 patients with metastatic RCC who underwent either complete or incomplete metastasectomy, showing a significant survival advantage for those with complete resection (109.8 vs. 31.9 months, $P < 0.001$). These findings underscore the recognized value of complete metastasectomy, when feasible, despite the extent of disease burden.

Retrospective studies of this type are inherently biased, often favoring healthier patients with a lower disease burden. In many cases, incomplete resections are performed as palliative measures, which can significantly distort the results due to selection bias. Zaid et al. [83] conducted a meta-analysis that made a focused effort to address these biases. Their comparison of overall survival (OS) in patients undergoing complete metastasectomy, stratified by performance status, revealed no significant differences [83]. Moreover, the analysis of pooled data from eight studies yielded a hazard ratio (HR) of 2.37 (95% CI, 2.10–2.87; $P < 0.001$) for complete metastasectomy, underscoring the survival benefit of complete resection when it is feasible [83].

While complete metastasectomy has gained widespread acceptance, the value of incomplete resection in metastatic disease remains controversial. Numerous studies have shown that incomplete metastasectomy is a significant negative prognostic indicator for survival [78, 79, 83, 104, 105]. Reported median survival times for patients who underwent complete versus incomplete resection range from 4.8 to 9.1 years and 1.3 to 2.7 years, respectively [79, 104, 105]. Nevertheless, some research has sought to compare outcomes between patients who had incomplete resections and those who underwent no surgical intervention at all. For instance, in the study by Alt et al. [79] discussed earlier, not only did complete metastasectomy offer a 5-year cancer-specific survival (CSS) benefit (49.4%), but incomplete resection also provided a survival advantage over no resection (23.7% vs. 8.9%, $P < 0.001$). Identifying patients who might benefit from incomplete resection and determining the optimal integration of targeted therapy and immune checkpoint inhibitors will require further focused research.

With advancements in systemic treatments for metastatic RCC, the combination of targeted therapies and immune checkpoint inhibitors with surgical resection has become standard practice and is likely to remain so in the foreseeable future. Reports on metastasectomy following targeted therapies are available but involve a limited number of patients [22, 106–108]. In one study, Karam et al. [106] analyzed 22 patients who underwent targeted therapy followed by complete metastasectomy at multiple sites. The study found a 50% tumor recurrence rate, with all but one patient alive at a median follow-up of 109 weeks. The single reported death occurred roughly 2 years after metastasectomy. The highest perioperative complication rates were observed in patients undergoing retroperitoneal resections, with complications including chylous ascites, atrial fibrillation, and prolonged ileus. Additionally, 9 out of the 22 patients received adjuvant targeted therapy. The KEYNOTE-564 trial, designed to evaluate adjuvant pembrolizumab monotherapy versus placebo in patients with localized RCC following nephrectomy, or after nephrectomy and metastasectomy in those with M1 rendered NED, demonstrated a significant improvement with the use of adjuvant pembrolizumab. The study showed a significant improvement in disease-free survival (DFS) compared to placebo, with a hazard ratio of 0.63 (95% CI 0.50–0.80), solidifying its role as an effective postoperative treatment in high-risk RCC [22]. Vascular endothelial growth factor receptor (VEGFR) inhibitors, such as pazopanib, have also been evaluated, but the results have been less than encouraging. In a randomized, double-blind phase III trial comparing pazopanib to placebo in patients with metastatic renal cell carcinoma (mRCC) who were no evidence of disease (NED) following metastasectomy, Appleman et al. aimed to increase disease-free survival (DFS) from 25% to 45% at 3 years. However, the study failed to meet its primary endpoint, with a 3-year DFS of 27.4% (95% CI, 17.9–41.17) for pazopanib compared to 21.9% (95% CI, 13.3–36.2) for placebo. The 3-year overall survival (OS) was 81.9% (95% CI, 72.7–92.2) for pazopanib and 91.4% (95% CI, 84.4–98.9) for placebo, with a noted decline in health-related quality of life among patients receiving pazopanib [109].

Conclusion

Careful patient selection is crucial in the surgical management of locally recurrent and metastatic RCC to ensure that the appropriate therapy is applied at the optimal time. Isolated local recurrence after a well-executed radical nephrectomy, partial nephrectomy, or tumor ablation is relatively uncommon. Surgical resection following either radical or partial nephrectomy is technically demanding and carries a significant risk of morbidity. However, with careful patient selection, excellent oncologic outcomes can be achieved. A multidisciplinary approach at a high-volume referral center is essential for the successful management of these cases.

In instances of local recurrence after ablation, it is critical to confirm recurrence through biopsy before considering a complex resection, which is more challenging than primary renal surgery. Proper surgical planning and realistic expectations are vital. Metastasectomy, when performed in appropriately selected patients, appears to be associated with prolonged disease-free survival. Currently, ideal candidates for metastasectomy are those with good performance status and disease that is completely resectable. Future evaluations of this approach will need to be integrated with ongoing assessments of the therapeutic benefits of targeted systemic therapies.

References

1. Cancer Facts & Figures: American Cancer Society; 2024. https://www.cancer.org/cancer/types/kidney-cancer/about/key-statistics.html.
2. Attalla K, Weng S, Voss MH, Hakimi AA. Epidemiology, risk assessment, and biomarkers for patients with advanced renal cell carcinoma. Urol Clin North Am. 2020;47(3):293–303.
3. Chin AI, Lam JS, Figlin RA, Belldegrun AS. Surveillance strategies for renal cell carcinoma patients following nephrectomy. Rev Urol. 2006;8(1):1–7.
4. Leopold Z, Srivastava A, Singer EA. Predictors of recurrence for T3a RCC: a recurring conundrum. Diagnostics (Basel). 2020;10(11):983.
5. Esrig D, Ahlering TE, Lieskovsky G, Skinner DG. Experience with fossa recurrence of renal cell carcinoma. J Urol. 1992;147(6):1491–4.
6. Levy DA, Slaton JW, Swanson DA, Dinney CP. Stage specific guidelines for surveillance after radical nephrectomy for local renal cell carcinoma. J Urol. 1998;159(4):1163–7.
7. Sandock DS, Seftel AD, Resnick MI. A new protocol for the followup of renal cell carcinoma based on pathological stage. J Urol. 1995;154(1):28–31.
8. Bandi G, Wen CC, Moon TD, Nakada SY. Single center preliminary experience with hand-assisted laparoscopic resection of isolated renal cell carcinoma fossa recurrences. Urology. 2008;71(3):495–9; discussion 9–500.
9. Margulis V, McDonald M, Tamboli P, Swanson DA, Wood CG. Predictors of oncological outcome after resection of locally recurrent renal cell carcinoma. J Urol. 2009;181(5):2044–51.
10. Master VA, Gottschalk AR, Kane C, Carroll PR. Management of isolated renal fossa recurrence following radical nephrectomy. J Urol. 2005;174(2):473–7; discussion 7.
11. Yohannan J, Feng T, Berkowitz J, Connolly SS, Pierorazio P, Allaf ME. Laparoscopic resection of local recurrence after previous radical nephrectomy for clinically localized renal-cell carcinoma: perioperative outcomes and initial observations. J Endourol. 2010;24(10):1609–12.
12. Liu NW, Khurana K, Sudarshan S, Pinto PA, Linehan WM, Bratslavsky G. Repeat partial nephrectomy on the solitary kidney: surgical, functional and oncological outcomes. J Urol. 2010;183(5):1719–24.
13. Autorino R, Khalifeh A, Laydner H, Samarasekera D, Rizkala E, Eyraud R, et al. Repeat robot-assisted partial nephrectomy (RAPN): feasibility and early outcomes. BJU Int. 2013;111(5):767–72.
14. Huang J, Wang Y, Zhang C, Hu X, Wang P, Shi G, et al. Surgical management and oncologic outcomes for local retroperitoneal recurrence of renal cell carcinoma after radical nephrectomy. Clin Genitourin Cancer. 2023;21(2):315e1–7.
15. Di Lorenzo G, Autorino R, Sternberg CN. Metastatic renal cell carcinoma: recent advances in the targeted therapy era. Eur Urol. 2009;56(6):959–71.
16. Heng DY, Xie W, Regan MM, Warren MA, Golshayan AR, Sahi C, et al. Prognostic factors for overall survival in patients with metastatic renal cell carcinoma treated with vascular endothelial growth factor-targeted agents: results from a large, multicenter study. J Clin Oncol. 2009;27(34):5794–9.
17. Escudier B, Porta C, Schmidinger M, Rioux-Leclercq N, Bex A, Khoo V, et al. Renal cell carcinoma: ESMO clinical practice guidelines for diagnosis, treatment and follow-up. Ann Oncol. 2019;30(5):706–20.
18. Mejean A, Ravaud A, Thezenas S, Chevreau C, Bensalah K, Geoffrois L, et al. Sunitinib alone or after nephrectomy for patients with metastatic renal cell carcinoma: is there still a role for cytoreductive nephrectomy? Eur Urol. 2021;80(4):417–24.
19. McIntosh AG, Umbreit EC, Holland LC, Gu C, Tannir NM, Matin SF, et al. Optimizing patient selection for cytoreductive nephrectomy based on outcomes in the contemporary era of systemic therapy. Cancer. 2020;126(17):3950–60.
20. Bex A, Albiges L, Ljungberg B, Bensalah K, Dabestani S, Giles RH, et al. Updated European Association of Urology guidelines for cytoreductive nephrectomy in patients with synchronous metastatic clear-cell renal cell carcinoma. Eur Urol. 2018;74(6):805–9.
21. Motzer RJ, Russo P. Cytoreductive nephrectomy—patient selection is key. N Engl J Med. 2018;379(5):481–2.
22. Powles T, Tomczak P, Park SH, Venugopal B, Ferguson T, Symeonides SN, et al. Pembrolizumab versus placebo as post-nephrectomy adjuvant therapy for clear cell renal cell carcinoma (KEYNOTE-564): 30-month follow-up analysis of a multicentre, randomised, double-blind, placebo-controlled, phase 3 trial. Lancet Oncol. 2022;23(9):1133–44.

23. Siegel RL, Miller KD, Jemal A. Cancer statistics, 2020. CA Cancer J Clin. 2020;70(1):7–30.
24. Thomas AZ, Adibi M, Borregales LD, Hoang LN, Tamboli P, Jonasch E, et al. Surgical management of local retroperitoneal recurrence of renal cell carcinoma after radical nephrectomy. J Urol. 2015;194(2):316–22.
25. Psutka SP, Heidenreich M, Boorjian SA, Bailey GC, Cheville JC, Stewart-Merrill SB, et al. Renal fossa recurrence after nephrectomy for renal cell carcinoma: prognostic features and oncological outcomes. BJU Int. 2017;119(1):116–27.
26. Du Y, Grullich C, Hadaschik B, Hatiboglu G, Hohenfellner M, Pahernik S. Local recurrence after curative surgical treatment of renal cell cancer: a study of 91 patients. Clin Genitourin Cancer. 2016;14(4):e379–85.
27. Marchioni M, Sountoulides P, Furlan M, Mir MC, Aretano L, Rubio-Briones J, et al. Management of local recurrence after radical nephrectomy: surgical removal with or without systemic treatment is still the gold standard. Results from a multicenter international cohort. Int Urol Nephrol. 2021;53(11):2273–80.
28. Abu-Ghanem Y, Ramon J, Berger R, Kaver I, Fridman E, Leibowitz-Amit R, et al. Positive surgical margin following radical nephrectomy is an independent predictor of local recurrence and disease-specific survival. World J Surg Oncol. 2017;15(1):193.
29. El Hajj A, Thanigasalam R, Molinie V, Massoud W, Fourati M, Girard F, et al. Feasibility and oncological outcomes of laparoscopic treatment for local relapse of renal cell carcinoma. BJU Int. 2013;112(4):E307–13.
30. Vitagliano G, Ameri C, Castillo O, Rozanec J. Laparoscopic resection of isolated fossa recurrence of renal cell carcinoma after open nephrectomy: report of 6 cases and literature review. Arch Esp Urol. 2014;67(3):277–83.
31. Smaldone MC, Cannon GM Jr, Hrebinko RL. Resection of recurrent inferior vena cava tumor after radical nephrectomy for renal cell carcinoma. Urology. 2006;67(5):1084e5–7.
32. Minervini A, Salinitri G, Lera J, Caldarelli C, Caramella D, Minervini R. Solitary floating vena caval thrombus as a late recurrence of renal cell carcinoma. Int J Urol. 2004;11(4):239–42.
33. Finkelstein MP, Drinis S, Tortorelis DG, Lafaro RJ, Konno S, Choudhury MS. Recurrence of renal cell carcinoma with extensive vena caval thrombus three years after radical nephrectomy. Urol Int. 2002;68(3):199–201.
34. D'Arrigo L, Pennisi M, Pepe P, Scolaro A, Lomeo A, Aragona F. Isolated local recurrence of renal neoplasm with caval involvement 16 years after radical nephrectomy. Arch Esp Urol. 2005;58(10):1093–4.
35. Paparel P, Bigot P, Matillon X, Bensalah K, Salomon L, Baumert H, et al. Local recurrence after radical nephrectomy for kidney cancer: management and prediction of outcomes. A multi-institutional study. J Surg Oncol. 2014;109(2):126–31.
36. Choueiri TK, Tomczak P, Park SH, Venugopal B, Ferguson T, Symeonides SN, et al. Overall survival with adjuvant Pembrolizumab in renal-cell carcinoma. N Engl J Med. 2024;390(15):1359–71.
37. Campbell SC, Uzzo RG, Karam JA, Chang SS, Clark PE, Souter L. Renal mass and localized renal cancer: evaluation, management, and follow-up: AUA guideline: part II. J Urol. 2021;206(2):209–18.
38. Finelli A, Ismaila N, Bro B, Durack J, Eggener S, Evans A, et al. Management of small renal masses: American Society of Clinical Oncology clinical practice guideline. J Clin Oncol. 2017;35(6):668–80.
39. Ljungberg B, Albiges L, Abu-Ghanem Y, Bedke J, Capitanio U, Dabestani S, et al. European Association of Urology guidelines on renal cell carcinoma: the 2022 update. Eur Urol. 2022;82(4):399–410.
40. Motzer RJ, Jonasch E, Agarwal N, Alva A, Bagshaw H, Baine M, et al. NCCN guidelines(R) insights: kidney cancer, version 2.2024. J Natl Compr Canc Netw. 2024;22(1):4–16.
41. Wood EL, Adibi M, Qiao W, Brandt J, Zhang M, Tamboli P, et al. Local tumor bed recurrence following partial nephrectomy in patients with small renal masses. J Urol. 2018;199(2):393–400.
42. Shuch B, Linehan WM, Bratslavsky G. Repeat partial nephrectomy: surgical, functional and oncological outcomes. Curr Opin Urol. 2011;21(5):368–75.
43. Kreshover JE, Richstone L, Kavoussi LR. Renal cell recurrence for T1 tumors after laparoscopic partial nephrectomy. J Endourol. 2013;27(12):1468–70.
44. Thompson RH, Atwell T, Schmit G, Lohse CM, Kurup AN, Weisbrod A, et al. Comparison of partial nephrectomy and percutaneous ablation for cT1 renal masses. Eur Urol. 2015;67(2):252–9.
45. Hafez KS, Fergany AF, Novick AC. Nephron sparing surgery for localized renal cell carcinoma: impact of tumor size on patient survival, tumor recurrence and TNM staging. J Urol. 1999;162(6):1930–3.
46. Khalifeh A, Kaouk JH, Bhayani S, Rogers C, Stifelman M, Tanagho YS, et al. Positive surgical margins in robot-assisted partial nephrectomy: a multi-institutional analysis of oncologic outcomes (leave no tumor behind). J Urol. 2013;190(5):1674–9.
47. Shah PH, Moreira DM, Okhunov Z, Patel VR, Chopra S, Razmaria AA, et al. Positive surgical margins increase risk of recurrence after partial nephrectomy for high risk renal tumors. J Urol. 2016;196(2):327–34.
48. Petros FG, Metcalfe MJ, Yu KJ, Keskin SK, Fellman BM, Chang CM, et al. Oncologic outcomes of patients with positive surgical margin after partial nephrectomy: a 25-year single institution experience. World J Urol. 2018;36(7):1093–101.
49. Yossepowitch O, Thompson RH, Leibovich BC, Eggener SE, Pettus JA, Kwon ED, et al. Positive surgical margins at partial nephrectomy: predictors and oncological outcomes. J Urol. 2008;179(6):2158–63.

50. Morrone A, Bentellis I, Bernhard JC, Bensalah K, Champy C, Bruyere F, et al. Positive surgical margin's impact on short-term oncological prognosis after robot-assisted partial nephrectomy (MARGINS study: UroCCR no 96). Sci Rep. 2022;12(1):18342.
51. Bensalah K, Pantuck AJ, Rioux-Leclercq N, Thuret R, Montorsi F, Karakiewicz PI, et al. Positive surgical margin appears to have negligible impact on survival of renal cell carcinomas treated by nephron-sparing surgery. Eur Urol. 2010;57(3):466–71.
52. Beksac AT, Carbonara U, Abou Zeinab M, Meagher M, Hemal S, Tafuri A, et al. Redo robotic partial nephrectomy for recurrent renal tumors: a multi-institutional analysis. J Endourol. 2022;36(10):1296–301.
53. Bratslavsky G, Liu JJ, Johnson AD, Sudarshan S, Choyke PL, Linehan WM, et al. Salvage partial nephrectomy for hereditary renal cancer: feasibility and outcomes. J Urol. 2008;179(1):67–70.
54. Okhawere KE, Grauer R, Zuluaga L, Meilika KN, Ucpinar B, Beksac AT, et al. Operative and oncological outcomes of salvage robotic radical and partial nephrectomy: a multicenter experience. J Robot Surg. 2023;17(4):1579–85.
55. Magera JS Jr, Frank I, Lohse CM, Leibovich BC, Cheville JC, Blute ML. Analysis of repeat nephron sparing surgery as a treatment option in patients with a solid mass in a renal remnant. J Urol. 2008;179(3):853–6.
56. Watson MJ, Sidana A, Diaz AW, Siddiqui MM, Hankins RA, Bratslavsky G, et al. Repeat robotic partial nephrectomy: characteristics, complications, and renal functional outcomes. J Endourol. 2016;30(11):1219–26.
57. Ghani KR, Sukumar S, Sammon JD, Rogers CG, Trinh QD, Menon M. Practice patterns and outcomes of open and minimally invasive partial nephrectomy since the introduction of robotic partial nephrectomy: results from the nationwide inpatient sample. J Urol. 2014;191(4):907–12.
58. Russo P, Blum KA, Weng S, Graafland N, Bex A. Outcomes for atypical tumor recurrences following minimally invasive kidney cancer operations. Eur Urol Open Sci. 2022;40:125–32.
59. Lee Z, Jegede OA, Haas NB, Pins MR, Messing EM, Manola J, et al. Local recurrence following resection of intermediate-high risk non metastatic renal cell carcinoma: an anatomical classification and analysis of the ASSURE (ECOG-ACRIN E2805) adjuvant trial. J Urol. 2020;203(4):684–9.
60. Kane CJ, Mallin K, Ritchey J, Cooperberg MR, Carroll PR. Renal cell cancer stage migration: analysis of the National Cancer DataBase. Cancer. 2008;113(1):78–83.
61. Campbell SC, Clark PE, Chang SS, Karam JA, Souter L, Uzzo RG. Renal mass and localized renal cancer: evaluation, management, and follow-up: AUA guideline: part I. J Urol. 2021;206(2):199–208.
62. Campbell S, Uzzo RG, Allaf ME, Bass EB, Cadeddu JA, Chang A, et al. Renal mass and localized renal cancer: AUA guideline. J Urol. 2017;198(3):520–9.
63. Pierorazio PM, Johnson MH, Patel HD, Sozio SM, Sharma R, Iyoha E, et al. Management of renal masses and localized renal cancer: systematic review and meta-analysis. J Urol. 2016;196(4):989–99.
64. Best SL, Park SK, Youssef RF, Olweny EO, Tan YK, Trimmer C, et al. Long-term outcomes of renal tumor radio frequency ablation stratified by tumor diameter: size matters. J Urol. 2012;187(4):1183–9.
65. Kunkle DA, Uzzo RG. Cryoablation or radiofrequency ablation of the small renal mass: a meta-analysis. Cancer. 2008;113(10):2671–80.
66. Hafez KS, Novick AC, Campbell SC. Patterns of tumor recurrence and guidelines for followup after nephron sparing surgery for sporadic renal cell carcinoma. J Urol. 1997;157(6):2067–70.
67. Eggener SE, Yossepowitch O, Pettus JA, Snyder ME, Motzer RJ, Russo P. Renal cell carcinoma recurrence after nephrectomy for localized disease: predicting survival from time of recurrence. J Clin Oncol. 2006;24(19):3101–6.
68. Capogrosso P, Capitanio U, La Croce G, Nini A, Salonia A, Montorsi F, et al. Follow-up after treatment for renal cell carcinoma: the evidence beyond the guidelines. Eur Urol Focus. 2016;1(3):272–81.
69. Stein AJ, Mayes JM, Mouraviev V, Chen VH, Nelson RC, Polascik TJ. Persistent contrast enhancement several months after laparoscopic cryoablation of the small renal mass may not indicate recurrent tumor. J Endourol. 2008;22(11):2433–9.
70. Donat SM, Diaz M, Bishoff JT, Coleman JA, Dahm P, Derweesh IH, et al. Follow-up for clinically localized renal neoplasms: AUA guideline. J Urol. 2013;190(2):407–16.
71. Nguyen CT, Lane BR, Kaouk JH, Hegarty N, Gill IS, Novick AC, et al. Surgical salvage of renal cell carcinoma recurrence after thermal ablative therapy. J Urol. 2008;180(1):104–9; discussion 9.
72. Karam JA, Wood CG, Compton ZR, Rao P, Vikram R, Ahrar K, et al. Salvage surgery after energy ablation for renal masses. BJU Int. 2015;115(1):74–80.
73. Abarzua-Cabezas FG, Sverrisson E, De La Cruz R, Spiess PE, Haddock P, Sexton WJ. Oncological and functional outcomes of salvage renal surgery following failed primary intervention for renal cell carcinoma. Int Braz J Urol. 2015;41(1):147–54.
74. Gandaglia G, Ravi P, Abdollah F, Abd-El-Barr AE, Becker A, Popa I, et al. Contemporary incidence and mortality rates of kidney cancer in the United States. Can Urol Assoc J. 2014;8(7–8):247–52.
75. Motzer RJ, Tannir NM, McDermott DF, Aren Frontera O, Melichar B, Choueiri TK, et al. Nivolumab plus Ipilimumab versus Sunitinib in advanced renal-cell carcinoma. N Engl J Med. 2018;378(14):1277–90.
76. Motzer RJ, Powles T, Burotto M, Escudier B, Bourlon MT, Shah AY, et al. Nivolumab plus cabozantinib versus sunitinib in first-line treatment for advanced

renal cell carcinoma (CheckMate 9ER): long-term follow-up results from an open-label, randomised, phase 3 trial. Lancet Oncol. 2022;23(7):888–98.
77. Motzer R, Alekseev B, Rha SY, Porta C, Eto M, Powles T, et al. Lenvatinib plus Pembrolizumab or Everolimus for advanced renal cell carcinoma. N Engl J Med. 2021;384(14):1289–300.
78. Kavolius JP, Mastorakos DP, Pavlovich C, Russo P, Burt ME, Brady MS. Resection of metastatic renal cell carcinoma. J Clin Oncol. 1998;16(6):2261–6.
79. Alt AL, Boorjian SA, Lohse CM, Costello BA, Leibovich BC, Blute ML. Survival after complete surgical resection of multiple metastases from renal cell carcinoma. Cancer. 2011;117(13):2873–82.
80. Eggener SE, Yossepowitch O, Kundu S, Motzer RJ, Russo P. Risk score and metastasectomy independently impact prognosis of patients with recurrent renal cell carcinoma. J Urol. 2008;180(3):873–8. discussion 8.
81. Wiechno P, Kucharz J, Sadowska M, Michalski W, Sikora-Kupis B, Jonska-Gmyrek J, et al. Contemporary treatment of metastatic renal cell carcinoma. Med Oncol. 2018;35(12):156.
82. Motzer RJ, Jonasch E, Agarwal N, Alva A, Baine M, Beckermann K, et al. Kidney cancer, version 3.2022, NCCN clinical practice guidelines in oncology. J Natl Compr Canc Netw. 2022;20(1):71–90.
83. Zaid HB, Parker WP, Safdar NS, Gershman B, Erwin PJ, Murad MH, et al. Outcomes following complete surgical metastasectomy for patients with metastatic renal cell carcinoma: a systematic review and meta-analysis. J Urol. 2017;197(1):44–9.
84. Kato S, Demura S, Murakami H, Tsuchiya H. Surgical metastasectomy for renal cell carcinoma: which patients are the real candidates for surgery? Ann Transl Med. 2019;7(Suppl 8):S273.
85. Lu Z, Yang C, He W, Zhou J, Xiang R. Nomogram to predict risk and prognosis of synchronous lung metastasis in renal cell carcinoma: a large cohort analysis. Medicine (Baltimore). 2022;101(27):e29764.
86. Agrawal A, Sahni S, Iftikhar A, Talwar A. Pulmonary manifestations of renal cell carcinoma. Respir Med. 2015;109(12):1505–8.
87. Meacci E, Nachira D, Zanfrini E, Evangelista J, Triumbari EKA, Congedo MT, et al. Prognostic factors affecting survival after pulmonary resection of metastatic renal cell carcinoma: a multicenter experience. Cancers (Basel). 2021;13(13):3258.
88. Kawashima A, Nakayama M, Oka D, Sato M, Hatano K, Mukai M, et al. Pulmonary metastasectomy in patients with renal cell carcinoma: a single-institution experience. Int J Clin Oncol. 2011;16(6):660–5.
89. Gilbert N. Surgical treatment of pulmonary metastases in metastatic renal cell carcinoma. Aktuelle Urol. 2020;51(3):271–4.
90. Murthy SC, Kim K, Rice TW, Rajeswaran J, Bukowski R, DeCamp MM, et al. Can we predict long-term survival after pulmonary metastasectomy for renal cell carcinoma? Ann Thorac Surg. 2005;79(3):996–1003.
91. Hofmann HS, Neef H, Krohe K, Andreev P, Silber RE. Prognostic factors and survival after pulmonary resection of metastatic renal cell carcinoma. Eur Urol. 2005;48(1):77–81; discussion –2.
92. Pfannschmidt J, Hoffmann H, Muley T, Krysa S, Trainer C, Dienemann H. Prognostic factors for survival after pulmonary resection of metastatic renal cell carcinoma. Ann Thorac Surg. 2002;74(5):1653–7.
93. Winter H, Meimarakis G, Angele MK, Hummel M, Staehler M, Hoffmann RT, et al. Tumor infiltrated hilar and mediastinal lymph nodes are an independent prognostic factor for decreased survival after pulmonary metastasectomy in patients with renal cell carcinoma. J Urol. 2010;184(5):1888–94.
94. Meimarakis G, Angele M, Staehler M, Clevert DA, Crispin A, Ruttinger D, et al. Evaluation of a new prognostic score (Munich score) to predict long-term survival after resection of pulmonary renal cell carcinoma metastases. Am J Surg. 2011;202(2):158–67.
95. Grunwald V, Eberhardt B, Bex A, Florcken A, Gauler T, Derlin T, et al. An interdisciplinary consensus on the management of bone metastases from renal cell carcinoma. Nat Rev Urol. 2018;15(8):511–21.
96. Xu C, Liu W, Yin C, Li W, Liu J, Sheng W, et al. Establishment and validation of a machine learning prediction model based on big data for predicting the risk of bone metastasis in renal cell carcinoma patients. Comput Math Methods Med. 2022;2022:5676570.
97. Huang Z, Du Y, Zhang X, Liu H, Liu S, Xu T. Clear cell renal cell carcinoma bone metastasis: what should be considered in prognostic evaluation. Eur J Surg Oncol. 2019;45(7):1246–52.
98. Shuch B, La Rochelle JC, Klatte T, Riggs SB, Liu W, Kabbinavar FF, et al. Brain metastasis from renal cell carcinoma: presentation, recurrence, and survival. Cancer. 2008;113(7):1641–8.
99. Siva S, Correa RJM, Warner A, Staehler M, Ellis RJ, Ponsky L, et al. Stereotactic ablative radiotherapy for >/=T1b primary renal cell carcinoma: a report from the international radiosurgery oncology consortium for kidney (IROCK). Int J Radiat Oncol Biol Phys. 2020;108(4):941–9.
100. Siva S, Ali M, Correa RJM, Muacevic A, Ponsky L, Ellis RJ, et al. 5-year outcomes after stereotactic ablative body radiotherapy for primary renal cell carcinoma: an individual patient data meta-analysis from IROCK (the international radiosurgery consortium of the kidney). Lancet Oncol. 2022;23(12):1508–16.
101. Ikushima H, Tokuuye K, Sumi M, Kagami Y, Murayama S, Ikeda H, et al. Fractionated stereotactic radiotherapy of brain metastases from renal cell carcinoma. Int J Radiat Oncol Biol Phys. 2000;48(5):1389–93.
102. Ippen FM, Mahadevan A, Wong ET, Uhlmann EJ, Sengupta S, Kasper EM. Stereotactic radiosurgery for renal cancer brain metastasis: prognostic factors

and the role of whole-brain radiation and surgical resection. J Oncol. 2015;2015:636918.
103. Ma J, Del Balzo L, Walch H, Khaleel S, Knezevic A, Flynn J, et al. Clinical outcomes and targeted genomic analysis of renal cell carcinoma brain metastases treated with stereotactic radiosurgery. Eur Urol Oncol. 2025;8:338.
104. Naito S, Kinoshita H, Kondo T, Shinohara N, Kasahara T, Saito K, et al. Prognostic factors of patients with metastatic renal cell carcinoma with removed metastases: a multicenter study of 556 patients. Urology. 2013;82(4):846–51.
105. Daliani DD, Tannir NM, Papandreou CN, Wang X, Swisher S, Wood CG, et al. Prospective assessment of systemic therapy followed by surgical removal of metastases in selected patients with renal cell carcinoma. BJU Int. 2009;104(4):456–60.
106. Karam JA, Rini BI, Varella L, Garcia JA, Dreicer R, Choueiri TK, et al. Metastasectomy after targeted therapy in patients with advanced renal cell carcinoma. J Urol. 2011;185(2):439–44.
107. Rini BI, Shaw V, Rosenberg JE, Kim ST, Chen I. Patients with metastatic renal cell carcinoma with long-term disease-free survival after treatment with sunitinib and resection of residual metastases. Clin Genitourin Cancer. 2006;5(3):232–4.
108. Thomas AA, Rini BI, Stephenson AJ, Garcia JA, Fergany A, Krishnamurthi V, et al. Surgical resection of renal cell carcinoma after targeted therapy. J Urol. 2009;182(3):881–6.
109. Appleman LJ, Kim SE, Harris WB, Pal SK, Pins MR, Kolesar J, et al. Randomized, double-blind phase III study of Pazopanib versus placebo in patients with metastatic renal cell carcinoma who have no evidence of disease after Metastasectomy: ECOG-ACRIN E2810. J Clin Oncol. 2024;42(17):2061–70.

Management of Renal Cell Carcinoma of Variant Histology

18

Kevin Kayvan Zarrabi, Mehmet Asim Bilen, Nizar M. Tannir, and Pedro C. Barata

Introduction

In 2024, over 81,000 Americans are expected to be diagnosed with cancer of the kidney and renal pelvis, and over 14,390 will die from their disease [1]. Over the last 35 years, the incidence of kidney cancer has steadily increased, and there has been an increasing trend in years of life lost due to renal cancer [2]. This translates to a lifetime cumulative mortality risk of 0.5% and 0.2% for men and women, respectively, in the developed world [3].

Surgical resection remains the primary treatment modality in early-stage renal cell carcinoma (RCC), irrespective of histological subtype, aside from renal medullary carcinoma where neoadjuvant chemotherapy can be considered. When technically feasible, partial nephrectomy is the preferred surgical treatment as it has been shown in most studies to be associated with improved overall survival and preserved renal function when compared with radical nephrectomy [4–6]. The role of routine lymphadenectomy is less clear. Patients with T1–T2 tumors without clinically apparent nodal metastases and in the absence of unfavorable features may be spared lymphadenectomy [7, 8].

Unfortunately, up to 30% of patients with localized disease will ultimately develop recurrence, and once renal cancer metastasizes to distant organs, the prognosis is universally poor [9]. Spontaneous responses of metastatic RCC can occur but are seen in less than 2% of patients treated with cytoreductive surgery; the true cause and effect remain debated [10]. Comparatively, at experienced centers, the mortality of cytoreductive surgery may be lower than 0.1% [11]. The role of cytoreductive surgery in variant histology RCC (vhRCC) has not been studied explicitly, and management should be considered in that context. In patients with clear cell RCC, cytoreductive nephrectomy prior to interferon-alpha-2b conferred a survival advantage over interferon-alpha-2b, alone [12], but without a full understanding of why cytoreductive surgery benefited patients; extrapolating this evidence to patients with vhRCC should be done only with caution. For example, in very

K. K. Zarrabi
Department of Medical Oncology, Sidney Kimmel Cancer Center, Thomas Jefferson University, Philadelphia, PA, USA
e-mail: kevin.zarrabi@jefferson.edu

M. A. Bilen
Department of Hematology and Medical Oncology, Emory University School of Medicine, Atlanta, GA, USA
e-mail: mehmet.a.bilen@emory.edu

N. M. Tannir
Genitourinary Medical Oncology, UT MD Anderson Cancer Center, Houston, TX, USA
e-mail: ntannir@mdanderson.org

P. C. Barata (✉)
Division of Solid Tumor Oncology, University Hospitals Seidman Cancer Center, Case Western Reserve University, Cleveland, OH, USA
e-mail: pedro.barata@uhhospitals.org

J. A. Libertino, J. R. Gee (eds.), *Renal Cancer*, https://doi.org/10.1007/978-3-031-97599-8_18

aggressive RCC, such as collecting duct carcinoma (CDC), renal medullary carcinoma (RMC), or RCC with sarcomatoid dedifferentiation, nephrectomy may only delay systemic therapy [13]. Conversely, in more indolent RCC, cytoreductive surgery or metastasectomy may offer clinical benefit.

Renal cell cancers have historically been considered radio-resistant [14], although this may no longer be the case with the ablative radiation doses currently achievable [15]. A dose–response relationship has been noted from experience with radiation treatment in the localized disease and palliative settings [16, 17]. The role of radiation treatment in vhRCC should be confined to palliative therapy for specific lesions, such as brain or symptomatic tumors (e.g., bone lesions), or in the case of localized disease, radiation therapy should ideally be considered as part of a clinical trial or after careful multidisciplinary discussion at an experienced center.

Renal cell carcinoma encompasses a pathologically diverse group of malignancies, including clear cell renal cell carcinoma (ccRCC, 70–80%), papillary renal cell carcinoma (pRCC, 10–15%), chromophobe renal cell carcinoma (chRCC, 5%), unclassified renal cell carcinoma (uRCC, 5%), collecting duct carcinoma (CDC, <1%), translocation RCC (<1%), and renal medullary carcinoma (RMC, <1%) [18, 19]. Owing to advances in molecular diagnostics and elucidation of underlying molecular mechanisms of disease, there have been significant changes to the World Health Organization (WHO) 2022 classification of urinary and male genital tumors (fifth edition) from the prior edition from 2016. Each subtype has its own unique histologic, cytogenetic, molecular, and clinical characteristics, and classification now relies less heavily on anatomic origin and tumor architecture and strengthens the role of molecular-based classification. Notable reclassifications surrounding new molecularly defined subsets of RCC include TFE3-rearranged RCC, TFEB-altered RCC, FH-deficient RCC, and ALK-rearranged RCC among others [20].

Sarcomatoid Dedifferentiation

Sarcomatoid RCC, an aggressive variant of renal cancer once believed to be a separate histologic entity, can arise from any histologic subtype and should be considered in that context [21]. Sarcomatoid dedifferentiation is found in approximately 5% of all RCC tumors but is present in up to 20% of patients with advanced disease [22]. Although the presence of sarcomatoid features seems to portend a poorer prognosis independent of tumor, node, metastasis (TNM) staging [23], the effect of the histologic subtype of RCC on prognosis remains unclear. In univariable analysis, histologic subtype seems to be a prognostic indicator but may or may not be preserved in multivariable analysis [24, 25]. ChRCC, however, is biologically a tumor of low malignant potential (particularly in the absence of sarcomatoid dedifferentiation) and is significantly associated with a better prognosis than other RCC subtypes, with 10-year survival reported as high as 90% [26]. Variant histologies of RCC may have diminished metastatic potential compared to ccRCC, but once metastatic, the prognosis between the two groups becomes similar [27, 28]. Histologic subtype may be predictive of response to immunotherapy, with vhRCC showing increased resistance compared with ccRCC [29, 30]. Potential treatment options for vhRCC are subtype-specific.

Anti-VEGF agents and mTOR inhibitors have limited efficacy in sarcomatoid disease, although it can be difficult to perform subtype-specific comparisons because the number of patients with vhRCC included in most clinical trials has been relatively small, and there may be anti-tumor activity in certain biologic subtypes [24, 31]. Tumors with sarcomatoid dedifferentiation have been demonstrated to express higher PD-L1 expression and are enriched with tumor-infiltrating lymphocytes [32, 33]. There is strong biologic rationale for employment on ICIs for tumors harboring sarcomatoid features, and indeed subgroup analyses from a number of studies have demonstrated improved outcomes with employment of immunotherapy in patients with sarcomatoid features compared to those without

[34, 35]. The most compelling data come from the CheckMate-214 study, which evaluated the role of ipilimumab and nivolumab in patients with clear cell histology. Progression-free survival (26.5 months vs. 5.1 months; $P = 0.009$), objective response rates (61% vs. 23%), complete response rate (19% vs. 3%), and durability of response with an overall survival of 48.6 months versus 14.2 months favored patients receiving ipilimumab with nivolumab over sunitinib [36]. Smaller subsets of patients from studies of vhRCC included patients with sarcomatoid features and demonstrated clinical activity of anti-VEGF agents in combination with ICIs, which may serve as an alternative to dual-ICI approaches if deemed necessary [37, 38]. Together, these data affirm ICI's as a favored approach for patients with sarcomatoid tumors, with data being more robust for the perceived improved efficacy in clear cell histology.

Papillary Renal Cell Carcinoma

Unlike ccRCC, vhRCC does not result from von Hippel–Lindau (*VHL*) inactivation, a gene that resides on chromosome 3p25. The loss of VHL function, either through mutation or inactivation by methylation, results in increased concentrations of hypoxia-inducible factor (HIF) within the affected cells [39, 40]. The over expression of HIF then leads to increased production of VEGF and erythropoietin, and impairs glucose metabolism, which leads to the clear cell appearance. Conversely, pRCC is characterized by dysregulation of the MET pathway [41, 42]. MET expression can be influenced by mutation, constitutive kinase activation, and genetic amplification [43]. Activation of the MET pathway can result in increased signaling via the hepatocyte growth factor receptor, which in turn can affect cell survival, cell adhesion, and invasion. MET mutations are found in most patients with hereditary pRCC and in 13% of sporadic cases [42]. Moreover, increased MET expression has been found in over 80% of sporadic pRCC, with a trend toward worse prognosis in those tumors with increased MET expression [44].

The optimal treatment strategy for metastatic pRCC is debatable. The pivotal trial of sunitinib excluded vhRCC [45, 46]. The subsequent expanded access trial was made up of 14% variant histology subtypes [47]. The overall response rate in the intention-to-treat population was 17% with a median progression-free survival of 10.9 months (95% CI, 10.3–11.2), and overall survival was 18.4 months (95% CI, 17.4–19.2). Sunitinib was less efficacious in vhRCC, with a response rate of 11%, but this may have resulted from the absence of a standardized procedure for measuring disease response, variable local practices, and lack of central pathology review. A phase II trial was conducted with sunitinib in 57 patients with advanced vhRCC (pRCC, 27; chRCC 5; uRCC, 8; sarcomatoid, 7; CDC/RMC, 6; others, 4) [48]. Median progression-free survival for 55 evaluable patients was 2.7 months (95% CI, 1.4 — 5.4000). Median progression-free survival for patients with pRCC was 1.6 months (95% CI, 1.4–5.4). Median overall survival for all 57 patients was 16.8 months (95% CI, 10.7–26.3). Only three patients (two with chRCC and one with uRCC) had a confirmed partial response for an overall objective response rate of 5%.

The ESPN trial was a randomized phase II trial of everolimus versus sunitinib in patients with metastatic vhRCC and no prior systemic therapy. Seventy-three patients were enrolled, including 14 patients in the sunitinib arm and 13 patients in the everolimus arm with pRCC. In an interim analysis, both overall survival and progression-free survival favored sunitinib, and the trial was closed to new patient enrollment. However, the final analysis was not powered to detect differences in overall survival, progression-free survival, or the overall response rate. The median overall survival for patients with pRCC was 16.6 months in the sunitinib arm and 14.9 months in the everolimus arm. The ESPN trial was the first study to compare a VEGFR-TKI with an mTOR inhibitor but was limited by small sample size and heterogeneity of histologic subtypes [49].

The ASPEN trial also compared everolimus versus sunitinib in patients with metastatic non-clear cell RCC. There was a weak trend towards an increase in progression-free survival with sunitinib compared with everolimus (hazard ratio 1.41, 95% CI 0.87–2.28, $P = 0.16$), and the analysis of overall survival was inconclusive (hazard ratio 1.12, 95% CI 0.7–2.1, $P = 0.6$). Overall radiographic responses were noted in 9/51 evaluable patients (18%) treated with sunitinib, and in 5/57 evaluable patients (9%) treated with everolimus. Thirty-three out of 51 patients (65%) in the sunitinib arm and 37 of 57 (65%) in the everolimus arm had pRCC. Of these patients, only four (sunitinib arm) and two (everolimus arm) had pRCC type 1. The overall response rate for patients with pRCC was 24% with sunitinib and 5% with everolimus. With regard to toxicity, 78% of patients in the sunitinib arm experienced serious adverse events (grade 3 or worse) compared to 60% of patients in the everolimus arm [50].

Given the role of MET mutations or activation in pRCC proliferation, inhibition of this pathway has naturally been leveraged as a useful therapeutic target. MET inhibition has been extensively tested in phase II trials. Foretinib, an oral multikinase inhibitor targeting MET, VEGF, RON, AXL, and TIE-2 receptors, has recently been studied in one of the largest clinical trials devoted exclusively to pRCC, with 74 patients enrolled. Overall response rate was only 13.5%, less than the pre-specified desired response rate of 25%, with a median duration of response of 18.5 months. The 1-year survival rate was 70%, and median overall survival has not yet been reached. Fatigue, hypertension, and diarrhea were the most frequently observed toxicities. Notably, non-fatal pulmonary embolism was observed in 11% of patients treated with foretinib [51]. Patients in this trial were stratified based on MET pathway activation status. The presence of germline MET mutations correlated with activity of foretinib and achievement of partial response. However, other measures of MET pathway activation were not predictive of response [52]. The highly selective MET tyrosine kinase inhibitor savolitinib was studied in the phase II trial of 109 patients with pRCC in which 40% of patients had MET-driven tumors, and MET status was unknown in 17%. The MET status was determined using next-generation sequencing of tumor samples. Eight patients (18%) with MET-driven tumors responded to treatment, and 0 patients with MET-independent tumors responded. Stable disease was reported in 50% of patients with MET-driven tumors and in 11% of those that were MET-independent. The progression-free survival in patients with MET-driven tumors was 6.2 months. In all study patients, the overall response rate was 7%. Nine patients (6%) discontinued savolitinib due to adverse events, but the side-effect profile of this therapy was generally mild, with few serious adverse events [53]. A phase II trial of savolitinib versus sunitinib in pRCC began in 2017 with an estimated enrollment of 180 patients in an open-label, parallel assignment.

The landmark phase II PAPMET trial evaluated cabozantinib, crizotinib, sunitinib, or the selective c-MET inhibitor savolitinib in previously treated patients with pRCC. The study was agnostic to MET-biomarker status. The savolitinib and crizotinib treatment arms were terminated at interim analysis given futility and underperformance, and the trial proceeded as a randomized two-arm study of cabozantinib and sunitinib. Patients treated with cabozantinib benefited from a progression-free survival benefit of 9.0 months compared to 5.6 months for those treated with sunitinib ($p = 0.019$). The objective response rate similarly favored cabozantinib over sunitinib (23% vs. 4%, $p = 0.010$) [54]. With a median follow-up of 17.5 months, the median overall survival was 21.5 months (95% CI, 12.0 to 28.1) with cabozantinib and 17.3 months (95% CI, 12.8 to 21.8) with sunitinib (hazard ratio, 0.83; 95% CI, 0.51 to 1.36; $P = 0.46$). Despite the lack of survival benefit, cabozantinib remains an ideal targeted therapy for patients with pRCC [55].

The role of ICIs is evolving with regard to management of pRCC. Cohort B from the KEYNOTE-427 trial was a multicenter, single-arm, phase II study in which front-line pembrolizumab was investigated in 165 patients with vhRCC, of whom 71.5% had pRCC. The ORR in the pRCC subgroup was 28.8% (95% CI,

20.8–37.9), and the disease control rate was 47.5%. The median progression free survival in this subgroup was 5.5 months (95% CI, 3.9–6.9), and median overall survival was 31.5 months (95% CI, 25.5—NR). Deep and durable responses were reported, and a 5.9% CR rate was observed among the papillary cohort [56]. The phase III/IV CheckMate-920 was a single-arm study evaluating ipilimumab and nivolumab in previously untreated patients with vhRCC, of whom 34.6% had pRCC. Modest activity was noted throughout the study. The objective response rate in the patients with pRCC was 11%, although nine patients with pRCC experienced a complete response [57]. The phase II SUNNIFORCAST study enrolled 309 patients with metastatic or locally advanced vhRCC and was stratified by papillary vs. non-papillary histology on central pathological review. There were 178 patients with pRCC included in the study. Patients were randomized to receive ipilimumab and nivolumab or investigators' choice of standard of care. Primary endpoint was overall survival at 12 months. Of enrolled patients, 87% in the standard of care arm received sunitinib. The objective response rate for the pRCC patients was 29.2% for ipilimumab and nivolumab, compared to 21% for standard of care. The 12-month overall survival rate for ipilimumab- and nivolumab-treated patients among the entire study population was 86.9% (95% CI, 80.2%–91.5%) compared to that of standard of care, which was 76.8% (95% CI, 68.6%–83.1%) (p = 0.014). Papillary and non-papillary RCC showed a similar benefit in overall survival rate for ipilimumab and nivolumab in the study [58].

Given the efficacy of both antiangiogenesis therapy and ICIs, investigators paralleled combination therapy studies that have shown success in the clear cell experience to patients with vhRCC. The KEYNOTE-B61 study was a single-arm, multicenter, phase II trial evaluating lenvatinib and pembrolizumab combination therapy in patients with vhRCC. Of the 158 patients enrolled, the most common histology was papillary RCC (59%). The results were provocative, considering the anti-VEGF targeting therapy employed did not target cMET. The objective response rate was an impressive 54%, of whom 9% of patients benefited from a complete response. Further, 33% of patients had stable disease as best response, and median duration of treatment on both lenvatinib and pembrolizumab was 9.7 months (IQR 4.2–14.0) [37].

Given the role of cMET as a molecular driver of pRCC tumorigenesis, a similarly designed single-arm, phase II basket study employing cabozantinib and nivolumab evaluated 40 patients with vhRCC, 80% of whom had pRCC (80%). An objective response rate was observed in 15 of 32 (47%, 95% CI, 29–65) patients with papillary histology [59]. No new safety signals were observed for either combination regimen in the vhRCC studies compared to the clear cell histology experience which has FDA approvals for use as frontline therapies. The CALYPSO trial evaluated the MET-specific TKI savolitinib with durvalumab in a single-arm trial of 41 patients, many of whom had previously treated disease. Amongst patients with MET-driven tumors (MET mutation or copy number amplification), the objective response rate was an impressive 53% [60].

Chromophobe Renal Cell Carcinoma

Chromophobe renal cell carcinoma (chRCC) is the third most common RCC histology and arises from the intercalated cells of the distal nephron and thus harbors a high density of mitochondria [61]. Recent molecular analysis from an international, multi-institutional, real-world cohort of patients with RCC who have undergone comprehensive molecular testing revealed genomic structural rearrangements involving the TERT promoter region, as well as diffusely increased mitochondrial function and mitochondrial DNA alterations. chRCC typically harbors multiple losses of chromosomes 1, 2, 6, 10, 13, 17, and 21, whereas TP53 and PTEN are the two most frequently mutated genes [33]. These tumors have a distinct morphologic appearance and unique molecular features with potential management implications. Unlike other RCC subtypes, chRCC stains readily for c-KIT due to the c-KIT proto-oncogene amplification [62]. ChRCC can also be defined by its hypodiploidy of multiple chromosomes, including 1, 2, 6, 10, 13, 17, and 21 [63, 64]. The two histologic chRCC subtypes are classic chRCC (characterized by pale cytoplasm) and eosinophilic chRCC (characterized by pink cytoplasm due to high mitochondrial density) [65]. Classic chRCC is more likely to demonstrate monosomy of chromosomes 1, 2, 6, 10, 13, 17, and 21 and to contain more somatic inactivating mutations in TP53 and PTEN [66]. Eosinophilic chRCC is more likely to harbor mutations in mitochondrial genes, particularly those involving complex 1 of the electron transport chain [33]. Furthermore, whole genome sequencing has revealed that chRCC, unique among RCCs, harbors genomic rearrangements in the TERT promoter region [66]. ChRCC can also be found in patients exhibiting the Burt–Hogg–Dube (BHD) syndrome of follicle tumors, lung cysts, and renal tumors; the BHD tumor-suppressor gene folliculin (FLCN) may play a role in chRCC development [67]. FLCN mutations can lead to deregulated cell proliferation via the interaction of FLCN with the mTOR pathway [68]. Most chRCC tumors associated with BHD will stain positive for CK7, Ksp-cadherin, and CD82, distinguishing them from other BHD-associated tumors [69]. However, patients can also develop ccRCC or pRCC in conjunction with FLCN mutations, so the role of this gene in the pathogenesis of chRCC specifically is unclear [70]. Of note, FLCN inactivation in sporadic renal cancers, including sporadic chRCC, is very infrequent [71]. Since most trials of vhRCC have not distinguished between the various subtypes, the clinical benefit of targeted therapy for chRCC is less clear, especially since its biologic characteristics are different. Antiangiogenesis targeted therapy, mTOR inhibitors, and immune checkpoint blockade have all included chRCC in their clinical trials [31, 47, 72]. In the sorafenib expanded access trial, the observed response rate was only 5%, but 90% of patients had stable disease. In one study that included 12 patients with chRCC, three patients (25%) achieved a response with either sorafenib (two patients) or sunitinib (one patient) [73]. In the single-arm phase II trial with everolimus plus bevacizumab, five patients with chRCC were treated with the combination, and three remained on treatment for more than 12 months. The results of this trial lend some support to the effectiveness of rapalog therapies in these patients [74].

MITF Translocation Renal Cancer

Translocation RCC was only originally recognized as a distinct clinical entity in the World Health Organization 2004 renal tumors classification and is now included in the molecularly defined renal carcinomas group within the WHO 2022 renal tumors classification [75]. Translocation carcinomas share histological characteristics with both ccRCC and pRCC and are often described as having features of both cell types. Consequently, the incidence of this tumor subtype is less clear and may have been previously misclassified. It now appears as though translocation renal cell carcinoma may represent 1–5% of all RCC cases when systematically examining pathology specimens for the presence of a defined translocation [76].

Although this renal cancer subtype may demonstrate various chromosomal abnormalities, the vast majority involve a break at Xp11, resulting in altered TFE3 transcription-factor gene expression [77–79]. The Xp11 translocation can be uncovered by molecular genetic analysis, but translocation RCC may also be diagnosed with immunohistochemistry utilizing nuclear antibodies to TFE3 and TFEB proteins, or fluorescence in situ hybridization (FISH) assays for the corresponding gene aberrations [80–82]. Translocations involving t(6;11) have also been described, causing altered TFEB function: a related protein of TFE3, with similar function [83, 84]. There are several similarities between these two subtypes of translocation RCC, and therefore, they were grouped together in the family of MiTF translocation RCC in the 2013 Vancouver Classification of Renal Neoplasia [85]. Both subtypes are more common in younger patients. The morphologies of these tumors may overlap with each other and with other RCC subtypes, but those with Xp11 translocations usually have clear cells and papillary architecture, while those with t(6;11) translocations may have a biphasic appearance and nodules of basement membrane material. Both subtypes express cytokeratin and epithelial membrane antigen (EMA) relative to other RCC subtypes [82, 86]. RCC with TFEB amplification was more recently identified and appears to be more common and confer a worse prognosis compared with t(6;11) TFEB translocation RCCs [82]. These TFEB-amplified RCCs arise as high-grade adenocarcinomas of the distal nephron, usually in the mid-to-late seventh decade of life with a slight male predominance [82]. Only a small proportion of the published cases of tumors with t(6;11) translocations developed metastases, but all translocation RCCs have the capacity to recur after many years. Therefore, careful long-term follow-up for these patients is essential [86].

Experience in the treatment of translocation carcinoma is limited. Anti-VEGF therapy with sunitinib, sorafenib, or bevacizumab may result in partial responses or disease stabilization. Of 15 patients studied in one retrospective review, three patients achieved a partial response, seven patients had stable disease, and five patients progressed through therapy [87]. Median progression-free survival was 7.1 months, while median overall survival was 14.3 months. In the first-line setting, targeted therapy appears to improve progression-free survival over cytokines [88]. The response rate with sunitinib may be as high as 27%, with the potential for complete responses. Based on data from tumor microarrays, the mTOR pathway seems to be upregulated upregulated in translocation RCC [77]. In the second-line setting, anti-VEGF tyrosine kinase inhibitors and mTOR inhibitors may produce progression-free survival in the range of 6–11 months, with sunitinib appearing to be the most efficacious agent. Translocation carcinoma may also respond to temsirolimus or everolimus even when resistant to anti-VEGF therapy [88]. Multiple retrospective analyses of ICI monotherapy and ICI in combination with anti-VEGF tyrosine kinase inhibitors outcomes demonstrate efficacy of ICI monotherapy or ICI with anti-angiogenesis in a subset of patients. Genomic sequencing may identify potential therapeutic targets for this malignancy that remains difficult to treat [89, 90].

Renal Medullary Carcinoma and Collecting Duct Renal Cell Carcinoma

Renal medullary carcinoma and collecting duct carcinoma are highly aggressive RCCs that arise from the distal nephron. RMC typically arising from the calyceal epithelium of the collecting duct, whereas CDC more commonly arising from collecting duct principal cells [91]. In contrast to most RCCs, RMC has a clear clinical association: sickle cell trait and other sickle hemoglobinopathies [92–95]. The typical RMC patient is a young male of African ancestry with sickle cell trait and presents with local and/or systemic symptoms. The median age at diagnosis is 28 years, although it can manifest in young adults and children as young as 9 years old [96]. RMC affects males over females in a 2:1 ratio and tends to be highly aggressive, with distant metastases often present at the time of diagnosis. The right kidney is involved in approximately 75% of cases, believed to be due to the underlying chronic renal medullary infarcts in the right kidney in the setting of sickle hemoglobinopathies and medullary hypoxia [95]. RMC is always characterized by loss of the tumor-suppressor gene SMARCB1, also known as INI1, hSNF5, or BAF47 [97, 98]. RMC is resistant to anti-VEGF targeted therapies and mTOR inhibitors, and these therapies should not be used in these patients [48, 96]. Renal cell carcinoma, unclassified with medullary phenotype (RCCU-MP), is a very rare SMARCB1-negative RMC subtype that is histopathologically and clinically similar to RMC but occurs in individuals without sickle hemoglobinopathies [99].

RMC and collecting duct carcinoma may be difficult to distinguish by light microscopy. However, RMC is more likely to contain reticular/yolk sac tumor-like patterns (85% of cases) compared with CDC (8% of cases) [99]. In addition, sickled erythrocytes will be found within the tumor specimens in RMC but not in CDC or RCCU-MP cases [99]. The most important distinguishing factor is the lack of expression of SMARCB1 in RMC and RCCU-MP cases, whereas CDC tumors will show positivity for SMARCB1 by immunohistochemistry. Collecting duct carcinoma is a diagnosis of exclusion, and cases where this histology is being considered should be reviewed at high-volume or expert centers.

Cytotoxic chemotherapy is the mainstay for the therapy of RMC. For RMC, platinum-based cytotoxic regimens are recommended, with carboplatin and paclitaxel being recommended as the preferred frontline therapy [100]. Alternative three-drug combinations of either cisplatin or carboplatin, combined with paclitaxel and gemcitabine, have been reported to produce responses [101] as has the combination of methotrexate, vinblastine, doxorubicin, and cisplatin (MVAC) [102, 103], among others as well. However, no platinum-based treatment regimen has shown superiority, and durable complete responses have been noted in 2 out of 22 (9%) patients with metastatic RMC treated with the relatively low-intensity regimen of carboplatin plus paclitaxel [96]. The vast majority (>90%) of patients with RMC will present with nodal and/or visceral metastases [96]. Even those few patients who present with localized disease on imaging will develop distant metastases, often within weeks. For this reason, upfront systemic therapy (platinum-based cytotoxic chemotherapy or clinical trial) should be used for most patients with newly diagnosed RMC [100]. The data is limited on treatment beyond the second-line setting. Owing to the high expression of topoisomerase II in RMC, targeting topoisomerase II may prove beneficial. A case report of doxorubicin and gemcitabine therapy in a patient with widespread metastatic RMC post gemcitabine/paclitaxel chemotherapy produced a significant response and progression-free survival for 9 months. Gene expression analysis confirmed that this patient's tumor over-expressed topoisomerase II [104]. There are retrospective reports demonstrating that erlotinib and bevacizumab can be active in patients with RMC who progressed on prior platinum-based chemotherapy and gemcitabine with doxorubicin [105].

To date, the best studied regimen for CDC consists of gemcitabine in combination with either cisplatin or carboplatin [106]. The response rate for this regimen is 26% (95% CI, 8–44), with a complete response rate of less than 5%. This translates to a median progression-free survival of 7.1 months (95% CI, 3–11.3) and overall survival of 10.5 months (95% CI, 3.8–17.1). Platinum-doublet therapy can also be combined with bevacizumab, which has been demonstrated as a feasible treatment strategy, although the observed toxicity may not warrant the modest improvement in outcomes [107].

An early report of three patients with CDC treated with cabozantinib noted partial response in one patient and stable disease in two patients [108]. The subsequent BONSAI study was a single-center phase II trial enrolling 23 patients with CDC nicely demonstrating the efficacy of cabozantinib and the role of antiangiogenesis in CDC. Cabozantinib demonstrated an objective response rate of 35%, including a patient who benefited from a complete response [109]. Other targeted approaches include utilization of a CDK4/6 inhibitors given the prognostic role of chromosome 9p and CDKN2A/B loss in CDC and also consideration for HER2-targeted therapies as HER2 amplification has been noted in up to 45% of CDC tumors. Literature on outcomes from these approaches, however, are limited to individual case reports [110].

Miscellaneous Renal Cancers

Other tumor subtypes of RCC are beginning to emerge from the previously unclassified category or from re-classification as new pathology techniques are developed. Mucinous tubular and spindle cell carcinoma (MTSCC) and tubulocystic renal cell carcinoma (tcRCC) are two examples of RCC that have only recently been described. MTSCC is an extremely rare malignancy that develops from either the collecting duct or the loop of Henle and, as its name implies, is defined by the presence of tubules, spindle-cells, and a mucinous stroma and foam cells [111]. MTSCC shows a female predominance [112] and may be associated with nephrolithiasis [113]. Immunohistochemical analysis for MTSCC resembles the staining pattern of papillary RCC and may represent an unusual variant of pRCC [114, 115]. Cytogenetic examination may reveal a host of abnormalities including loss or gain of all or parts of chromosomes 1–20, 22, X and Y [113]. Trisomies of chromosomes 7 and 17 have also been reported [116]. Deregulation of the Hippo pathway, with a low overall mutational burden and recurrent chromosomal losses, appears to be the defining molecular characteristic of MTSCC [117]. In general, MTSCC is considered an indolent tumor type, but it has been reported to metastasize to lymph nodes and distant organs [118]. Fluorodeoxyglucose positron emission tomography (FDG PET/CT) may be of diagnostic and clinical benefit in MTSCC [119]. Sarcomatoid dedifferentiation may also occur in conjunction with MTSCC, leading to a worse prognosis [120, 121]. The prognosis for MTSCC is generally favorable with few reported cases of recurrence after surgical resection or metastases [119]. TcRCC is a low-grade malignancy, with a male predominance and similar IHC and chromosomal abnormalities as pRCC and MTSCC [122]. It is identified by the presence of packed tubules and cysts [123]. tcRCC can rarely metastasize, and sunitinib has been shown to induce a partial response in some of these cases [124]. Sarcomatoid dedifferentiation is extremely rare but has been noted in one case report [125].

Follicular renal cell carcinoma has also been newly described as a type of RCC, which histologically resembles follicular carcinoma of the thyroid. Until recently, all reported cases were incidental findings, confined to the kidney, and cured with surgery alone [126–128]. Gene expression profiling has shown multiple abnormalities, including under-expression and over-expression of chromosomes 1, 2, 3, 5, 6, 10, 11, 16, and 17. A single case of thyroid-like follicular renal cell carcinoma presenting with lung and retroperitoneal lymph node metastasis has been reported. This patient was treated with sunitinib for 1 year followed by cytoreductive nephrectomy and retroperitoneal lymph node dissection. She had stable disease for at least 4 years after diagnosis.

There has been a rapid advance in our understanding of the molecular underpinnings and gene expression profiles of different RCC histologies, beyond that previously described from large prospective trials restricted to clear cell histology. Whole-exome sequencing of variant histology tumors reveals patterns of differentially expressed gene sets involved in key molecular pathways. Gene sets enriched in variant histologies compared to clear cell tumors include pathways particular to the cell cycle, fatty acid oxidation/AMPK signaling, and fatty acid synthesis/pentose phosphate signaling [33]. The fifth edition of the WHO classification of urogenital tumors now includes molecularly defined renal tumors, which are those recognized by having heterogeneous morphological aspects and can therefore not be diagnosed by morphology alone [129]. These include eosinophilic solid and cystic RCC that harbors gene alterations in the *TSC* gene, which can activate the mTOR pathway; ELOC-mutated RCC due to underlying *ELOC* (*TCEB1*) mutation; ALK-rearranged RCC; SMARCB1-deficient medullary RCC; and FH-deficient RCC with underlying *FH* loss or mutation, which may be associated with HLRCC.

Tuberous sclerosis complex (TSC) associated RCC is a complex entity that entails mTOR pathway-related alterations. The development of TSC-related RCC can occur due to germline inheritance of alterations producing a hereditary TSC syndrome or can occur with bi-allelic inactivation of genes in a classic "two-hit" paradigm [130]. TSC-related RCC encompasses a diverse morphologic and molecular spectrum of disease—with targets of increased expression of downstream targets of *MTOR* being a shared characteristic. The National Comprehensive Cancer Network and the American Urologic Association both have guideline recommendations for genetic risk evaluation of patients with RCC who have a potential hereditary component [131]. Such testing is vital, as the breadth of disease and manifestation of TSC-related RCC are heterogeneous, and nuances have treatment implications.

Fumarate Hydratase-Deficient Renal Cell Carcinoma

Fumarate hydratase-deficient RCC is a new pathologic entity and is considered rare, with a predominance of reported cases localized to Europe and the United States [132]. FH-deficient RCC was previously considered within the spectrum of papillary RCC, specifically papillary type II disease, prior to the updates in the WHO classification. The disease was initially named hereditary leiomyomatosis and renal cell cancer (HLRCC) syndrome, which is an autosomal-dominant condition encompassing a constellation of renal cell carcinoma, and both uterine and cutaneous leiomyomas. Now recognized as its own molecular entity and adopted by the WHO classification, FH-deficient RCC encompasses patients with germline mutations as well as sporadic FH-deficient tumors with biallelic somatic *FH* alterations. Both germline and sporadic disease can manifest early in life and are typically highly aggressive with early metastatic spread even when associated small primary renal tumors. Classic immunohistochemical findings from tumor tissue are PAX8 positivity, CK7 loss, FH deficiency (FH-), and S-(2-succino)-cysteine (2SC) positivity (2SC 2+). FH loss is less sensitive, as retained defective FH protein can be detected on tumor samples [133, 134].

The FH gene encodes an enzyme integral to the tricarboxylic acid cycle (TCA). Defective or absent FH leads to intracellular accumulation of fumarate—an oncometabolite that can drive tumorigenesis. FH inactivation and ineffective intracellular TCA cycle metabolism lead to a reliance on aerobic glycolysis, and subsequent inactivation of the NRF2 pathway [135, 136].

Prior to the histologic reclassification of disease, and given the metabolic alterations underlying HLRCC and potential susceptibility, a sentinel study was performed evaluating targeted therapy with a combination of bevacizumab and erlotinib. The study was performed in two parallel independent cohorts of (1) HLRCC and (2) sporadic pRCC to enrich for patients with FH deficiency. A total of 83 patients were enrolled, including 42 in the HLRCC cohort and 41 in the sporadic pRCC cohort. In the HLRCC cohort, the objective response rate was 64% (27/42; 95% CI, 49–77). The median progression-free survival was an impressive 21.1 months (95% CI, 15.6–26.6) [137].

The Role of Surgery in Metastatic Variant Histology Renal Cell Carcinoma

Limited data exist on the benefit of cytoreductive nephrectomy in patients with vhRCC. Kassouf et al. compared 92 patients with metastatic vhRCC with 514 patients with clear cell metastatic RCC [138]. Patients with vhRCC were noted to be younger (54 vs. 57 years), have more sarcomatoid features (23% vs. 14%), higher pathologic stage, and more nodal metastases (77% vs. 26%). By multivariable analysis, higher T stage (HR = 3.6, 95% CI 1.5–8.5), worse performance status (HR = 2.1, 95% CI 1.1–3.9), and sarcomatoid features (HR = 2.8, 95% CI 1.5–5.2) were independently associated with worse overall survival in patients with vhRCC treated with cytoreductive nephrectomy. Patients with vhRCC had worse disease-specific survival when compared with those with clear cell features (median DSS 9.7 vs. 20.3 months), which was confirmed even in the subgroups of patients with node-negative disease (median DSS 7.7 vs. 24.6 months) and in the absence of sarcomatoid features (median DSS 14 vs. 23.1 months). As a result of the poor survival and lack of effective systemic therapies in this patient population, some investigators have questioned the role of cytoreductive nephrectomy in the presence of known vhRCC [139]. In 2017, Marchioni et al. reported retrospectively that 68% of 851 patients with metastatic vhRCC underwent cytoreductive nephrectomy. Cancer-specific mortality at 2 years was 53% in the group that underwent nephrectomy and 78% in the group that did not, a significant clinical benefit [140]. Careful consideration should be given when faced with a patient with vhRCC, in order to decide if surgery should be done, and if so, how to time it with the administration of systemic therapy.

Role of Adjuvant Therapy in Localized Variant Histology Renal Cell Carcinoma

Nephrectomy remains the standard approach for localized disease, noting that careful observation of small renal masses or locally directed therapies such as cryoablation or SBRT are acceptable approaches in select cases. The KEYNOTE-564 study was a large randomized phase III study that evaluated the role of adjuvant pembrolizumab versus placebo and demonstrated an overall survival benefit in patients with intermediate-high or high risk of recurrence, or M1 no evidence of disease (hazard ratio for death, 0.62; 95% CI, 0.44 to 0.87; $P = 0.005$) [141]. The study led to regulatory approval of adjuvant pembrolizumab by the United States Food and Drug Administration for adjuvant therapy agnostic of RCC histology. However, the study was restricted to patients with clear cell RCC, and the data do not inform management of cases with vhRCC. The phase III EVERST trial was a randomized, double-blind, phase III trial evaluating adjuvant everolimus or placebo in patients with RCC who had undergone resection and were deemed to be at intermediate-high or very high risk of recurrence. Postoperative everolimus did not improve recurrence-free survival compared with placebo among patients enrolled in the study (5-year recurrence-free survival hazard ratio 0.85, 95% CI 0.72–1.00; $p = 0.051$) [142]. The EVEREST study was a basket trial with respect to RCC histology and included 109 patients with papillary RCC and 99 patients with chromophobe RCC. On subgroup analysis, adjuvant everolimus did not improve the recurrence-free survival for papillary histology (hazard ratio, 1.19; 95% CI, 0.61–2.33; $P = 0.61$) nor for patients with chromophobe histology (hazard ratio, 0.89; 95% CI, 0.37–2.13; $P = 0.79$). There remains an urgent and unmet need for high-level data to guide treatment decision-making in the adjuvant space for patients with vhRCC. While adjuvant pembrolizumab may be considered on the basis of extrapolated data, this remains an area of unmet need and requires further investigation before a foundation supporting widespread use can be established.

Conclusion

Variant histology RCC represents a heterogeneous group of tumors. Their varying underlying pathobiology and rarity complicate the design and execution of randomized clinical trials, leading to a paucity of high-level evidence. However, significant advances have been made in the understanding of variant histology RCC subtypes. Efficacious therapies from the clear cell RCC experience, including VEGF inhibitors, mTOR inhibitors, and ICIs, have been shown to have activity in many types of variant histology RCC subtypes, but definitive evidence for the optimal agents and sequencing is still lacking. More work is required to determine the optimal agent, or combination of treatments, for specific histologic subtypes. Integration of molecular profiles and genomics will inevitably advance our understanding of the disease subtypes and provide conduits for the employment of novel therapies. Participation in a clinical trial should still be considered a priority for the majority of patients with metastatic variant histology RCC. Further basic, translational, and clinical research is required to improve patient outcomes (Table 18.1).

Table 18.1 Notable ongoing clinical trials in variant histology RCC

NCI Trial ID	Histology	Treatment	Comments
NCT05220267	Variant histology RCC	Anlotinib + Sintilimab	*Not yet recruiting*
NCT05678673	Papillary, unclassified, translocation RCC	XL092 + Nivolumab vs. Sunitinib	*Recruiting*
NCT06053658	Papillary, chromophobe, oncocyticneoplasms, unclassified	Tivozanib + Nivolumab	*Recruiting*
NCT05124431	Variant histology RCC	Anlotinib + Everolimus	*Not yet recruiting*
NCT04413123	Variant histology RCC	Cabozantinib + Ipilimumab + Nivolumab	*Recruiting*
NCT05831891	Variant histology RCC	Fruquintinib + Serplulimab	*Not yet recruiting*
NCT06302569	Collecting duct and renal medullary carcinoma	Pembrolizumab + Enfortumab Vedotin	*Not yet recruiting*
NCT05411081	Papillary RCC	Cabozantinib + Atezolizumab vs. Cabozantinib	*Recruiting*
NCT05347212	Renal medullary carcinoma	Ipilimumab + Nivolumab	*Recruiting*
NCT05043090	Papillary RCC	Savolitinib + Durvalumab vs. Sunitinib vs. Durvalumab	*Recruiting*
NCT03587662	Renal medullary carcinoma	Ixazomib + Gemcitabine + Doxorubicin	*Recruiting*
NCT03595124	TFE/translocation renal cell carcinoma (tRCC)	Axitinib + Nivolumab vs. Nivolumab	*Active, not recruiting*
NCT05877820	FH-deficient RCC	Lenvatinib + Tislelizumab	*Recruiting*
NCT05286801	Relapsed or refractory SMARCB1 or SMARCA4 deficient tumors	Tiragolumab + Atezolizumab	*Recruiting*

References

1. Siegel RL, Giaquinto AN, Jemal A. Cancer statistics, 2024. CA Cancer J Clin. 2024;74(1):12–49.
2. Kamel MH, et al. Potential years of life lost due to urogenital cancer in the United States: trends from 1972 to 2006 based on data from the SEER database. J Urol. 2012;187(3):868–71.
3. Jemal A, et al. Global cancer statistics. CA Cancer J Clin. 2011;61(2):69–90.
4. Zini L, et al. Radical versus partial nephrectomy: effect on overall and noncancer mortality. Cancer. 2009;115(7):1465–71.
5. Antonelli A, et al. Elective partial nephrectomy is equivalent to radical nephrectomy in patients with clinical T1 renal cell carcinoma: results of a retrospective, comparative, multi-institutional study. BJU Int. 2012;109(7):1013–8.
6. Miller DC, et al. Renal and cardiovascular morbidity after partial or radical nephrectomy. Cancer. 2008;112(3):511–20.
7. Blom JH, et al. Radical nephrectomy with and without lymph-node dissection: final results of European Organization for Research and Treatment of cancer (EORTC) randomized phase 3 trial 30881. Eur Urol. 2009;55(1):28–34.
8. Capitanio U, et al. Lymph node dissection in renal cell carcinoma. Eur Urol. 2011;60(6):1212–20.
9. Giuliani L, et al. Radical extensive surgery for renal cell carcinoma: long-term results and prognostic factors. J Urol. 1990;143(3):468–73; discussion 473–4.
10. Walther MM, et al. Cytoreductive surgery before high dose interleukin-2 based therapy in patients with metastatic renal cell carcinoma. J Urol. 1997;158(5):1675–8.
11. Russo P, et al. Cytoreductive nephrectomy and nephrectomy/complete metastasectomy for metastatic renal cancer. ScientificWorldJournal. 2007;7:768–78.
12. Flanigan RC, et al. Nephrectomy followed by interferon alfa-2b compared with interferon alfa-2b alone for metastatic renal-cell cancer. N Engl J Med. 2001;345(23):1655–9.
13. Mejean A, et al. Is there a place for radical nephrectomy in the presence of metastatic collecting duct (Bellini) carcinoma? J Urol. 2003;169(4):1287–90.
14. Vaeth JM. Proceedings: cancer of the kidney—radiation therapy and its indications in non-Wilms' tumors. Cancer. 1973;32(5):1053–5.
15. Siva S, et al. Radiotherapy for renal cell carcinoma: renaissance of an overlooked approach. Nat Rev Urol. 2017;14(9):549–63.
16. Onufrey V, Mohiuddin M. Radiation therapy in the treatment of metastatic renal cell carcinoma. Int J Radiat Oncol Biol Phys. 1985;11(11):2007–9.
17. Siva S, et al. TROG 15.03 phase II clinical trial of focal ablative STereotactic radiosurgery for can-

cers of the kidney—FASTRACK II. BMC Cancer. 2018;18(1):1030.
18. Reuter VE. The pathology of renal epithelial neoplasms. Semin Oncol. 2006;33(5):534–43.
19. Motzer RJ, Bander NH, Nanus DM. Renal-cell carcinoma. N Engl J Med. 1996;335(12):865–75.
20. Lobo J, et al. WHO 2022 landscape of papillary and chromophobe renal cell carcinoma. Histopathology. 2022;81(4):426–38.
21. de Peralta-Venturina M, et al. Sarcomatoid differentiation in renal cell carcinoma: a study of 101 cases. Am J Surg Pathol. 2001;25(3):275–84.
22. Keskin SK, et al. Outcomes of patients with renal cell carcinoma and Sarcomatoid dedifferentiation treated with nephrectomy and systemic therapies: comparison between the cytokine and targeted therapy eras. J Urol. 2017;198(3):530–7.
23. Cheville JC, et al. Sarcomatoid renal cell carcinoma: an examination of underlying histologic subtype and an analysis of associations with patient outcome. Am J Surg Pathol. 2004;28(4):435–41.
24. Patard JJ, et al. Prognostic value of histologic subtypes in renal cell carcinoma: a multicenter experience. J Clin Oncol. 2005;23(12):2763–71.
25. Beck SD, et al. Effect of papillary and chromophobe cell type on disease-free survival after nephrectomy for renal cell carcinoma. Ann Surg Oncol. 2004;11(1):71–7.
26. Amin MB, et al. Chromophobe renal cell carcinoma: histomorphologic characteristics and evaluation of conventional pathologic prognostic parameters in 145 cases. Am J Surg Pathol. 2008;32(12):1822–34.
27. Amin MB, et al. Prognostic impact of histologic subtyping of adult renal epithelial neoplasms: an experience of 405 cases. Am J Surg Pathol. 2002;26(3):281–91.
28. Leibovich BC, et al. Histological subtype is an independent predictor of outcome for patients with renal cell carcinoma. J Urol. 2010;183(4):1309–15.
29. Motzer RJ, et al. Survival and prognostic stratification of 670 patients with advanced renal cell carcinoma. J Clin Oncol. 1999;17(8):2530–40.
30. Ronnen EA, et al. Treatment outcome for metastatic papillary renal cell carcinoma patients. Cancer. 2006;107(11):2617–21.
31. Hudes G, et al. Temsirolimus, interferon alfa, or both for advanced renal-cell carcinoma. N Engl J Med. 2007;356(22):2271–81.
32. Kawakami F, et al. Programmed cell death ligand 1 and tumor-infiltrating lymphocyte status in patients with renal cell carcinoma and sarcomatoid dedifferentiation. Cancer. 2017;123(24):4823–31.
33. Barata P, et al. Renal cell carcinoma histologic subtypes exhibit distinct transcriptional profiles. J Clin Invest. 2024;134(11):e178915.
34. Motzer RJ, et al. Nivolumab plus Ipilimumab versus Sunitinib in advanced renal-cell carcinoma. N Engl J Med. 2018;378(14):1277–90.
35. Choueiri TK, et al. Updated efficacy results from the JAVELIN renal 101 trial: first-line avelumab plus axitinib versus sunitinib in patients with advanced renal cell carcinoma. Ann Oncol. 2020;31(8):1030–9.
36. Rini BI, et al. Long-term outcomes with nivolumab plus ipilimumab versus sunitinib in first-line treatment of patients with advanced sarcomatoid renal cell carcinoma. J Immunother Cancer. 2022;10(12):e005445.
37. Albiges L, et al. Pembrolizumab plus lenvatinib as first-line therapy for advanced non-clear-cell renal cell carcinoma (KEYNOTE-B61): a single-arm, multicentre, phase 2 trial. Lancet Oncol. 2023;24(8):881–91.
38. McGregor BA, et al. Results of a multicenter phase II study of Atezolizumab and bevacizumab for patients with metastatic renal cell carcinoma with variant histology and/or sarcomatoid features. J Clin Oncol. 2020;38(1):63–70.
39. Kaelin WG Jr. The von Hippel-Lindau tumor suppressor protein and clear cell renal carcinoma. Clin Cancer Res. 2007;13(2 Pt 2):680s–4s.
40. Kim WY, Kaelin WG. Role of VHL gene mutation in human cancer. J Clin Oncol. 2004;22(24):4991–5004.
41. Lubensky IA, et al. Hereditary and sporadic papillary renal carcinomas with c-met mutations share a distinct morphological phenotype. Am J Pathol. 1999;155(2):517–26.
42. Schmidt L, et al. Germline and somatic mutations in the tyrosine kinase domain of the MET proto-oncogene in papillary renal carcinomas. Nat Genet. 1997;16(1):68–73.
43. Boccaccio C, Comoglio PM. Invasive growth: a MET-driven genetic programme for cancer and stem cells. Nat Rev Cancer. 2006;6(8):637–45.
44. Sweeney P, et al. Biological significance of c-met over expression in papillary renal cell carcinoma. J Urol. 2002;168(1):51–5.
45. Motzer RJ, et al. Overall survival and updated results for sunitinib compared with interferon alfa in patients with metastatic renal cell carcinoma. J Clin Oncol. 2009;27(22):3584–90.
46. Motzer RJ, et al. Sunitinib versus interferon alfa in metastatic renal-cell carcinoma. N Engl J Med. 2007;356(2):115–24.
47. Gore ME, et al. Safety and efficacy of sunitinib for metastatic renal-cell carcinoma: an expanded-access trial. Lancet Oncol. 2009;10(8):757–63.
48. Tannir NM, et al. A phase 2 trial of sunitinib in patients with advanced non-clear cell renal cell carcinoma. Eur Urol. 2012;62(6):1013–9.
49. Tannir NM, et al. Everolimus versus Sunitinib prospective evaluation in metastatic non-clear cell renal cell carcinoma (ESPN): a randomized multicenter phase 2 trial. Eur Urol. 2016;69(5):866–74.
50. Armstrong AJ, et al. Everolimus versus sunitinib for patients with metastatic non-clear cell renal cell carcinoma (ASPEN): a multicentre, open-label, randomised phase 2 trial. Lancet Oncol. 2016;17(3):378–88.

51. Choueiri TK, et al. Phase II and biomarker study of the dual MET/VEGFR2 inhibitor foretinib in patients with papillary renal cell carcinoma. J Clin Oncol. 2013;31(2):181–6.
52. Srinivasan R, et al. Correlation of germline <i>MET</i> mutation with response to the dual Met/VEGFR-2 inhibitor foretinib in patients with sporadic and hereditary papillary renal cell carcinoma: results from a multicenter phase II study (MET111644). J Clin Oncol. 2012;30(5_suppl):372.
53. Choueiri TK, et al. Biomarker-based phase II trial of Savolitinib in patients with advanced papillary renal cell cancer. J Clin Oncol. 2017;35(26):2993–3001.
54. Pal SK, et al. A comparison of sunitinib with cabozantinib, crizotinib, and savolitinib for treatment of advanced papillary renal cell carcinoma: a randomised, open-label, phase 2 trial. Lancet. 2021;397(10275):695–703.
55. Barata P, et al. Final overall survival analysis of S1500: a randomized, phase II study comparing Sunitinib with Cabozantinib, Crizotinib, and Savolitinib in advanced papillary renal cell carcinoma. J Clin Oncol. 2024;42(33):3911–6.
56. McDermott DF, et al. Open-label, single-arm, phase II study of Pembrolizumab monotherapy as first-line therapy in patients with advanced non-clear cell renal cell carcinoma. J Clin Oncol. 2021;39(9):1029–39.
57. Tykodi SS, et al. Safety and efficacy of nivolumab plus ipilimumab in patients with advanced non-clear cell renal cell carcinoma: results from the phase 3b/4 CheckMate 920 trial. J Immunother Cancer. 2022;10(2):e003844.
58. Bergmann L, Albiges MAL, Goupil MG, Boleti E, Gravis G, Flechon A, Grimm MJ, Rausch S, Barthelemy P, Gauna DEC, Gonzalez BM, Ivanyi P, Floercken A, Rodriguez CS, Rey JPM, Gruenwald V, Burkholder I, Hartmann A, Haanen JBAG. LBA75—Prospective randomised phase-II trial of ipilimumab/nivolumab versus standard of care in non-clear cell renal cell cancer: results of the SUNNIFORECAST trial. In: European Society of Medical Oncology Congress 2024; 2024.
59. Lee CH, et al. Phase II trial of Cabozantinib plus Nivolumab in patients with non-clear-cell renal cell carcinoma and genomic correlates. J Clin Oncol. 2022;40(21):2333–41.
60. Suarez C, et al. Phase II study investigating the safety and efficacy of Savolitinib and Durvalumab in metastatic papillary renal cancer (CALYPSO). J Clin Oncol. 2023;41(14):2493–502.
61. Fleming S. Distal nephron neoplasms. Semin Diagn Pathol. 2015;32(2):114–23.
62. Yamazaki K, et al. Overexpression of KIT in chromophobe renal cell carcinoma. Oncogene. 2003;22(6):847–52.
63. Speicher MR, et al. Specific loss of chromosomes 1, 2, 6, 10, 13, 17, and 21 in chromophobe renal cell carcinomas revealed by comparative genomic hybridization. Am J Pathol. 1994;145(2):356–64.
64. Akhtar M, et al. Chromophobe cell carcinoma of the kidney. A clinicopathologic study of 21 cases. Am J Surg Pathol. 1995;19(11):1245–56.
65. Haake SM, Rathmell WK. Renal cancer subtypes: should we be lumping or splitting for therapeutic decision making? Cancer. 2017;123(2):200–9.
66. Davis CF, et al. The somatic genomic landscape of chromophobe renal cell carcinoma. Cancer Cell. 2014;26(3):319–30.
67. Nickerson ML, et al. Mutations in a novel gene lead to kidney tumors, lung wall defects, and benign tumors of the hair follicle in patients with the Birt-Hogg-Dube syndrome. Cancer Cell. 2002;2(2):157–64.
68. Baba M, et al. Folliculin encoded by the BHD gene interacts with a binding protein, FNIP1, and AMPK, and is involved in AMPK and mTOR signaling. Proc Natl Acad Sci U S A. 2006;103(42):15552–7.
69. Kato I, et al. Fluorescent and chromogenic in situ hybridization of CEN17q as a potent useful diagnostic marker for Birt-Hogg-Dube syndrome-associated chromophobe renal cell carcinomas. Hum Pathol. 2016;52:74–82.
70. Schmidt LS, et al. Germline BHD-mutation spectrum and phenotype analysis of a large cohort of families with Birt-Hogg-Dube syndrome. Am J Hum Genet. 2005;76(6):1023–33.
71. Khoo SK, et al. Inactivation of BHD in sporadic renal tumors. Cancer Res. 2003;63(15):4583–7.
72. Stadler WM, et al. Safety and efficacy results of the advanced renal cell carcinoma sorafenib expanded access program in North America. Cancer. 2010;116(5):1272–80.
73. Choueiri TK, et al. Efficacy of sunitinib and sorafenib in metastatic papillary and chromophobe renal cell carcinoma. J Clin Oncol. 2008;26(1):127–31.
74. Voss MH, et al. Phase II trial and correlative genomic analysis of Everolimus plus bevacizumab in advanced non-clear cell renal cell carcinoma. J Clin Oncol. 2016;34(32):3846–53.
75. Alaghehbandan R, Siadat F, Trpkov K. What's new in the WHO 2022 classification of kidney tumours? Pathologica. 2022;115(1):8–22.
76. Zhong M, et al. Translocation renal cell carcinomas in adults: a single-institution experience. Am J Surg Pathol. 2012;36(5):654–62.
77. Argani P, et al. Xp11 translocation renal cell carcinoma (RCC): extended immunohistochemical profile emphasizing novel RCC markers. Am J Surg Pathol. 2010;34(9):1295–303.
78. Clark J, et al. Fusion of splicing factor genes PSF and NonO (p54nrb) to the TFE3 gene in papillary renal cell carcinoma. Oncogene. 1997;15(18):2233–9.
79. Argani P, et al. Primary renal neoplasms with the ASPL-TFE3 gene fusion of alveolar soft part sarcoma: a distinctive tumor entity previously included among renal cell carcinomas of children and adolescents. Am J Pathol. 2001;159(1):179–92.
80. Argani P, et al. Aberrant nuclear immunoreactivity for TFE3 in neoplasms with TFE3 gene fusions: a

sensitive and specific immunohistochemical assay. Am J Surg Pathol. 2003;27(6):750–61.
81. Argani P, et al. Renal carcinomas with the t(6;11)(p21;q12): clinicopathologic features and demonstration of the specific alpha-TFEB gene fusion by immunohistochemistry, RT-PCR, and DNA PCR. Am J Surg Pathol. 2005;29(2):230–40.
82. Skala SL, et al. Detection of 6 TFEB-amplified renal cell carcinomas and 25 renal cell carcinomas with MITF translocations: systematic morphologic analysis of 85 cases evaluated by clinical TFE3 and TFEB FISH assays. Mod Pathol. 2018;31(1):179–97.
83. Davis IJ, et al. Cloning of an alpha-TFEB fusion in renal tumors harboring the t(6;11)(p21;q13) chromosome translocation. Proc Natl Acad Sci U S A. 2003;100(10):6051–6.
84. Kuiper RP, et al. Upregulation of the transcription factor TFEB in t(6;11)(p21;q13)-positive renal cell carcinomas due to promoter substitution. Hum Mol Genet. 2003;12(14):1661–9.
85. Srigley JR, et al. The International Society of Urological Pathology (ISUP) Vancouver classification of renal neoplasia. Am J Surg Pathol. 2013;37(10):1469–89.
86. Argani P. MiT family translocation renal cell carcinoma. Semin Diagn Pathol. 2015;32(2):103–13.
87. Choueiri TK, et al. Vascular endothelial growth factor-targeted therapy for the treatment of adult metastatic Xp11.2 translocation renal cell carcinoma. Cancer. 2010;116(22):5219–25.
88. Malouf GG, et al. Targeted agents in metastatic Xp11 translocation/TFE3 gene fusion renal cell carcinoma (RCC): a report from the juvenile RCC network. Ann Oncol. 2010;21(9):1834–8.
89. Alhalabi O, et al. Immune checkpoint therapy combinations in adult advanced MiT family translocation renal cell carcinomas. Oncologist. 2023;28(5):433–9.
90. Bakouny Z, et al. Integrative clinical and molecular characterization of translocation renal cell carcinoma. Cell Rep. 2022;38(1):110190.
91. Dizman N, Philip EJ, Pal SK. Genomic profiling in renal cell carcinoma. Nat Rev Nephrol. 2020;16(8):435–51.
92. Davis CJ Jr, Mostofi FK, Sesterhenn IA. Renal medullary carcinoma. The seventh sickle cell nephropathy. Am J Surg Pathol. 1995;19(1):1–11.
93. Sathyamoorthy K, Teo A, Atallah M. Renal medullary carcinoma in a patient with sickle-cell disease. Nat Clin Pract Urol. 2006;3(5):279–83; quiz 289.
94. Baig MA, et al. Renal medullary carcinoma. J Natl Med Assoc. 2006;98(7):1171–4.
95. Msaouel P, Tannir NM, Walker CL. A model linking sickle cell Hemoglobinopathies and SMARCB1 loss in renal medullary carcinoma. Clin Cancer Res. 2018;24(9):2044–9.
96. Shah AY, et al. Management and outcomes of patients with renal medullary carcinoma: a multicentre collaborative study. BJU Int. 2017;120(6):782–92.
97. Margol AS, Judkins AR. Pathology and diagnosis of SMARCB1-deficient tumors. Cancer Genet. 2014;207(9):358–64.
98. Cheng JX, et al. Renal medullary carcinoma: rhabdoid features and the absence of INI1 expression as markers of aggressive behavior. Mod Pathol. 2008;21(6):647–52.
99. Sirohi D, et al. Renal cell carcinoma, unclassified with medullary phenotype: poorly differentiated adenocarcinomas overlapping with renal medullary carcinoma. Hum Pathol. 2017;67:134–45.
100. Msaouel P, et al. Updated recommendations on the diagnosis, management, and clinical trial eligibility criteria for patients with renal medullary carcinoma. Clin Genitourin Cancer. 2019;17(1):1–6.
101. Strouse JJ, et al. Significant responses to platinum-based chemotherapy in renal medullary carcinoma. Pediatr Blood Cancer. 2005;44(4):407–11.
102. Noguera-Irizarry WG, Hibshoosh H, Papadopoulos KP. Renal medullary carcinoma: case report and review of the literature. Am J Clin Oncol. 2003;26(5):489–92.
103. Rathmell WK, Monk JP. High-dose-intensity MVAC for advanced renal medullary carcinoma: report of three cases and literature review. Urology. 2008;72(3):659–63.
104. Schaeffer EM, et al. Renal medullary carcinoma: molecular, pathological and clinical evidence for treatment with topoisomerase-inhibiting therapy. BJU Int. 2010;106(1):62–5.
105. Wiele AJ, et al. Efficacy and safety of bevacizumab plus Erlotinib in patients with renal medullary carcinoma. Cancers (Basel). 2021;13(9):2170.
106. Oudard S, et al. Prospective multicenter phase II study of gemcitabine plus platinum salt for metastatic collecting duct carcinoma: results of a GETUG (Groupe d'Etudes des Tumeurs Uro-Genitales) study. J Urol. 2007;177(5):1698–702.
107. Pecuchet N, et al. Triple combination of bevacizumab, gemcitabine and platinum salt in metastatic collecting duct carcinoma. Ann Oncol. 2013;24(12):2963–7.
108. Martinez Chanza N, et al. Cabozantinib in advanced non-clear-cell renal cell carcinoma: a multicentre, retrospective, cohort study. Lancet Oncol. 2019;20(4):581–90.
109. Procopio G, et al. Cabozantinib as first-line treatment in patients with metastatic collecting duct renal cell carcinoma: results of the BONSAI trial for the Italian network for research in urologic-oncology (meet-URO 2 study). JAMA Oncol. 2022;8(6):910–3.
110. Bronchud MH, et al. HER2 blockade in metastatic collecting duct carcinoma (CDC) of the kidney: a case report. Onkologie. 2012;35(12):776–9.
111. Ferlicot S, et al. Mucinous tubular and spindle cell carcinoma: a report of 15 cases and a review of the literature. Virchows Arch. 2005;447(6):978–83.
112. Zhao M, He XL, Teng XD. Mucinous tubular and spindle cell renal cell carcinoma: a review of clinicopathologic aspects. Diagn Pathol. 2015;10:168.

113. Hes O, et al. Spindle and cuboidal renal cell carcinoma, a tumour having frequent association with nephrolithiasis: report of 11 cases including a case with hybrid conventional renal cell carcinoma/ spindle and cuboidal renal cell carcinoma components. Histopathology. 2002;41(6):549–55.
114. Paner GP, et al. Immunohistochemical analysis of mucinous tubular and spindle cell carcinoma and papillary renal cell carcinoma of the kidney: significant immunophenotypic overlap warrants diagnostic caution. Am J Surg Pathol. 2006;30(1):13–9.
115. Shen SS, et al. Mucinous tubular and spindle cell carcinoma of kidney is probably a variant of papillary renal cell carcinoma with spindle cell features. Ann Diagn Pathol. 2007;11(1):13–21.
116. Cossu-Rocca P, et al. Renal mucinous tubular and spindle carcinoma lacks the gains of chromosomes 7 and 17 and losses of chromosome Y that are prevalent in papillary renal cell carcinoma. Mod Pathol. 2006;19(4):488–93.
117. Mehra R, et al. Biallelic alteration and dysregulation of the hippo pathway in mucinous tubular and spindle cell carcinoma of the kidney. Cancer Discov. 2016;6(11):1258–66.
118. Thway K, et al. Metastatic renal mucinous tubular and spindle cell carcinoma. Atypical behavior of a rare, morphologically bland tumor. Ann Diagn Pathol. 2012;16(5):407–10.
119. Furuya S, et al. Renal mucinous tubular and spindle cell carcinoma shows a high uptake on (18)F-FDG PET/CT. Intern Med. 2018;57(8):1131–4.
120. Pillay N, et al. Mucinous tubular and spindle cell carcinoma with aggressive histomorphology—a sarcomatoid variant. Hum Pathol. 2008;39(6):966–9.
121. Dhillon J, et al. Mucinous tubular and spindle cell carcinoma of the kidney with sarcomatoid change. Am J Surg Pathol. 2009;33(1):44–9.
122. Zhou M, et al. Renal tubulocystic carcinoma is closely related to papillary renal cell carcinoma: implications for pathologic classification. Am J Surg Pathol. 2009;33(12):1840–9.
123. Amin MB, et al. Tubulocystic carcinoma of the kidney: clinicopathologic analysis of 31 cases of a distinctive rare subtype of renal cell carcinoma. Am J Surg Pathol. 2009;33(3):384–92.
124. Mego M, et al. Sunitinib in the treatment of tubulocystic carcinoma of the kidney. A case report. Ann Oncol. 2008;19(9):1655–6.
125. Bhullar JS, Thamboo T, Esuvaranathan K. Unique case of tubulocystic carcinoma of the kidney with sarcomatoid features: a new entity. Urology. 2011;78(5):1071–2.
126. Jung SJ, et al. Thyroid follicular carcinoma-like tumor of kidney: a case report with morphologic, immunohistochemical, and genetic analysis. Am J Surg Pathol. 2006;30(3):411–5.
127. Sterlacci W, et al. Thyroid follicular carcinoma-like renal tumor: a case report with morphologic, immunophenotypic, cytogenetic, and scintigraphic studies. Virchows Arch. 2008;452(1):91–5.
128. Amin MB, et al. Primary thyroid-like follicular carcinoma of the kidney: report of 6 cases of a histologically distinctive adult renal epithelial neoplasm. Am J Surg Pathol. 2009;33(3):393–400.
129. Powles T, et al. Renal cell carcinoma: ESMO clinical practice guideline for diagnosis, treatment and follow-up. Ann Oncol. 2024;35(8):692–706.
130. Shah RB, Mehra R. Renal cell carcinoma associated with TSC/MTOR genomic alterations: an update on its expanding spectrum and an approach to clinicopathologic work-up. Adv Anat Pathol. 2024;31(2):105–17.
131. Motzer RJ, et al. NCCN guidelines(R) insights: kidney cancer, version 2.2024. J Natl Compr Canc Netw. 2024;22(1):4–16.
132. Lv Y, Song L, Hu M. Fumarate hydratase-deficient renal cell carcinoma: a case report and review of the literature. J Med Case Reports. 2023;17(1):182.
133. Trpkov K, et al. Fumarate hydratase-deficient renal cell carcinoma is strongly correlated with fumarate hydratase mutation and hereditary Leiomyomatosis and renal cell carcinoma syndrome. Am J Surg Pathol. 2016;40(7):865–75.
134. Chen YB. Update on selected high-grade renal cell carcinomas of the kidney: FH-deficient, ALK-rearranged, and medullary carcinomas. Adv Anat Pathol. 2024;31(2):118–25.
135. Zarrabi K, Walzer E, Zibelman M. Immune checkpoint inhibition in advanced non-clear cell renal cell carcinoma: leveraging success from clear cell histology into new opportunities. Cancers (Basel). 2021;13(15):3652.
136. Ooi A. Advances in hereditary leiomyomatosis and renal cell carcinoma (HLRCC) research. Semin Cancer Biol. 2020;61:158–66.
137. Srinivasan R, et al. Results from a phase II study of bevacizumab and erlotinib in subjects with advanced hereditary leiomyomatosis and renal cell cancer (HLRCC) or sporadic papillary renal cell cancer. J Clin Oncol. 2020;38(15_suppl):5004.
138. Kassouf W, et al. Cytoreductive nephrectomy for metastatic renal cell carcinoma with nonclear cell histology. J Urol. 2007;178(5):1896–900.
139. Abel EJ, Wood CG. Cytoreductive nephrectomy for metastatic RCC in the era of targeted therapy. Nat Rev Urol. 2009;6(7):375–83.
140. Marchioni M, et al. Survival after cytoreductive nephrectomy in metastatic non-clear cell renal cell carcinoma patients: a population-based study. Eur Urol Focus. 2019;5(3):488–96.
141. Choueiri TK, et al. Overall survival with adjuvant Pembrolizumab in renal-cell carcinoma. N Engl J Med. 2024;390(15):1359–71.
142. Ryan CW, et al. Adjuvant everolimus after surgery for renal cell carcinoma (EVEREST): a double-blind, placebo-controlled, randomised, phase 3 trial. Lancet. 2023;402(10407):1043–51.

19 Surgical Management for Transitional Cell Carcinoma of the Upper Tract

Jason R. Gee

Epidemiology

According to the National Center for Health Statistics, upper tract malignancies are relatively uncommon, with an estimated annual incidence of 1–4 per 100,000 [1–3]. An increase in incidence of 1.5% annually in the United States has been noted for kidney cancer [4]. In contrast, the incidence has risen sharply in other parts of the world, such as the Netherlands, where greater than a 50% rise in the incidence of upper urinary tract urothelial cancer (UTUC) has been identified between 1993 and 2017 [5]. A more modest increase of 3.86% in Korea was reported by Cho et al spanning 22 years from 1999 to 2020 [6]. Renal pelvic tumors account for 15% of all renal tumors, whereas ureteral cancers comprise 1–2% of urologic cancers [7, 8]. The incidence of UTUC has been found to vary by region [9]. For instance, the incidence of UTUC in the Balkan endemic nephropathy region has been reported to account for 65% of kidney cancers [10]. While the vast majority of these cancers are urothelial in origin, up to 10% may feature squamous histology [11]. Relatively rare histologic variants include adenocarcinoma, small cell carcinoma, and micropapillary urothelial carcinoma [12–14], and benign pathology such as fibroepithelial polyps and glomus tumors may also be encountered [15, 16]. Upper tract urothelial carcinoma is more prevalent in Caucasians and males [17, 18]. However, women who are diagnosed with upper tract urothelial cancers have a 25% higher risk of death from this disease, which for unclear reasons is gender-specific [19]. This has been confirmed by a more recent multi-institutional study in which a statistically significant association was identified between female gender and both disease recurrence (hazard ratio [HR] 1.7, $p = 0.03$) and cancer-specific mortality (HR 2 = 0.009) [20].

Patients with Lynch Syndrome (LS) are also at risk for developing UTUC. Interestingly, Wischhusen et al established clinical factors that can reliably predict patients with LS who are at risk for developing UTUC. In their analysis, male gender, harboring of germline EPCAM/MSH2 variants, and family history of UTUC were factors of which at least one was noted in 143/158 (90.5%) of patients with LS that were diagnosed with UTUC. Conversely, no LS carriers were found to have UTUC without at least one of these factors [21]. Further characterization of five mutational subtypes of UTUC has revealed correlations with prognosis and tumor histology. For instance, the FGFR3 mutation subtype was identified in patients with improved survival rates harboring low-grade UTUC, whereas the RAS-mutated subtype of UTUC was associated with

J. R. Gee (✉)
Associate Professor of Urology, Tufts University School of Medicine, Department of Urology, Tufts University Medical Center, Boston, MA, USA

Department of Urology, MGH Cancer Center, Emerson Hospital, Concord, MA, USA
e-mail: JGee@Emersonhosp.org

J. A. Libertino, J. R. Gee (eds.), *Renal Cancer*, https://doi.org/10.1007/978-3-031-97599-8_19

high-grade tumors and squamous cell histology. The most aggressive tumors harbored TP53/MDM2 mutations, whereas a 'triple negative subtype' featured a similar prognosis. A hypermutated subtype was also identified in this study in which MMR mutations characteristic of LS were identified [22].

The incidence of renal pelvic cancer has been correlated with socioeconomic status as well. In a Canadian study by Tope et al, lower income status, both individual and regional, has been associated with a higher incidence of renal pelvic cancer [23]. Additionally, Valencia et al studied the relationship between Social Vulnerability Index (SVI) and time to surgery as well as survival following surgery for kidney cancer. SVI was developed by the Centers for Disease Control and Prevention using 16 census criteria to help predict the ability of a community to survive and thrive when subjected to disaster. In this study of Hispanics and American Indians living in Arizona, a high SVI was associated with both longer time to surgery and decreased survival [24].

Patients who are at the highest risk of developing upper tract urothelial malignancy are those who have been diagnosed with bladder tumors. With 5-year follow-up, the estimated risk of developing upper tract disease following diagnosis of bladder cancer ranges from 2% to 4% [25]. More significantly, patients who are diagnosed with upper tract tumors are at high risk for developing bladder cancer. As justification for regular cystoscopic surveillance, an estimated incidence of 25–75% of these patients can develop bladder cancer [26–29].

More recent studies have focused on the stratification of patients with UTUC in predicting their risk of bladder cancer recurrence (BCR). For instance, in a multicenter study, Fradet et al. identified clinical parameters including age, tumor location within the renal pelvis versus ureter, extravesical ureterectomy, and treatment with adjuvant systemic chemotherapy as significant factors in predicting BCR following nephroureterectomy [30]. Pathologic parameters, including lymphovascular invasion and papillary histology, have also been reported as factors affecting BCR [31]. However, yet other investigators have identified parameters including tumor grade and stage, location, and gender as significant in determining the risk for BCR, suggesting that discrepancies among these studies exist. The presently accepted clinical factors for BCR risk stratification by the European Association of Urology include gender (male), history of bladder cancer, preoperative renal disease, and smoking status. Additionally, the presence of tumor invasion, necrosis, and multifocality, as well as ureteral tumor location and a positive urine cytology, have been determined to be significant tumor-related risk factors for BCR. And technical aspects of treatment, including positive surgical margins and an extravesical approach to bladder cuff removal via laparoscopy, have also been implicated as risk factors for BCR [32]. A trial currently underway will evaluate the role of preoperative intravesical mitomycin C in reducing the risk of BCR. This study, the REBACARE-trial, is significant given the concern that instillation of mitomycin C immediately following radical nephroureterectomy may result in toxicity due to extravesical extravasation of this medication [33].

Fortunately, synchronous and metachronous involvement of the upper tracts occurs uncommonly in only 5% of patients with this disease [34].

Biology

In general, the prognosis associated with upper tract urothelial malignancies tends to be worse than that of bladder cancers, in that >60% of these patients present with invasive disease at the time of diagnosis. In contrast, 25–30% of patients with bladder cancer are initially diagnosed with muscle invasion [35, 36]. A more recent review of the Surveillance, Epidemiology, and Results (SEER) Database by Park also noted that the likelihood of disease progression was greater for UTUC than UCB, and among patients with UTUC, the overall metastasis rate associated with renal pelvis cancer was worse than that of ureteral cancer [37]. Conversely, a review of patients with UTUC from the National Cancer

Database revealed ureteral cancers to be associated with a worse prognosis than renal pelvic cancers. While the reason for this discrepancy is unclear, the authors postulate this could be due to a lower incidence of radical nephroureterectomy for patients with ureteral cancers [38].

However, these differences in outcome may also be due to the biology of these cancers as a function of primary tumor origin. Since the first edition of this chapter, much work has been done in this area.

In 2016, a genomic comparison of germline and tumor DNA from UTUC (n = 83) and UCB (n = 102) was reported by Sfakianos and colleagues. In this significant and well-designed study, they actually identified a similar array of genetic alterations between UTUC and UCB. However, significant differences were seen in the prevalence of recurrent gene mutations for HRAS ($p = 0.001$), TP53 ($p < 0.001$), and RB-1 ($p < 0.001$). Furthermore, mutations in the FGFR3 gene, known to occur in association with low-grade UCB, were also identified in low-grade UTUC in 22 of 23 specimens. Surprisingly, no RB-1 mutations were identified in this UTUC cohort, whereas they were identified with a frequency of 18.6% in UCB [39]. Table 19.1

In contrast, Lee and colleagues reported their findings for UTUC and UCB by genomic profiling of commonly mutated genes for urothelial carcinoma. As has been established by The Cancer Genome Atlas (TCGA) [40] and others, the primary molecular alterations for both UTUC and UBC were identified for TP53, PIK3CA, and FGFR3 genes. However, the frequency of mutations between both UTUC (n = 31) and UBC (n = 61) was not statistically different ($p = 0.13$). One notable exception was that again no RB-1 mutations were identified in UTUC, as compared to 19.7% RB-1 mutations found in UCB ($p = 0.02$) [41].

Table 19.1 Significant differences in oncogene and tumor suppressor mutation rates between UTUC and UCB [39]

	UTUC	UCB	
FGFR3	35.6%	21.6%	p=0.065
HRAS	13.6%	1.0%	p=0.001
CDKN2B	15.3%	3.9%	p=0.016
ARID1A	13.6%	27.5%	p=0.050
RB1	None	18.6%	p<0.001
TP53	25.4%	57.8%	p<0.001
TP53/MDM2	35.6%	62.7%	p=0.001

A more recent genomic profiling study featuring cohorts of larger sample size (UCB n = 1984, UTUC n = 479) revealed significant differences in genomic alterations (GA) of multiple genes in which gene mutations, rearrangements, alteration in copy number, and short insertions/deletions were compared. In this study, among other significant findings the investigators verified a greater GA frequency of RB-1 in UCB as compared to UTUC (21% vs. 7.8%, $p < 0.001$). In addition, significant differences in GAs between UCB and UTUC, respectively, were also identified for FGFR3 (19% vs. 26%, $p = 0.02$) and HRAS (2.8% vs. 6.9%, $p = 0.006$) [42].

Other research would imply that molecular urothelial expression profiles of upper tract urothelium differ from that of bladder urothelium. Microsatellite alterations have been identified in urothelium, which are specific to the upper tract as compared to the bladder [43]. Furthermore, uroplakin is a urothelium-specific marker that has been identified in bladder and upper tract disease and has been utilized in transgenic mice capable of spontaneously generating urothelial tumors [44]. However, multiple subtypes of uroplakin exist, and recent studies have revealed that upper tract urothelium expresses a different uroplakin expression profile as compared to bladder urothelium [45]. As such, differences in cellular and biologic properties do exist based on the location of native benign urothelium in the urinary tract, which may explain differences in tumor biology that have been reported based on location [46–49].

Given the similar histopathology of UTUC and urothelial bladder cancer (UBC) and relative rarity of UTUC, treatment of UTUC is typically based on our available data and experience in treating patients with UBC [50, 51]. However, in more recent studies, identification of biomarkers elucidating the biology of UTUC has been reported. For instance, elevated levels of B2-microglobulin in the urine have been associated with disease progression in patients with UTUC [52]. These efforts will hopefully permit tailoring of treatment specific to UTUC, given its relatively unfavorable biology. These biomarkers are particularly of interest as potential targets for molecular-based therapies.

Other markers include HER2 and other mediators of PI3K/AKT pathway activation, p53, and Ki-67 among others. Human epidermal growth factor receptor 2 (HER2), a biomarker that has been found to be aberrantly overexpressed in UBC and is a known target for tyrosine kinase inhibitor therapy, has also been found to be overexpressed in high-grade UTUC, whereas the vast majority of low-grade tumors were negative (94% vs 6%). These findings would imply that UTUC overexpressing HER2 may be amenable to HER2-targeted (Herceptin) treatment [53]. Furthermore, activating mutations of PIK3CA and loss of PTEN expression have been identified in UTUC, which in turn lead to activation of the PI3K/AKT pathway. This signaling cascade can in turn mediate cellular proliferation and resistance to apoptosis [54].

Aberrant expression of p53 has been well established for UBC, and likewise overexpression of this gene in UTUC has been associated with higher tumor stage and grade [55]. Significant differences in survival (overall and cancer specific) have been identified in association with overexpression of p53 in UTUC [55–57]. Significant work on the role of p53 in tumorigenesis of UTUC has been accomplished in patients with Balkan endemic nephropathy, in that aristolochic acid (AA)-p53 DNA adducts have been implicated in cell cycle dysregulation. Specifically, point mutations in p53 have been confirmed in this group of UTUC patients as a molecular signature of AA exposure [58].

Ki-67 is a mediator of cell proliferation, which has been found to be overexpressed in UTUC and associated with grade, stage, and lymphovascular invasion (LVI) [59]. Overexpression of this biomarker has also been found to correlate with bladder recurrence and adverse prognosis in multiple studies [60, 61]. And a recent large-scale meta-analysis by the International Upper Tract Urothelial Carcinoma Collaboration revealed that LVI, higher tumor stage and nodal metastasis, tumor necrosis and sessile tumor features, and the presence of carcinoma in situ were all significantly associated with the overexpression of Ki-67 [62]. The importance of LVI as a prognostic factor was also established for renal pelvic cancer by Danzig et al [63]. In this study, a significantly lower 5-year survival was identified for patients with T3 renal pelvic cancer with LVI, which was comparable to T4 renal pelvic cancer without LVI. Gene promoter hypermethylation has also been described for renal pelvic cancers. Hypermethylation in turn is a mechanism whereby oncogene and tumor suppressor gene expression may be regulated [64].

Additionally, tissue-based microRNA signatures have been found to hold prognostic significance in urothelial carcinoma. In a multi-institutional tissue-based analysis by Summerhayes and colleagues, miRNA-20 and miRNA-200 have been identified in association with invasive urothelial carcinoma of the bladder [65]. Similarly, Montalbo et al. have identified the significance of miRNA in upper tract urothelial carcinoma, in which miRNA-151b has been correlated with disease progression and cancer-specific survival [66]. In 2022, Chung et al identified low tissue expression levels of MiR-226a-5p in UTUC as compared to adjacent normal urothelium. Furthermore, inhibition of WNT5A/β--catenin signaling as well as downregulation of NF-kB and Matrixmetalloproteinase (MMP)-9 were observed with restoration of MiR-26a-5p expression in stably transfected BFTC-909 UTUC cells in vitro, consistent with a tumor suppressor role for this microRNA in that the phenotype resulting from epithelial-to-mesenchymal transition (EMT) may be reversed [67].

Carcinogenesis

The development of urothelial carcinoma of the upper tract is attributed to carcinogen exposure in a manner similar to bladder cancer. Tobacco exposure remains a primary contributing factor, in which aromatic amines including benzopyrene, dimethylbenzanthracene, and arylamines have been implicated. These carcinogens are metabolized into less toxic derivatives by multiple enzymes including CYP1A1, glutathione S-transferase, and N-acetyl transferase. Genetic mutations of these genes have been attributed to differing susceptibility to these carcinogens [68]. Aromatic amines in industrial dyes have also been implicated [69]. Analgesic consumption has also been identified as a risk factor in the development of upper tract TCC. Phenacetin, for instance, was noted to induce mutations and to also cause papillary necrosis, which can trigger the development of upper tract tumors [70]. And as discussed earlier in this chapter, region-specific susceptibility has also been identified with Balkan endemic nephropathy [71, 72]. Interestingly, in China, the regular consumption of Chinese herbs containing aristolochic acid (AA) has been associated with specific mutations of upper tract cancer and may prove to be a common factor in the development of this disease in individuals who consume these herbs [73–75]. And as mentioned above, recent work in this area has revealed AA-DNA adducts resulting in A:T point mutations involving the p53 gene. The carcinogenic effects of AA have also been hypothesized to be based on metabolic susceptibility. Specifically, this could be due to pharmacogenomic differences and specific genetic polymorphisms affecting the expression/function of CYP1A1/2 and other enzymes, which have been shown in laboratory studies to affect AA metabolism [58].

Recent studies have identified an association between certain occupations and an increased risk of renal pelvis cancer. These include occupations involving work at sea and occupations involving exposures to welding fumes, heavy metals, and asbestos [9, 76]. While in vivo research has identified increased levels of copper, manganese, zinc, and chromium in renal tissue following exposure to welding fumes, further study establishing specific carcinogenic pathways for renal pelvis cancer is warranted [77].

Diagnosis and Clinicopathologic Risk Factors

Patients with a history of bladder cancer are at the highest risk of developing upper tract tumors. Guidelines for surveillance of the upper tracts following diagnosis of bladder cancer vary but have been based primarily on risk stratification [78–80]. For instance, patients who have high-grade or invasive bladder tumors are at the highest risk of developing upper tract recurrence, in which upper tract surveillance is recommended every 1–2 years. Carcinoma in situ of the bladder, in particular, has been shown to be a significant risk factor for upper tract recurrence [81, 82]. Intermediate-risk patients with low-grade bladder tumors with either multiple recurrences or high-volume disease should undergo upper tract surveillance every 1–2 years. However, upper tract surveillance is typically not recommended for the lowest risk patients with low-grade, small-volume tumors [80]. Following radical cystectomy, the majority of early recurrences can be detected through routine oncologic surveillance [83]. However, long-term recurrences may only be detected following the development of symptoms [84]. This is significant in that flank pain on presentation has been correlated with non-organ-confined disease [85].

Retrograde pyelography and excretory urography have traditionally been the standard radiologic imaging modalities in evaluating the upper urinary tracts for evidence of tumor. A ureteral tumor is typically visualized as a filling defect corresponding to the tumor within the ureter. This is classically referred to as a 'goblet sign' as shown in Figs. 19.1 and 19.2. Infundibular tumors may yield the appearance of calyceal amputation. In either case, a stipple sign may be observed in which contrast is caught among papillary fronds of tumor [86]. An example of a stipple pattern by CT scan for a papillary calyceal tumor is shown in Fig. 19.3.

With the advent of CT urography, excretory urography is being utilized less frequently. Reasons for this change are that CT urography with enhanced sensitivity can provide much more detailed anatomic information in regard to the primary tumor and may reveal the presence of locoregional or distant metastasis as well. Whereby the sensitivity of CT scan imaging has previously been reported to be as low as 50% [87], with newer helical CT and multidetector computed tomogra-

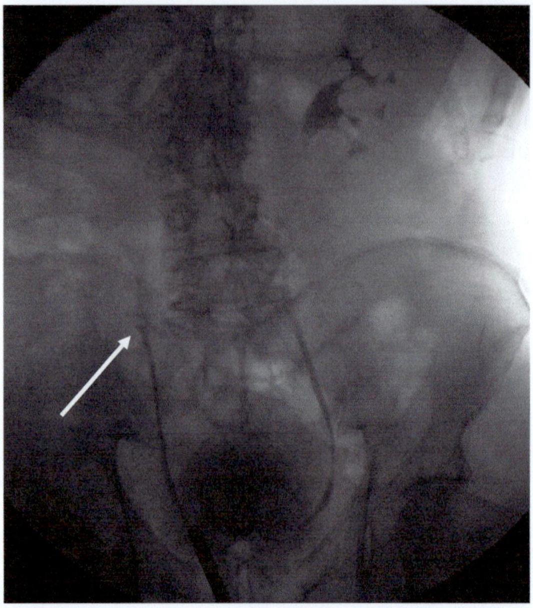

Fig. 19.1 Patient with a right mid-ureteral tumor exhibiting a "goblet sign" by retrograde pyelography

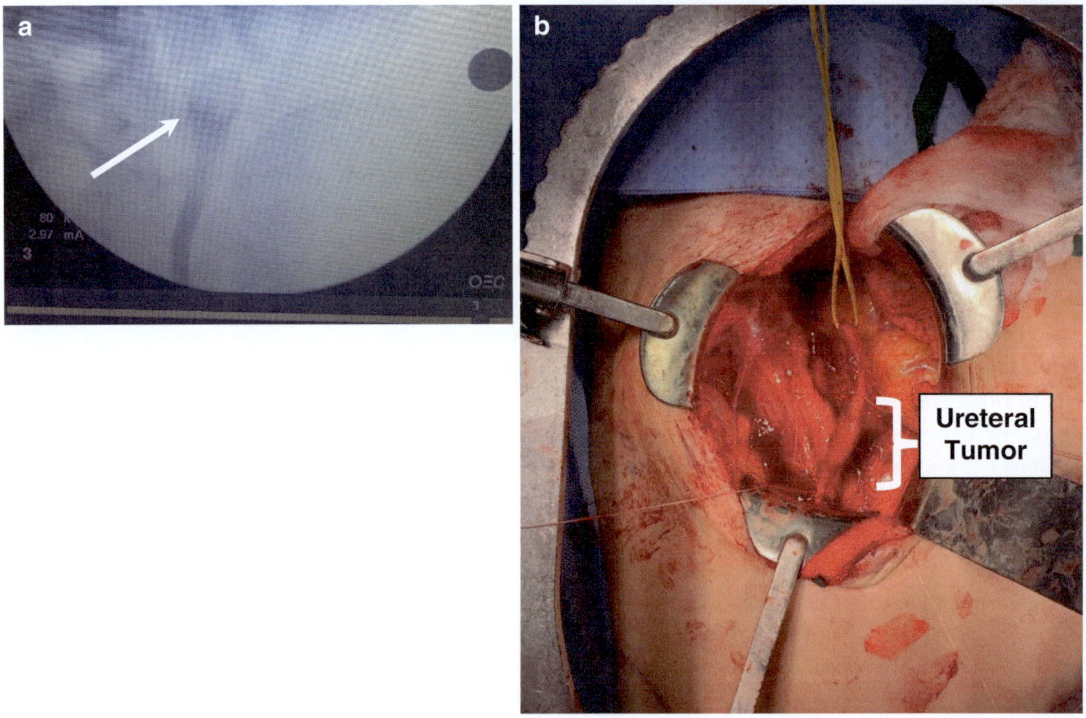

Fig. 19.2 Left ureteral tumor in a 65yo woman with Muir-Torre Syndrome. (a) Goblet sign seen on left retrograde pyelogram. (b) Mobilized left ureter with tumor isolated between vicryl ties, prior to segmental resection

phy (MDCT) technology, a recent meta-analysis revealed a sensitivity and specificity of 96% and 99%, respectively [88]. This compares much more favorably to the reported sensitivity of excretory urography of 50% [89].

MRI may also be utilized for patients for whom the use of iodine-based intravenous contrast is contraindicated, although MR urography remains an evolving technique. The reason for this is that the resolution is inferior to that of CT urography, and motion artifacts secondary to breathing and peristalsis can occur. Nevertheless, MRI can also provide detailed anatomic information and is considered to be comparable to CT urography [86].

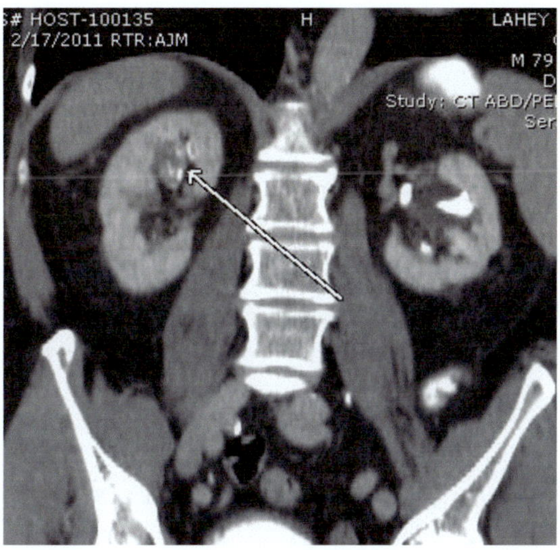

Fig. 19.3 Upper calyx papillary tumor with a stippled contrast pattern

Diagnostic Ureteroscopy: Biopsy When Feasible

Ureteroscopy is typically performed when evaluating an upper tract radiologic abnormality concerning for a urothelial tumor. For instance, a filling defect identified by retrograde pyelography or a renal pelvic or centrally located lesion by CT scan would be indications for upper tract endoscopy, at which time a biopsy may be performed. It can be challenging to obtain sufficient biopsy tissue for histopathology. As such, in instances where an obvious upper tract tumor is seen, and biopsies of upper tract lesions are either nondiagnostic or are not performed for other reasons, surgical removal may be performed on the basis of the visible tumor itself (Fig. 19.4).

Recently, Mertens et al found that the use of diagnostic URS prior to RN-U has been associated with an increased risk of intravesical recur-

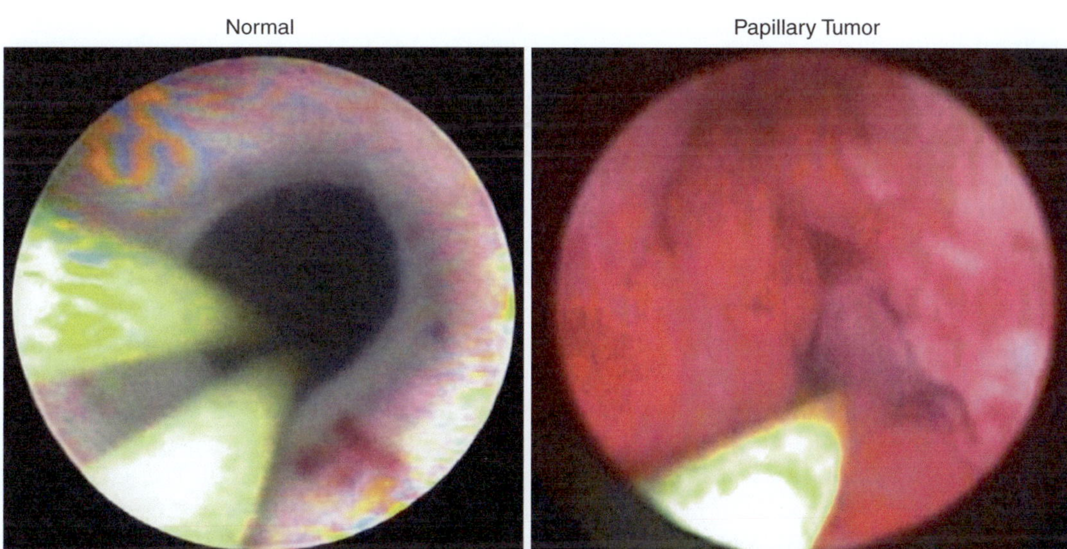

Fig. 19.4 Ureteroscopic evaluation of the upper tract with normal mucosa versus obvious papillary tumor

rence [90]. Furthermore, others have reported that ureteroscopic biopsy in particular has been correlated with subsequent bladder recurrence. However, given at least 3-fold higher rates of benign pathology on RN-U for patients not undergoing diagnostic ureteroscopic biopsy preoperatively, the value of pathologic diagnosis prior to RN-U versus the higher risk of intravesical recurrence must be carefully considered [91].

Clinicopathologic Prognostic Factors

Ureteral tumor location has been correlated with a worse prognosis. One hypothesis associated with this finding is that the ureteral adventitia is relatively thin and has a more extensive network of blood vessels and lymphatic drainage, which contribute to the potential for invasion and metastasis. Another hypothesis is that the renal parenchyma can act as a protective barrier to tumor spread in some instances [38, 92]. However, this remains controversial as there are conflicting studies to suggest renal pelvic tumors portend a more severe prognosis than ureteral tumors [49]. And in yet other research, investigators have reported no difference in tumor aggressiveness between ureteral and renal pelvic tumors [93, 94]. Clearly, biomarkers seem more promising than tumor location as a definitive prognostic tool.

More reliable predictors of cancer-specific survival for upper tract urothelial carcinoma have been established. Among these, the pathologic stage is presently one of the most important [95]. The most recent TNM staging criteria for these tumors are shown in Table 19.2 [96]. Multiple series have validated the pathologic stage as an indicator of metastatic potential and prognosis [97–99]. Accordingly, investigators have also identified tumor grade and architecture as prognostic factors [100]. Lymphovascular invasion, tumor necrosis, and the presence of hydronephrosis have also been identified as indicators of worse prognosis in patients with these tumors [99, 101–103]. Various predictive tools based on established prognostic markers have been described [104].

Table 19.2 TNM staging

TNM stage	Disease extent
Ta	Noninvasive papillary carcinoma that is confined to urothelium and projecting toward the lumen
Tis	Carcinoma in situ: flat tumor with high-grade histologic features that is confined to urothelium
T1	Tumor invades subepithelial connective tissue (lamina propria)
T2	Tumor invades muscularis
T3	Renal pelvis: tumor invades beyond the muscularis into the peripelvic fat or renal parenchyma
	Ureter: tumor invades beyond the muscularis into the periureteric fat
T4	Tumor invades adjacent organs or through the kidney into the perinephric fat
N0	No regional lymph node metastases
N1	Metastasis to a single lymph node that is <2 cm in greatest dimension
N2	Metastasis to a single lymph node that is more than 2 cm in greatest dimension or to multiple lymph nodes
M0	No distant metastasis
M1	Distant metastasis

TNM staging of upper urinary tract transitional cell carcinoma (Adapted from Ref. [96])

Endoscopic Approaches to Treatment

Upper tract TCC features, multifocality, and recurrence of these cancers tend to be ipsilateral, with only 1–5.8% developing tumors in the contralateral kidney [105]. Given this natural history, nephroureterectomy has been traditionally considered the gold standard in treating upper tract TCC for over 60 years [106]. However, in patients in whom nephroureterectomy will lead to dialysis, nephron-sparing treatment options may be preferred. Since the concept of nephron-sparing surgery for upper tract TCC was introduced by Vest in 1945, endoscopic resection was reported infrequently in the 1950s and 1960s but did not gain wider acceptance until the mid-1980s [107–109]. The development of better rigid and flexible scopes, with more maneuverability and better optics, has resulted in the emergence of endoscopic procedures in the diagnosis and treatment of upper tract TCC.

In terms of diagnosis, ureteroscopy permits direct visualization of upper tract tumors. Furthermore, washings for cytologic analysis and tumor tissue may also be obtained for pathologic evaluation. While staging of upper tract tumors by ureteroscopy has been reported to be inaccurate [110], tumor grading by cytology is accurate with 90% correlation with that of final pathology of the tumor specimen [111]. Furthermore, both CT and MRI imaging of these tumors have been shown to be accurate such that tumors that are noninvasive and low grade may be reliably selected for endoscopic management [111, 112].

Endoscopic management of upper tract TCC has traditionally been reserved for patients with a solitary kidney, bilateral involvement, or renal insufficiency. The currently accepted indications for endoscopic management of upper tract TCC include renal insufficiency, solitary kidney, bilateral disease, severe medical comorbidities, palliation, and low-grade, papillary tumors (Table 19.3) [113].

More recently, however, endoscopic treatment of upper tract TCC has been effectively utilized in patients with a normal contralateral kidney. In a series by Elliott et al. [114], patients with a normal contralateral kidney who had limited upper tract disease were managed endoscopically. Inclusion criteria for this study included tumors with a papillary/superficial appearance, tumor size <2 cm in diameter, complete tumor visualization and resection, lack of CT evidence of invasion, and close postoperative surveillance. A recent large-scale meta-analysis underscores this strategy, in which selected patients with low-grade disease appear to have favorable short-term (5-year) outcomes, although long-term (10-year) outcomes are still less certain, and therefore in many instances, the advantages of renal preservation and endoscopic surgery need to be weighed against the increased risk of tumor recurrence and progression as compared to radical nephroureterectomy. And following their review of contemporary studies of endoscopic management of upper tract urothelial carcinoma, high-grade disease continues to be a relative contraindication [115].

Table 19.3 Currently accepted indications for endoscopic management of upper tract TCC

(a) Renal insufficiency
(b) Solitary kidney
(c) Bilateral disease
(d) Severe medical comorbidities
(e) Palliation
(f) Low-grade, papillary tumors

With the development of smaller ureteroscopes with better optics, upper tract tumor ablation may be achieved safely and accurately. Rigid ureteroscopy may be ideal for distal and mid-ureteral tumors in which scope deflection is not necessarily required in accessing the tumor. The working channel of these scopes is somewhat larger as well, which can facilitate specimen acquisition. Tumor tissue may be excised with the Piranha (Boston Scientific) ureteroscopic biopsy forceps. However, more recently, the BIGopsy forceps (Cook) has been designed for the purpose of obtaining larger tissue samples [116].

When more maneuverability is required in the proximal ureter and renal pelvis, flexible ureteroscopy may be employed. Electrocautery may be utilized for tumor ablation with a 2-French Bugbee electrode. However, laser energy is more frequently used, in which a 200 uM fiber provides the least reduction in scope deflection. Both the holmium (Ho:YAG) and neodymium (Nd:YAG) lasers are effective in tumor ablation, although given deeper tissue penetration with Nd:YAG, there is a higher risk of ureteral stricture [117]. Nevertheless, Nd:YAG can be useful in treating bulky, vascular tumors. A ureteral stent can be left following this procedure to facilitate drainage or should a staged procedure be necessary in removing more extensive tumor [118].

Complications associated with ureteroscopic management of upper tract tumors tend to be less significant than that of percutaneous resection [119]. These include ureteral perforation (0–10%) and ureteral stricture (5–14%) [120]. Dissemination of tumor cells outside of the urinary tract or seeding of uninvolved urothelium is also a potential risk, although this is considered by some to be theoretical [118].

Percutaneous resection has also been utilized for larger tumors of the renal pelvis. This procedure is generally reserved for patients who are unable to undergo nephroureterectomy for the reasons stated above and have tumors larger than 1.5–2 cm. This approach can also be utilized for upper tract recurrence following radical cystectomy in which a retrograde approach to the upper tract is not feasible. Another advantage of the percutaneous technique is that deeper and more extensive biopsies can be obtained [121]. Once access is obtained, the tumor can be completely ablated by any of a number of modalities that have been described including monopolar and bipolar cautery, laser ablation, and electrovaporization [122]. The entire tumor should be ablated, and flexible nephroscopy can be subsequently performed to inspect the tumor bed and remaining renal pelvis [123].

A major concern regarding percutaneous resection of upper tract tumors remains the risk of seeding of the nephrostomy tract and/or retroperitoneum. However, in a series of 36 percutaneous procedures, no tract seeding was observed [124]. Bleeding with transfusion requirement is a significant risk of percutaneous surgery. This can be attributed to the vascularity of the kidney, and renal vein injury during percutaneous resection has been reported as well [125].

Treatment with Topical Agents

Topical treatment of upper tract tumors can be utilized either as primary treatment or adjuvant therapy following tumor ablation. For this purpose, installation of BCG or chemotherapeutics such as mitomycin C and thiotepa has been shown to be effective in which these agents can be administered via an indwelling nephrostomy tube. Following ureteroscopy, retrograde instillation of the upper tracts can be achieved by placing an indwelling ureteral stent into the affected ureter(s) prior to bladder instillations. Mitomycin C is most commonly utilized following ureteroscopy in which 40 mg of mitomycin C diluted in 100 ml saline can be delivered over 1 h via a retrograde catheter [126]. While the distal ureter may be treated effectively in this fashion, delivery of medication to the proximal upper tract may be less certain. A more direct approach would consist of retrograde catheterization via cystoscopy with each installation. This has been described by O'Donnell and colleagues in which 1/3 to 1/10 strength BCG combined with 50–100 million units interferon-alpha 2b can be instilled in the office setting following cystoscopic placement of a ureteral stent for upper tract instillation [127]. In their experience, a 70% response rate was achieved, with the greatest response occurring in patients with carcinoma in situ [128]. Also utilizing this approach, Katz et al. report 80% complete response to BCG-interferon retrograde installation [129]. A recent issue with this approach has been the business decision by Merck, the sole supplier of interferon alpha-2b, to cease manufacture of this agent, rendering this treatment no longer possible [130].

Another approach to delivery of topical agents described by Patel and Fuchs avoids the need for repeated cystoscopy and stent placement, in which the distal end of a single-J stent is brought out through a percutaneous cystostomy and secured to the skin [131]. However, Studer et al. [132] prefer antegrade installation of topical agents via a nephrostomy tract to achieve optimal delivery even when percutaneous access is not otherwise required. Given a paucity of randomized trials, the benefit of adjuvant BCG following resection remains unclear. One comparison study failed to demonstrate benefit with the exception of a lower recurrence rate in patients with low-grade tumors who received BCG versus those who did not [133].

A novel mode of delivery of topical mitomycin involves the use of UGN-101, a reverse thermal gel containing this agent. This was evaluated in the OLYMPUS trial for the treatment of tumors involving the renal pelvis and calyces, in which 59% of patients experienced a complete response, which was sustained in 70% of patients undergoing this treatment [134]. Evaluation of this agent for ureteral tumors was promising as well with a 47.8% complete response rate. However, ureteral stenosis was found to be an issue for patients undergoing treatment with this agent, with a

37.8% ureteral stenosis rate for patients with ureteral tumors as compared to a 16.5% ureteral stenosis rate for patients with pyelocalyceal tumors. However, in their analysis, the investigator found the ureteral stenosis rate to be significantly lower at 5.4% when patients with prior hydronephrosis or ureteral stenosis were excluded [135].

Topical treatment has also been found to minimize the risk of bladder cancer recurrence (BCR) following treatment of UTUC. In patients undergoing nephroureterectomy randomized to receive mitomycin-C versus standard care, a single postoperative bladder instillation of mitomycin C on removal of the Foley catheter has been shown to reduce the risk of subsequent BCR (16% versus 27%, $p = 0.03$) [136]. However, despite established safety [137], this practice appears to be underutilized [138].

Disease-related outcomes following ureteroscopic treatment of upper tract tumors are favorable. In a series of 23 patients with these tumors and a normal contralateral kidney, 100% disease-specific survival was reported with 83% organ sparing [139]. In another series of 21 patients without imperative indications for endoscopic management, a 38% recurrence rate was reported, whereas there was an organ preservation rate of 81% and no death resulted from conservative treatment [114]. Survival rates ranging from 86% to 93% have been reported in studies with shorter follow-up, whereas recurrence rates range from 30 to 40% with ureteroscopic ablation [140–143]. Despite significant recurrence rates, survival does not appear to be adversely impacted by ureteroscopic management of upper tract tumors.

Cancer-related outcomes following percutaneous resection of upper tract tumors are typically a function of tumor grade and stage. For instance, recurrence rates ranging from 18% to 28% have been reported for low-grade disease, whereas approximately 50% of high-grade tumors can recur [144]. Jabbour et al. found in a series of 54 patients that stage Ta tumors were associated with a recurrence rate of 30% and disease-related survival of 93%. Conversely, 57% of patients with stage T1 disease recurred and a disease-specific survival of 64% was observed [133]. Percutaneous tract seeding remains a concern, although only two cases to date have been reported [145, 146]. Furthermore, many other clinical series have reported no tract seeding with this technique [133, 142, 147–150].

Nephroureterectomy

Radical nephroureterectomy has been the gold standard for treating upper tract urothelial cancer. This was first performed in 1898 by Le Dentu and Albarran [151]. This was based on the observation of frequent recurrence in the remnant distal ureter in patients who do not undergo removal of the entire ureter [152, 153]. In select patients with both upper tract tumors and locally advanced bladder cancer, a nephroureterectomy en bloc with radical cystectomy is sometimes necessary. This can be achieved best via an extended midline incision (Fig. 19.5). In most patients undergoing open nephroureterectomy, however, a flank incision and ipsilateral Gibson incision for the bladder cuff resection are typically performed.

In addition to locally advanced cancer, tumors associated with congenital variant anatomy may be best managed by open nephroureterectomy. Two examples below illustrate patients with a left-sided duplicate vena cava and ipsilateral renal pelvic tumor (Fig. 19.6), as well as a patient with a retrocaval ureter (Fig. 19.7).

While the open nephroureterectomy with bladder cuff excision has been the standard approach upon which other procedures are compared, this procedure can involve considerable morbidity with two incisions. The advent of laparoscopic nephrectomy has reduced this morbidity with port incisions, and as a result, patients have in general had faster recovery and less blood loss. Oncologic outcomes also appear to be similar to that of the open approach, although longer term follow-up studies are needed to further establish oncologic efficacy. Nevertheless, regardless of which approach is used, oncologic outcomes are based primarily on grade and stage of disease. This was demonstrated by Hall et al., in which 5-year cancer-specific survival rates were 100% for Ta/cis, 92% for T1, 73% for T2, and 41% for stage T3 cancers, and less than 5% for stage T4

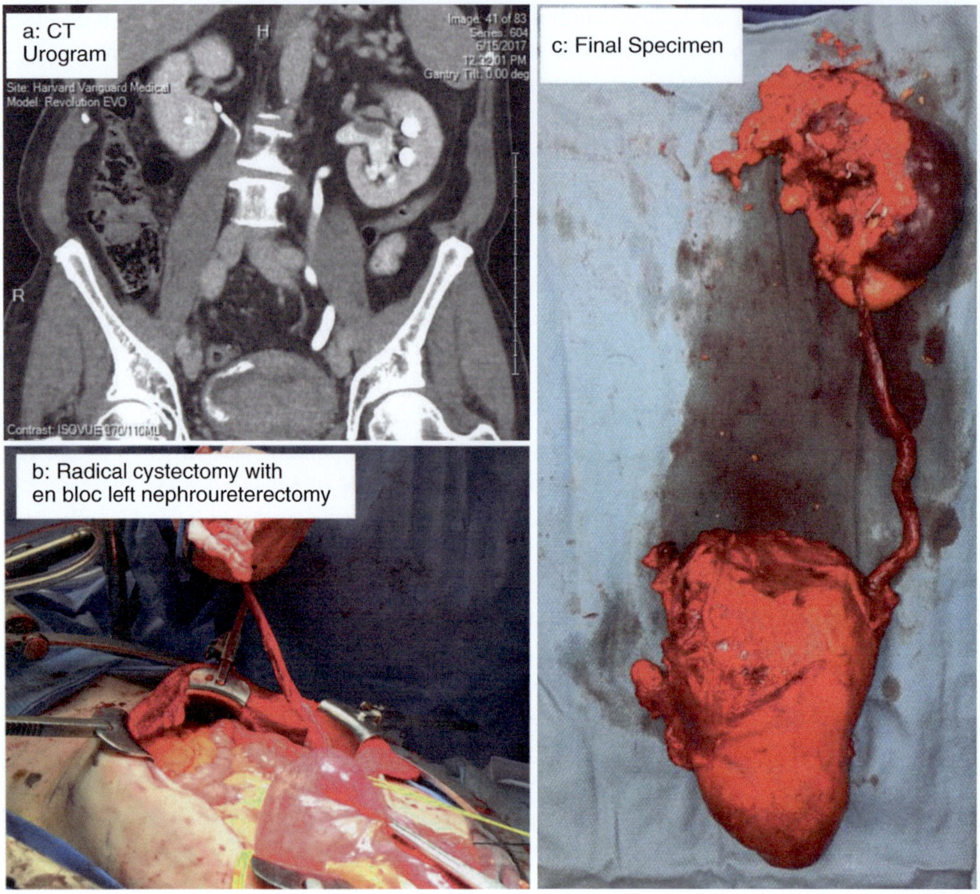

Fig. 19.5 A patient with locally advanced bladder cancer and left renal pelvic cancer managed by left nephroureterectomy with en bloc radical cystectomy via a midline approach

Fig. 19.6 Left-sided duplicate vena cava and ipsilateral renal pelvic tumor

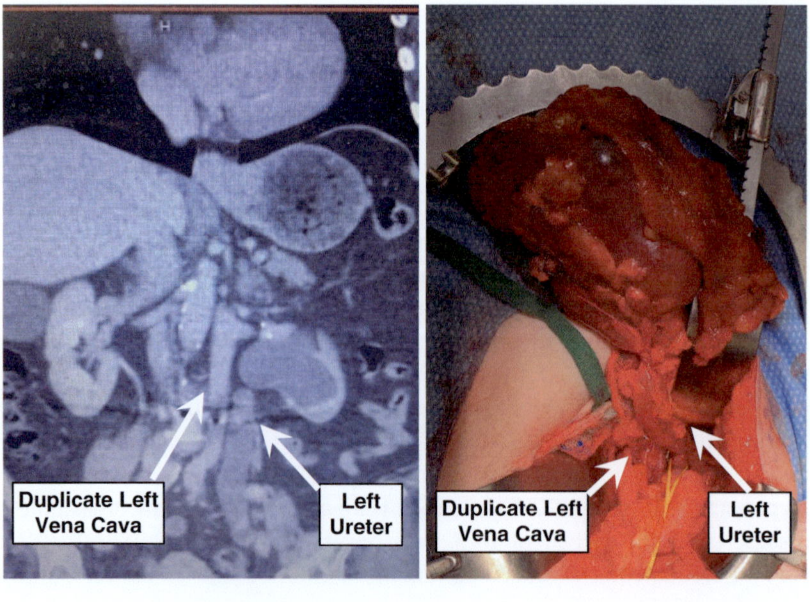

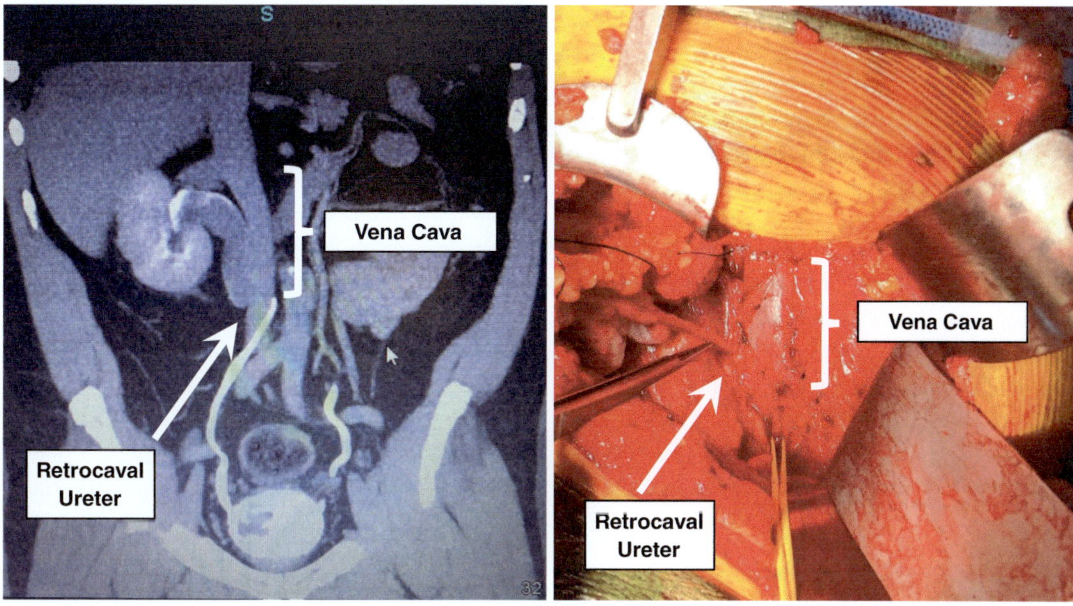

Fig. 19.7 Right renal pelvic and ureteral tumor with retrocaval ureter (yellow vessel loop encircles lower right ureter medial to vena cava)

cancer with a median survival of only 6 months [154]. Earlier studies have also revealed a direct correlation between prognosis and tumor stage [155, 156].

Now that laparoscopy is well established in renal surgery, major medical centers utilize this approach on a regular basis. This approach has been shown to be associated with less morbidity, less blood loss, and acceptable oncologic outcomes with limited follow-up. The debate has switched from whether or not to utilize laparoscopy to which approach should be utilized for the distal ureter.

Bladder Cuff Removal

Open Technique

Following the nephroureterectomy portion of the operation, the ureter is mobilized to the level of the pelvic brim. Dissection of the distal ureter and bladder cuff is then performed through a Gibson incision or lower abdominal incision. The intact specimen can then be retrieved through this incision. Hand-assisted laparoscopic nephrectomy was described by Nakada et al. [157], and more recently, adaptation of this technique for nephroureterectomy has been described in which the hand-port incision can also be utilized for bladder cuff dissection and specimen retrieval [158].

Intussusception

Intussusception was described by Clayman and colleagues in 1983 as an endoscopic method of managing the distal ureter, thereby avoiding the need for two incisions for open nephroureterectomy [159]. As recently reported in a large series of patients with renal pelvic cancer and proximal ureteral tumors, the ureter is divided following nephrectomy, and a negative surgical margin is confirmed by frozen section. Subsequently, a 7-French ureteral catheter is advanced antegrade through the ureter, into the bladder, and directed distally out of the urethra. The ureteral catheter is secured to the proximal ureter with a suture. The distal ureter is then deeply cauterized circumferentially, and the catheter is then advanced into the ureter proximally while the catheter is simultaneously pulled distally, thereby intussuscepting the ureter, which is then detached from the bladder. The mucosal defect overlying the trigone is then cauterized [160].

Oncologic outcomes were similar in a comparison of patients undergoing bladder cuff removal versus intussusception in a retrospective study by Hara et al. [160]. When evaluating recurrence outside of the urinary tract, 5-year recurrence-free survival for patients undergoing bladder cuff removal was 71.4% versus 74.8% for patients undergoing intussusception ($p = 0.766$, log rank). Five-year urinary tract recurrence-free survival at 65.0% versus 76.6%, respectively, actually favored the intussusception group, although this was not statistically significant ($p = 0.089$, log rank) [160].

Pluck Technique

Another method that has been utilized to avoid a lower abdominal incision for removal of the distal ureter is commonly referred to as the 'pluck' technique. Following nephrectomy, the ipsilateral ureteral orifice is resected deeply into perivesical fat, such that the ureter could then be avulsed with the removal of the entire specimen through the nephrectomy incision. More recently, ureteral catheterization has been utilized to facilitate distal resection. However, this procedure has been criticized by some in terms of oncologic efficacy, with reports of local seeding following this procedure [161–163].

Transvesical Approach

Gill and colleagues have also reported the transvesical approach, in which two 5 mm cystotomy trocars are placed to permit endoscopic bladder cuff dissection through the bladder. A resectoscope is also utilized for visualization, and with distal traction on the ureter, extravesical dissection of 3–4 cm of extravesical ureter is also performed through the bladder wall defect utilizing the resectoscope. Early oncologic efficacy comparison between this approach and open bladder cuff excision revealed similar outcomes, although follow-up was limited [164].

Unroofing Technique

The unroofing technique refers to initial mobilization of the intramural ureter and bladder cuff via a cystoscopic approach. Following placement of a 7-French ureteral dilation balloon within the intramural ureter via fluoroscopy, the balloon is instilled with dilute contrast to less than 1 atmosphere of pressure. The ureter is then unroofed with an electrosurgical knife, thereby exposing the intramural tunnel. The balloon is then removed, and the floor of the intramural ureter is cauterized with the rollerball electrode. A 7-French ureteral balloon catheter is then placed into the renal pelvis and placed to gravity drainage to prevent tumor seeding during dissection and mobilization of the kidney and proximal ureter. With extended follow-up, a comparison study of open nephroureterectomy versus laparoscopic nephroureterectomy utilizing the unroofing technique revealed similar tumor recurrence rates [165, 166].

Segmental Ureteral Resection

While nephroureterectomy remains the standard of treatment of upper tract urothelial carcinoma, endoscopic ablation of ureteral tumors has also been effective in select patients and can be preferable in terms of nephron sparing for low-grade, low-volume disease. Accordingly, ureteral tumors that are too large to treat endoscopically may be removed by segmental ureteral resection when nephron sparing is critical. In properly selected patients, this procedure has been shown to be an effective surgical option for ureteral tumors [167, 168].

Autotransplantation

Patients with upper tract urothelial carcinoma involving a solitary kidney face nephroureterectomy with resulting hemodialysis and therefore pose a significant treatment challenge. While contraindicated in patients with a normal contralateral kidney, open excision/partial nephrectomy/

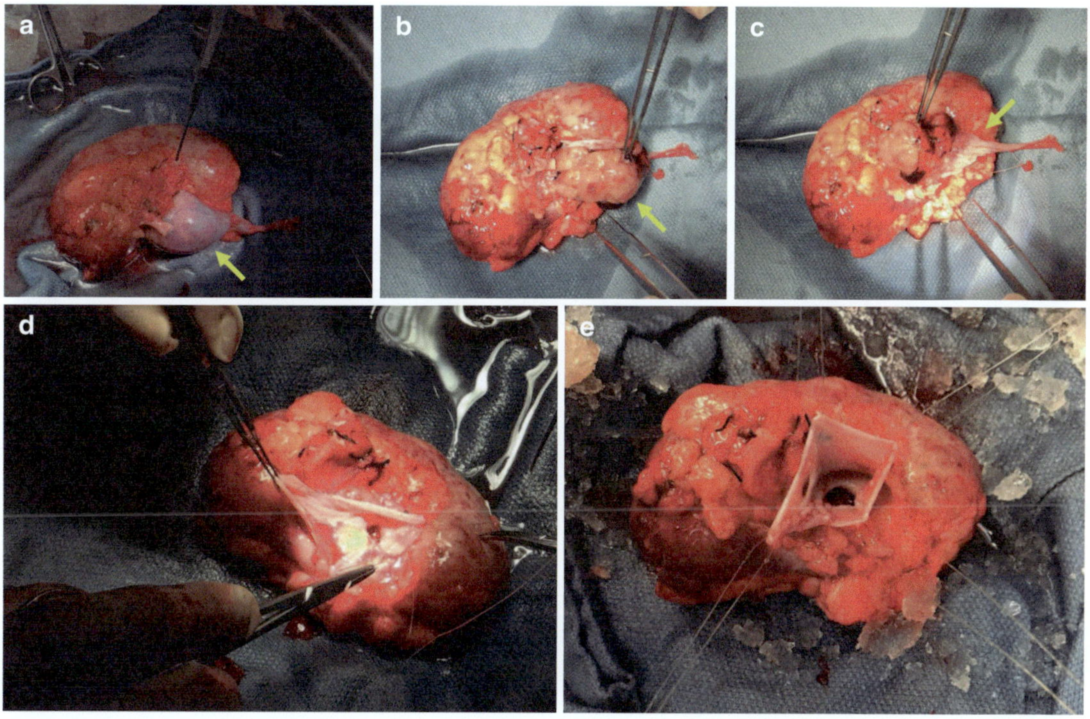

Fig. 19.8 Renal autotransplantation: ex vivo kidney bench surgery (Courtesy J. Libertino, MD)

open excision of ureteral and/or renal pelvic tumor with autotransplantation of the solitary kidney is feasible and has been described in select patients. Following the removal of the kidney and infusion of University of Wisconsin solution, the kidney is placed on ice, and bench surgery is performed to resect the tumor. Figure 19.8 illustrates bench surgery with resection of a renal pelvic tumor and surgical reconstruction of the renal pelvis. In these instances, pyelovesicostomy has been described [169], in which direct access to the renal pelvis via cystoscopy with fulguration of recurrent renal pelvic tumors is feasible. Another advantage is the proximity of renal pelvic mucosa for direct instillation of intravesical agents. However, reports of long-term freedom from recurrence with this procedure are sporadic, and eventual metastatic recurrence with transplantectomy and hemodialysis has been described for other patients. Nevertheless, two patients with high-grade noninvasive renal pelvic disease had long-term freedom from recurrence following this operation [170]. However, it is difficult to know whether these outcomes were due to biology of their disease as opposed to this technique based on more robust data, and there is consensus that this technique should be considered in the rarest of cases in which endoscopic management is not feasible [171].

Role of Lymphadenectomy

The role of lymphadenectomy in upper tract TCC remains controversial. Part of the reason for this is that there is a paucity of data, and reports of lymphadenectomy for upper tract urothelial carcinoma are typically retrospective. However, one clear advantage of lymphadenectomy is that these patients may be more accurately staged. This is important given that patients with nodal involvement have significantly worse survival as compared to patients with pN0 status [98, 172]. Indeed, the 5-year cancer-specific survival of these patients ranges from 0% to 39% and therefore these high-risk patients should be identified as they may benefit from adjuvant therapies [173]. Depending on the imaging modality utilized (PET, MRI, or CT), nodal metastases may be missed in 20–50% of cases, which further justifies the use of lymphadenectomy for staging [173–175].

Relatively few studies regarding staging lymphadenectomy for UTUC are available in the literature. Bobjer et al recently reported their experience in systematic lymphadenectomy for patients with clinical stage T2–4 or nodal involvement for renal pelvic and proximal ureteral cancers. A template was standardized for LND for right versus left renal pelvic and proximal ureteral cancers, emulating a testicular retroperitoneal lymphadenectomy (RPLND) template extended above the renal hilum. Interestingly, right renal pelvic tumors were more frequently associated with LN metastases. Given the relative accuracy with a higher sensitivity and specificity, PET-CT scans were utilized more commonly during the latter part of the study [176].

While it is postulated that selected patients with limited nodal involvement (pN1/pN2) are potentially cured by lymphadenectomy [175, 177], a clear survival advantage for patients undergoing lymphadenectomy has not been demonstrated [178, 179]. Part of the criticism of these studies, in addition to their retrospective nature, is that a dissection template is not uniformly applied. While renal pelvic tumors drain preferentially to the hilar lymph nodes, the lymphatic drainage of ureteral tumors varies depending on location. For instance, right-sided, upper, and mid-ureteral tumors drain to the retrocaval and interaortocaval nodes, whereas left-sided ureteral tumors drain to the para-aortic nodes. Lower ureteral tumors drain to their respective common and internal iliac nodal beds in the pelvis [180, 181].

Another aspect of lymphadenectomy, which has also been explored in bladder cancer, is whether patients undergoing lymphadenectomy without nodal involvement (pN0) have a survival advantage as compared to those patients who do not undergo lymphadenectomy (pNx). The hypothesis is that micrometastatic disease to lymph nodes may be removed with lymphadenectomy, and therefore, a survival advantage is conferred. In a multi-institutional study, Roscingo and colleagues reported a survival advantage for patients undergoing lymphadenectomy (HR 0.7, $p = 0.007$) [182]. Furthermore, Abe et al. reported that locoregional recurrence as well as distant metastasis was higher in patients with pT2 or greater disease who did not undergo lymphadenectomy [183]. However, most other studies have not measured a survival advantage [184], including a large population-based study utilizing the SEER database in which multivariate analysis revealed no significant survival difference between pN0 and pNx patients (HR = 0.99, p = 0.9) [185]. In summary, while the advantages of lymphadenectomy have been reported for other genitourinary cancers, the role of lymphadenectomy in upper tract urothelial cancer remains to be determined.

Role of Neoadjuvant Versus Adjuvant Chemotherapy

The role of perioperative chemotherapy for urothelial carcinoma has been described primarily for bladder cancer. In a large randomized trial of MVAC, neoadjuvant chemotherapy was found to confer a benefit in terms of disease-free survival [186].

An encouraging study of cisplatin-based neoadjuvant chemotherapy has revealed significant downstaging with an overall response rate of 53% and complete remission in 2 of 15 (13%) patients [187]. Other more recent studies of either cisplatin- or carboplatin-based neoadjuvant chemotherapy for UTUC have also demonstrated benefit in terms of pathological response and survival [188–190]. And in a non-randomized study of patients undergoing cisplatin-based neoadjuvant chemotherapy as compared to surgery alone, Kohada et al observed a significant improvement in progression-free survival (p = 0.012), pathologic stage (p = 0.007) and presence of LVI (p = 0.002) with neoadjuvant systemic therapy. This benefit was realized specifically for patients with primary renal pelvic cancer as opposed to primary ureteral tumors [191].

Adjuvant chemotherapy has also been found to be effective in this disease [192]. In upper tract urothelial carcinoma, adjuvant chemotherapy has been used selectively in patients with high-risk disease, whereas minimal benefit has been reported, particularly for patients with unresectable or metastatic disease [193, 194]. In fact, an earlier multi-institutional study revealed no significant survival benefit for adjuvant chemotherapy [195].

As such, limited efficacy, and concern for toxicity including nephrotoxicity, has prevented widespread use of this strategy. Nevertheless, others have reported benefits with less toxic regimens. For instance, Bamias et al. demonstrated that four cycles of paclitaxel and carboplatin were well tolerated in a study of 36 patients with high-risk UTUC (defined as >=T3 or with nodal involvement). The 5-year disease-free survival was 40.2%, and the rate of distant metastasis was reduced in this study [196].

More recently, the perioperative chemotherapy versus surveillance in upper tract urothelial cancer (POUT) trial was completed, in which patients with pT2-T4 pN0–N3 M0 or pT(any) pN1–3 M0 UTUC were treated with adjuvant platinum-based chemotherapy (cisplatin or carboplatin) following RN-U, in comparison to postoperative surveillance alone. Patients undergoing adjuvant chemotherapy with gemcitabine/cisplatin experienced 71% 3-year disease-free survival as compared to 46% for the surveillance arm. As such, a 55% reduction in relative risk of recurrence of disease or death was observed for patients undergoing adjuvant chemotherapy ($p = 0.0001$) [197].

A recent breakthrough, the immune checkpoint inhibitor (ICI) nivolumab was reported with the Checkmate 274 clinical trial. In this study, patients with muscle-invasive urothelial carcinoma were found to have an improved progression-free survival with adjuvant nivolumab as compared to placebo. However, this benefit appeared to pertain primarily to patients with primary bladder cancer as opposed to upper tract cancer on subgroup analysis [198].

While perioperative chemotherapy is commonly offered to patients with advanced upper tract urothelial cancer, more effective therapies and better patient selection will hopefully lead to a defined survival benefit with this strategy.

References

1. National Cancer Institute. Annual cancer statistics review: including cancer trends: 1950–1985, NIH Publication no 88-2789. Bethesda, MD: US Department of Health and Human Services; 1987.
2. Rouprêt M, Babjuk M, Compérat E, Zigeuner R, Sylvester RJ, Burger M, Cowan NC, Böhle A, Van Rhijn BW, Kaasinen E, Palou J, Shariat SF. European Association of Urology guidelines on upper urinary tract urothelial carcinoma: 2015 update. Eur Urol. 2015;68(5):868–79.
3. Siegel R, Miller KD, Jemal A. Cancer statistics, 2018. CA Cancer J Clin. 2018;68:7–30.
4. Siegel RL, Giaquinto AN, Jemal A. Cancer statistics, 2024. CA Cancer J Clin. 2024;74(1):12–49.
5. van Doeveren T, van der Mark M, van Leeuwen PJ, Boormans JL, Aben KKH. Rising incidence rates and unaltered survival rates for primary upper urinary tract urothelial carcinoma: a Dutch population-based study from 1993 to 2017. BJU Int. 2021;128(3):343–51. https://doi.org/10.1111/bju.15389. Epub 2021 May 4
6. Cho S, Park WJ. Twenty-two-year incidence trend of urological cancers in the Republic of Korea: 1999-2020. Investig Clin Urol. 2024;65(1):23–31.
7. Guinan P, Vogelzang NJ, Randazzo R, Sener S, Chmiel J, Fremgen A, Sylvester J. Renal pelvic cancer: a review of 611 patients treated in Illinois 1975–1985: Cancer Incidence and End Results Committee. Urology. 1992;40:393–9.
8. Huben RP. Tumor markers in bladder cancer. Urology. 1984;23:10–7.
9. Soualhi A, Rammant E, George G, Russell B, Enting D, Nair R, Van Hemelrijck M, Bosco C. The incidence and prevalence of upper tract urothelial carcinoma: a systematic review. BMC Urol. 2021;21(1):110.
10. Samardzic J, Hasukic S. Upper urinary tract urothelial cancer in Croatian and Bosnian endemic nephropathy regions. Med Arch. 2017;71(6):430–3.
11. Bhandari A, Alassi O, Rogers C, MacLennan GT. Squamous cell carcinoma of the renal pelvis. J Urol. 2010;183(5):2023–4. Epub 2010 Mar 19
12. Ho CH, Lin WC, Pu YS, Yu HJ, Huang CY. Primary mucinous adenocarcinoma of renal pelvis with carcinoembryonic antigen production. Urology. 2008;71:e7–8.
13. Ouzzane A, Ghoneim TP, Udo K, Verhasselt-Crinquette M, Puech P, Betrouni N, Rouprêt M, Villers A, Leroy X, Colin P. Small cell carcinoma of the upper urinary tract (UUT-SCC): report of a rare entity and systematic review of the literature. Cancer Treat Rev. 2011;37(5):366–72.
14. Munakata S, Tahara H, Kojima K, Kishimoto T. Micropapillary urothelial carcinoma of the renal pelvis: report of a case and review of the literature. Med Sci Monit. 2007;13(4):CS47–52

15. Romesburg JW, Stein RJ, Desai MM, Lagwinski N, Ross JH. Treatment of child with bilateral ureteropelvic junction obstruction due to fibroepithelial polyps and review of the literature. Urology. 2009;73(4):929.e9–11.
16. Herawi M, Parwani AV, Edlow D, Smolev JK, Epstein JI. Glomus tumor of renal pelvis: a case report and review of the literature. Hum Pathol. 2005;36(3):299–302.
17. Devesa SS, Silverman DT, McLaughlin JK, Brown CC, Connelly RR, Fraumeni JF Jr. Comparison of the descriptive epidemiology of urinary tract cancers. Cancer Causes Control. 1990;1(2):133–41.
18. Fernández MI, Shariat SF, Margulis V, Bolenz C, Montorsi F, Suardi N, Remzi M, Wood CG, Roscigno M, Kikuchi E, Oya M, Zigeuner R, Langner C, Weizer A, Lotan Y, Koppie TM, Raman JD, Karakiewicz P, Bensalah K, Schultz M, Bernier P. Evidence-based sex-related outcomes after radical nephroureterectomy for upper tract urothelial carcinoma: results of large multicenter study. Urology. 2009;73:142–6.
19. Jemal A, Tiwari RC, Murray T, Ghafoor A, Samuels A, Ward E, Feuer EJ, Thun MJ. American Cancer Society. Cancer statistics, 2004. CA Cancer J Clin. 2004;54:8–29.
20. Rink M, Xylinas E, Trinh QD, Lotan Y, Margulis V, Raman JD, Fisch M, Lee RK, Chun FK, Abdennabi J, Seitz C, Pycha A, Zlotta AR, Karakiewicz PI, Babjuk M, Scherr DS, Shariat SF. Gender-specific effect of smoking on upper tract urothelial carcinoma outcomes. BJUI. 2013;112:623–37.
21. Wischhusen JW, Ukaegbu C, Dhingra TG, Uno H, Kastrinos F, Syngal S, Yurgelun MB. Clinical factors associated with urinary tract cancer in individuals with Lynch syndrome. Cancer Epidemiol Biomarkers Prev. 2020 January;29(1):193–9.
22. Fujii Y, Sato Y, Suzuki H, Kakiuchi N, Yoshizato T, Lenis AT, Maekawa S, Yokoyama A, Takeuchi Y, Inoue Y, Ochi Y, Shiozawa Y, Aoki K, Yoshida K, Kataoka K, Nakagawa MM, Nannya Y, Makishima H, Miyakawa J, Kawai T, Morikawa T, Shiraishi Y, Chiba K, Tanaka H, Nagae G, Sanada M, Sugihara E, Sato TA, Nakagawa T, Fukayama M, Ushiku T, Aburatani H, Miyano S, Coleman JA, Homma Y, Solit DB, Kume H, Ogawa S. Molecular classification and diagnostics of upper urinary tract urothelial carcinoma. Cancer Cell. 2021;39:793–809.
23. Tope P, Morais S, El-Zein M, Franco EL, Malagón T. Differences in site-specific cancer incidence by individual- and area-level income in Canada from 2006 to 2015. Int J Cancer. 2023;153(10):1766–83.
24. Valencia C, Wightman P, Morrill KE, Hsu C, Arif-Tiwari H, Kauffman E, Gachupin FC, Chipollini J, Lee BR, Garcia DO, Batai K. Neighborhood social vulnerability and disparities in time to kidney cancer surgical treatment and survival in Arizona. Cancer Med. 2024 Feb;13(3):e7007.
25. Solsona E, Iborra I, Ricós JV, Monrós JL, Dumont R, Almenar S. Extravesical Involvement in patients with bladder carcinoma in situ: biological and therapy implications. J Urol. 1996;155:895–9. discussion 899–900
26. Holmäng S, Hedelin H, Anderström C, Holmberg E, Johansson SL. Long–term follow-up of a bladder carcinoma cohort: routine follow-up urography is not necessary. J Urol. 1998;160:45–8.
27. Abercrombie GF, Eardley I, Payne SR, Walmsley BH, Vinnicombe J, Modified nephro-ureterectomy. Long-term follow-up with particular reference to subsequent bladder tumours. Br J Urol. 1988;61(3):198–200.
28. Huben RP, Gaeta J. Pathology and its importance in evaluating outcome in patients with superficial bladder cancer. Semin Urol Oncol. 1996;14(1 Suppl 1):23–9. Review
29. Cho YH, Seo YH, Chung SJ, Hwang I, Yu HS, Kim SO, Jung SI, Kang TW, Kwon DD, Park K, Hwang JE, Heo SH, Kim GS, Hwang EC. Predictors of intravesical recurrence after radical Nephroureterectomy for upper urinary tract urothelial carcinoma: an inflammation-based prognostic score. Korean J Urol. 2014;55:453–9.
30. Fradet V, Mauermann J, Kassouf W, Rendon R, Jacobsen N, Fairey A, Izawa J, Kapoor A, Black P, Tanguay S, Chin J, So A, Lattouf JB, Bell D, Saad F, Sheyegan B, Drachenberg D, Cagiannos I, Lacombe L. Risk factors for bladder cancer recurrence after nephroureterectomy for upper tract urothelial tumors: results from the Canadian Upper Tract Collaboration. Urol Oncol. 2014;32:839–45.
31. Ishioka J, Saito K, Kijima T, Nakanishi Y, Yoshida S, Yokoyama M, Matsuoka Y, Numao N, Koga F, Masuda H, Fujii Y, Sakai Y, Arisawa C, Okuno T, Nagahama K, Kamata S, Sakura M, Yonese J, Morimoto S, Noro A, Tsujii T, Kitahara S, Gotoh S, Higashi Y, Kihara K. Risk stratification for bladder recurrence of upper urinary tract urothelial carcinoma after radical nephroureterectomy. BJUI. 2015;115:705–12.
32. Rouprêt M, Babjuk M, Compérat E, Zigeuner R, Sylvester RJ, Burger M, Cowan NC, Gontero P, Van Rhijn BWG, Mostafid AH, Palou J, Shariat SF. European Association of Urology guidelines on upper urinary tract urothelial carcinoma: 2017 update. Eur Urol. 2018;73:111–22.
33. van Doeveren T, van Leeuwen PJ, Aben KKH, van der Aa M, Barendrecht M, Boevé ER, Cornel EB, van der Heijden AG, Hendricksen K, Hirdes W, Kooistra A, Kroon B, Leliveld AM, Meijer RP, van Melick H, Merks B, de Reijke TM, de Vries P, Wymenga LFA, Wijsman B, Boormans JL. Reduce bladder cancer recurrence in patients treated for upper urinary tract urothelial carcinoma: the REBACARE-trial. Contemp Clin Trials Commun. 2018;9:121–9.
34. Murphy DM, Zincke H, Furlow WL. Management of high grade transitional cell cancer of the upper urinary tract. J Urol. 1981;125(1):25–9.

35. Leow JJ, Chong KT, Chang SL, et al. Upper tract urothelial carcinoma: a different disease entity in terms of management. ESMO Open. 2017;1:e000126.
36. Cha EK, Shariat SF, Kormaksson M, et al. Predicting clinical outcomes after radical nephroureterectomy for upper tract urothelial carcinoma. Eur Urol. 2012;61:818–25.
37. Park HK. Do histology and primary tumor location influence metastatic patterns in bladder cancer? Curr Oncol. 2023;30(10):9078–89.
38. Lwin AA, Hsu CH, Chipollini J. Urothelial carcinoma of the renal pelvis and ureter: does location make a difference? Clin Genitourin Cancer. 2020;18:45–9.
39. Sfakianos John P, Cha Eugene K, Iyer G, et al. Genomic characterization of upper tract urothelial carcinoma. Eur Urol. 2015;68(6):970–7.
40. Cancer Genome Atlas Research Network. Comprehensive molecular characterization of urothelial bladder carcinoma. Nature. 2014;507:315–22.
41. Lee JY, Kim K, Sung HH, et al. Molecular characterization of urothelial carcinoma of the bladder and upper urinary tract. Transl Oncol. 2018;11:37–42.
42. Necchi A, Madison R, Pal SK, Ross JS, Agarwal N, Sonpavde G, Joshi M, Yin M, Miller VA, Grivas P, Chung JH, Ali SM. Comprehensive Genomic Profiling of Upper-tract and Bladder Urothelial Carcinoma. Eur Urol Focus. 2021 Nov;7(6):1339–46.
43. Takahashi T, Kakehi Y, Mitsumori K, Akao T, Terachi T, Kato T, Ogawa O, Habuchi T. Distinct microsatellite alterations in upper urinary tract tumors and subsequent bladder tumors. J Urol. 2001;165(2):672–7.
44. Zhang ZT, Pak J, Shapiro E, Sun TT, Wu XR. Urothelium-specific expression of an oncogene in transgenic mice induced the formation of carcinoma in situ and invasive transitional cell carcinoma. Cancer Res. 1999;59(14):3512–7.
45. Riedel I, Liang FX, Deng FM, Tu L, Kreibich G, Wu XR, Sun TT, Hergt M, Moll R. Urothelial umbrella cells of human ureter are heterogeneous with respect to their uroplakin composition: different degrees of urothelial maturity in ureter and bladder? Eur J Cell Biol. 2005;84(2–3):393–405.
46. Park S, Hong B, Kim CS, Ahn H. The impact of tumor location on prognosis of transitional cell carcinoma of the upper urinary tract. J Urol. 2004;171:621–5.
47. Ouzzane A, Colin P, Xylinas E, Pignot G, Ariane MM, Saint F, Hoarau N, Adam E, Azemar MD, Bensadoun H, Cormier L, Cussenot O, Houlgatte A, Karsenty G, Bruyère F, Maurin C, Nouhaud FX, Phe V, Polguer T, Roumiguié M, Ruffion A, Rouprêt M, French Collaborative National Database, on UUT-UC. Ureteral and multifocal tumours have worse prognosis than renal pelvic tumours in urothelial carcinoma of the upper urinary tract treated by nephroureterectomy. Eur Urol. 2011;60(6):1258–65. Epub 2011 Jun 7
48. Akdogan B, Dogan HS, Eskicorapci SY, Sahin A, Erkan I, Ozen H. Prognostic significance of bladder tumor history and tumor location in upper tract transitional cell carcinoma. J Urol. 2006;176:48–52.
49. van der Poel HG, Antonini N, van Tinteren H, Horenblas S. Upper urinary tract cancer: location is correlated with prognosis. Eur Urol. 2005;48(3):438–44.
50. Szarvas T, Modos O, Horvath A, et al. Why are upper tract urothelial carcinoma two different diseases? Transl Androl Urol. 2016;5:636–47.
51. Rouppret M, Zigeuner R, Palou J, et al. European guidelines for the diagnosis and management of upper urinary tract urothelial cell carcinomas: 2011 update. Eur Urol. 2011;59:584–94.
52. Han JH, Jeong S, Kim SH, Yuk HD, Jeong CW, Kwak C, Ku JH. Increased urinary B2-microglobulin is associated with poor prognosis of upper tract urothelial carcinoma. Eur Urol Focus. 2021;7(6):1339–46.
53. Ehsani L, Osunkoya AO. Human epidermal growth factor receptor 2 expression in urothelial carcinoma of the renal pelvis: correlation with clinicopathologic parameters. Int J Clin Exp Pathol. 2014;7(5):2544–50.
54. Cantley LC. The phosphoinositide 3-kinase pathway. Science. 2002;296:1655–7.
55. Ku JH, Byun SS, Jeong H, Kwak C, Kim HH, Lee SE. The role of p53 on survival of upper urinary tract urothelial carcinoma: a systematic review and meta-analysis. Clin Genitourin Cancer. 2013;11:221–8.
56. Rey A, Lara PC, Redondo E, Valdes E, Apolinario R. Overexpression of p53 in transitional cell carcinoma of the renal pelvis and ureter. Relation to tumor proliferation and survival. Cancer. 1997;79:2178–85.
57. Missaoui N, Bdioui A, Baccouche A, Belkacem O, Hmida W, Mokni M, Hmissa S. Significance of p53, p27, Ki-67, E-cadherin, and HER2 expression in upper urinary tract urothelial carcinoma. J Egypt Natl Canc Inst. 2020;32(1):36.
58. Stiborova M, Arlt VM, Schmeiser HH. DNA adducts formed by aristolochic acid are unique biomarkers of exposure and explain the initiation phase of upper urothelial cancer. Int J Mol Sci. 2017;18:2144.
59. Kamijima S, Tobe T, Suyama T, Ueda T, Igarashi T, Ichikawa T, et al. The prognostic value of p53, Ki-67 and matrix metalloproteinases MMP-2 and MMP-9 in transitional cell carcinoma of the renal pelvic and ureter. Int J Urol. 2005;12:941–7.
60. Krabbe LM, Bagrodia A, Lotan Y, Gayed BA, Darwish OM, Youssef RF, et al. Prospective analysis of Ki-67 as an independent predictor of oncologic outcomes in patients with high grade upper tract urothelial carcinoma. J Urol. 2014;191:28–34.
61. Joung JY, Yang SO, Jeong IG, Han KS, Seo HK, Chung J, et al. Identification of immunohistochemical factors that predict the synchronous or metachronous development of bladder tumors in patients with upper tract tumors. Urol Int. 2008;81:306–11.
62. Krabbe LM, Bagrodia A, Haddad AQ, Kapur P, Khalil D, Hynan LS, et al. Multi-institutional validation of the predictive value of Ki-67 in patients with

high grade urothelial carcinoma of the upper urinary tract. J Urol. 2015;193:1486–93.
63. Danzig MR, Mallin K, McKiernan JM, Stadler WM, Sridhar SS, Morgan TM, Bochner BH, Lee CT. Prognostic importance of lymphovascular invasion in urothelial carcinoma of the renal pelvis. Cancer. 2018;124(12):2507–14.
64. Fang D, Shiming H, Xiong G, Singla N, Cao Z, Zhang L, Li X, Zhou L. Comparison of clinicopathologic characteristics, epigenetic biomarkers and prognosis between renal pelvic and ureteral tumors in upper tract urothelial carcinoma. BMC Urol. 2018;18:22.
65. Lenherr SM, Tsai S, Neto BS, Sullivan TB, Cimmino CB, Logvinenko T, Gee J, Huang W, Libertino JA, Summerhayes IC, Rieger-Christ KM. MicroRNA expression profile identifies high grade, non-muscle-invasive bladder tumors at elevated risk to progress to an invasive phenotype. Genes (Basel). 2017;8(2):77.
66. Montalbo R, Izquierdo L, Ingelmo-Torres M, Lozano JJ, Capitán D, Alcaraz A, Mengual L. Prognostic value of circulating mi-RNAs in upper tract urinary carcinoma. Oncotarget. 2018;9:16691–700.
67. Chung Y, Cheng Y, Kao Y, Tsai W, Huang G, Chen Y, Shen Y, Tai M, Chiang P. MiR-26a-5p as a useful therapeutic target for upper tract urothelial carcinoma by regulating WNT5A/β-catenin signaling. Sci Rep. 2022;12(1):6955.
68. Yang MH, Chen KK, Yen CC, Wang WS, Chang YH, Huang WJ, Fan FS, Chiou TJ, Liu JH, Chen PM. Unusually high incidence of upper urinary tract urothelial carcinoma in Taiwan. Urology. 2002;59:681–7.
69. Shinka T, Miyai M, Sawada Y, Inagaki T, Okawa T. Factors affecting the occurrence of urothelial tumors in dye workers exposed to aromatic amines. Int J Urol. 1995;2(4):243–8.
70. Stewart JH, Hobbs JB, McCredie MR. Morphologic evidence that analgesic-induced kidney pathology contributes to the progression of tumors of the renal pelvis. Cancer. 1999;86:1576–82.
71. Colin P, Koenig P, Ouzzane A, Berthon N, Villers A, Biserte J, Rouprêt M. Environmental factors involved in carcinogenesis of urothelial cell carcinomas of the upper urinary tract. BJUI. 2009;104:1436–40.
72. Arlt VM, Stiborová M, vom Brocke J, Simões ML, Lord GM, Nortier JL, Hollstein M, Phillips DH, Schmeiser HH. Aristolochic acid mutagenesis: molecular clues to the aetiology of Balkan endemic nephropathy-associated urothelial cancer. Carcinogenesis. 2007;28:2253–61.
73. Lord GM, Cook T, Arlt VM, Schmeiser HH, Williams G, Pusey CD. Urothelial malignant disease and Chinese herbal nephropathy. Lancet. 2001;358:1515–6.
74. Laing C, Hamour S, Sheaff M, Miller R, Woolfson R. Chinese herbal uropathy and nephropathy. Lancet. 2006;368:338.
75. Debelle FD, Vanherweghem JL, Nortier JL. Aristolochic acid nephropathy: a worldwide problem. Kidney Int. 2008;74:158–69.
76. Michalek IM, Martinsen JI, Weiderpass E, Kjaerheim K, Lynge E, Sparen P, Tryggvadottir L, Pukkala E. Occupation and risk of cancer of the renal pelvis in Nordic countries. BJU Int. 2019 Feb;123(2):233–8.
77. Zeidler-Erdely PC, Battelli LA, Salmen-Muniz R, et al. Lung tumor production and tissue metal distribution after exposure to manual metal ARC-stainless steel welding fume in A/J and C57BL/6J mice. J Toxicol Environ Health A. 2011;74:728–36.
78. Babjuk M, Oosterlinck W, Sylvester R, Kaasinen E, Bohle A, Palou-Redorta J. EAU guidelines on non-muscle-invasive urothelial carcinoma of the bladder. Eur Urol. 2008;54:303–14.
79. Hall MC, Chang SS, Dalbagni G, Pruthi RS, Seigne JD, Skinner EC, et al. Guideline for the management of nonmuscle invasive bladder cancer (stages Ta, T1, and Tis): 2007 update. J Urol. 2007;178:2314–30.
80. Montie JE, Bahnson RR, Cohen SM. Bladder cancer. Clinical practice guidelines in oncology. J Natl Compr Cancer Netw. 2005;3(1):19–34.
81. Solsona E, Iborra I, Ricos JV, Dumont R, Casanova JL, Calabuig C. Upper urinary tract involvement in patients with bladder carcinoma in situ (Tis): Its impact on management. Urology. 1997;49:347–52.
82. Youssef RF, Shariat SF, Lotan Y, Wood CG, Sagalowsky AI, Zigeuner R, Langner C, Montorsi F, Bolenz C, Margulis V. Prognostic effect of urinary bladder carcinoma in situ on clinical outcome of subsequent upper tract urothelial carcinoma. Urology. 2011;77(4):861–6.
83. Slaton JW, Swanson DA, Grossman HB, Dinney CP. A stage specific approach to tumor surveillance after radical cystectomy for transitional cell carcinoma of the bladder. J Urol. 1999;162:710–4.
84. Solsona E, Iborra I, Rubio J, Casanova J, Dumont R, Monros JL. Late oncological occurrences following radical cystectomy in patients with bladder cancer. Eur Urol. 2003;43:489–94.
85. Yeh HC, Jan HC, Wu WJ, et al. Concurrent preoperative presence of hydronephrosis and flank pain independently predicts worse outcome of upper tract urothelial carcinoma. PLoS One. 2015;10:e0139624.
86. Browne RF, Meehan CP, Colville J, Power R, Torreggiani WC. Transitional cell carcinoma of the upper urinary tract: spectrum of imaging findings. Radiographics. 2005;25(6):1609–27.
87. McCoy JG, Honda H, Reznicek M, Williams RD. Computerized tomography for detection and staging of localized and pathologically defined upper tract urothelial tumors. J Urol. 1991;146(6):1500–3.
88. Chlapoutakis K, Theocharopoulos N, Yarmenitis S, Damilakis J. Performance of computed tomographic urography in diagnosis of upper urinary tract urothelial carcinoma, in patients presenting with hematuria: systematic review and meta-analysis. Eur J Radiol. 2010;73(2):334–8. Epub 2008 Dec 6

89. Albani JM, Ciaschini MW, Streem SB, Herts BR, Angermeier KW. The role of computerized tomographic urography in the initial evaluation of hematuria. J Urol. 2007;177(2):644–8.
90. Mertens LS, Sharma V, Matin SF, Boorjian SA, Thompson RH, van Rhijn BW, Masson-Lecomte A. Bladder Recurrence Following Upper Tract Surgery for Urothelial Carcinoma: A Contemporary Review of Risk Factors and Management Strategies. Eur Urol Open Sci. 2023 Jan;28(49):60–6.
91. Sharma V, Miest TS, Juvet TS, Toussi A, Packiam V, Chamie K, Matin SF, Boorjian SA, Thompson RH, Frank I, Tollefson MK, Potretzke AM. The impact of upper tract urothelial carcinoma diagnostic modality on intravesical recurrence after radical nephroureterectomy: a single institution series and updated meta-analysis. J Urol. 2021;206:558–67.
92. Park J, Ha SH, Min GE, et al. The protective role of renal parenchyma as a barrier to local tumor spread of upper tract transitional cell carcinoma and its impact on patient survival. J Urol. 2009;182:894–9.
93. Raman JD, Ng CK, Scherr DS, Margulis V, Lotan Y, Bensalah K, Patard JJ, Kikuchi E, Montorsi F, Zigeuner R, Weizer A, Bolenz C, Koppie TM, Isbarn H, Jeldres C, Kabbani W, Remzi M, Waldert M, Wood CG, Roscigno M, Oya M, Langner C, Wolf JS, Ströbel P, Fernández M, Karakiewcz P, Shariat SF. Impact of tumor location on prognosis for patients with upper tract urothelial carcinoma managed by radical nephroureterectomy. Eur Urol. 2010;57:1072–9.
94. Catto JW, Yates DR, Rehman I, Azzouzi AR, Patterson J, Sibony M, Cussenot O, Hamdy FC. Behavior of urothelial carcinoma with respect to anatomical location. J Urol. 2007;177:1715–20.
95. Margulis V, Youssef RF, Karakiewicz PI, Lotan Y, Wood CG, Zigeuner R, Kikuchi E, Weizer A, Raman JD, Remzi M, Roscigno M, Montorsi F, Bolenz C, Kassouf W, Shariat SF. Upper Tract Urothelial Carcinoma Collaborative Group. Preoperative multivariable prognostic model for prediction of nonorgan confined urothelial carcinoma of the upper urinary tract. J Urol. 2010;184(2):453–8. Epub 2010 Jun 17
96. Brierley JD, Gospodarowicz M, Wittekind C. TNM classification of malignant tumours. 8th ed. Chichester, UK: Wiley-Blackwell; 2016.
97. Langner C, Hutterer G, Chromecki T, Winkelmayer I, Rehak P, Zigeuner R. pT classification, grade, and vascular invasion as prognostic indicators in urothelial carcinoma of the upper urinary tract. Mod Pathol. 2006;19(2):272–9.
98. Novara G, De Marco V, Gottardo F, Dalpiaz O, Bouygues V, Galfano A, Martignoni G, Patard JJ, Artibani W, Ficarra V. Independent predictors of cancer-specific survival in transitional cell carcinoma of the upper urinary tract: multi-institutional dataset from 3 European centers. Cancer. 2007;110(8):1715–22.
99. Kim DS, Lee YH, Cho KS, Cho NH, Chung BH, Hong SJ. Lymphovascular invasion and pT stage are prognostic factors in patients treated with radical nephroureterectomy for localized upper urinary tract transitional cell carcinoma. Urology. 2010;75(2):328–32.
100. Remzi M, Haitel A, Margulis V, Karakiewicz P, Montorsi F, Kikuchi E, Zigeuner R, Weizer A, Bolenz C, Bensalah K, Suardi N, Raman JD, Lotan Y, Waldert M, Ng CK, Fernández M, Koppie TM, Ströbel P, Kabbani W, Murai M, Langner C, Roscigno M, Wheat J, Guo CC, Wood CG, Shariat SF. Tumour architecture is an independent predictor of outcomes after nephroureterectomy: a multi-institutional analysis of 1363 patients. BJU Int. 2009;103(3):307–11.
101. Zigeuner R, Shariat SF, Margulis V, Karakiewicz PI, Roscigno M, Weizer A, Kikuchi E, Remzi M, Raman JD, Bolenz C, Bensalah K, Capitanio U, Koppie TM, Kassouf W, Sircar K, Patard JJ, Fernández MI, Wood CG, Montorsi F, Ströbel P, Wheat JC, Haitel A, Oya M, Guo CC, Ng C, Chade DC, Sagalowsky A, Langner C. Tumour necrosis is an indicator of aggressive biology in patients with urothelial carcinoma of the upper urinary tract. Eur Urol. 2010;57(4):575–81.
102. Cho KS, Hong SJ, Cho NH, Choi YD. Grade of hydronephrosis and tumor diameter as preoperative prognostic factors in ureteral transitional cell carcinoma. Urology. 2007;70(4):662–6.
103. Chung SD, Wang SM, Lai MK, Huang CY, Liao CH, Huang KH, Pu YS, Chueh SC, Yu HJ. Lymphovascular invasion predicts poor outcome of urothelial carcinoma of renal pelvis after nephroureterectomy. BJU Int. 2009;103(8):1047–51.
104. Mbeutcha A, Mathieu R, Roupret M, Gust KM, Briganti A, Karakiewicz PI, Shariat SF. Predictive models and prognostic factors for upper tract urothelial carcinoma: a comprehensive review of the literature. Transl Androl Urol. 2016;5(5):720–34.
105. Kang CH, Yu TJ, Hsieh HH, Yang JW, Shu K, Huang CC, Chiang PH, Shiue YL. The development of bladder tumors and contralateral upper urinary tract tumors after primary transitional cell carcinoma of the upper urinary tract. Cancer. 2003;98:1620–6.
106. Blute ML, Segura JW, Patterson DE, Benson RC Jr, Zincke H. Impact of endourology on diagnosis and management of upper urinary tract urothelial cancer. J Urol. 1989;141:1298–301.
107. Colston JA, Arcadi JA. Bilateral renal papillomas: transpelvic electro-resection with preservation of kidney; contralateral nephrectomy; four-year survival. J Urol. 1955;73:460–7.
108. Gibson TE. Local excision in transitional cell tumors of the upper urinary tract. J Urol. 1967;97:619–22.
109. Huffman JL, Bagley DH, Lyon ES, Morse MJ, Herr HW, Whitmore WF Jr. Endoscopic diagnosis and treatment of upper-tract urothelial tumors. A preliminary report. Cancer. 1985;55:1422–8.
110. Daneshmand S, Quek ML, Huffman JL. Endoscopic management of upper urinary tract transitional

cell carcinoma: long-term experience. Cancer. 2003;98:55–60.
111. Adamis S, Varkarakis J, Jarrett TW. Endoscopic treatment of urothelial tumours of the renal pelvis and ureter. Arch Esp Urol. 2011;64(2):89–96.
112. Badalament RA, Bennett WF, Bova JG, Kenworthy PR, Wise HA 2nd, Smith S, Perez J. Computed tomography of primary transitional cell carcinoma of upper urinary tracts. Urol. 1992;40:71–5.
113. Mills IW, Laniado ME, Patel A. The role of endoscopy in the management of patients with upper urinary tract transitional cell carcinoma. BJU Int. 2001;87:150–62.
114. Elliott DS, Segura JW, Lightner D, Patterson DE, Blute ML. Is nephroureterectomy necessary in all cases of upper tract transitional cell carcinoma? Long-term results of conservative endourologic management of upper tract transitional cell carcinoma in individuals with a normal contralateral kidney. Urology. 2001;58:174–8.
115. Cutress ML, Stewart GD, Zakikhani P, Phipps S, Thomas BG, Tolley DA. Ureteroscopic and percutaneous management of upper tract urothelial carcinoma (UTUC): systematic review. BJU Int. 2012;110(5):614–28. https://doi.org/10.1111/j.1464-410X.2012.11068.x.
116. Ritter M, Bolenz C, Bach T, Strobel P, Hacker A. Standardized ex vivo comparison of different upper urinary tract biopsy devices: impact on ureterorenoscopes and tissue quality. World J Urol. 2012;31(4):907–12. Epub ahead of print
117. Schmeller NT, Hofstetter AG. Laser treatment of ureteral tumors. J Urol. 1989;141:840–3.
118. Johnson GB, Grasso M. Ureteroscopic management of upper urinary tract transitional cell carcinoma. Curr Opin Urol. 2005;15:89–93.
119. Potter SR, Chow GK, Jarrett TW. Percutaneous endoscopic management of urothelial tumors of the renal pelvis. Urol. 2001;58:457–9.
120. Chen GL, Bagley DH. Ureteroscopic surgery for upper tract transitional-cell carcinoma: complications and management. J Endourol. 2001;15:399–404.
121. Varkarakis I, Jarrett T. Percutaneous approach to upper urinary tract tumors. In: Nakada S, Pearle M, editors. Advanced endourology. Totowa: Humana Press; 2006. p. 253–66.
122. Nakada S, Clayman RV. Percutaneous electrovaporization of upper tract transitional cell carcinoma in patients with functionally solitary kidneys. Urology. 1995;46:751–5.
123. Chew BH, Pautler SE, Denstedt JD. Percutaneous management of upper tract transitional cell carcinoma. J Endourol. 2005;19:658–64.
124. Jarrett TW, Sweetser PM, Weiss GH, Smith AD. Percutaneous management of transitional cell carcinoma of the renal collecting system: 9-year experience. J Urol. 1995;154:1629–35.
125. Goel MC, Roberts JG. Percutaneous resection of renal transitional carcinoma: venous injury and its conservative management. Urol Int. 2001;67:170–2.
126. Keeley F-XJ, Bagley DH. Adjuvant mitomycin C following endoscopic treatment of upper tract transitional cell carcinoma. J Urol. 1997;158:2074.
127. Nepple KG, Joudi FN, O'Donnell MA. Review of topical treatment of upper tract urothelial carcinoma. Adv Urol. 2009;2009(472831):1–6.
128. Burns JA. Williams RD. O'Donnell MA. The treatment of upper tract transitional cell carcinoma with BCG plus interferon-alpha. In Proceedings of the North Central Section of the American Urological Association Annual Meeting, Cancun, Mexico: Hedican SP; October 2001.
129. Katz MH, Lee MW, Gupta M. Setting a new standard for topical therapy of upper-tract transitional-cell carcinoma: BCG and interferon-a2B. J Endourol. 2007;21(4):374–7.
130. Wheeler M. Current Drug Shortages – 1/10/2022 Interferon alfa-2b Injection. ASHP (2022, January 10). www.ashp.org/drug-shortages/current-shortages/drug-shortage-detail.aspx?id=724&loginreturnUrl=SSOCheckOnly
131. Patel A, Fuchs GJ. New techniques for the administration of topical adjuvant therapy after endoscopic ablation of upper urinary tract transitional cell carcinoma. J Urol. 1998;159:71–5.
132. Studer UE, Casanova G, Kraft R, Zingg EJ. J Urol. 1989;142:975–7.
133. Jabbour ME, Smith AD. Primary percutaneous approach to upper urinary tract transitional cell carcinoma. Urol Clin North Am. 2000;27:739–50.
134. Kleinmann N, Matin S, Lerner S, et al. Primary chemoablation of low-grade upper tract urothelial carcinoma using UGN-101, a mito-mycin-containing reverse thermal gel (OLYMPUS): An open-label, single-arm, phase 3 trial. Lancet Oncol. 2020;21(6):776–85.
135. Jacob JM, Woldu SL, Linehan J, Labbate C, Rose KM, Sexton WJ, Tachibana I, Kaimakliotis H, Nieder A, Bjurlin MA, Humphreys M, Ghodoussipour SB, Quek ML, Johnson B, O'Donnell M, Eisner BH, Feldman AS, Murray KS, Matin SF, Lotan Y, Dickstein RJ. First analysis of the safety and efficacy of UGN-101 in the treatment of ureteral tumors. Urol Oncol. 2024 Jan;42(1):20.e17–23.
136. O'Brien T, Ray E, Singh R, Coker B, Beard R. Prevention of bladder tumours after nephroureterectomy for primary upper urinary tract urothelial carcinoma: a prospective, multicentre, randomised clinical trial of a single postoperative intravesical dose of mitomycin C (the ODMIT-C Trial). Eur Urol. 2011;60(4):703–10.
137. Gallioli A, Boissier R, Territo A, Vila Reyes H, Sanguedolce F, Gaya JM, Regis F, Subiela JD, Palou J, Breda A. Adjuvant Single-Dose Upper Urinary Tract Instillation of Mitomycin C After Therapeutic Ureteroscopy for Upper Tract Urothelial Carcinoma: A Single-Centre Prospective Non-Randomized Trial. J Endourol. 2020;34(5):573–80.
138. Lu DD, Boorjian SA, Raman JD. Intravesical chemotherapy use after radical nephroureterectomy: A

national survey of urologic oncologists. Urol Oncol. 2017;35(3):113.e1–7.
139. Chen GL, Bagley DH. Ureteroscopic management of upper tract transitional cell carcinoma in patients with normal contralateral kidneys. J Urol. 2000;164:1173.
140. Ho KV, Chow GK. Ureteroscopic resection of upper-tract transitional-cell carcinoma. J Endourol. 2005;19:841–8.
141. Tawfiek ER, Bagley DH. Upper-tract transitional cell carcinoma. Urology. 1997;50:321–9.
142. Martinez-Pineiro JA, Matres MJ, Martinez-Pineiro L. Endourological treatment of upper-tract urothelial carcinomas: analysis of a series of 59 tumors. J Urol. 1996;156:377–85.
143. Elliott DS, Blute ML, Patterson DE, Bergstralh EJ, Segura JW. Long-term follow-up of endoscopically treated upper urinary tract transitional cell carcinoma. Urology. 1996;47:819–25.
144. Deligne E, Colombel M, Badet L, Taniere P, Rouviere O, Dubernard JM, Lezrek M, Gelet A, Martin X. Conservative management of upper tract tumors. Eur Urol. 2002;42:43–8.
145. Huang A, Low RK, White R. Case reports: nephrostomy tract tumor seeding following percutaneous manipulation of a ureteral carcinoma. J Urol. 1995;153:1041–2.
146. Sharma NK, Nicol A, Powell CS. Tract infiltration following percutaneous resection of renal pelvic transitional cell carcinoma. Br J Urol. 1994;73:597–8.
147. Liatsikos EN, Dinlenc CZ, Kapoor R, Smith AD. Transitional-cell carcinoma of the renal pelvis: ureteroscopic and percutaneous approach. J Endourol. 2001;15:377–83.
148. Patel A, Soonawalla P, Shepherd SF, Dearnaley DP, Kellett MJ, Woodhouse CR. Long-term outcome after percutaneous treatment of transitional cell carcinoma of the renal pelvis. J Urol. 1996;155:868–74.
149. Lee BR, Jabbour ME, Marshall FF, Smith AD, Jarrett TW. 13-year survival comparison of percutaneous and open nephroureterectomy approaches for management of transitional cell carcinoma of renal collecting system: equivalent outcomes. J Endourol. 1999;13:289–94.
150. Plancke HR, Strijbos WE, Delaere KP. Percutaneous endoscopic treatment of urothelial tumours of the renal pelvis. Br J Urol. 1995;75:736–9.
151. Haupt G. Editorial comment: transitional-cell carcinoma of the ureter. J Endourol. 2001;15:409.
152. Babaian RJ, Johnson DE. Primary carcinoma of the ureter. J Urol. 1980;123:357–9.
153. Zincke H, Neves RJ. Feasibility of conservative surgery for transitional cell cancer of the upper urinary tract. Urol Clin North Am. 1984;11:717–24.
154. Hall MC, Womack S, Sagalowsky AI, Carmody T, Erickstad MD, Roehrborn CG. Prognostic factors, recurrence, and survival in transitional cell carcinoma of the upper urinary tract: a 30-year experience in 252 patients. Urology. 1998;52:594–601.
155. Heney NM, Nocks BN, Daly JJ, Blitzer PH, Parkhurst EC. Prognostic factors in carcinoma of the ureter. J Urol. 1981;125:623–6.
156. Batata MA, Whitmore WF, Hilaris BS, Tokita N, Grabstald H. Primary carcinoma of the renal pelvis: a prognostic study. Cancer. 1975;35:1626.
157. Nakada SY, Moon TD, Gist M, Mahvi D. Use of Pneumosleeve as an adjunct in laparoscopic nephrectomy. Urology. 1997;49:612–3.
158. Chen J, Chueh SC, Hsu WT, Lai MK, Chen SC. Modified approach of hand-assisted laparoscopic nephroureterectomy for transitional cell carcinoma of the upper urinary tract. Urology. 2001;58:930–4.
159. Clayman RV, Garske GL, Lange PH. Total nephroureterectomy with ureteral intussusception and transurethral ureteral detachment and pull-through. Urology. 1983;21:482.
160. Hara N, Kitamura Y, Saito T, Wakatsuki S, Sakata Y, Komatsubara S. Nephrectomy plus endoscopy-assisted intussusception ureterectomy for patients with renal pelvic cancer: long term oncologic outcomes in comparison with nephroureterectomy plus bladder cuff removal. J Endourol. 2011;25(4):691–7.
161. Hetherington JW, Ewing R. Modified nephroureterectomy: a risk of tumour implantation. Br J Urol. 1986;58:368–70.
162. Jones DR, Moisey CU. A cautionary tale of the modified "pluck" nephroureterectomy. Br J Urol. 1993;71:486.
163. Arango O, Bielsa O, Carles J, Gelabert-Mas A. Massive tumor implantation in the endoscopic resected area in modified nephroureterectomy. J Urol. 1997;157:1839.
164. Gill IS, Sung GT, Hobart MG, Savage SJ, Meraney AM, Schweizer DK, Klein EA, Novick AC. Laparoscopic radical nephroureterectomy for upper tract transitional cell carcinoma: the Cleveland Clinic experience. J Urol. 2000;164:1513–22.
165. McDougall EM, Clayman RV, Elashry O. Laparoscopic nephroureterectomy for upper tract transitional cell cancer: the Washington University experience. J Urol. 1995;154:975–80.
166. Shalhav AL, Dunn MD, Portis AJ, Elbahnasy AM, McDougall EM, Clayman RV. Laparoscopic nephroureterectomy for upper tract transitional cell cancer: the Washington University experience. J Urol. 2000;163:1100–4.
167. Thompson RH, Krambeck AE, Lohse CM, Elliott DS, Patterson DE, Blute ML. Elective endoscopic management of transitional cell carcinoma first diagnosed in the upper urinary tract. BJU Int. 2008;102(9):1107–10.
168. Jeldres C, Lughezzani G, Sun M, Isbarn H, Shariat SF, Budaus L, Lattouf JB, Widmer H, Graefen M, Montorsi F, Perrotte P, Karakiewicz PI. Segmental ureterectomy can safely be performed in patients with transitional cell carcinoma of the ureter. J Urol. 2010;183(4):1324–9.

169. Pettersson S, Brynger H, Johansson S, Nilsson AE. Extracorporeal surgery and autotransplantation for carcinoma of the pelvis and ureter. Scand J Urol Nephrol. 1979;13:89–93.
170. Holmang S, Johansson SL. Tumours of the ureter and renal pelvis treated with resection and renal autotransplantation: a study with up to 20 years of follow-up. BJU Int. 2005;95:1201–5.
171. Steffens J, Humke U, Alloussi S, Ziegler M, Siemer S. Partial nephrectomy and autotransplantation with pyelovesicostomy for renal urothelial carcinoma in solitary kidneys: a clinical update. BJU Int. 2007;99:1020–3.
172. Oosterlinck W, Solsona E, van der Meijden AP, Sylvester R, Böhle A, Rintala E, Lobel B, European Association of Urology. EAU guidelines on diagnosis and treatment of upper urinary tract transitional cell carcinoma. Eur Urol. 2004;46:147.
173. Kundu SD, Eggener SE. Retroperitoneal lymph nodes in transitional cell carcinoma of the kidney and ureter. Adv Urol. 2009;2009:181927. Epub 2009 Jan 26
174. Jensen TK, Holt P, Gerke O, Riehmann M, Svolgaard B, Marcussen N, Bouchelouche K. Preoperative lymph-node staging of invasive urothelial bladder cancer with 18F-fluorodeoxyglucose positron emission tomography/computed axial tomography and magnetic resonance imaging: correlation with histopathology. Scand J Urol Nephrol. 2011;45:122.
175. Komatsu H, Tanabe N, Kubodera S, Maezawa H, Ueno A. The role of lymphadenectomy in the treatment of transitional cell carcinoma of the upper urinary tract. J Urol. 1997;157:1622.
176. Bobjer J, Gerdtsson A, Abrahamsson J, Baseckas G, Bergkvist M, Bläckberg M, Brändstedt J, Jancke G, Hagberg O, Kollberg P, Lundström KJ, Löfgren A, Nyberg M, Rian Mårtensson L, Saemundsson Y, Ståhl E, Sörenby A, Warnolf Å, Liedberg F. Location of Retroperitoneal Lymph Node Metastases in Upper Tract Urothelial Carcinoma: Results from a Prospective Lymph Node Mapping Study. Eur Urol Open Sci. 2023 Sep;27(57):37–44.
177. Abe T, Shinohara N, Harabayashi T, Sazawa A, Ishikawa S, Kubota K, Matsuno Y, Osawa T, Shibata T, Shinno Y, Kamota S, Minami K, Sakashita S, Takeuchi I, Kumagai A, Mori T, Togashi M, Nonomura K. The role of lymph-node dissection in the treatment of upper urinary tract cancer: a multi-institutional study. BJU Int. 2008;102(5):576–80.
178. Kondo T, Nakazawa H, Ito F, Hashimoto Y, Toma H, Tanabe K. Impact of the extent of regional lymphadenectomy on the survival of patients with urothelial carcinoma of the upper urinary tract. J Urol. 2007;178(4 Pt 1):1212–7.
179. Roscigno M, Shariat SF, Margulis V, Karakiewicz P, Remzi M, Kikuchi E, Langner C, Lotan Y, Weizer A, Bensalah K, Raman JD, Bolenz C, Guo CC, Wood CG, Zigeuner R, Wheat J, Kabbani W, Koppie TM, Ng CK, Suardi N, Bertini R, Fernández MI, Mikami S, Isida M, Michel MS, Montorsi F. Impact of lymph node dissection on cancer specific survival in patients with upper tract urothelial carcinoma treated with radical nephroureterectomy. J Urol. 2009;181:2482.
180. Kondo T, Nakazawa H, Ito F, Hashimoto Y, Toma H, Tanabe K. Primary site and incidence of lymph node metastases in urothelial carcinoma of upper urinary tract. Urology. 2007;69(2):265–9.
181. Kondo T, Tanabe K. The role of lymph node dissection in the management of urothelial carcinoma of the upper urinary tract. Int J Clin Oncol. 2011;16:170–8.
182. Roscigno M, Cozzarini C, Bertini R, Scattoni V, Freschi M, Da Pozzo LF, Briganti A, Gallina A, Capitanio U, Colombo R, Giorgio G, Montorsi F, Rigatti P. Prognostic value of lymph node dissection in patients with muscle-invasive transitional cell carcinoma of the upper urinary tract. Eur Urol. 2008;53:794–802.
183. Abe T, Shinohara N, Muranaka M, Sazawa A, Maruyama S, Osawa T, Harabayashi T, Kubota K, Matsuno Y, Shibata T, Toyada Y, Shinno Y, Minami K, Sakashita S, Kumagai A, Takada N, Togashi M, Sano H, Mori T, Nonomura K. Role of lymph node dissection in the treatment of urothelial carcinoma of the upper urinary tract: multi-institutional relapse analysis and immunohistochemical re-evaluation of negative lymph nodes. Eur J Surg Oncol. 2010;36:1085–91.
184. Weight C, Gettman MT. The emerging role of lymphadenectomy in upper tract urothelial carcinoma. Urol Clin N Am. 2011;38:429–37.
185. Lughezzani G, Jeldres C, Isbarn H, Shariat SF, Sun M, Pharand D, Widmer H, Arjane P, Graefen M, Montorsi F, Perrotte P, Karakiewicz PI. A critical appraisal of the value of lymph node dissection at nephroureterectomy for upper tract urothelial carcinoma. Urology. 2010;75:118.
186. Grossman HB, Natale RB, Tangen CM, Speights VO, Vogelzang NJ, Trump DL, deVere White RW, Sarosdy MF, Wood DP Jr, Raghavan D, Crawford ED. Neoadjuvant chemotherapy plus cystectomy compared with cystectomy alone for locally advanced bladder cancer. N Engl J Med. 2003;349(9):859–66.
187. Igawa M, Urakami S, Shiina H, Kishi H, Himeno Y, Ishibe T, Kadena H, Usui T. Neoadjuvant chemotherapy for locally advanced urothelial cancer of the upper urinary tract. Urol Int. 1995;55(2):74–7.
188. Kim DK, Lee JY, Kim JW, Hah YS, Cho KS. Effect of neoadjuvant chemotherapy on locally advanced upper tract urothelial carcinoma: A systematic review and meta-analysis. Crit Rev Oncol Hematol. 2019 Mar;135:59–65.
189. Gregg RW, Vera-Badillo FE, Booth CM, Mahmud A, Brundage M, Leveridge MJ, Hanna TP. Perioperative chemotherapy for urothelial carcinoma of the upper urinary tract: A systematic review and meta-analysis. Crit Rev Oncol Hematol. 2018 Aug;128:58–64.
190. Kubota Y, Hatakeyama S, Tanaka T, Fujita N, Iwamura H, Mikami J, Yamamoto H, Tobisawa Y, Yoneyama T, Yoneyama T, Hashimoto Y, Koie T, Ito

H, Yoshikawa K, Sasaki A, Kawaguchi T, Ohyama C. Oncological outcomes of neoadjuvant chemotherapy in patients with locally advanced upper tract urothelial carcinoma: a multicenter study. Oncotarget. 2017;8(60):101500–8.
191. Kohada Y, Hayashi T, Takemoto K, Miyamoto S, Babasaki T, Kobatake K, Kitano H, Ikeda K, Goto K, Hieda K, Honda Y, Sentani K, Oue N, Awai K, Hinata N. The Efficacy of Neoadjuvant Gemcitabine and Cisplatin Chemotherapy for cT3N0M0 Upper Tract Urothelial Carcinoma: The Impact of Tumor Location. Urol J. 2023;21(02):98–106.
192. Millikan R, Dinney C, Swanson D, Sweeney P, Ro JY, Smith TL, Williams D, Logothetis C. Integrated therapy for locally advanced bladder cancer: final report of a randomized trial of cystectomy plus adjuvant M-VAC versus cystectomy with both preoperative and postoperative M-VAC. J Clin Oncol. 2001;19(20):4005–13.
193. Kwak C, Lee SE, Jeong IG, Ku JH. Adjuvant systemic chemotherapy in the treatment of patients with invasive transitional cell carcinoma of the upper urinary tract. Urology. 2006;68(1):53–7.
194. Lee SE, Byun SS, Park YH, Chang IH, Kim YJ, Hong SK. Adjuvant chemotherapy in the management of pT3N0M0 transitional cell carcinoma of the upper urinary tract. Urol Int. 2006;77(1):22–6.
195. Hellenthal NJ, Shariat SF, Margulis V, Karakiewicz PI, Roscigno M, Bolenz C, Remzi M, Weizer A, Zigeuner R, Bensalah K, Ng CK, Raman JD, Kikuchi E, Montorsi F, Oya M, Wood CG, Fernandez M, Evans CP, Koppie TM. Adjuvant chemotherapy for high risk upper tract urothelial carcinoma: results from the Upper Tract Urothelial Carcinoma Collaboration. J Urol. 2009;182(3):900–6.
196. Bamias A, Deliveliotis C, Fountzilas G, Gika D, Anagnostopoulos A, Zorzou MP, Kastritis E, Constantinides C, Kosmidis P, Dimopoulos MA. Adjuvant chemotherapy with paclitaxel and carboplatin in patients with advanced carcinoma of the upper urinary tract: a study by the Hellenic Cooperative Oncology Group. J Clin Oncol. 2004;22(11):2150–4.
197. Birtle A, Johnson M, Chester J, Jones R, Dolling D, Bryan RT, Harris C, Winterbottom A, Blacker A, Catto JWF, Chakraborti P, Donovan JL, Elliott PA, French A, Jagdev S, Jenkins B, Keeley FX Jr, Kockelbergh R, Powles T, Wagstaff J, Wilson C, Todd R, Lewis R, Hall E. Adjuvant chemotherapy in upper tract urothelial carcinoma (the POUT trial): a phase 3, open-label, randomised controlled trial. Lancet. 2020;395(10232):1268–77.
198. Bajorin DF, Witjes JA, Gschwend JE, Schenker M, Valderrama BP, Tomita Y, Bamias A, Lebret T, Shariat SF, Park SH, Ye D, Agerbaek M, Enting D, McDermott R, Gajate P, Peer A, Milowsky MI, Nosov A, Neif Antonio J Jr, Tupikowski K, Toms L, Fischer BS, Qureshi A, Collette S, Unsal-Kacmaz K, Broughton E, Zardavas D, Koon HB, Galsky MD. Adjuvant Nivolumab versus Placebo in muscle-invasive urothelial carcinoma. N Engl J Med. 2021;384(22):2102–14.

Postoperative Surveillance Protocols for Renal Cell Carcinoma

20

Elizabeth E. Ellis, Brittney H. Cotta, Megan M. Merrill, and Jose A. Karam

Introduction

Cancers of the kidney and renal pelvis accounted for approximately 4–5% of all malignancies diagnosed in the United States in 2024, with 81,610 new cases and 14,390 deaths [1]. The majority of these cancers are renal cell carcinomas (RCC). The incidence of RCC continues to rise, increasing by 2% per year, in part secondary to the increasing use of abdominal imaging resulting in the incidental finding of renal masses. Despite the potential advantage of identifying and treating asymptomatic patients at earlier disease stages, 20–30% of patients will eventually develop local or distant recurrence following surgical extirpation [2–4].

Prognosis of patients with untreated recurrent disease is poor, with 5-year survival rates of 3–9% [5, 6]. If identified early, however, metastasectomy with or without systemic therapy has been shown to improve overall survival [7–10]. Further, patients with recurrence who underwent treatment were almost four times less likely to die of their disease. Therefore, the use of surveillance to effectively identify those at risk for recurrence is of paramount importance.

This chapter reviews the recurrence patterns of RCC and the prognostic factors associated with the risk of recurrence as a rationale for the establishment of surveillance protocols. Although there is no single consensus on the optimal guidelines for follow-up, there are several evidence-based recommendations and reviews that are currently being used in the postoperative setting, following radical and partial nephrectomy as well as ablative therapies for RCC. Routine surveillance beyond 5 years is controversial, and the rationale for each argument will also be discussed in this chapter.

Natural History of RCC and Recurrence Patterns

Renal cell carcinoma originates from the proximal tubular epithelium and typically grows slowly, forming discrete focal lesions. Local disease progression occurs by invasion through the renal capsule into Gerota's fascia and further local extension to surrounding structures. In addition, renal cell carcinoma spreads to distant sites through both hematogenous and lymphatic routes. The lung, bone, and liver are the most common sites of metastasis, although RCC can also metastasize to the brain, contralateral kidney, adrenal gland, and soft tissues [11]. Involvement of lymph nodes without distant

E. E. Ellis · B. H. Cotta · J. A. Karam (✉)
Department of Urology, The University of Texas MD Anderson Cancer Center, Houston, TX, USA
e-mail: EEEllis@mdanderson.org; BHCotta@mdanderson.org; JAKaram@mdanderson.org

M. M. Merrill
Department of Urology, Kaiser Permanente South Sacramento, Sacramento, CA, USA

J. A. Libertino, J. R. Gee (eds.), *Renal Cancer*, https://doi.org/10.1007/978-3-031-97599-8_20

metastases is uncommon, although disease progression can be unpredictable secondary to the variable lymphatic drainage of the kidneys [12]. Synchronous metastasis is defined as metastasis diagnosed at the same time as the primary tumor, while metachronous metastasis develops during follow-up. Synchronous metastasis portends a worse prognosis. There are multiple subtypes of RCC with the most common being clear cell RCC, papillary RCC, and chromophobe RCC. Each subtype has a different genetic basis and prognoses between subtypes differs with clear cell RCC generally having a worse prognosis.

Distant Recurrence

Lung

The most common site of metastasis from RCC is the lung, with a reported incidence of 3–16% [13–17]. Median time to development of pulmonary recurrence is correlated with tumor stage, with an earlier time to recurrence for higher stage disease. One series reports the median time to metastasis to be 53 months for pT1 disease, 31 months for pT2 disease, and 14 months for pT3 disease. In this same observational study, none of the patients with pT1 disease were symptomatic at diagnosis of recurrence, 11% with pT2 disease were symptomatic, and only 9% with pT3 disease presented with symptoms [14].

Symptoms associated with pulmonary metastasis include pleuritic chest pain, hemoptysis, cough, dyspnea, and weight loss. Multiple other studies have confirmed the low rates of symptomatic lung recurrences, with pulmonary lesions being found in over 90% of asymptomatic patients with metastases undergoing routine surveillance imaging [16, 18, 19].

A meta-analysis reviewing post-nephrectomy pulmonary metastasis reports the latest pulmonary lesion discovered at 67 months for pT1 tumors, 97 months for pT2 tumors, and 138 months for pT3 tumors, emphasizing the importance of surveillance up to at least 5 years postoperatively and ideally longer [14–16, 20].

The high percentage of asymptomatic recurrences for all stages of disease has led to recommendations for routine chest imaging in the form of CXR or chest CT for all stages of disease with emphasis on the first 3–5 years postoperatively. However, there is no consensus between the EAU and other guideline panels on whether the use CXR instead of CT is acceptable for lower stage disease. CXR is preferred in stages where the risk of pulmonary metastasis is <5% due to the lower likelihood of incidental findings, decreased radiation exposure, and cost benefits, while CT chest is more likely to detect metastasis earlier. According to the EAU guidelines, the sensitivity of CXR is significantly lower than CT-scans, and therefore recommends using CT chest in their surveillance protocols. In a retrospective study of 249 patients with T1-T3N0 who underwent radical or partial nephrectomy, 10/19 pulmonary metastasis were not detected by CXR. In another study evaluating the utility of CXR in postoperative surveillance of T1a disease, pulmonary metastasis developed in 1.2%, and CXR did not detect the metastasis in one of the three patients. Despite underdetection of a very small proportion of chest metastases, the AUA, NCCN, and CAU recommend utilizing CXR for low- and intermediate-risk disease.

Bone

Bone metastasis occurs in approximately 2–8% of all patients after nephrectomy for RCC and comprises 16–27% of patients with recurrent disease [14–16, 19]. Although reported to be less common for patients with pT1 disease (0–25%), bone metastasis for patients with pT2 and pT3 disease occurs in 17.6–45% and 16–26.5%, respectively. Recurrence is at a median time of 39 months for pT1 disease, 24–40 months for pT2 disease, and 7–20 months for pT3 disease [14–16, 20].

As with pulmonary metastasis, tumor stage is correlated with median time to recurrence. In contrast to pulmonary recurrence, however, most patients with bone metastasis present with symptoms. Bone pain is reported in 67–90% of patients, and alkaline phosphatase levels are elevated in 33–55% [14, 19, 20]. In a study by Shvarts et al., 68% of patients with bone metastasis were also found to have extraosseous metastasis, and 95.5% had an ECOG performance status of 1 or more [21]. Given these data, routine surveillance with nuclear scintigraphy is not warranted in the absence of symptoms or an elevated alkaline phosphatase level.

Liver

The reported incidence of liver metastasis is between 1% and 7%. It is rarely reported for patients with pT1 disease, with an incidence of 0 in several studies [14–16, 20]. In one series, an incidence of 12% is reported for patients with pT2 disease and 9% for pT3 disease, with a median time to recurrence of 53–83 months and 5–67 months, respectively [14, 20]. Most patients (pT2, 60–100%; pT3, 73–100%) were diagnosed after presenting with abdominal pain and/or elevated liver function tests (LFTs).

Brain

Brain metastasis occurs in 2–4% of all patients after nephrectomy [19], but this is likely underestimated as this rate captures only patients with symptomatic brain metastases. Data derived from a meta-analysis by Skolarikos et al. report the incidence of brain metastasis for pT1 tumors to be from 0% to 12%. However, the 12% was derived from a single study in which one patient with pT1 disease in a cohort of 8 developed brain metastasis [14]. For pT2 and pT3 disease, the reported incidence ranges from 0% to 15% and 4% to 11%, respectively. All patients who developed brain metastasis presented with symptoms such as headache, mental status change, or other neurologic deficits [14–16, 20]. For this reason, routine imaging has not been recommended in the absence of focal or new-onset neurological symptoms. However, requisite brain imaging for clinical trial participation has identified asymptomatic brain metastasis, which excludes patients from trial enrollment. Early detection significantly alters the treatment plan for the patient and should be considered routinely. Additionally, in other malignancies, such as melanoma diagnosis of asymptomatic brain metastasis, portend a better prognosis than symptomatic metastases. A retrospective study using the Canadian Kidney Cancer Information System database evaluated outcomes of asymptomatic (N = 106, 40%) versus symptomatic (N = 161, 60%) brain metastases. Thirty five patients were found to have isolated brain metastases. The high rate of asymptomatic lesions can partially be attributed to reporting bias in this retrospective study. There was no significant difference between median overall survival between symptomatic and asymptomatic metastasis in this cohort. In a review of patients being evaluated for clinical trial eligibility across 68 clinical trials, asymptomatic brain metastases were identified in 4.3% of patients with metastatic RCC. 63% of the metastases were solitary lesions, and 40% were greater than 1 cm in size. 92% of patients harbored lung metastases. Median overall survival was 10.3 months. Risk factors for brain metastasis include white race, clear cell histology, sarcomatoid differentiation, T2–T4 disease, tumor size > 10 cm, and node-positive disease. Based on these findings, revision of screening algorithms to include routine screening for brain metastases are needed for earlier identification which will enable earlier intervention.

Lymph Nodes

Development of new lymph node metastasis was identified in up to 25% of patients with pT2 and pT3 disease. In all cases, patients were asymptomatic, diagnosed by routine CT scans, and found to have concomitant sites of recurrent disease [14, 16]. Lymph node positivity portends worse survival outcomes. While the American Joint Committee on Cancer staging considers pT1-T3N1M0 RCC patients as stage III, survival with node-positive disease is worse than T3N0M0 disease and similar to stage IV disease in multiple studies. One study cites cancer specific survival of pT3N0M0, pT1-T3N1M0, and pT1-T3N0/xM1 as >10.2 years, 2.8 years, and 2.1 years, respectively. There is a discrepancy between clinical lymph node and true pathologic lymph node status. In two studies of patients with lymphadenopathy who underwent lymph node dissection, only 20% and 29% of the patients suspected to have node-positive disease on imaging were confirmed to be pathologically node positive. A newer imaging modality using lymphotropic nanoparticle-enhanced MRI has demonstrated 100% sensitivity and 96% specificity in diagnosing pathologic node positive disease.

Local Recurrence After Radical Nephrectomy

Local recurrence involving the renal fossa, ipsilateral adrenal gland, or axial musculoskeletal anatomy is rare, and incidence varies between 3% and 27% depending on the literature reviewed [14, 22, 23]. A retrospective study from the Mayo Clinic published in 2000 followed 1737 node-negative patients who underwent nephrectomy for RCC. Authors reported a 1.8% incidence of isolated renal fossa recurrence at 5 years, with 60% of patients being symptomatic upon diagnosis [24].

An updated cohort from the Mayo Clinic that included 2502 patients with localized RCC reported the overall incidence of isolated renal fossa recurrence to be 1.3%, with a median time to recurrence of 1.5 years [25]. In this study, published in 2017, the authors found advanced pathologic stage and coagulative necrosis in the primary tumor to be independently associated with increased risk of developing an isolated renal fossa recurrence. They also reported significantly better oncologic outcomes for patients treated with local definitive therapy, including metastasectomy, ablation or radiation, versus systemic therapy, or observation (3-year cancer-specific survival 64% versus 50% versus 28%, respectively).

Margulis et al. reviewed 2945 patients who had a radical nephrectomy with curative intent and reported an isolated local recurrence in 54 (1.8%) of those patients [26]. Local recurrence was defined as any RCC, proven by pathologic evaluation, and localized in the renal fossa, ipsilateral adrenal gland, or ipsilateral retroperitoneal lymph nodes. Consistent with the Mayo Clinic series, 61.2% of patients were symptomatic (28 patients with local symptoms and 5 with systemic symptoms) at presentation. In this population, the authors identified five risk factors that portend poor prognosis: size >5 cm, positive surgical margins, presence of sarcomatoid elements, abnormal LDH, and abnormal alkaline phosphatase. Patients with none of these risk factors ($N = 34$) had a median survival of 111 months. Patients with only 1 risk factor ($N = 9$) had a median survival of 40 months, while patients with more than 1 risk factor ($N = 11$) had a median survival of only 8 months after resection. Tumor size was a poor prognostic indicator, suggesting that earlier detection of such recurrence could lead to improved resectability and achieving negative surgical margins, decreased surgical morbidity, and ultimately improved survival.

Recurrence After Partial Nephrectomy

Historically, there was a concern of increased risk of local recurrence in the ipsilateral kidney following partial nephrectomy. However, multiple studies over the past decade have found recurrence rates to be similar to radical nephrectomy despite the utilization of a nephron-sparing approach. A study from the Cleveland Clinic reviewed 327 patients who underwent partial nephrectomy and demonstrated a local recurrence rate of 4% and a metastatic recurrence rate of 7.6% over 55.6 months [13]. A follow-up study from the same group observed 107 patients over 10 years and found no local recurrence for patients with localized pT1 and pT2 disease. For patients with pT3a and pT3b disease, local recurrence rates were 10% and 12%, respectively. Distant metastatic disease occurred in 2%, 29%, 0%, 33%, and 53% of patients with pT1a, pT1b, pT2, pT3a, and pT3b, respectively [27].

In more recent years, the size threshold for renal masses amenable to partial nephrectomy has been expanded to include masses up to 7 cm and in some cases >7 cm when technically feasible and clinically indicated. The feasibility of partial nephrectomy in larger renal masses has come with concern regarding long-term oncological outcomes [28]. The group from the Mayo Clinic studied 5-year survival rates for patients with renal masses 4–7 cm who underwent either partial or radical nephrectomy. They concluded that after controlling for stage, grade, tumor necrosis, and histological subtype, there was no statistical difference in cancer-specific survival or distant metastatic-free survival for those undergoing partial or radical nephrectomy [29].

Aside from the influence of size on recurrence patterns after partial nephrectomy, the effect of positive surgical margins (PSMs) has also been investigated. A study conducted by Memorial Sloan Kettering Cancer Center (MSKCC) and the Mayo Clinic reviewed 1344 patients who underwent partial nephrectomy at one of these institutions between 1972 and 2005 [30]. A total of 77 patients (5.5%) were noted to have PSMs. 63% were clear cell RCC, 25% were papillary RCC, 9% were chromophobe, and 3% were unclassified or miscellaneous. Of the entire cohort, 39 patients had local recurrence and 57 had progression to metastatic disease. For patients with PSMs, the 5-year freedom from local recurrence was 98% and from metastatic progression 95%. There was no significant difference in freedom from local recurrence or metastatic progression between patients with positive surgical margins and negative surgical margins [30].

A retrospective multi-institutional review collected data from 26 centers throughout Europe and North America and reported similar results [31]. They identified 119 positive surgical margins following partial nephrectomy. A negative surgical margin cohort was obtained from a multi-institutional database and was matched for surgical indication, tumor size, and Fuhrman grade. There was no difference in recurrence-free survival between patients with negative surgical margins and those with positive surgical margins. Rates of cancer-specific survival and overall survival were comparable for both groups [31].

Contrary to previous literature, a study from MD Anderson Cancer Center reported a significantly higher rate of local tumor bed recurrence following partial nephrectomy for patients who had positive surgical margins (15.9% versus 3% in a matched control group). Consistent with other publications, they reported a 1.9% incidence of local tumor bed recurrence following partial nephrectomy in a contemporary cohort of 2256 patients undergoing surgery between 2000 and 2014 [32]. On multivariate analysis, male gender, a solitary kidney, positive surgical margins, more than two tumors excised, pT3 tumors, and RENAL nephrometry score of 10 or greater were variables that predicted a shorter time to local tumor bed recurrence. The authors suggest that the higher rate of local tumor bed recurrence for patients with positive surgical margins in this series could be influenced by the inclusion of higher stage tumors (23% pT3) and potentially more challenging partial nephrectomies with higher nephrometry scores (53% score 7–9).

Collectively, these data indicate that recurrence and survival rates are similar following partial and radical nephrectomy regardless of tumor size and positive surgical margins. As such, contemporary surveillance strategies for the two groups have not markedly differed.

Surveillance Following Radical or Partial Nephrectomy

Rationale for Surveillance

According to observational data from the National Cancer Data Base for patients diagnosed with RCC between 2001 and 2002, the 5-year overall survival rates are 81% for stage T1, 74% for T2, 53% for T3, and 8% for T4 [33]. Contemporary recurrence rates for patients with clear cell RCC pT1 disease are 9.2%, pT2 is 32%, and pT3 is 49%. Long-term follow-up of the RECUR database in Europe evaluated long-term outcomes of clear cell RCC. Recurrence risk at 5 years for low risk was 7.2%, 23.2 for intermediate risk, and 61.6% for high-risk disease. Highest risk of cancer-related death occurred in younger and higher risk patients. This study suggests an age, comorbidity, and risk-score-dependent follow-up approach.

Given that complete metastasectomy grants a survival benefit in select patients, early detection of metastatic disease is imperative to improving clinical outcomes. In early stages, chest and abdominal metastases are usually asymptomatic, with symptoms only appearing in advanced stages [14]. In patients with surgically resectable metastases, early intervention in the absence of symptoms when complete resection is still possible could result in higher survival rates [34]. The Mayo Clinic reported that complete metastasectomy confers a cancer-specific survival (CSS) advantage in patients who present with multiple synchronous and asynchronous metastatic lesions. Alt et al. reviewed 887 patients who underwent nephrectomy for renal cell carcinoma and were diagnosed with metastatic disease [35]. One hundred twenty-five (125) patients underwent complete surgical metastasectomy and were found to have an improved median CSS compared to patients who did not undergo metastasectomy (4.8 versus 1.3 years). Patients with pulmonary metastasis who underwent complete surgical resection had a 5-year CSS of 73% versus 19% for those who did not have complete metastasectomy. Patients with multiple, nonpulmonary lesions also benefited from complete resection compared to those who did not undergo complete resection (5-year CSS 32.5% versus 12.4%). A survival advantage was seen following metastasectomy for both patients with localized disease who developed synchronous or asynchronous metastasis and patients who initially presented with metastatic disease and then developed asynchronous metastasis [35].

Components of Surveillance

There is currently no consensus on the optimal surveillance protocol following surgical resection or ablative therapy for the treatment of RCC. Historically, surveillance has included history, physical examination, laboratory work, and periodic chest and abdominal imaging studies at intervals based on established recurrence patterns.

A thorough history and physical examination is important for promptly identifying signs and symptoms that suggest disease recurrence and warrant further investigation. Constitutional symptoms such as fever, weight loss, and fatigue are concerning for metastatic disease. A complete review of systems should be performed to identify the presence of weight loss, night sweats, pleuritic chest pain, dyspnea, hemoptysis, epistaxis, abdominal pain, flank pain, bone pain, dermatologic involvement, change in mental status, musculoskeletal pain, weakness, or focal neurologic deficits. Physical exam findings such as a palpable abdominal mass or abdominal wall mass, groin and supraclavicular or axillary lymphadenopathy, and lower extremity swelling are also concerning for metastatic disease and should elicit further workup.

Current National Comprehensive Cancer Network (NCCN) guidelines recommend lab work to include a comprehensive metabolic panel (CMP), which consists of liver function, LDH, calcium, electrolytes, BUN, and creatinine studies. The AUA guidelines also recommend obtaining urinalysis annually to evaluate for proteinuria, hematuria, or inflammatory changes. Close monitoring of renal function is paramount to intervene early with risk modifications and referral to a nephrologist if renal function declines should occur.

Routine blood work plays a prognostic role in surveillance of oncological as well as nononcological parameters. Motzer et al. identified that a lactate dehydrogenase level > 1.5 times the upper limit of normal, a hemoglobin level < lower limit of normal, a corrected serum calcium level > 10 mg/dL, a Karnofsky performance score ≤ 70, and an interval of less than 1 year from the original diagnosis to start of systemic therapy predicted short survival in patients with advanced renal cell carcinoma. In this study, patients with three or more of these factors had a poor prognosis, with a median survival of 5 months and a 1-, 2-, and 3-year survival rate of

20%, 6%, and 2% [36]. Patients with elevated liver function studies should be evaluated with abdominal imaging, and those with elevated alkaline phosphatase should receive a nuclear bone scan to evaluate for metastatic disease.

Aside from monitoring lab work that relates to oncological outcomes, it is also important to follow kidney function parameters including creatinine, estimated glomerular filtration rate (eGFR), and urinalysis. Chronic kidney disease (CKD) is defined as eGFR < 60 ml/min or the presence of factors that suggest kidney damage, such as albuminuria or abnormal renal imaging, occurring for 3 months or greater [37]. CKD has been shown to be associated with a higher risk of morbidity and mortality [38]. Early identification of worsening serum creatinine, eGFR, and development of proteinuria identifies patients who are developing chronic kidney disease following surgery and allows for early referral to a nephrologist, who will work with the patient to control medical comorbidities and optimize renal function.

Modalities of Abdominal Imaging

Computed tomography (CT) without and with intravenous contrast is the most common imaging modality being utilized in the postoperative setting for surveillance of disease progression in patients with renal cell carcinoma. With the number of diagnostic CT scans dramatically increasing in the United States over the past several decades, there has been a growing concern over radiation exposure and risk of developing a secondary malignancy [98, 99]. The National Council on Radiation Protection and Measurements (NCRP) reported that radiation exposure associated with medical technology has risen sixfold since the 1980s from 0.5 to 3.0 mSv [100]. In 2007, Brenner et al. estimated that as many as 1.5–2% of cancers could be a result of radiation from CT scans [98]. In response to these worrisome trends, the Food and Drug Administration (FDA) launched an initiative in 2010 to reduce radiation exposure from medical imaging and increase patient awareness about the risks of frequent exposure [100].

According to the AUA guidelines, CT or MRI pre- and post-IV contrast are both feasible imaging modalities for follow-up. After 2 years, the panel states that abdominal ultrasound alternating with cross sectional imaging can be considered in low-risk and intermediate-risk groups. The EAU guidelines approve both CT and MRI pre and post contrast, however does not recommend abdominal ultrasound in the use of follow-up due to poor sensitivity. The CAU guidelines recommend CT or MRI pre and post contrast for all risk groups or ultrasound for low and intermediate risk groups. The NCCN guidelines recommend CT or MRI without and with contrast for all stages but note that MRI is the preferred imaging modality. The guidelines provide the option for contrast-enhanced ultrasound for follow up after ablative therapies or stage III disease.

F-18 fluorodeoxyglucose positron emission tomography (FDG-PET) CT scans should not be routinely obtained due to false positives due to post-surgical scarring or inflammation. Newer agents such as [^{89}Zr]Zr-DFO-girentuximab-PET/CT are being tested in ongoing clinical trials that have demonstrated increased lesion detection compared to CT alone. We may see their emergence in the clinical setting in the future.

Prognostic Factors Influencing Recurrence

Pathologic stage is the most important prognostic factor in determining RCC recurrence. Early recommendations for surveillance have been guided mostly by the correlation of tumor stage with time to recurrence and site of recurrence [14–16, 20]. The likelihood of developing metastatic disease has been shown to be greatest in the first 3 years after nephrectomy and directly correlates with tumor stage. In one series, the risk of metastatic disease was 7.1% for those with T1 disease, 26.5% for T2 disease, and 39.4% for T3 disease [14]. Chae et al. reviewed patterns of tumor recurrence in 194 patients and found that 21% of patients recurred in a mean time of 17 months. Eighty-three percent of those who recurred were diagnosed within the first 2 years after surgery, and the rate of recurrence was higher for patients with tumor size of >5 cm [39].

Literature published in 2013 demonstrated the impact of length of survival on future survival probability, otherwise known as conditional survival [40]. In this series, 42,090 patients from the Surveillance, Epidemiology, and End Results (SEER) database who underwent nephrectomy from 1988 to 2008 were reviewed, and the 5-year cancer-specific survival rate immediately following surgery was reported to be 83.5%. For those patients surviving ≥1, ≥2, ≥3, ≥4, and ≥ 5 years after nephrectomy, the probabilities of surviving an additional 5 years were 87.0%, 89.6%, 90.9%, 92.0%, and 92.3%. Even patients with advanced disease had a more favorable prognosis if they had already survived 1–2 years. However, other findings suggest relapses occur more than 5 years post-operatively, and patients with lower risk disease are more likely to have a later recurrence. Stewart and colleagues sought to assess the guidelines to capture 100% of recurrences with appropriate surveillance duration. Using the 2014 AUA recommendations and 2014 NCCN recommendations, 66.9% and 68.2% of recurrences would have been detected at a median follow up of 9 years. The authors found that to capture 95% of stage pT1 recurrences, patients would need to be followed for 15 years after a partial nephrectomy, 21 years after a radical nephrectomy, and they would have to be surveilled for 14 years to capture 95% of recurrences in patients with pT2-4 N0–1 disease.

This should be balanced with cost, patient expectations, and life expectancy or competing comorbidities. The Medicare cost of surveillance of a patient with pT1 disease using the 2014 NCCN surveillance guidelines is $2131.52 in 2014, and to capture 95% of recurrences, the surveillance cost would escalate to $9856.82 in 2014.

Over the last decade, data have emerged that support the addition of other important prognostic factors to models that predict postoperative recurrence of RCC. In 2001, Kattan and colleagues at MSKCC constructed a nomogram to predict 5-year disease-free survival rates following radical or partial nephrectomy. In addition to tumor stage, tumor size, histology, and symptomatic presentation were analyzed for 601 patients and determined to be important prognostic factors influencing disease recurrence [41].

Tumor size has been demonstrated to be an independent predictor of disease-free survival [42–44]. Five-year survival rates in one publication were reported to be 84% for tumors less than 5 cm, 50% for tumors 5–10 cm, and 0% in tumors greater than 10 cm [45]. In a follow-up study, the MSKCC group also confirmed the importance of tumor size in predicting disease recurrence independent of pathologic stage [46].

Histology by itself has also been shown to predict disease-specific survival and effect recurrence patterns. Of the four most common subtypes of RCC, chromophobe RCC confers a better prognosis than conventional (clear cell) RCC or papillary RCC [47]. Papillary type II, however, has been shown to independently predict poor survival [48, 49]. The presence of sarcomatoid dedifferentiation on final pathology indicates poor prognosis and has been utilized in risk-stratification algorithms to predict disease recurrence [50, 51]. A subgroup analysis of the phase 3 ECOG-ACRIN E2805 trial evaluated patterns of recurrence for patients with high-risk non-clear cell renal cell carcinoma. Patients enrolled in this trial had complete resection of their localized disease and received adjuvant therapy with sunitinib, sorafenib, or placebo. Although 5-year recurrence rates were similar between patients with ccRCC and non-clear cell RCC, patients with non-clear cell RCC had higher rates of abdominal recurrences and were less likely to recur in the chest [52].

The MSKCC group published an externally validated postoperative nomogram in 2004 that analyzed a cohort of 701 patients diagnosed specifically with clear cell RCC. The prognostic factors in this nomogram included tumor size, symptomatic presentation, pathologic stage, Fuhrman grade, presence of necrosis, and presence of microvascular invasion [46]. Both Fuhrman grade and microvascular invasion were predictive of disease-free survival on multivariate analysis.

Other literature has also confirmed the importance of Fuhrman grade, microvascular invasion, and necrosis in predicting disease recurrence [42, 53, 54]. The group from Mayo Clinic constructed a scoring system, SSIGN, based on tumor stage, tumor size, Fuhrman grade, and presence of tumor necrosis. All four factors were predictive of cancer-specific survival on multivariate analysis and used in an algorithm to predict clinical outcomes [53].

Authors from University of California Los Angeles (UCLA) demonstrated the importance of the Eastern Cooperative Oncology Group (ECOG) performance status score in predicting overall survival. Based on stage, grade, and ECOG performance status, they established a risk classification system predicting 2- and 5-year survival rates [55]. This model was later used to create a surveillance strategy that has been recommended by the NCCN and is widely used today [22].

A preoperative nomogram from MSKCC and Mayo clinic was published in 2008, which was developed after reviewing clinicopathologic factors and outcomes of 2517 patients. Gender, symptomatic presentation, lymphadenopathy by imaging, tumor necrosis, and tumor size were used to create a preoperative nomogram predicting disease-free recurrence at 12 years [54].

Other nomograms and predictive tools have been previously reported and will be the subject of a separate chapter in this book.

Surveillance Following Radical or Partial Nephrectomy in Patients with Sporadic RCC

Since the early 1990s, multiple investigators have used their institutional databases to put forth recommendations for postoperative surveillance for patients with RCC. These will be described in detail in this section and summarized in Table 20.1.

In 1994, Montie et al. proposed a 5-year surveillance protocol that included physical exam,

Table 20.1 Surveillance guidelines after nephrectomy and partial nephrectomy

	Clinical assessment (history, physical exam, laboratory studies)	Chest X-ray	Abdominal CT
pT1			
Sandock (1995) [16]	Not specified	Not recommended	Not recommended
Hafez (1997) [13]	Yearly	Not recommended	Not recommended
Levy (1998) [14]	Yearly	Yearly	Not recommended
Ljunberg (1999)[a] [15]	Not recommended	Not recommended	Not recommended
Mickisch (2001) [56]	Every 6 months for 3 years, then yearly from years 3 to 5	Every 6 months for 3 years, then yearly from years 3 to 5	Not recommended
Stephenson (2004) [57]	Yearly	Yearly	Not recommended
Novick (2005) [58]	Yearly	Not recommended	Not recommended
Kassouf (2009) [59]	Yearly	Yearly	At years 2, 5 (optional at 3 months)
pT2			
Sandock (1995) [16]	Every 6 months for 3 years, then yearly	Every 6 months for 3 years and then yearly	Not recommended
Hafez (1997) [13]	Yearly	Yearly	Every 2 years
Levy (1998) [14]	Every 6 months for 3 years, then yearly	Every 6 months for 3 years and then yearly	At years 2, 5
Ljunberg (1999)[b] [15]	At 3 and 6 months and then every 6 months until 3 years and then yearly	At 3 and 6 months, then every 6 months until 3 years, and then yearly	Not recommended

(continued)

Table 20.1 (continued)

	Clinical assessment (history, physical exam, laboratory studies)	Chest X-ray	Abdominal CT
Mickisch (2001) [56]	Every 6 months for 3 years and then yearly from years 3 to 5	Every 6 months for 3 years and then yearly from years 3 to 5	Not recommended
Stephenson (2004) [57]	Yearly	Yearly	Not recommended
Novick (2005) [58]	Yearly	Yearly	Every 2 years
Kassouf (2009) [59]	Every 6 months for 3 years and then yearly	Every 6 months for 3 years and then yearly	12, 36, 60, 80, and 108 months
pT3			
Sandock (1995) [16]	Every 6 months for 3 years and then yearly	Every 6 months for 3 years and then yearly	Not recommended
Hafez (1997) [13]	Yearly	Yearly	Every 6 months until 2 years and then every 2 years
Levy (1998) [14]	At 3 and 6 months, then every 6 months until 3 years, and then yearly	At 3 and 6 months, then every 6 months until 3 years, and then yearly	At years 2, 5
Ljunberg (1999) [15]	At 3 and 6 months, then every 6 months until 3 years, and then yearly	At 3 and 6 months, then every 6 months until 3 years, and then yearly	At 6 and 12 months (optional)
Mickisch (2001) [56]	Every 6 months for 3 years and then yearly from years 3 to 10	Every 6 months for 3 years and then yearly from years 3 to 10	Every 6 months for 3 years and then yearly from years 3 to 10
Stephenson (2004) [57]	Every 6 months for 3 years and then yearly	Every 6 months for 3 years and then yearly	At 6, 12, 24, and 36 months and then every 2 years
Novick (2005) [58]	Yearly	Yearly	Every 6 months for 2 years and then every 2 years
Kassouf (2009) [59]	Every 6 months for 3 years and then yearly	Every 6 months for 3 years and then yearly	At 6, 12, 18, 24, 36, and 60 months and then every 2 years
UCLA risk groups [22]			
Low risk	Yearly	Yearly for 5 years	At years 2, 4
Intermediate risk	Every 6 months for 3 years and then yearly until 10 years	Every 6 months for 3 years and then yearly until 10 years	At years 1 and 2 and then every 2 years for 10 years
High risk	Every 6 months for 3 years and then yearly until 10 years	Every 6 months for 3 years and then yearly until 10 years	Every 6 months for 2 years, then yearly until 5 years, and then every 2 years until 10 years
Nodal disease	At 3, 6, 12, 18, and 24 months and then yearly	At 3, 6, 12, 18, and 24 months and then yearly	At 3, 6, 12, 18, and 24 months and then yearly

[a] Includes pT1 tumors < 5 cm, pT1 diploid, and pT2 diploid
[b] Includes pT1 > 5 cm aneuploid/ploidy not assessed or pT2 aneuploid/ploidy not assessed

laboratory studies, and CXR every 6 months as well as an abdominal CT at 12, 24, and 48 months, independent of pathologic stage after nephrectomy [60]. While more metastases are potentially detected using this unselected schedule, one has to keep in mind the cost-effectiveness of such an approach, as well as potential radiation risk.

In 1995, in order to sub-select surveillance tools based on stage, Sandock and colleagues [16] from Case Western Reserve University retrospectively reviewed 137 patients without nodal or metastatic disease at presentation who underwent radical nephrectomy between 1979 and 1993. Nineteen patients were pT1 and had no recurrence at a mean follow-up of 44.4 months. Eighty-two patients were pT2 and 15.9% recurred at mean of 29.5 months. Thirty-six patients were pT3 and 52.8% recurred at mean of 22 months. Of those patients who experienced recurrence, chest metastases occurred in 53.8% (7 of 13) of patients with pT2 and 63.2% (12 of 19) with pT3. For patients with pT2 and pT3 disease, 71% (5 of 7) and 75% (9 of 12), respectively, were specifically symptomatic with dyspnea, cough, hemoptysis, and/or pleuritic chest pain. Abdominal metastases occurred in 38.5% (5 of 13) of patients with pT2 and 42.1% (8 of 19) of patients with pT3. Twelve of these 13 patients with abdominal metastases (liver 8, local 3, both 2) had signs or symptoms of metastatic disease. Bone metastases developed in 38.5% (5 of 13) patients with pT2 and 26.4% (5 of 19) patients with pT3, and all 10 patients with bone metastases presented with bone pain that prompted further workup. Brain metastases developed in two patients with pT2 and four patients with pT3. In all six patients, brain metastases were symptomatic with headaches or mental status changes. Lymphadenopathy occurred in 25% (3 of 13) patients with pT2 and 25% (5 of 19) patients with pT3, and all 8 recurrences were not isolated but were associated with other findings. Most recurrences (85%) occurred in the first 3 years after radical nephrectomy. From the authors' dataset, only 1 of the 137 patients they studied benefited from a routine CT scan. The authors concluded that bone scans and CT scans should not be routinely performed, and that follow-up should include only a history and physical examination in patients with pT1 disease. For patients with pT2 and pT3 disease, they recommended a history, physical examination, liver function tests, and chest X-rays every 6 months for the first 3 years and then yearly thereafter.

In 1997, Hafez et al. from Cleveland Clinic reported oncological outcomes for 327 patients who underwent partial nephrectomy prior to December 1994. Mean follow-up was 54 months and recurrence developed in a total of 38 patients (11.6%). Thirteen patients (4%) had local recurrence, of which seven also had distant metastatic disease. Twenty-five patients (7.6%) presented with metastatic disease in the absence of local recurrence. Incidences for local recurrence and metastatic disease by stage were 0 and 4.4% for T1, 2.0 and 5.3% for T2, 8.2 and 11.5% for T3a, and 10.6 and 14.9% for T3b. Local recurrence was most often diagnosed from 6 to 24 months and after 48 months. Based on these data, the authors recommended that all patients should undergo a yearly history, physical exam, and lab work. No imaging was recommended for patients with T1 disease since the risk of recurrence was found to be low; however, a yearly chest X-ray was recommended for patients with T2 and T3 disease as metastasis to the lung was more common in these groups. Occasional follow-up every 2 years with CT abdomen was suggested for patients with T2 disease, and since local recurrence is highest in T3 disease, the authors recommend CT abdomen every 6 months for the first 2 years and then every 2 years thereafter [13].

In 1998, Saidi and colleagues [61] from Columbia University reported on 45 patients that were enrolled in an adjuvant autolymphocyte therapy trial for N + M0 high-risk patients. Twelve patients were T2, 30 were T3, and 3 were T4. Sixty-four percent recurred after radical nephrectomy (29 of 45) at a mean of 14.9 months. Fourteen recurred in the retroperitoneal nodes at 13.9 months, eleven in the lung at 14.4 months, five in the liver at 14.9 months, five in the bone at 11.9 months, four in the mediastinal nodes at 11.8 months, three in the renal fossa at 6.9 months, and two in the brain at 20.7 months. Of those who had disease progression, 31% did so by 6 months, 59% by 12 months, 83% by 24 months, and 93% by 36 months. As such, the authors recommended routine chest X-ray and CT abdomen at least every 6 months for the first 3 years and then yearly. Given that this study involved very high-risk patients (node-positive), the follow-up recommended cannot be necessarily applied to the general population of patients with renal cell carcinoma treated with surgery.

In 1998, Levy and colleagues [14] from MD Anderson Cancer Center proposed postoperative surveillance guidelines stratified by stage and based on 286 patients who were surgically treated for renal cell carcinoma without nodal or distant metastases between 1985 and 1994. At a median follow-up of 23 months, 68 patients developed metastatic disease in a total of 92 sites. Eight of 113 patients with pT1, 17 of 64 patients with pT2, and 43 of 109 patients with pT3 developed metastases at a median of 38 months, 32 months, and 17 months, respectively. Sixty-four percent (59 of 92) of the metastases were asymptomatic (32 detected on chest X-ray and 12 on routine laboratory studies). Only six patients (9%) had an isolated intraabdominal metastasis without associated symptoms. All brain metastases presented with neurological symptoms that prompted further evaluation. In the eight pT1 patients with recurrent disease, four were in the chest (lung), two in the bone, and one each in the brain and uvula. In the 17 pT2 patients with recurrence, 9 were in the chest (lung), 5 in the abdomen (liver 2, lymph node 1, adrenal 1, pancreas 1), 3 in the bone, and 1 in the brain. In the 43 pT3 patients, 18 were in the chest (lung, 18% diagnosed <6 months after surgery), 10 in the abdomen (local 4, liver 4, adrenal 2), 7 in the bone, 5 in the lymph nodes (detected on physical examination), and 3 in the brain. Eleven of the pT3 patients were diagnosed with metastases <6 months after surgery. The authors suggested starting with abdominal CTs no earlier than 24 months after surgery, as in their experience, all 344 CT scans done in the first 24 months of surveillance did not yield any useful information. For patients with pT2 disease the authors recommended history, physical exam, laboratory studies, and chest X-ray at 12, 24, 36, 48, and 60 months after surgery for pT1 and history, physical exam, laboratory studies, and chest X-ray at 6, 12, 18, 24, 30, 36, 48, and 60 months and CT abdomen at 24 and 60 months for pT2. Recommended follow-up for pT3 was similar to pT2, with the addition of history, physical exam, laboratory studies, and chest X-ray at 3 months after surgery.

In 1999, Ljundberg and colleagues [15] from Umeå University in Sweden developed a surveillance protocol based on stage, tumor size, and DNA ploidy. They retrospectively reviewed 187 patients with no clinical nodal or distant metastases treated with radical nephrectomy between 1982 and 1997. Fifty-six patients developed a total of 98 metastases at a median of 14.5 months after radical nephrectomy. Thirty-seven were in the chest (lung), 24 were in the bone, 21 were intraabdominal (11 liver, 7 local or retroperitoneal, 3 abdominal), 4 were in the brain, 3 were in the skin, and 9 in other sites. In 43% of the 56 patients, the metastases were discovered in the first year, in 70% in the first 2 years, in 80% in the first 3 years, and in 93% in the first 5 years after surgery. Seven percent (5 of 70) of patients with T1 experienced a recurrence at a median of 40 months; however, all these patients had tumors larger than 5 cm in size. 14% (6 of 43) of patients with pT2 recurred at median of 8 months, 55% (26 of 48) of patients recurred at median of 12 months, and 73% (19 of 26) recurred at a median of 15 months. Of the 11 recurrences in patients with pT1 and pT2, 6 were in the lung (only 1 symptomatic) and 5 were in the bone (all symptomatic). In patients with pT3, only 1 of 24 lung recurrences was symptomatic, while all 10 bones, all 5 livers, and both liver recurrences were symptomatic. Patients with pT1–T2 homogenously diploid tumors did not experience a recurrence, while ploidy did not affect patient outcomes in patients with stage pT3. Based on these findings, the authors recommend no follow-up for patients with pT1 tumors <5 cm, pT1 diploid, and pT2 diploid. Physical examination, laboratory studies, and chest X-ray at 3, 6, 12, 18, 24, 30, 36, 48, and 60 months were recommended for patients with pT1 > 5 cm aneuploid/ploidy not assessed or pT2 aneuploid/ploidy not assessed and a similar follow-up as the latter category with the addition of optional CT abdomen and bone scan at 6 and 12 months for patients with pT3 or N1 disease.

In 2001, Mickisch and colleagues [56] from Erasmus University Rotterdam reviewed multiple publications [13, 14, 16] and established a follow-up protocol. For patients with pT1 and pT2 disease, the authors recommended history, physical exam, laboratory studies, and a chest

X-ray every 6 months for the first 3 years and then yearly until 5 years. Abdominal CT was not recommended for this group. More intense follow-up for a longer period of time was recommended for patients with pT3 disease. A clinical assessment, chest X-ray, and abdominal CT were recommended every 6 months for the first 3 years then yearly up to 10 years [56].

In 2003, Frank and colleagues [62] from Mayo clinic retrospectively reviewed 1864 patients treated with partial or radical nephrectomy in the absence of distant metastases and defined recurrence locations into four major categories: chest, abdomen, bone, and brain. 16% (300 patients) recurred in the chest at a median of 1.6 years, 10% (185 patients) recurred in the abdomen at a median of 1.7 years, 7% (134 patients) recurred in bone at a median of 1.5 years, and 4% (81 patients) recurred in the brain at a median of 2.5 years. The authors then used analyses that included different combinations of risk factors (positive surgical margins, tumor stage, nodal status, size >10 cm, nuclear grade, tumor necrosis, sarcomatoid features, cystic architecture, and multifocality) to devise scoring systems that predicted the risk of metastases into each of these four locations. One important finding, in line with other studies, is that 98.2% of brain metastases and 90.5% of bone metastases were symptomatic at presentation, obviating the need for routine surveillance for these sites in the absence of specific symptoms. The authors, however, did not recommend a particular surveillance schedule based on these findings and recommended that the clinician should decide on the appropriate follow-up scheme on an individual basis that considers the scoring system as well as individual patient characteristics such as age and comorbidities among others.

In 2004, Stephenson and colleagues [57] retrospectively reviewed 495 patients who underwent partial or radical nephrectomy in five Canadian centers. Sixty-seven patients had a recurrence after surgery (63 distant, and 12 local), and only 4 patients had an isolated local recurrence. 16 of 303 patients with pT1 relapsed at a median of 35 months, with 15 of these relapses being solitary. Thirteen patients had symptoms with or without a chest recurrence that would have been found on physical examination or chest X-ray. There were three asymptomatic (two after partial nephrectomy and one after radical nephrectomy) and one symptomatic abdominal recurrence. 14 of 84 patients with pT2 recurred at a median of 25 months. All these 14 patients had symptoms with or without a chest recurrence, and only 10 of 14 recurrences were solitary. 23 of 74 patients with pT3a recurred at 14 months (only 16 recurrences were solitary), and 14 of 34 patients with pT3b recurred at 8 months (only 8 recurrences were solitary). Based on their findings, the authors recommended annual history, physical examination, and chest X-ray in patients with pT1 or pT2 disease. They recommended that patients with pT3a or pT3b should be followed up every 6 months for the first 3 years with history, physical examination, and chest X-ray and then annual follow-up while obtaining CT abdomen at 6, 12, 24, and 36 months after surgery and then every 2 years afterward.

In 2005, Lam and colleagues from University of California Los Angeles [22] developed a postoperative surveillance protocol (UISS), an integrated risk stratification model that incorporates the 1997 TNM staging, Fuhrman grade, and ECOG status into five categories—and have been shown to predict outcomes in patients post-nephrectomy for RCC [55] (Fig. 20.1). This UISS model has been validated in subsequent studies [63, 64]. In this retrospective study [22], 559 patients with nonmetastatic RCC treated between 1988 and 2003 were reviewed and risk stratified according to the established UISS model (low risk, intermediate risk, high risk, and node positive). Recurrence patterns were then analyzed, and a surveillance protocol was constructed based on their findings. 92.8% of patients had localized disease, and 70% underwent radical nephrectomy. Median follow-up was 26 months (Fig. 20.2). Patients identified as low risk (N = 196) had an overall 5-year recurrence rate of 9.6%, with a median time to recurrence of 28.9 months. 87.5% (7 of 8) had a solitary recurrence. The chest was the most common site of recurrence in the low-risk group, accounting for 75% of the overall recurrences in this cohort.

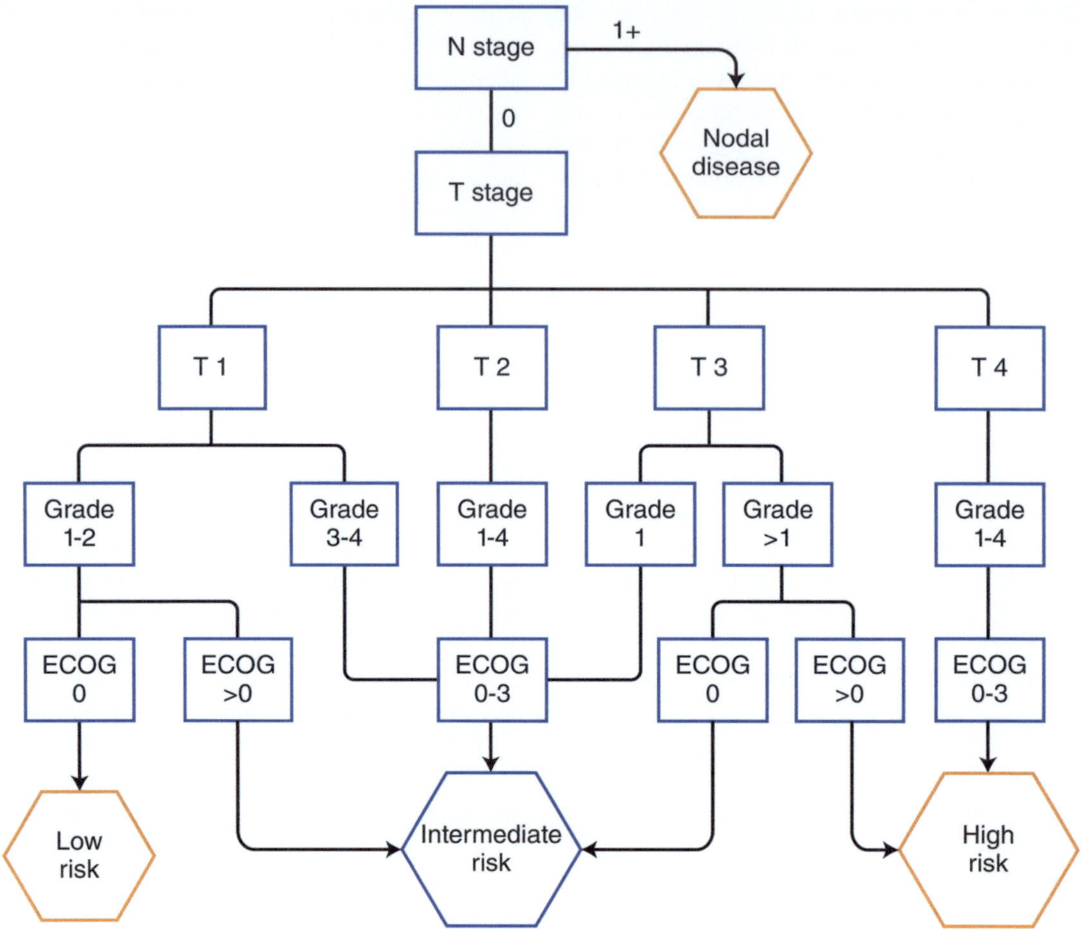

Fig. 20.1 Flowchart for UISS risk group assignment of patients with localized and locally advanced RCC. Progress from top to bottom using 1997 UICC N stage and T stage, Fuhrman grade, and ECOG-PS. (Reprinted from Lam et al. [22], with permission from Elsevier)

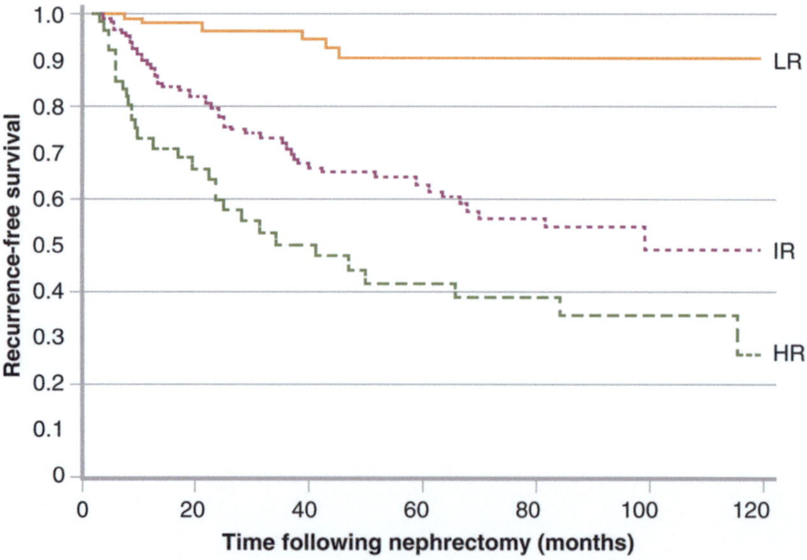

Fig. 20.2 Kaplan–Meier estimate of recurrence-free survival following nephrectomy among UISS risk groups. (Reprinted from Lam et al. [22], with permission from Elsevier)

Recurrence was most common in the first 3 years following nephrectomy with a median time to recurrence of 23.6 months. No pulmonary recurrences were diagnosed after 5 years. Abdominal recurrences comprised 37.5% of the recurrences with a median time to recurrence of 32 months. None of the abdominal recurrences in the low-risk group occurred before 20 months or after 5 years. For the intermediate risk group (*N*, 251), the 5-year recurrence rate was 38.2% at median time of 17.8 months. 40.5% (25 of 62) had solitary recurrence, 77.4% of the recurrences were discovered in the chest, and 58.1% in the abdomen. 41.7% of patients with chest metastasis were diagnosed in the first year, and of those, 70% were diagnosed between 6 months and 1-year post-nephrectomy and 58% of the abdominal recurrences were diagnosed within the first year, of which 66.6% were discovered between 6 months and 1 year after nephrectomy. 44% of the bone recurrences occurred within the first year, while 33% occurred after 5 years. Brain recurrences in this group were rare. Patients classified as high risk ($N = 72$) had a 5-year recurrence rate of 58.1% at a median time of 9.5 months. 74.2% (23 of 31) of the recurrences were solitary. The chest was the most frequent site of recurrence accounting for 45.5% of the recurrences. 50% of chest recurrences were diagnosed in the first year and 42.8% of those within the first 6 months after surgery. Seven percent of the chest recurrences were found on routine imaging after 5 years of follow-up. Abdominal recurrences including the renal fossa, liver, and other abdominal organs together comprised 68.2% of recurrences. Of these, 62% occurred within the first year and 61.5% of those within the first 6 months. Only 5% of abdominal recurrences were diagnosed after 5 years. Patients with lymph node-only metastasis experienced a 64% 5-year recurrence after surgery. Of those who recurred, 58.8% had a chest recurrence and 76.5% had an abdominal recurrence. In patients who recurred in the chest, recurrence occurred in 25%, 12.5%, 25%, and 37.5% at months 0–3, 3–6, 6–12, and 12–24 after surgery, respectively. In patients who recurred in the abdomen, recurrence occurred in 28.6%, 21.4%, and 28% at months 0–3, 3–6, and 12–24 after surgery, respectively. Based on these data, a surveillance protocol was constructed [19], outlining the optimal follow-up for patients post-nephrectomy as risk stratified according to the UISS model (Fig. 20.3).

A more recent publication assessed the accuracy of the UISS model in predicting postoperative recurrences by comparing it to a similar model that also incorporated patient age and tumor histology [65]. While patient age had no association with recurrence patterns, the average risk of recurrence within the first year of surgery significantly decreased across all UISS risk groups for patients with low-risk tumor types (papillary type 1 and chromophobe). Their data suggest that low-risk histology is a more

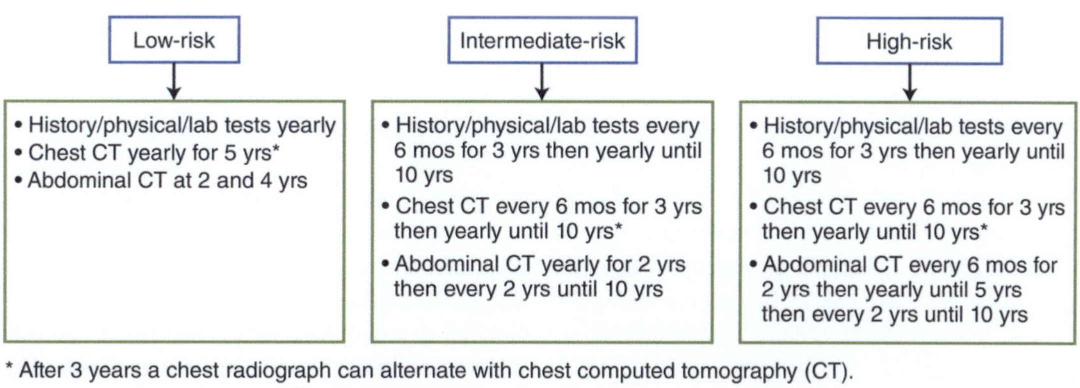

Fig. 20.3 Surveillance protocol following nephrectomy for localized renal cell carcinoma using the University of California Los Angeles Integrated Staging System. (Copyright © MedReviews®, LLC. Reprinted with permission of MedReviews®, LLC. Chin et al. [19]. *Reviews in Urology* is a copyrighted publication of MedReviews®, LLC. All rights reserved)

important predictor of recurrence than overall risk group and that these patients do not require the same degree of surveillance as patients with conventional clear cell renal cell carcinoma [65].

In 2005, Chae and colleagues from Asan Medical Center in Korea retrospectively reviewed 194 patients treated with surgery [39]. Twenty-one percent of patients experience disease recurrence at a mean of 17 months. Tumor recurred within 2 years after surgery in 34 (83%) patients. Disease recurrence occurred in the lung in 29, bone in 13, nephrectomy bed in 7, brain in 6, mediastinal lymph nodes in 5, liver in 5, contralateral kidney in 4, and the neck in 2. Patient with tumors >5 cm, stage III, or Fuhrman grade 3–4 had a higher risk of recurrence. With the lung being the most common site of metastasis in their series, the authors recommended that chest CT should be done every 6 months during the first 2 years after surgery and then annually for 2 years in patients with a high risk for tumor recurrence [39].

In 2009, Kassouf and colleagues from McGill University reviewed multiple series [2, 13–16, 20] before establishing the Canadian Urological Association guidelines for postoperative surveillance after nephrectomy [59]. The authors decided on a stage-based protocol to include a yearly history, physical exam, laboratory studies, and a chest X-ray for patients with pT1 disease. They recommend abdominal CT in this group at years 2 and 5, with an optional abdominal CT at 3 months and/or optional abdominal ultrasound yearly for patients who underwent partial nephrectomy. For patients with pT2 disease, history, physical exam, laboratory studies, and a chest X-ray were recommended every 6 months for 3 years and then yearly. Abdominal CT was recommended in this group at 12, 36, 60, 84, and 108 months postoperatively. Guidelines recommend the same follow-up in regard to clinical assessment and chest X-ray in patients with pT3 disease; however, abdominal CT should be done at 6, 12, 18, 24, 36, and 60 months and then continues every 2 years. For patients with node-positive disease, the authors recommended clinical assessment, chest X-ray, and abdominal CT at 3 and 6 months, every 6 months for 3 years, and then yearly [59].

In 2009, Siddiqui and colleagues from the Mayo Clinic [66] updated their prior surveillance protocol and included histological subtype as one of the additional risk factors for recurrence (in addition to the previously reported 1864 patients, the authors added 357 patients with papillary and 118 patients with chromophobe RCC). As such, tumor stage, grade, nodal status, margin status, and tumor necrosis were accounted for when recommending specific follow-up protocols. In addition, the authors recommended particular imaging at specific time intervals (Table 20.2), which was not provided in the prior manuscript in 2003 [62].

Stewart-Merrill et al. from the Mayo Clinic evaluated the performance of the 2014 NCCN and AUA guidelines at capturing recurrences after partial or radical nephrectomy. Despite guidelines being updated from previous versions to reflect a more risk-adapted approach, approximately one-third of recurrences were still missed [67]. The authors reviewed 1088 recurrences in patients who underwent partial or radial nephrectomy for RCC between 1970 and 2008 and determined that the 2014 NCCN guidelines would have detected 68.2% of recurrences, while the AUA guidelines would have detected only 66.9% of recurrences. They also estimated the cost of surveillance using both sets of guidelines and found that the older 2013 NCCN guidelines yielded a lower cost of $1228.79 (versus $3700.87 for the higher-risk patients using the 2014 NCCN guidelines); however captured only 35.9% of recurrences if strictly followed [67].

After exploring the performance of existing guidelines, the same group from the Mayo Clinic in 2015 proposed a risk-adapted individualized surveillance strategy. Using a median follow-up of 9 years, the authors identified 676 patients of 2511 who underwent surgery from 1990 to 2008 and had developed recurrence. By utilizing a competing-risk model, they found significant differences between patients depending on age, disease stage, comorbidities, and location of recurrence [68]. For example, patients age 80 or older with pT1Nx-0 disease and minimal comor-

Table 20.2 Postoperative surveillance guidelines based on histological subtype—Siddiqui 2009

	Clinical assessment (history, physical exam, laboratory studies)	Chest X-ray or CT	Abdominal CT or US
Clear cell RCC			
Low risk	Yearly	Every 6 months until year 2 and then yearly	CT at 18, 24, and 30 months and then year 5, 7, 10 US at year 3, 4, 6, 8, 9
Intermediate risk	Yearly	Every 3 months	CT at 6, 9, 12, 15, 24, 27, and 30 months and then yearly from years 4 to 10; US year 3
High risk	Yearly	Every 3 months for 1 year and then at years 2, 5	CT every 3 months until year 2, then every 6 months for 1 year, and then yearly from years 3 to 10
Papillary RCC			
Low risk	Yearly	Not recommended	CT at years 1, 2; US at 6, 9 months
Intermediate risk	Yearly	At 12, 18, 30, and 36 months and then yearly	CT year 3; US 6, 24 months and then every 2 years
High risk	Yearly	At 6, 9, 12, 18, and 24 months	CT at 6, 9, 12, 18, and 24 months and then every 2 years
Chromophobe RCC			
Low risk	Yearly	Not recommended	Not recommended
Intermediate risk	Yearly	Not recommended	CT year 3, 7; US year 5, 10
High risk	Yearly	At 6, 9, and 15 months	CT 3, 6 months and at year 7; US at year 3, 5, 10

bidities were at higher risk of an abdominal recurrence as compared with non-RCC death for 6 months after surgery but not after that time period, suggesting that follow-up beyond 6 months may not be warranted for this cohort. Conversely, for younger patients with the same stage disease and the same number of comorbidities, the risk of abdominal recurrence remained as high as the risk of non-RCC death, suggesting this patient population requires prolonged follow-up.

In 2018, a multicenter study used the European Association of Urology RECUR database to evaluate long-term outcomes in patients with localized RCC (PMID: 29525381). They also concluded that a better risk-adapted approach should be incorporated into contemporary surveillance protocols. The authors identified 131 potentially curable recurrences and 155 probably incurable recurrences in 1265 patients. The 5-year cumulative risk of recurrence for low-, intermediate-, and high-risk disease was 7.2%, 23.2%, and 61.6%, respectively. Of the high-risk patients that recurred, only 30.5% were potentially curable. Competing risk analysis revealed the highest risk of death in young and high-risk patients; however, comorbidities were not available for analysis. These findings highlight the need for more sophisticated surveillance modeling to capture potentially curable recurrences expeditiously while limiting over-imaging in patients with low risk of recurrence (PMID: 29525381).

Current NCCN, AUA, EAU and CUA Guidelines

Because pathologic stage has proven to be the most important prognostic factor for RCC to date, all four guideline panels have broken down surveillance recommendations into risk groups based on stage. High-quality studies are lacking; therefore, the follow-up recommendations are based on expert opinions. While the NCCN, AUA, and CUA guidelines classify all subtypes based on stage, the EAU uses different externally validated risk scoring systems for clear cell RCC and non-clear cell RCC, the 2003 Leibovich score and the UISS scoring systems (mentioned previously), respectively. Low-risk includes Leibovich score of 0–2 for clear cell RCC and a low-risk UISS score (T1N0M0 grade 1–2, ECOG performance status = 0) for non-clear cell RCC. Intermediate risk includes a Leibovich score of 3–5 for clear cell RCC and UISS intermediate risk disease. High-risk disease includes Leibovich score ≥6 for clear cell RCC or a high-risk UISS score (T3N0M0 grade 2–4, ECOG performance status ≥1 or T4N0M0) for non-clear cell RCC.

The NCCN guidelines [69] divide risk recommendations after partial or radical nephrectomy by stage I, II, and III. The CUA guidelines and AUA guidelines [70] have divided risk categories into four groups. The CUA guidelines divide groups by T stage and nodal status: Low risk is pT1, intermediate risk is pT2, high risk is pT3–4, very high risk is lymph node positive disease. The AUA guidelines divides risk categories by T stage, grade, and nodal status: Low risk is pT1, grade 1–2 disease; intermediate risk is pT1 grade 3–4 or pT2 disease; high risk is pT3, very high risk is pT4 or N1 disease or sarcomatoid or rhabdoid pathologic features or macroscopic positive margin. Each risk group has a progressively worse recurrence rate of 9.2%, 32%, 49% for low, intermediate, and high risk, respectively. Tumors with sarcomatoid features have a recurrence rate of 72% with a median time to recurrence of 26.2 months. The AUA panel also states that in the case of positive microscopic surgical margins, the surveillance protocol should follow one risk group higher than otherwise diagnosed and exercise increased clinical vigilance. The recurrence rate for a microscopic positive margin is 15.9% versus 3% in matched controls.

The components of surveillance including history and physical exam, laboratory studies, and chest and abdominal imaging are discussed previously. The follow-up schedule varies by risk group and by guideline. The NCCN guidelines recommend for stage I: annual history and physical, annual labs, baseline cross sectional imaging within 3–12 months postoperatively and then annually for 5 years. Follow up for stage II disease includes annual history and physical and laboratory studies, baseline cross sectional imaging every 6 months for 2 years then annually for 5 years. CXR or CT chest should be performed annually for 5 years for both stage I and II disease. More rigorous follow up is suggested for both stage I and II disease in the setting of positive margins, high grade disease (grades 3–4) or sarcomatoid features. The recommended follow up for stage III RCC includes history and physical and laboratory studies every 3–6 months for 3 years then annually for 5 years, baseline cross sectional imaging within 3–6 months followed by surveillance imaging every 3–6 months for 3 years, then annually for 5 years. A CT chest should be performed within 3–6 months then every 3–6 months for 3 years and annually for up to 5 years. The NCCN emphasizes no single follow-up schedule is appropriate for every patient.

The EAU guidelines for low-risk disease recommend follow-up with evaluation of renal function studies and cardiovascular risk factors, and CT scan of the abdomen and chest at 6 months, 18, months, and 30 months. After 3 years, the panel recommends stopping surveillance or obtaining follow up every 2 years. For intermediate risk of recurrence, the panel recommends follow up with the above at 6 months, 12 months, 24, months, 36 months, annually from 3–5 years. After 5 years the panel recommends stopping surveillance or continuing with follow-up every 2 years. For high risk of recurrence, the panel recommends follow up with the above at 3 months, 6 months, 12 months, 18 months, 24 months, and 36 months. After 3 years, they recommend yearly follow-up until 5 years and obtaining follow up every 2 years thereafter.

The CAU guidelines recommended surveillance for the low-risk group includes history and physical, blood test and CXR annually, and abdominal imaging at 24 and 60 months. For the intermediate risk group, they recommend history and physical, laboratory studies, and CXR or CT chest every 6 months for 3 years, then annually until 5 years, and abdominal imaging annually for 5 years. For the high-risk group, the panel recommends history and physical, laboratory studies, CXR or CT chest and cross sectional abdominal imaging every 6 months for 2 years, then history and physical and laboratory and chest imaging at 30, 36, 48, and 60 months and abdominal imaging every other year for 5 years. For the very high-risk group the panel recommends follow up with history and physical, laboratory studies, CXR or CT chest, and cross sectional abdominal imaging at 3 and 6 months, then every 6 months for the first 3 years, then annually until 5 years.

The AUA guidelines follow up schedule for low-risk disease is at 12, 24, 48, and 60 months followed by every other year for 10 years. For intermediate risk disease the panel recommends follow up at 6 and 12 months and then annually for 5 years and every other year for 10 years. For high risk of recurrence groups, the panel recommends follow-up every 6 months for 3 years, then annually for 5 years and every 2 years for 10 years. For the very high-risk group, the panel recommends follow-up every 3 months for 2 years, every 6 months for the third year, annually for 5 years, and every 2 years for 10 years. For low- and intermediate-risk groups, the panel recommends chest imaging with CXR and for high and very high-risk groups, the panel recommends CT chest for the first 5 years and after 5 years surveillance a CXR is acceptable given most pulmonary metastasis presents within 5 years.

When to Stop Surveillance

The length of surveillance is currently under scrutiny. 30% of recurrences are diagnosed after 60 months and surveillance for 10 years will detect 90% of recurrences [31]; therefore surveillance after 5 years may be valuable in select patients. Additionally, patients with lower risk disease are more likely to relapse later. The AUA guidelines provide a suggested surveillance schedule for up to 10 years but state that informed decision-making should guide surveillance after 5 years. The NCCN guidelines suggest that after 5 years a clinician considers continuing surveillance with increasing intervals of abdominal imaging for all stages and chest imaging for higher stage disease at increasing intervals based on competing sources for mortality, performance status, risk factors, and patient preference. A history and physical and laboratory studies to evaluate renal function should be performed by a primary care physician annually. The EAU guidelines recommend terminating oncological follow-up for low-risk profiles >3 years and intermediate risk >5 years post-operatively, but the decision should be based on assessing comorbidities, life expectancy, and patient preferences. The CAU guidelines state surveillance beyond 5 years is optional and can be risk-adapted at the physician's discretion.

Surveillance for Hereditary RCC

Patients with familial forms of renal cell carcinoma have a high risk of recurrence and often require multiple nephron-sparing surgeries to treat their disease process. Steinbach et al. [71] conducted a multi-institutional study that reviewed 65 patients with von Hippel-Lindau (VHL) disease. Sixteen patients underwent radical nephrectomy and 49 underwent partial nephrectomy with a mean follow-up of 68 months. Fifty-one percent of patients who underwent partial nephrectomy had local recurrence in the ipsilateral kidney at a mean follow-up of 99 months and required further surgical intervention. Given the high risk of recurrence in patients with hereditary forms of RCC and the potential for multiple further surgeries, the relationship between tumor size and risk of developing metastatic disease was evaluated. Duffey et al. [72] reported metastatic disease occurring in 27% of patients who had renal masses >3 cm, whereas no patients with tumors <3 cm were found to have evidence of metastasis. Therefore, active surveillance in this patient population has been recommended without surgical intervention until the largest tumor size approaches 3 cm. In patients who are diagnosed specifically with VHL, screening for other manifestations of their disease process is also warranted. The NIH recommends checking urinary catecholamines every 1–2 years from age 2, yearly ophthalmoscopy starting from birth, contrast-enhanced MR imaging of the brain and spine every 2 years starting at age 11 and then every 3–5 years from age 60, abdominal ultrasound yearly from age 11, and then CT abdomen every 1–2 years after age 20 [73].

Surveillance Following Ablative Therapies for RCC

As an increasing number of elderly patients with multiple medical comorbidities are diagnosed with renal masses, minimally invasive nephron-sparing ablative therapies have become more popular as an alternative to partial nephrectomy. Ablative technologies include radiofrequency ablation (RFA), cryoablation, microwave, high-intensity focused ultrasound, laser interstitial thermotherapy, and radiotherapy [74–77].

The two most established ablative modalities being utilized for the definitive treatment of small renal masses are RFA and cryoablation. Data exist to support good short-term cancer control following ablative therapy, and literature reports promising intermediate-term outcomes [33, 78–82]. Oncological success following ablative therapy is defined as a lack of contrast enhancement and absence of tumor growth on follow-up CT or MRI imaging. Currently, a universal protocol for post-ablation imaging is undefined. Surveillance strategies following ablative therapies for RCC are therefore at the discretion of the individual physician and vary based on the institution or according to individual patient characteristics.

Radiofrequency Ablation

Contrast imaging with CT or MRI is used post-ablation to monitor oncological success of treatment. Initially, following therapy, the lesion visualized on CT is slightly larger. Over time, the lesions decrease in size at a rate slower than seen in lesions treated with cryoablation [83]. Unenhanced areas seen on CT correlate with tissue necrosis, and often a hyperattenuating halo around the defect can also be seen [84]. On MRI, the lesion is also initially larger with some minimal decrease in size over time, when compared to the original tumor size. T2-weighted images reveal the ablation defect to be hypointense, and on T1, it appears hyperintense relative to the renal cortex. There can also be a slight rim of enhancement seen initially on contrast-enhanced T1-weighted imaging; however, this becomes barely present after 3 months. Any persistent enhancement on gadolinium-enhanced MRI after 3 months or increase in tumor size is consistent with residual disease until proven otherwise [84, 85].

Despite promising data reporting favorable oncological outcomes, some studies have questioned the effectiveness of radiofrequency ablation. Rendon et al. compared pathological outcomes after RFA in 10 patients with a mean tumor size of 2.4 cm. Partial or radical nephrectomy was performed in four patients with five renal masses immediately following intraoperative RFA of the renal mass. Six patients underwent percutaneous RFA and then delayed nephrectomy 7 days later. Pathologic evaluation of the nephrectomy specimens revealed residual viable tumor in four of five specimens in the acute group and three of six specimens in the delayed group [86]. The group from Cleveland Clinic also investigated the presence of residual viable tumor following RFA. They discovered that 46% of patients in their cohort had a positive biopsy 6 months following RFA despite the lack of enhancement demonstrated on CT or MRI [87]. The discrepancy between radiographic imaging and pathologic findings following RFA has made it difficult to determine the success of therapy based on imaging alone. However, accurate interpretation of the pathologic specimen has also been questioned and surmised to be time-dependent (i.e. not all positive pathology following RFA indicates true presence of disease). RFA causes heat fixation of tumor cells—a process that preserves atypical cellular architecture and delays degeneration and can make it difficult to distinguish treatment effect from viable tumor [88]. The time period in which cellular degeneration is complete is debated in the literature, and further study is needed to reconcile these inconsistencies. Most investigators agree that biopsies should be done at least 6 months after RFA, when clinically indicated, to minimize false-positive results and avoid misinterpretation. However, there are currently no guidelines to support routine biopsy following RFA when recurrence or residual disease is not suspected radiographically [87].

Cryoablation

Since cryoablation does not uniformly freeze the lesion, most clinicians use a 1 cm margin beyond the tumor edge to ensure the entire tumor reaches the critical temperature for successful treatment [89]. Unlike RFA, histologic evaluation post-cryoablation reveals a fibrotic scar with inflammatory changes, and there is no preservation of tumor or normal renal parenchymal cellular architecture [33].

On CT imaging immediately following cryoablation, the lesion appears as a larger hypoattenuating defect. Over time, lesions decrease in size at a rate faster than that of RFA-treated lesions. Cryoablated tumors appear isointense to hyperintense on T1-weighted MR images and hypointense on T2 images [84]. It is not uncommon to see complete resolution of the ablation defect on follow-up imaging. Rukstalis et al. described 20 of 23 patients as having complete resolution of the treated mass or small residual scar on MRI at 3 months [90]. Gill et al. reported a 75% reduction in defect size over 3 years, with no evidence of scar detected in 38% of patients [91].

As many institutions began to incorporate minimally invasive ablative therapies into their treatment modalities for small renal masses, the accuracy of follow-up imaging to detect disease recurrence and the optimal timing of surveillance came into question. As with radiofrequency ablation, several groups set out to validate the definition of radiographic success following cryoablation. Weight et al. [87] investigated the correlation of radiographic imaging and histopathology following ablative therapy for renal masses. One hundred percent of the cryoablation cohort who had no evidence of enhancement on post-ablation imaging also had negative biopsies. A total of six positive biopsies were obtained from the cryoablation cohort, and all of these came from tumors that demonstrated some degree of enhancement. Peripheral enhancement was observed in 26 lesions at 6-month follow-up and of those only 2 yielded positive biopsies. There were 11 centrally enhancing lesions identified on imaging at 6 months and positive biopsies were found in 4 of those patients. The sensitivity of central enhancement on 6-month follow-up to predict a positive biopsy following cryoablation was 77.8%, with 95% specificity, 63.4% PPV, and 97.7% NPV [87].

A series by Beemster et al. concluded that at 6 months following cryoablation, persistent rim enhancement occurred in 20% of cryolesions with a size reduction of 38% despite negative histopathological diagnosis. The rim enhancement disappeared on further follow-up imaging, and the authors concluded that persistent rim enhancement is common in the first few months following cryoablation and routine biopsies are not justified [92].

Recommendations for Surveillance Following Radiofrequency Ablation or Cryoablation

Given the variation in follow-up protocols after ablative therapy and the lack of a universal surveillance strategy, Matin et al. conducted a multi-institutional study with the objective of providing evidence-based recommendations [93]. In this retrospective review of data from seven institutions (Table 20.3), recurrence patterns were reviewed for 616 patients who underwent RFA or cryoablation. Residual disease was defined as enhancement seen on the first CT or MRI following ablative therapy. Recurrent disease was any enhancement demonstrated after an initial negative imaging study. Residual or recurrent disease occurred in a total of 63 patients, 55 of 410 (13.4%) undergoing RFA and 8 of 206 (3.9%) undergoing cryoablation. Approximately, 70% of residual or recurrent disease was detected within the first 3 months of surveillance imaging, and

Table 20.3 Examples of surveillance protocols following ablative therapy of renal masses

	Preferred imaging modality and schedule	Technology used and year started	Access route	Routine biopsy on follow-up
Case Western Reserve University	MRI Week 2, month 3, 6, 9, 12, and then biannually	RFA, 1999	Percutaneous	No
Cleveland Clinic	MRI Day 1, month 1, 3, 6, 12, and then yearly	Cryoablation, 1999; RFA, 2002;	Percutaneous; laparoscopic	Yes; at 6 months
Fox Chase Cancer Center	CT Month 1, 3, 6, 12 and then every 6 months	RFA and cryoablation, 2002	Percutaneous and laparoscopic	No
Massachusetts General Hospital	CT Month 1, 3, 6 and 12 and then every 6–12 months	RFA, 1998	Percutaneous	No
M. D. Anderson Cancer Center	CT Month 1, 3, 6, 12 and then every 6–12 months	RFA, 2001; cryoablation, 2002	Percutaneous and laparoscopic	No
Southwestern Medical Center	CT Week 6, month 6, 12, and then yearly	RFA, 2001	Percutaneous and laparoscopic	No
Wake Forest University	CT Month 2, 8 and then every 6 months	RFA, 2000	Percutaneous	No

Reprinted from Matin et al. [93], with permission from Elsevier

92% was detected within the first year of surveillance following ablative therapy. Of the 63 patients who had residual or recurrent disease, 46 underwent salvage ablative therapy and 37 patients had no further evidence of disease on follow-up imaging. Metastasis-free survival for the patients who had recurrent or residual disease following ablative therapy was 97.4% at 2 years. Survival did not differ based on type of approach (laparoscopic versus percutaneous) or ablative modality utilized (RFA versus cryoablation) [93].

Based on these findings, a minimum schedule of three–four imaging studies was recommended in the first year following ablative therapy for renal masses. A CT scan or MRI without and with intravenous contrast is recommended in months 1, 3, 6 (optional), and 12.

Multiple guideline panels have established follow-up protocols after ablative therapies. The NCCN guidelines recommend an annual history and physical, laboratory data, and abdominal CT or MRI without and with IV contrast or contrast-enhanced ultrasound at 1–3 months post-procedure, 6 months, 12 months then annually. Chest imaging with CXR or CT chest is recommended yearly for 5 years if the disease is biopsy proven low-risk disease (grade 1–2) and harbors no sarcomatoid features, or if it was a non-diagnostic biopsy, or if no biopsy was performed. The CAU guideline panel recommends history and physical, laboratory studies and abdominal imaging at 3, 6, and 12 months, then annually for up to 5 years and annual CXR for 5 years. The AUA guideline panel recommends obtaining abdominal cross sectional imaging with and without IV contrast within 6 months post-operatively, and subsequent surveillance follows the protocol for intermediate risk disease.

The Future of Surveillance

The Incorporation of Molecular Markers into Surveillance Strategies

In the current era of targeted therapy, research efforts have focused on the molecular biology of renal cell carcinoma and the impact of individual molecular markers on diagnosis, prognostication, and surveillance. Several prognostic algorithms exist based on clinicopathologic factors that predict disease progression and survival with acceptable accuracy [94]. The addition of molecular markers to clinicopathologic factors has been shown, in limited studies, to improve accuracy of these prognostic models.

Many molecular biomarkers have been identified and demonstrated to predict cancer-specific survival as well as disease progression in patients with renal cell carcinoma. To name a few, Nogueria and Kim provide a thorough review of all prognostic molecular markers [95], and Crispen et al. evaluated the markers IMP-3, CXCR3, p53, Survivin, cIAP1, B7-H1, and B7-H4 that specifically predict disease progression following nephrectomy [94]. However, these are not in routine clinical use and are mainly limited to research studies. On the other hand, clinically available markers, such as C-reactive protein, have been shown to have potential in identifying patients at risk of recurrence after definitive surgery [96] and should be further validated in external cohorts. Recently, in 2014, Abel et al. evaluated immunohistochemical staining of a tissue microarray for 216 patients with renal cell carcinoma who underwent partial or radical nephrectomy. The authors reported Ki-67 to be an independent predictor of metastatic disease recurrence [97]. PTEN, Bcl-2, E-cadherins, microRNAs (miR-21 and miR-126) have also demonstrated potential prognostic utility. Other studies that have evaluated biomarkers as prognostic factors will be covered in a separate chapter.

Despite the valuable prognostic information that molecular markers confer, they also have several limitations in clinical practice. Most biomarkers that have been identified require histopathologic examination of the tumor specimen. In addition, the cost, reproducibility, need for special expertise, commercial availability of the antibodies, and lack of large-scale external validation limit the use of these biomarkers in clinical practice at present. Future research efforts should focus on identifying important molecular markers in the serum or urine that could potentially play a valuable role in identifying early diagnosis of disease recurrence as well as measure response of individuals to systemic therapy [94].

Cost of Surveillance

In the current economic climate, increasing healthcare utilization and cost has been extensively scrutinized. The goal of an ideal surveillance protocol is to accurately detect the presence of disease progression in a timely fashion while minimizing the cost and radiation risk associated with unnecessary over-imaging. Levy et al. reviewed the number and cost of CT scans performed 24 months following nephrectomy in 286 patients. A total of 344 CT scans were completed in the first 2 years following nephrectomy, 95 CT scans for patients with pT1 disease, 102 for patients with pT2 disease, and 147 for those with pT3 disease. Each CT was estimated to cost $1200 for a total cost of $412,800 [14].

Dion et al. performed a cost analysis comparison of two surveillance strategies in a Canadian cohort [101]. The authors compared the follow-up practices performed at their own institution with a projected cost of surveillance had they followed the 2009 Canadian Urological Association (CUA) guidelines. Mean follow-up was 31 months for 75 patients who had undergone nephrectomy for localized renal cell carcinoma. They concluded that total medical costs, in Canadian dollars, were higher for their institutional strategy than the CUA guidelines ($181,861 versus $135,054). Interestingly, when analyzing cost by tumor stage, the cost to survey patients with pT1 tumors at the authors' institution was more expensive than the calculated cost based on the CUA guidelines, whereas the cost to survey patients with pT3 tumors was more expensive as estimated by the CUA guidelines than their institutional strategy. This was likely secondary to over-imaging patients with pT1 tumors who may have had little indication for CT scan with low risk of abdominal recurrence [101].

Siddiqui et al. [66] performed cost analysis comparing the Mayo surveillance protocol to a traditional scheme, as well as other published work [14–16, 22] using Medicare part B reimbursement estimates. They reported that the Mayo algorithm was more expensive than stage-based algorithms for patients with clear cell RCC, while it resulted in more savings compared to traditional protocols and the UCLA protocol in patients with papillary and chromophobe RCC.

In 2016, Lobo et al. compared the cost differences, radiation exposure, and cancer outcomes in the following CUA, AUA, EAU, and NCCN guidelines for patients who underwent partial nephrectomy by using a Monte Carlo simulation model. The results of their model estimated the 5-year cost of surveillance for low-risk patients to be $587 (CUA), $1076 (AUA), $1705 (EAU), and $1768 (NCCN), while for high-risk patients, the cost was $903 (CUA), $2525 (EAU), and $3904 (AUA and NCCN) [102]. The EAU and CUA guidelines detected the highest numbers of recurrences in low-risk patients while all guidelines captured more than 92% of recurrences in the high-risk population.

A study from 2018 further supports a risk-adapted approach to surveillance that adheres to established national guidelines. Dabestani et al. evaluated outcomes of 1889 patients in the multicenter European database RECUR who underwent nephrectomy for localized RCC. Authors reported that patients who underwent more intensive follow-up, defined as greater than twice the recommended imaging by EAU guidelines, did not have an improved overall survival after a recurrence was detected [103, 104].

The Medicare cost of surveillance of a patient with pT1 disease using the 2014 NCCN surveillance guidelines is $2131.52 in 2014 and based on the previously mentioned study by Stewart and colleagues to capture 95% of recurrences the surveillance cost would escalate to $9856.82 in 2014. While longer surveillance protocols are more costly, this should be balanced with patient expectations, life expectancy and competing comorbidities.

Conclusion

Patients with renal cell carcinoma are at risk of recurrence, even after definitive surgical therapy, and should be carefully monitored to detect recurrences early enough to allow for meaningful intervention that could lead to prolonged survival. While the existing surveillance guidelines are based on expert opinion, the clinician must consider many aspects of a patient's life including competing risks of death, life expectancy, risk of disease recurrence, cost, psychological aspects of long-term surveillance, and the benefit of future therapeutic interventions to tailor the guidelines to the individual. The continued goal of these surveillance protocols is to capture the most recurrences while considering cost. Hopefully, advances in genomic sciences and molecular markers will lead to the development of more robust and individualized follow-up schemas for patients in the future.

References

1. Siegel R, Giaquinto AN, Jemal A. Cancer statistics, 2024. CA Cancer J Clin. 2024;74(1):12–49.
2. Janzen NK, Kim HL, Figlin RA, Belldegrun AS. Surveillance after radical or partial nephrectomy for localized renal cell carcinoma and management of recurrent disease. Urol Clin North Am. 2003;30(4):843–52.
3. Rabinovitch RA, Zelefsky MJ, Gaynor JJ, Fuks Z. Patterns of failure following surgical resection of renal cell carcinoma: implications for adjuvant local and systemic therapy. J Clin Oncol. 1994;12(1):206–12.
4. Ramon J, Goldwasser B, Raviv G, Jonas P, Many M. Long-term results of simple and radical nephrectomy for renal cell carcinoma. Cancer. 1991;67(10):2506–11.
5. Maldazys JD, deKernion JB. Prognostic factors in metastatic renal carcinoma. J Urol. 1986;136(2):376–9.
6. Negrier S, Escudier B, Gomez F, Douillard JY, Ravaud A, Chevreau C, Bucion M, Perol D, Lasset C. Prognostic factors of survival and rapid progression in 782 patients with metastatic renal carcinomas treated by cytokines: a report from the Groupe Francais d' Immunotherapie. Ann Oncol. 2002;13(9):1460–8.
7. Motzer RJ, Rini BI, Bukowski RM, Curti BD, George DJ, Hudes GR, Redman BG, Margolin

KA, Merchan JR, Wilding G, Ginsberg MS, Bacik J, Kim ST, Baum CM, Michaelson MD. Sunitinib in patients with metastatic renal cell carcinoma. JAMA. 2006;295(21):2516–24.
8. Hofmann HS, Neef H, Krohe K, Andreev P, Silber RE. Prognostic factors and survival after pulmonary resection of metastatic renal cell carcinoma. Eur Urol. 2005;48(1):77–81.
9. Baloch KG, Grimer RJ, Carter SR, Tillman RM. Radical surgery for the solitary bony metastasis from renal cell carcinoma. J Bone Joint Surg Br. 2000;82(1):62–7.
10. Sandhu SS, Symes A, A'Hern R, Sohaib SA, Eisen T, Gore M, Christmas TJ. Surgical excision of isolated renal-bed recurrence after radical nephrectomy for renal cell carcinoma. BJU Int. 2005;95(4):522–5.
11. Chawla SN, Crispen PL, Hanlon AL, Greenberg RE, Chen DY, Uzzo RG. The natural history of observed enhancing renal masses: metaanalysis and review of the world literature. J Urol. 2006;175(2):425–31.
12. Johnsen JA, Hellsten S. Lymphatogenous spread of renal cell carcinoma: an autopsy study. J Urol. 1997;157(2):450–3.
13. Hafez KS, Novick AC, Campbell SC. Patterns of recurrence and guidelines for follow-up after nephron-sparing surgery for sporadic renal cell carcinoma. J Urol. 1997;157(6):2067–70.
14. Levy DA, Slaton JW, Swanson DA, Dinney CP. Stage specific guidelines for surveillance after radical nephrectomy for local renal cell carcinoma. J Urol. 1998;159(4):1163–7.
15. Ljungberg B, Alamdari FI, Rasmuson T, Roos G. Follow-up guidelines for nonmetastatic renal cell carcinoma based on the occurrence of metastases after radical nephrectomy. BJU Int. 1999;84(4):405–11.
16. Sandock DS, Seftel AD, Resnick MI. A new protocol for the followup of renal cell carcinoma based on pathological stage. J Urol. 1995;154(1):28–31.
17. Stephenson AJ, Chetner MP, Rourke K, Gleave ME, Signaevsky M, Palmer B, Kuan J, Brock GB, Tanguay S. Guidelines for the surveillance of localized renal cell carcinoma based on the patterns of relapse after nephrectomy. J Urol. 2004;172(1):58–62.
18. Lam JS, Leppert JT, Figlin RA, Belldegrun AS. Surveillance following radical or partial nephrectomy for renal cell carcinoma. Curr Urol Rep. 2005;6(1):7–18.
19. Chin AI, Lam JS, Figlin RA, Belldegrun AS. Surveillance strategies for renal cell carcinoma patients following nephrectomy. Rev Urol. 2006;8(1):1–7.
20. Skolarikos A, Alivizatos G, Laguna P, de la Rosette J. A review on follow-up strategies for renal cell carcinoma after nephrectomy. Eur Urol. 2007;51(6):1490–500.
21. Shvarts O, Lam JS, Kim HL, Han KR, Figlin R, Belldegrun A. Eastern cooperative oncology group performance status predicts bone metastasis in patients presenting with renal cell carcinoma: implication for preoperative bone scans. J Urol. 2004;172(3):867–70.
22. Lam JS, Shvarts O, Leppert JT, Pantuck AJ, Figlin RA, Belldegrun AS. Postoperative surveillance protocol for patients with localized and locally advanced renal cell carcinoma based on a validated prognostic nomogram and risk group stratification system. J Urol. 2005;174(2):466–72.
23. Breda A, Konijeti R, Lam JS. Patterns of recurrence and surveillance strategies for renal cell carcinoma following surgical resection. Expert Rev Anticancer Ther. 2007;7(6):847–62.
24. Itano NB, Blute ML, Spotts B, Zincke H. Outcome of isolated renal cell carcinoma fossa recurrence after nephrectomy. J Urol. 2000;164(2):322–5.
25. Psutka SP, Heidenreich M, Boorjian SA, Bailey GC, Cheville JC, Stewart-Merrill SB, Lohse CM, Atwell TD, Costello BA, Leibovich BC, Thompson RH. Renal fossa recurrence after nephrectomy for renal cell carcinoma: prognostic features and oncological outcomes. BJU Int. 2017;119:116–27.
26. Margulis V, McDonald M, Tamboli P, Swanson DA, Wood CG. Predictors of oncological outcome after resection of locally recurrent renal cell carcinoma. J Urol. 2009;181(5):2044–51.
27. Fergany AF, Hafez KS, Novick AC. Long-term results of nephron-sparing surgery for localized renal cell carcinoma: 10-year followup. J Urol. 2000;163(2):442–5.
28. Campbell SC, Novick AC, Belldegrun AS, Blute ML, Chow GK, Derweesh IH, Faraday MM, Kaouk JH, Leveillee RJ, Matin SF, Russo P, Uzzo RG. Guideline for management of the clinical T1 renal mass. J Urol. 2009;182(4):1271–9.
29. Leibovich BC, Blute M, Cheville JC, Lohse CM, Weaver AL, Zincke H. Nephron sparing surgery for appropriately selected renal cell carcinoma between 4 and 7 cm results in outcome similar to radical nephrectomy. J Urol. 2004;171(3):1066–70.
30. Yossepowitch O, Thompson RH, Leibovich BC, Eggener SE, Pettus JA, Kwon ED, Herr HW, Blute ML, Russo P. Positive surgical margins at partial nephrectomy: predictors and oncological outcomes. J Urol. 2008;179:2158–63.
31. Bensalah K, Pantuck AJ, Rioux-Leclercq N, Thuret R, Montorsi F, Karakiewicz PI, Mottet N, Zini L, Bertini R, Salomon L, Villers A, Soulie M, Bellec L, Rischmann P, De La Taille A, Avakian R, Crepel M, Ferriere JM, Bernhard JC, Dujardin T, Pouliot F, Rigaud J, Pfister C, Albouy B, Guy L, Joniau S, Van Poppel H, Lebret T, Culty T, Saint F, Zisman A, Raz O, Lang H, Spie R, Wille A, Roigas J, Aguilera A, Rambeaud B, Pineiro LM, Nativ O, Farfara R, Richard F, Roupret M, Doehn C, Bastian PJ, Muller SC, Tostain J, Belldegrun AS, Patard JJ. Positive surgical margin appears to have negligible impact on survival of renal cell carcinoma treated by nephron-sparing surgery. Eur Urol. 2010;57:466–73.
32. Wood EL, Adibi M, Qiao W, Brandt J, Zhang M, Tamboli P, Matin SF, Wood CG, Karam JK. Local

tumor bed recurrence following partial nephrectomy in patients with small renal masses. J Urol. 2018;199(2):393–400.
33. Desai MM, Gill IS. Current status of cryoablation and radiofrequency ablation in the mangagement of renal tumors. Curr Opin Urol. 2002;12(5):387–93.
34. Karam JA, Wood CG. The role of surgery in advanced renal cell carcinoma: cytoreductive nephrectomy and metastasectomy. Hematol Oncol Clin North Am. 2011;25(4):753–64.
35. Alt AL, Boorjian SA, Lohse CM, Costello BA, Leibovich BC, Blute ML. Survival after complete surgical resection of multiple metastases from renal cell carcinoma. Cancer. 2011;117(13):2873–82.
36. Motzer RJ, Bacik J, Murphy BA, Russo P, Mazumdar M. Interferon-alfa as a comparative treatment for clincal trials of new therapies against advanced renal cell carcinoma. J Clin Oncol. 2002;20(1):289–96.
37. Levey AS, Coresh J, Balk E, Kausz AT, Levin A, Steffes MW, Hogg RJ, Perrone RD, Lau J, Eknoyan G, National Kidney Foundation. National Kidney Foundation practice guidelines for chronic kidney disease: evaluation, classification, and stratification. Ann Intern Med. 2003;139(2):137–47.
38. Go AS, Chertow GM, Fan D, McCulloch CE, Hsu CY. Chronic kidney disease and the risks of death, cardiovascular events, and hospitalization. N Engl J Med. 2004;351(13):1296–305.
39. Chae EJ, Kim JK, Kim SH, Bae SJ, Cho KS. Renal cell carcinoma: analysis of postoperative recurrence patterns. Radiology. 2005;234:189–96.
40. Bianchi M, Becker A, Hansen J, Trinh Q, Tian Z, Abdollah F, Briganti A, Shariat SF, Perrotte P, Montorsi F, Karakiewicz PI, Sun M. Conditional survival after nephrectomy for renal cell carcinoma (RCC): changes in future survival probability over time. BJU Int. 2013;111(8):E283–9.
41. Kattan MW, Reuter V, Motzer R, Katz J, Russo P. A postoperative prognostic nomogram for renal cell carcinoma. J Urol. 2001;166(1):63–7.
42. Rini BI, Vogelzang NJ. Prognostic factors in renal carcinoma. Semin Oncol. 2000;27(2):213–20.
43. Delahunt B, Kittelson JM, McCredie MR, Reeve AE, Stewart JH, Bilous AM. Prognostic importance of tumor size for localized conventional (clear cell) renal cell carcinoma: assessment of TNM T1 and T2 tumor categories and comparison with other prognostic parameters. Cancer. 2002;94(3):658–64.
44. Cheville JC, Blute ML, Zincke H, Lohse CM, Weaver AL. Stage pT1 conventional (clear cell) renal cell carcinoma: pathological features associated with cancer specific survival. J Urol. 2001;166(2):453–6.
45. Giuliani L, Giberti C, Martorana G, Rovida S. Radical extensive surgery for renal cell carcinoma: long-term results and prognostic factors. J Urol. 1990;143(3):468–73.
46. Sorbellini M, Kattan MW, Snyder ME, Reuter V, Motzer R, Goetzi M, McKiernan J, Russo P. A postoperative prognostic nomogram predicting recurrence for patients with conventional clear cell renal cell carcinoma. J Urol. 2005;173(1):48–51.
47. Delahunt B, Eble J, McCredie MR, Bethwaite PB, Stewart JH, Bilous AM. Morphologic typing of papillary renal cell carcinoma: comparison of growth kinetics and patient survival in 66 cases. Hum Pathol. 2001;32(6):590–5.
48. Amin MB, Amin MB, Tamboli P, Javidan J, Stricker H, de Peralta Venturina M, Deshpande A, Menon M. Prognostic impact of histologic subtyping of adult renal epithelial neoplasms: an experience of 405 cases. Am J Surg Pathol. 2002;26(3):281–91.
49. Patard JJ, Leray E, Rioux-Leclercq N, Cindolo L, Ficarra V, Zisman A, De La Taille A, Tostain J, Artibani W, Abbou CC, Lobel B, Guille F, Chopin DK, Mulders PF, Wood CG, Swanson DA, Figlin RA, Belldegrun AS, Pantuck AJ. Prognostic value of histologic subtypes in renal cell carcinoma: a multicenter experience. J Clin Oncol. 2005;23(12):2763–71.
50. Abel EJ, Culp SH, Meissner M, Matin SF, Tamboli P, Wood CG. Identifying the risk of disease progression after surgery for localized renal cell carcinoma. BJU Int. 2010;106(9):1277–83.
51. Sella A, Logothetis CJ, Ro JY, Swanson DA, Samuels ML. Sarcomatoid renal cell carcinoma. A treatable entity. Cancer. 1987;60(6):1313–8.
52. Narayan V, Puligandla M, Haas NB, Subramanian P, DiPaola RS, Uzzo R. Patterns of relapse and implications for post-nephrectomy surveillance for patients with high-risk non-clear cell renal cell carcinoma: subgroup analysis of the phase 3 ECOG-ACRIN E2805 trial. J Urol. 2019;201(1):62–8.
53. Frank I, Blute ML, Cheville JC, Lohse CM, Weaver AL, Zincke H. An outcome prediction model for patients with clear cell renal cell carcinoma treated with radical nephrectomy based on tumor stage, size, grade and necrosis: the SSIGN score. J Urol. 2002;168(6):2395–400.
54. Raj GV, Thompson RH, Leibovich BC, Blute ML, Russo P, Kattan MW. Preoperative nomogram predicting 12-year probability of metastatic renal cancer. J Urol. 2008;179(6):2146–51.
55. Zisman A, Pantuck AJ, Dorey F, Said JW, Shvarts O, Quintana D, Gitlitz BJ, deKernion JB, Figlin RA, Belldegrun AS. Improved prognostication of RCC using an integrated staging system (UISS). J Clin Oncol. 2001;19(6):1649–57.
56. Mickisch G, Carballido J, Hellsten S, Schulze H, Mensink H. Guidelines on renal cell cancer. Eur Urol. 2001;40:252–5.
57. Stephenson AJ, Chetner MP, Rourke K, Gleave ME, Signaevsky M, Palmer B, et al. Guidelines for the surveillance of localized renal cell carcinoma

based on the patterns of relapse after nephrectomy. J Urol [Research Support, Non-US Gov't Research Support, US Gov't, PHS]. 2004;172(1):58–62.
58. Novick AC, Derweesh I. Open partial nephrectomy for renal tumours: current status. BJU Int. 2005;95(Suppl 2):35–40.
59. Kassouf W, Siemens R, Morash C, Lacombe L, Jewett M, Goldenberg L, Chin J, Chetner M, Wood CG, Tanguay S, Aprikian AG. Follow-up guidelines after radical or partial nephrectomy for localized and locally advanced renal cell carcinoma. Can Urol Assoc J. 2009;3(1):73–6.
60. Montie JE. Follow-up after partial or total nephrectomy for renal cell carcinoma. Urol Clin North Am. 1994;21(4):589–92.
61. Saidi JA, Newhouse JH, Sawczuk IS. Radiologic follow-up of patients with T1-3a,b,c or T4N+M0 renal cell carcinoma after radical nephrectomy. Urology [Clinical Trial Randomized Controlled Trial Research Support, Non-US Gov't]. 1998;52(6):1000–3.
62. Frank I, Blute ML, Cheville JC, Lohse CM, Weaver AL, Leibovich BC, et al. A multifactorial postoperative surveillance model for patients with surgically treated clear cell renal cell carcinoma. J Urol. 2003;170(6 Pt 1):2225–32.
63. Antonelli A, Cozzoli A, Zani D, Zanotelli T, Nicolai M, Cunico SC, Simeone C. The follow-up management of non-metastatic renal cell carcinoma: definition of a surveillance protocol. BJU Int. 2006;99(2):296–300.
64. Patard JJ, Kim HL, Lam JS, Dorey FJ, Pantuck AJ, Zisman A, Ficarra V, Han KR, Cindolo L, De La Taille A, Tostain J, Artibani W, Dinney CP, Wood CG, Swanson DA, Abbou CC, Lobel B, Mulders PF, Chopin DK, Figlin RA, Belldegrun AS. Use of the University of California Los Angeles integrated staging system to predict survival in renal cell carcinoma: an international multicenter study. J Clin Oncol. 2004;22(16):3316–22.
65. Capogrosso P, Larcher A, Sjoberg DD, Vertosick EA, Cianflone F, Dell'Oglio P, Carenzi C, Salonia A, Vickers AJ, Montorsi F, Bertini R, Capitanio U. Risk based surveillance after surgical treatment of renal cell carcinoma. J Urol. 2018;200(1):61–7.
66. Siddiqui SA, Frank I, Cheville JC, Lohse CM, Leibovich BC, Blute ML. Postoperative surveillance for renal cell carcinoma: a multifactorial histological subtype specific protocol. BJU Int. 2009;104(6):778–85.
67. Stewart-Merrill SB, Thompson RH, Psutka SP, Cheville JC, Lohse CM, Boorjian SA, Leibovich BC. Evaluation of the National Comprehensive Cancer Network and American urological association renal cell carcinoma surveillance guidelines. J Clin Oncol. 2014;32(36):4059–65.
68. Stewart-Merrill SB, Thompson RH, Boorjian SA, Psutka SP, Lohse CM, Cheville JC, Leibovich BC, Frank I. Oncologic surveillance after surgical resection for renal cell carcinoma: a novel risk-based approach. J Clin Oncol. 2015;33(35):4151–7.
69. NCCN Clinical Practice Guidelines in Oncology (NCCN Guidelines®) for Kidney Cancer (V.4.2018) © 2018 National Comprehensive Cancer Network, Inc. NCCN.org. Accessed 21 Aug 2018. To view the most recent and complete version of the NCCN Guidelines®, go on-line to NCCN.org.
70. AUA Clincal Practice Guidelines: follow-up for clinically localized renal neoplasms. 2013. auanet.org. Accessed 21 Aug 2018.
71. Steinbach F, Novick AC, Zincke H, Miller DP, Williams RD, Lund G, Skinner DG, Esrig D, Richie JP, Dekernion JB, et al. Treatment of renal cell carcinoma in von Hippel-Lindau disease: a multicenter study. J Urol. 1995;153(6):1812–6.
72. Duffey BG, Choyke PL, Glenn G, Grubb RL, Venzon D, Linehan WM, et al. The relationship between renal tumor size and metastases in patients with von Hippel-Lindau disease. J Urol. 2004;172(1):63–5.
73. Meister M, Choyke P, Anderson C, Patel U. Radiological evaluation, management, and surveillance of renal masses in von hippel-Lindau disease. Clin Radiol. 2009;64(6):589–600.
74. Lotfi MA, McCue P, Gomella LG. Laparoscopic interstitial contact laser ablation of renal lesions: an experimental model. J Endourol. 1994;8:153–6.
75. Yoshimura K, Okubo K, Ichioka K, Terada N, Matsuta Y, Arai Y. Laparoscopic partial nephrectomy with a microwave tissue coagulator for small renal tumor. J Urol. 2001;165:1893–6.
76. Vallancien G, Chartier-Kastler E, Chopin D, Veillon B, Brisset JM, Andre-Bougaran J. Focussed extracorporeal pyrotherapy: experimental results. Eur Urol. 1991;20:211–9.
77. Watkin NA, Morris SB, Rivens IH, ter Haar GR. High-intensity focused ultrasound ablation of the kidney in a large animal model. J Endourol. 1997;11:191–6.
78. Klatte T, Mauermann J, Heinz-Peer G, Waldert M, Weibi P, Klingler HC, Remzi M. Perioperative, oncologic, and functional outcomes of laparoscopic renal cryoablation and open parital nephrectomy: a matched pair analysis. J Endourol. 2011;25(6):991–7.
79. Guazzoni G, Cestari A, Buffi N, Lughezzani G, Nava L, Cardone G, Balconi G, Lazzeri M, Montorsi F, Rigatti P. Oncologic results of laparoscopic renal cryoablation for clinical T1a tumors: 8 years of experience in a single institution. Urology. 2010;76(3):624–9.

80. Aron M, Kamoi K, Remer E, Berger A, Desai M, Gill IS. Laparoscopic renal cryoablation: 8-year, single surgeon outcomes. J Urol. 2010;183(3):889–95.
81. El Dib R, Touma NJ, Kapoor A. Cryoablation vs radiofrequency ablation for the treatment of renal cell carcinoma: a meta-analysis of case series studies. BJU Int. 2012;110(4):510–6.
82. Tracy CR, Raman JD, Donnally C, Trimmer CK, Cadeddu JA. Durable oncologic outcomes after radiofrequency ablation: experience from treating 243 small renal masses over 7.5 years. Cancer. 2010;116(13):3135–42.
83. Matsumoto ED, Watumull L, Johnson DB, Ogan K, Taylor GD, Joseph S, Cadeddu JA. The radiographic evolution of radio frequency ablated renal tumors. J Urol. 2004;172(1):45–8.
84. Kawamoto S, Permpongkosol S, Bluemke DA, Fishman EK, Solomon SB. Sequential changes after radiofrequency ablation and cryoablation of renal neoplasms: role of CT and MR imaging. Radiographics. 2007;27(2):343–55.
85. Svatek RS, Sims R, Anderson JK, Abdel-Aziz K, Cadeddu JA. Magnetic resonance imaging characteristics of renal tumors after radiofrequency ablation. Urology. 2006;67(3):508–12.
86. Rendon RA, Kachura JR, Sweet JM, Gertner MR, Sherar MD, Robinette M, Tshlias J, Trachtenberg J, Sampson H, Jewett MA. The uncertainty of radio frequency treatment of renal cell carcinoma: findings at immediate and delayed nephrectomy. J Urol. 2002;167(4):1587–92.
87. Weight CJ, Kaouk JH, Hegarty NJ, Remer EM, O'Malley CM, Lane BR, Gill IS, Novick AC. Correlation of radiographic imaging and histopathology following cryoablation and radio frequency ablation for renal tumors. J Urol. 2008;179(4):1277–81.
88. Cadeddu JA. Correlation of radiographic imaging and histopathology following cryoablation and radio frequency ablation for renal tumors—editorial comment. J Urol. 2008;179:1281–2.
89. Campbell SC, Krishnamurthi V, Chow G, Hale J, Myles J, Novick AC. Renal cryosurgery: experimental evaluation of treatment parameters. Urology. 1998;52(1):33–4.
90. Rukstalis DB, Khorsandi M, Garcia FU, Hoenig DM, Cohen JK. Clinical experience with open renal cryoablation. Urology. 2001;172:1267–70.
91. Gill IS, Remer EM, Hasan WA, Strzempkowski B, Spaliviero M, Steinberg AP, Kaouk JH, Desai MM, Novick AC. Renal cryoablation: outcome at 3 years. J Urol. 2005;173(6):1903–7.
92. Beemster P, Phoa S, Wijkstra H, de la Rosette J, Laguna P. Follow-up of renal masses after cryosurgery using computed tomography; enhancement patterns and cryolesion size. BJU Int. 2008;101(10):1237–42.
93. Matin SF, Ahrar K, Cadeddu JA, Gervais DA, McGovern FJ, Zagoria RA, Uzzo RG, Haaga J, Resnick MI, Kaouk J, Gill IS. Residual and recurrent disease following renal energy ablative therapy: a multi-institutional study. J Urol. 2006;176(5):1973–7.
94. Crispen PL, Boorjian SA, Lohse CM, Leibovich BC, Kwon ED. Predicting disease progression after nephrectomy for localized renal cell carcinoma: the utility of prognostic models and molecular biomarkers. Cancer. 2008;113(3):450–60.
95. Nogueira M, Kim HL. Molecular markers for predicting prognosis of renal cell carcinoma. Urol Oncol. 2008;26(2):113–24.
96. Johnson TV, Abbasi A, Owen-Smith A, Young AN, Kucuk O, Harris WB, et al. Postoperative better than preoperative C-reactive protein at predicting outcome after potentially curative nephrectomy for renal cell carcinoma. Urology. 2010;76(3):766.e1–5.
97. Abel JE, Bauman TM, Weiker M, Shi F, Downs TM, Jarrard DF, Huang W. Analysis and validation of tissue biomarkers for renal cell carcinoma using automated high-throughput evaluation of protein expression. Hum Pathol. 2014;45(5):1092–9.
98. Brenner DJ, Hall EJ. Computed tomography–an increasing source of radiation exposure. N Engl J Med. 2007;357(22):2277–84.
99. Smith-Bindman R. Is computed tomography safe? N Engl J Med. 2010;363(1):1–4.
100. Society RR. Radiation exposures in medicine: biological and public health significance American statistical association conference on radiation and health. Annapolis, Maryland, June 13-16, 2010. Radiat Res. 2010;175(1):131–42.
101. Dion M, Martínez CH, Williams AK, Chalasani V, Nott L, Pautler SE. Cost analysis of two follow-up strategies for localized kidney cancer: a Canadian cohort comparison. Can Urol Assoc J. 2010;4(5):322–6.
102. Lobo JM, Nelson M, Nandanan N, Krupski TL. Comparison of renal cell carcinoma surveillance guidelines: competing trade-offs. J Urol. 2016;195(6):1664–70.
103. Dabestani S, Beisland C, Stewart GD, Bensalah K, Gudmundsson E, Lam TB, Gietzmann W, Zakikhani P, Marconi L, Fernandéz-Pello S, Monagas S, Williams SP, Torbrand C, Powles T, Van Werkhoven E, Meijer R, Volpe A, Staehler M, Ljungberg B, Bex A. Long-term outcomes of follow-up for initially localised clear cell renal cell carcinoma: RECUR database analysis. Eur Urol Focus. 2019;5(5):857–66. https://doi.org/10.1016/j.euf.2018.02.010.
104. Dabestani S, Beisland C, Stewart GD, Bensalah K, Gudmundsson E, Lam TB, Gietzmann W, Zakikhani P, Marconi L, Fernandéz-Pello S, Monagas S, Williams SP, Torbrand C, Powles T, Van Werkhoven E, Meijer R, Volpe A, Staehler M, Ljungberg B, Bex A. Intensive imaging-based follow-up of surgically treated localised renal cell carcinoma does not improve post-recurrence survival: results from a European multicentre database (RECUR). Eur Urol. 2019;75(2):261–4.

21 Role of Radiation Therapy in Renal Cancer

Andrea McKee, Arul Mahadevan, and Chad Tang

Introduction

Discussions of the role of radiation therapy (RT) in the treatment of renal cell carcinoma (RCC) frequently begin by paying homage to the dogma that RCC is a radioresistant neoplasm. Indeed, Deschavanne [1] found RCC to be the least radiosensitive cell type of 76 different cell types in a review of studies of human cell radiosensitivity when treated with low doses (2 Gy) in vitro. However, as time has passed, authors have less vigorously stressed these observations, and words like "relatively" and "variably" have begun to find themselves preceding "radioresistant" in more recent reviews [2, 3]. During this same period, technological advances have provided the ability to deliver larger doses of radiation with far greater precision. These ablative therapies are referred to as stereotactic radiosurgery (SRS) when delivered in a single fraction and stereotactic ablative radiation (SABR) or stereotactic body radiation therapy (SBRT) when administered over 3–5 fractions. Nonetheless, surgical resection justifiably remains the gold standard in the treatment of primary RCC [4–6], and the overall role of radiation therapy in the definitive treatment of RCC has historically been minimal but its use continuously grows [7]. In this chapter, we will review the literature for radiation in the upfront management of primary RCC and the treatment of adjuvant, oligometastatic, and palliative settings.

A. McKee (✉) · A. Mahadevan
Department of Radiation Oncology, Massachusetts General Cancer Center at Wentworth Douglass Hospital, Dover, NH, USA
e-mail: abmckee@mgb.org; amahadevan1@mgb.org

C. Tang
Department of Genitourinary Radiation Oncology, MD Anderson Cancer Center, Houston, TX, USA
e-mail: CTang1@mdanderson.org

Preoperative Neoadjuvant Radiation

Irradiation of human RCC before its transplantation into NMRI nu/nu mice yielded significantly lower acceptance rates than those for nonirradiated tumors (1/7 as compared to 13/13) [8]. These findings suggested a potential role for preoperative neoadjuvant radiation to lower the risk of intraoperative seeding of tumor cells [9]. A number of anecdotal accounts also suggested easier resectability as a result of tumor shrinkage and vessel sclerosis following radiation [10, 11]. Correspondingly, several retrospective series conducted prior to modern staging, surgery, and radiation therapy techniques reported positive outcomes following preoperative external beam radiation [12, 13].

Disappointingly, the two prospective randomized trials undertaken as a result of this prior research found little benefit. The Rotterdam Trial [14] examined 141 patients with carcinoma of the kidney, randomized either to preoperative

J. A. Libertino, J. R. Gee (eds.), *Renal Cancer*, https://doi.org/10.1007/978-3-031-97599-8_21

radiation (30 Gy in 15 fractions) and nephrectomy or to nephrectomy alone. There was no significant difference in 5-year survival between either group, regardless of P-category, an older staging system. Nonetheless, interesting differences were observed between P-categories. Those with P-3 disease (tumor infiltrating intrarenal, extrarenal veins, or lymph vessels) who were not randomized to preoperative radiation suffered incomplete tumor removal more frequently than other patients in the study. The study's authors reported that the survival of patients with residual disease was poor compared to those who enjoyed complete removal. After initial analysis, the trial was continued at a higher dose of 40 Gy, but continued to fail to show survival benefit at the primary endpoint [15]. Increased resectability was not a prespecified endpoint in the trial's design and represents an area potentially deserving of future research. Due to the lack of data at present, it has been suggested that patients with unresectable tumors should be considered for preoperative radiation therapy of 45 Gy in an effort to increase tumor resectability [2].

The Swedish Trial [16] examined 88 patients with renal carcinoma who were randomized to either radiation (33 Gy in 15 fractions) followed by nephrectomy or nephrectomy alone. Patients were analyzed according to histological subtype in addition to P-category. No significant difference was found between study arms, even upon subgroup analysis, although tumor cells from these patients showed a marked loss of proliferative capacity on tissue culture after preoperative irradiation. The 5-year survival rate for the preoperative radiation and nephrectomy group, as compared to that of nephrectomy alone, was 47% and 63%, respectively. Even less encouraging was the discrepancy between study arms among patients with high-grade malignancy, 13% and 36%, respectively.

Currently under investigation is the value of SBRT, discussed elsewhere in the chapter, as neoadjuvant treatment in locally advanced RCC [17]. Figure 21.1 is an example of a patient with a right upper pole renal mass treated with preoperative stereotactic body radiation therapy (on protocol), with pathology showing complete necrosis with normal surrounding renal parenchyma. A recently completed study utilizing neoadjuvant SBRT in patients with IVC thrombus demonstrated safety, decreased cancer cell proliferation, and evidence of immune activation [18]. Such approaches may facilitate complete resection of technically challenging locally advanced disease.

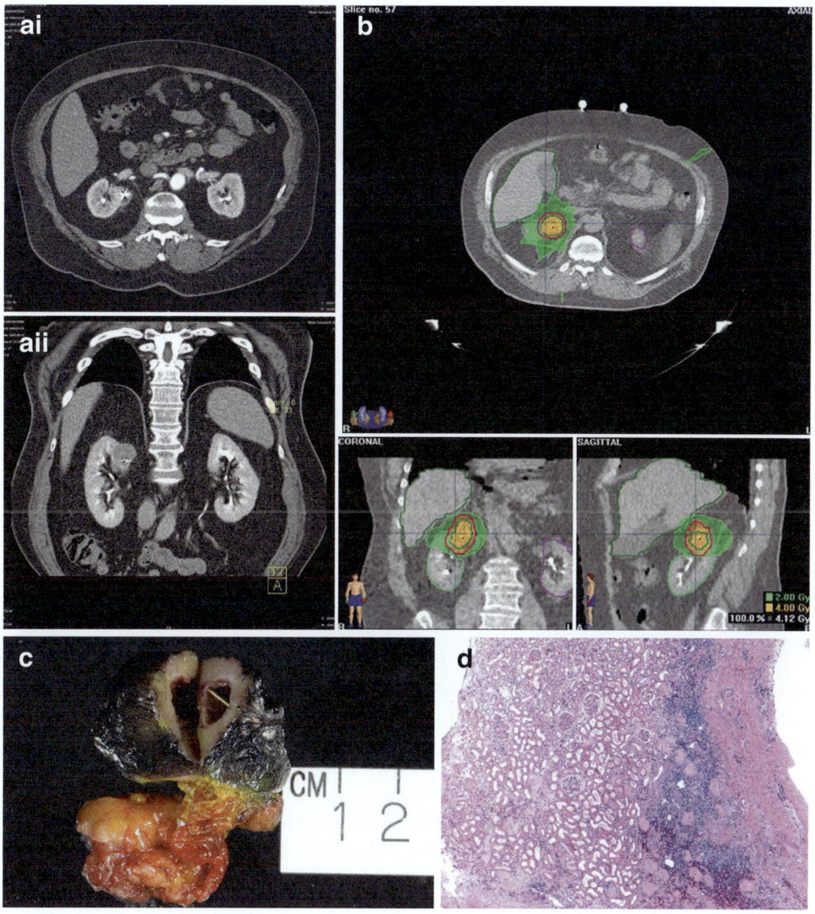

Fig. 21.1 (**ai**) A kidney lesion (clear cell type) with fiducial for SBRT—axial and (**aii**) coronal. (**b**) SBRT isodose plan (600 cGy × 4 fractions in 2 days—twice daily). (**c**) Laparoscopic partial nephrectomy specimen with fiducial. (**d**) Pathology showing complete necrosis at the site of tumor (*right*) with normal surrounding renal parenchyma (*left*)

Postoperative Adjuvant Radiation

Early retrospective data from the 1950s and 1960s reported improved survival at both 5 and 10 years following postoperative external beam radiation (EBRT) [12, 13, 19]. In a larger retrospective cohort, Rafla et al. found significantly improved survival and local control among those receiving postoperative radiation [20]. However, no information regarding dose or patient selection was offered by the investigators. Several years later, a prospective series failed to demonstrate survival benefit or improved secondary endpoints such as greater local control following postoperative adjuvant radiation [21]. Most discouraging was the Copenhagen Renal Cancer Study [22], a prospective trial where patients with stage II or III renal cell carcinoma were randomized to nephrectomy alone or nephrectomy followed by postoperative radiation (50 Gy in 20 fractions to the kidney bed, regional ipsilateral, and contralateral lymph nodes). The 5-year survival for those who received postoperative radiation was 38% as compared to the control group, whose 5-year survival was 63%. The decision was made to close the study to further patient accrual in light of the number of complications associated with radiation therapy. Forty-four percent of patients experienced significant complications involving radiation-related toxicity affecting the stomach, duodenum, or liver. Most disturbingly, toxicity from radiation was deemed responsible for 19% of the deaths in the study.

A number of questions regarding both the safety and efficacy of postoperative radiation for renal cell carcinoma remained unanswered by these trials. In the Copenhagen trial, for instance, both the control and postoperative radiation groups exhibited very low local recurrence (0% and 1%, respectively). However, in a Memorial Sloan-Kettering series of 172 surgically treated patients, the actuarial local failure was 5% [23]. This fact suggests that the selection of Copenhagen Study participants (ideally, those who would stand to benefit from radiation therapy) was far less than ideal. Additionally, 2.5 Gy per fraction represents an aggressive dose for an often wide and non-conformal radiation plan, and the resulting toxicity, superimposed upon a study in which participants from the outset had an extremely low risk of local recurrence, left very little room to find benefit. In response to these concerns, there have been a number of more recent retrospective trials reexamining the administration of postoperative radiation in patients at greater risk for local recurrence [24–27]. These studies all demonstrated improved local control with adjuvant radiation but failed to produce any evidence of benefit to overall survival. A 2010 meta-analysis from Tunio [28] agrees that postoperative radiation significantly reduces locoregional failure but has no effect on overall survival or disease-free survival and concludes that due to the frequent poor patient selection and heterogeneous and outdated radiation therapy techniques, there is a need for new trials to evaluate postoperative adjuvant therapy using modern radiation techniques.

Intraoperative Radiation

Clinicians from the Mayo Clinic, University Clinic of Navarra at Pamplona, the University of Heidelberg, and the University of California, San Francisco have investigated aggressive approaches utilizing adjuvant intraoperative electron irradiation (IOERT).

At the Mayo Clinic, 49 patients between 1983 and 1994 received IOERT as a component of therapy for locally advanced unresectable genitourinary (GU) malignancies [29, 30]. The site of primary origin was the kidney in the majority [26] of these cases. Maximum resection and IOERT were either preceded or followed by EBRT (median dose 49.9 Gy; range 5–56 Gy) in 42 of the 49 patients. Electrons with energy ranging from 6 to 18 MeV were used to deliver a median dose of 15 Gy (range 7.5–30 Gy) intraoperatively. Ten patients received chemotherapy either concurrently with EBRT or following all other treatments. The 15 surviving patients were followed for a median of 3 years, while all other participants were followed until death. Survival among RCC patients was significantly better than that of the patients diagnosed with malignancies of other GU sites (5-year survival—37% vs. 16%). Two patients (4%) suffered grade 3 toxicity associated with IOERT.

In Pamplona, at the University Clinic of Navarra, 11 patients with stage III (5 patients), IV (3 patients), or lumbar fossa recurrence (3 patients) of renal cancer were treated with IOERT and surgical resection [30]. Histological confirmation of clear cell adenocarcinoma was available in 10 of the 11 cases. Electrons with energy ranging from 9 to 20 MeV were used to deliver a dose ranging from 15 to 20 Gy. Seven patients received additional EBRT ranging from 30 to 45 Gy. With a median follow-up period of 8 months, upon the case series' initial publication, 3 patients were reported with a distant relapse. One of the 3 also suffered local recurrence at 7 months (no EBRT had been administered in this case). Further follow-up analysis revealed long-term survivors without evidence of recurrent disease (three patients with greater than 3 years of follow-up). The investigators detected no early or late radiation-associated toxicity.

A multicenter study conducted by Paly and colleagues from 1985 to 2010 reported results with the use of IOERT in patients with locally advanced RCC (28% of the cohort) or local recurrence in the renal fossa (72% of the cohort) [31]. Negative margins, small tumor size, and absence of sarcomatous features were found to be favorable prognostic variables in this high-risk group of patients who experienced a median survival time of 3.5 years.

At the University of Heidelberg, another series of 11 patients with RCC (locally advanced primary—3, locally recurrent—8) received treatment consisting of surgical resection, IOERT (15–20 Gy with 6–10 MeV), and postoperative

EBRT (40 Gy in 20 fractions). After a mean follow-up of 24 months, distant metastases occurred in five patients. Local control for the entire group was 100%. Overall and disease-free survival at 4 years were 47% and 34%, respectively. No late adverse effects associated with IOERT were detected [30].

At the University of California, San Francisco, 14 patients with local recurrence of RCC underwent subsequent surgical resection, with 10 of the 14 also receiving IOERT [30, 32]. Survival was 40% at 2 years and 30% at 5 years from surgery. Investigators found no difference in survival due to IOERT.

In a 2011 joint statement, the studies' authors concluded, "The addition of IOERT to surgery and EBRT is associated with a high rate of local control and acceptable toxicity. The best candidates are untreated patients with large tumor volume with risk of positive margins after radical nephrectomy, and patients with local recurrences. Distant relapse is common, especially in patients with recurrent disease. Accordingly, future treatment strategies should evaluate a systemic component of treatment (new targeted therapies)" [30]. However recent utilization of adjuvant pembrolizumab following nephrectomy in high risk patients as a result of the successful Keynote 564 study [33, 34] and improved technologic capabilities allowing us to target nephrectomy bed recurrences with SBRT will modify the utility of IOERT.

Stereotactic Body Radiotherapy (SBRT) as Definitive Treatment

Renal cancer (*see* Stereotactic body radiotherapy (SBRT)) cells have been historically classified as radioresistant to fractionated conventional radiation therapy, and molecular mechanisms to explain this were recently published [35]. However, several recent clinical reports have observed excellent tumor control rates with high-dose stereotactic body radiation therapy (SBRT—five or fewer fractions) or radiosurgery (SRS—single fraction) [36]. Molecular and biological mechanisms to explain these excellent results have recently been proposed. Studies by Fuks [37] have indicated that single high-dose radiation exposure (greater than 8 Gy) engages a microvascular apoptotic component in tumor response by inducing a vascular collapse within the endothelium. This pathway does not appear to be engaged in fractionated regimens because the individual doses are too low to invoke this apoptotic stimulus on endothelial cells.

Investigators at Brown University agreed with Deschavanne [1] that of the various classes of tumor cells exposed to conventional EBRT doses, RCC could be categorized to fall in the more radioresistant group along with primary brain tumors, breast, prostate, ovarian, and head and neck cancers [38]. However, they also noted that there was no correlation between this original taxonomy and the degree of radiosensitivity among different histological classes of neoplasms at single high doses (SRS). Adding some encouragement for stereotactic treatment, Walsh [39] reported quite recently that nude mice transfected with A498 human renal cell carcinoma cells exhibited a sustained decrease in tumor volume following high-dose-per-fraction radiation (3 fractions for a total dose of 48 Gy).

In the clinic, the ability to deliver high-dose radiation therapy in a single (SRS) or multifraction (SBRT) regimen relies on robust tumor and normal tissue localization, patient immobilization, multibeam intensity-modulated treatment planning, and image guidance. These modifications result in highly conformal, steep gradient dose delivery to the target with maximal sparing of nearby normal tissue organs at risk (OARs).

The radiation techniques employed in the delivery of SRS and SBRT have revolutionized the field of radiation oncology. Not surprisingly, the use of these modalities in the management of RCC has risen dramatically over the past decade. Haque et al. queried the National Cancer Database (NCDB) for cT1a/bN0Mo RCC patients receiving definitive treatment in the years 2004–2013 [7]. Of all patients in the database, 57,924 (41.8%) underwent partial nephrectomy and 67,168 (48.5%) radical nephrectomy, while only 308 (0.2%) received EBRT, including SBRT. These findings were in a follow up study by Grant et al. [40]. The proportion of RT-treated patients receiving SBRT increased from 2.5% in 2004 to 95.4% in 2013. Similarly, the use of ablative radiation therapy in the management of metastasis-directed treatment for metastatic RCC has steadily increased over that time frame [41].

In an attempt to examine the efficacy of definitive radiation treatment, Beitler [42] reported a series of nine patients with nonmetastatic renal cell carcinoma who refused definitive surgery. Patients received 40 Gy in 5 fractions using conformal EBRT. With a median follow-up of 27 months, four of the 9 patients were alive. The survivors' minimum follow-up was 48 months. In 2005, Wersall [43] reported on 58 patients with renal cell carcinoma who received stereotactic radiotherapy. Fifty of the patients received treatment for metastatic disease. However, eight received treatment for inoperable primary lesions or inoperable recurrent local disease following nephrectomy. High-dose-per-fraction SBRT (40 Gy in 5 fractions) was delivered with patients placed in a stereotactic body frame. Seven of the eight patients achieved local control. Six of eight were alive at publication. Median survival time was 58+ months. Local control rate was greater than 90% for the entire cohort of 58 patients.

Since then, there have been numerous retrospective and a few prospective trials evaluating the efficacy of ablative radiotherapy in primary RCC, most with small numbers of patients, utilizing a variety of different fractionation and dosing schedules. A systematic review of ten studies (seven retrospective and three prospective) compiled 126 patients with inoperable RCC treated with SBRT was shed in 2012 [44]. This review demonstrated excellent local control of 92.9% at a median follow-up of 2–3 years. Toxicity was acceptable at 3.8% grade 3 or greater.

The FASTRACK study was a prospective trial of 37 inoperable patients published in 2017 by Siva et al. continuing to demonstrate greater than 90% local control with limited grade 3 or greater toxicity of 3% [45, 46]. These findings were confirmed in the follow up FASTRACK II study, an international non-randomized phase 2 trial published on 70 patients with predominantly T1b or larger disease to receive 26Gy in single fraction or. 42Gy in 3 fractions. The authors reported local control at 12 months of 100% with 10% grade 3 treatment-related adverse events [47]. Both FASTRACK studies assessed local GFR through radiotracer imaging andnoted a dose response to GFR decline. For every 10 Gy of physical dose delivered, an exponential decline in affected kidney GFR was observed at 1-year follow-up. In FASTRACK, a 39% decrease in GFR of the affected kidney when treatment was delivered in one fraction (SRS) of 26 Gy was observed, and a 25% GFR loss for those receiving 42 Gy over three fractions. No patient required dialysis at 1-year follow-up [45]. These findings were confirmed in the FASTRACK II study demonstrating 39% and 62% decrease in the affected kidney at 2 years when treatment was delivered in single and multiple fractions [48].

In the absence of randomized controlled clinical trials or extensive clinical evidence, a consensus statement from eight international centers with expertise in SBRT for RCC has summarized current treatment recommendations [49]. The International Society of Stereotactic Radiosurgery (ISRS) published a systematic review of 36 studies consisting of 822 medically inoperable patients or those who declined surgery. Subjects received 25-26Gy in 1 or 42–48 Gy in 4 fractions. Median LC was 94.1% and 5-year OS 77.2%. The practice guideline concluded that SBRT for renal cell carcinoma is safe and effective for solitary kidney treatment, and that post treatment biopsy is not recommended. CT of the chest and abdomen q 6 months is the recommended surveillance follow up [50]. Before SBRT for primary RCC can be considered a standard of care multicenter prospective clinical trials are necessary and currently underway in several countries [51, 52].

Palliative Radiotherapy

Brain metastases are diagnosed in approximately 10% of patients with metastatic renal cell carcinoma [53, 54]. In a survey of patients treated at Massachusetts General Hospital for CNS metastases from renal cell carcinoma, Halperin [55] reported a disappointing response to conventionally fractionated radiation (30% response). At M.D. Anderson Cancer Center, the median survival time for 119 patients receiving whole brain radiation therapy for renal carcinoma metastases was 4.4 months following diagnosis [54]. Similarly, poor results over approximately the same time period (1976–1986) were reported at Memorial Sloan-Kettering [56]. More encouraging results have been reported following the advent of stereotactic techniques. Median survival with stereotactic treatment in a series of 29 patients from 1991 to 1998 at the Cleveland Clinic was 10 months [57]. Only 9% suffered CNS recurrence. The addition of whole-brain radiotherapy yielded no improvement in local control. However, patients presenting with multiple CNS lesions are twice as likely to develop distant brain failure and merit consideration for whole brain and stereotactic radiotherapy combined. In a similar series reported by Amendola [58], local control following radiosurgical treatments was 98.5%, with 18 of 21 patients dying of non-neurologic causes. A number of similar studies confirming efficacy and providing reassurance in regard to side effects emerged shortly thereafter [59, 60]. In 2003, Sheehan [61] reported an even more impressive median survival length of 15 months in a retrospective review of 69 patients following stereotactic radiosurgery. Local control was observed in 96% of patients. Recent studies suggest that radiosurgery has significantly reshaped the course of the illness. Early significant tumor response from high-dose stereotactic radiosurgery predicted improved survival for patients [62]. The patients were classified into the good response group when the sum of the volume of the brain metastases decreased to less than 75% of the original volume at the 1-month follow-up MRI. The good response group survived significantly longer than the poor response group (median survival times of 18 months and 9 months, respectively; $p = 0.025$). Staehler [63] recently reported that in a series of 51 patients, a treatment combination consisting of sunitinib and hypofractionated high-dose radiotherapy resulted in not a single death attributable to cerebral metastasis.

Osseous metastases are not an uncommon occurrence in patients with renal cancer. The most common site of these metastases is the spine. In fact, 30% of patients with renal cell carcinoma will ultimately develop spinal metastases [64]. In 1983, Halperin [55] reported that radiation produced good pain control (77% response) for patients with metastatic bone pain. Time-dose-fractionation (TDF) equivalent ranged from 45 to 85. No correlation between response and TDF was observed. A larger series following 86 patients with painful osseous metastases found a 65% response rate for TDF ≥ 70 in comparison to 25% for TDF < 70, leading the authors to recommend that the lesions be treated to higher doses to obtain maximum response rates [65]. As we have mentioned before, stereotactic radiation offers the capability of delivering higher doses with a great amount of precision, the utility of which is particularly relevant in the context of treating bony lesions adjacent to the spinal cord. Gerszten [64] found spinal radiosurgery to relieve pain in 89% of patients treated for RCC spinal metastases. Similarly, favorable results confirming the safety and efficacy of stereotactic treatment of spinal metastases have been reported by a number of other authors [66, 67]. A retrospective review of 105 extracranial metastatic lesions from renal cell carcinoma treated with either a single-dose, image-guided, intensity-modulated radiosurgery of 18–24 Gy or SBRT (less than 5 fractions) dose of 20–30 Gy reported local progression-free survival of 80% for high single dose (24 Gy) versus 21% and 17% for the low single dose (<24 Gy) or hypofractionated regimens [68]. Multivariate analysis revealed that 24 Gy vs. a lower dose ($p = 0.009$) and a single dose vs. hypofractionation ($p = 0.008$) were significant predictors of improved local progression-free survival.

A 2017 systematic review of the radiosurgery literature for spine disease from metastatic RCC compiled the results of nine published series [69]. The studies analyzed revealed improvement in pain for 41–95% of patients with excellent local control of 71–85.7% at 1 year. Vertebral body compression fractures (VCF) were seen in 16–27.5% with single fraction therapy increasing the VCF risk [69].

A highly morbid and often fatal condition in RCC are inferior vena cava (IVC) thrombi. IVC thrombus results from tumor growth into the slow flowing IVC. The hypercoagulable growing tumor promotes coagulation resulting in a thrombi composed of both malignant and bland components. Such a thrombus result can obstruct the portal venous system resulting in Budd-Chiari syndrome, IVC flow causing lower extremity edema, and directly extend into the heart which can compromise cardiac output. The standard of care is surgical resection or thrombectomy. However, in widely metastatic patients with extensive tumors and/or in older patients with poor performance status such interventions are often not feasible. Recent retrospective studies have utilized SBRT to target the tumor component of the IVC thrombus and demonstrated promising results. A multinational retrospective review of 15 patients demonstrating receiving SBRT for inoperable IVC thrombus identified radiographic response in 58% of patients with all recording symptom relief [70]. Given the intravascular location of IVC thrombi and its proximity to radiation sensitive organs such as the duodenum and heart, utilization of onboard MRI to visualize and track tumor motion has demonstrated success. A five patient case series, a MRI linear accelerator was utilized to treat IVC thrombi and demonstrated excellent visualization of the tumor thrombus, and at last follow up all patients with symptoms experienced resolution without any evidence of disease recurrence [71].

There are few reports in the literature on the use of SBRT as an alternative to cytoreductive nephrectomy in patients with metastatic disease. A prospective phase 1 dose-escalation trial of SABR as an alternative to cytoreductive nephrectomy for inoperable patients reported acceptable toxicity, renal function preservation, and stable quality of life in 12 patients with metastatic RCC [72]. Three successive dose cohorts were assessed: 25 Gy/3 fractions, 30 Gy/3 fractions, and 35 Gy/3 fractions. No dose-limiting toxicities were found at the 35 Gy dose level. Median primary tumor size reduction was 17.3% at a median follow-up of 5.3 months. All patients progressed systemically and median overall survival was 6.7 months. The authors concluded that 35 Gy in 5 fractions yielded acceptable results in inoperable metastatic RCC, with further prospective investigation warranted [72]. With the recent conflicting results of CARMENA [73], which demonstrated no benefit of surgical cytoreductive nephrectomy in metastatic RCC patients treated with sunitinib, there has been renewed interest in SBRT for this role. Three ongoing trials are currently investigating the role of definitive SBRT to the primary lesion in metastatic RCC: Cytoshrink (NCT#04090710), Samurai (NCT#05327686), and ITALIC-RCC (EU CT#2024-517789-41-00).

It seems reasonable to believe that the palliative role of radiation therapy, especially stereotactic and hypofractionated RT, will continue to develop in the coming years. Figures 21.2 and 21.3 are representative examples of current radiation therapy techniques including stereotactic body radiation therapy for recurrent renal fossa mass (Fig. 21.2) and spinal radiosurgery for a spinal metastasis (Fig. 21.3).

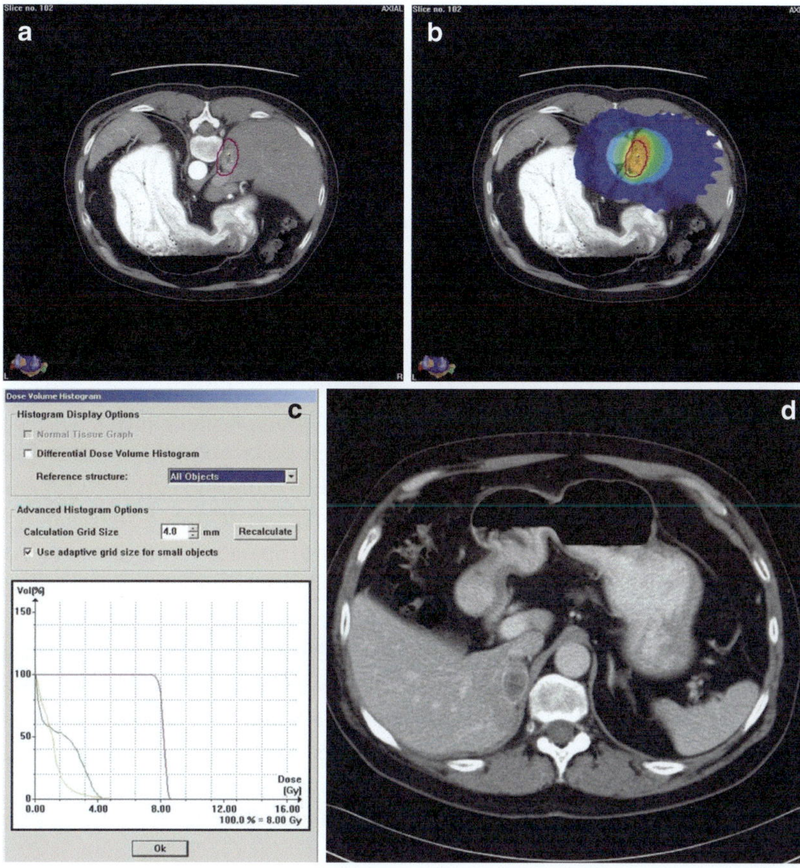

Fig. 21.2 (**a**) A 55-year-old male with history RCC s/p radical nephrectomy in 2002, s/p right lower and middle lobectomy for 1.5 cm RCC lung oligometastasis in 2004, presented in 2006 with local recurrence in right nephrectomy bed. Target delineated with 4D CT scan and treatment planning allowing for respiratory motion. (**b**) Color dose distribution. Prescription dose in *orange*, 30% dose in *dark blue*. (**c**) Dose-volume histogram (DVH) demonstrates nephrectomy bed mass (*purple*) received 32 Gy (8 Gy × 4) bowel (*green*) and spinal cord (*yellow*) were protected. (**d**) Posttreatment CT with increased conspicuity of the treated lesion due to central hypoattenuation seen at 4 months post treatment. The patient is now 6 years post-SBRT and NED

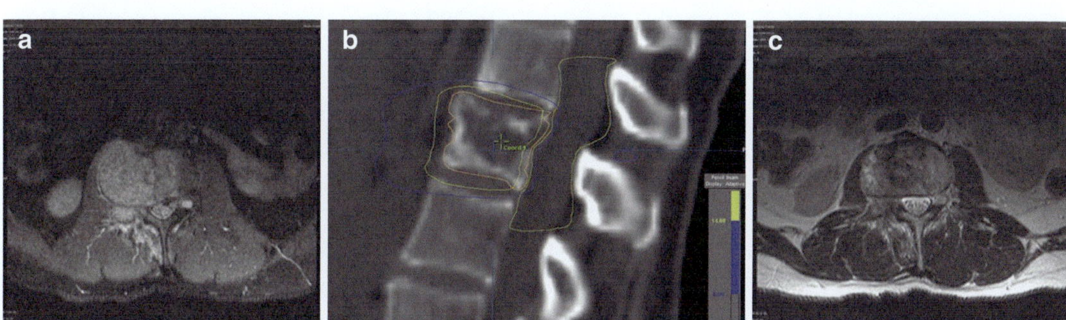

Fig. 21.3 (**a**) A 61-year-old male with severe back pain. MRI revealed spinal metastasis with paraspinal mass and mild thecal compression—biopsy metastatic RCC. (**b**) Isodose plan sagittal view. (**c**) Six months post SRS—regression of paraspinal mass and thecal compression. Patient pain-free at this site

Stereotactic Radiosurgery and Stereotactic Body Radiotherapy for Oligometastatic Disease

Oligometastatic disease is variably defined in the literature as having up to three or five metastases. In patients with RCC, metastases-directed therapy (MDT) including surgical metastasectomy, thermal ablation, and ablative radiation represent potentially curative options for individuals with oligometastatic RCC [41]. Alternatively, MDT has been proposed to defer systemic therapy, which has benefits in preserving quality of life and reducing healthcare expenditures [74, 75]. In patients receiving systemic therapy, the emergence of resistant clones, noted as a few areas of progressive metastatic deposits, is termed oligoprogression. Based on good initial reported outcomes, SBRT has been delivered to patients with oligometastatic and oligoprogressive disease with curative intent [76, 77].

The University of Texas Southwestern reported excellent local control with limited toxicity in its extracranial series utilizing SABR to treat 175 lesions in the spine (24%) and nonspine (76%) locations [78]. In this series, 75 of the 175 targeted lesions were treated with curative intent.

In 2021 Tang et al. published a single-arm prospective trial of serial SBRT in lieu of systemic therapy in 30 patients oligometastatic clear cell RCC and up to 5 metastases. Results were promising with no recorded deaths, and a median progression free survival of 22.7 months. At the time of study reporting only 7 of 30 patients had begun systemic therapy [75]. These results were confirmed in a similar prospective trial by Hannan et al. who once again investigated serial SBRT in 23 patients without systemic therapy, reporting 1 year freedom from systemic therapy of 91.3% and 1-year PFS not amenable to further SBRT at 82.6% [79]. The strategy of SBRT alone is being tested in a prospective ECOG-ACRIN EA8211 (SOAR) trial in which patients are being randomized to serial SBRT without systemic therapy versus frontline systemic therapy (NCT#05863351). In addition, the ASTROs trial is randomizing patients to maintenance 1-year pembrolizumab monotherapy after SBRT versus SBRT followed by surveillance to test whether pembrolizumab monotherapy will prolong time to progression (NCT#06004336).

Similarly, Meyer et al. recently published a retrospective compilation of 252 tumors treated with curative intent SABR in 188 patients from 6 French referral centers [80]. Among patients treated for oligometastatic disease, the median 2-year PFS and OS were 8.6 and 23 months, respectively. For those with oligoprogressive disease, the 2-year median PFS and OS were 7.6 and 33.9 months, respectively.

High-dose ablative RT has been combined with TKI inhibitors by several investigators to treat metastatic brain and spine disease sites with no apparent increase in risk of adverse effects from RT or targeted antiangiogenic agents [63, 81].

In 2017, Dewolf et al. reported the first phase I dose escalation trial combining high-dose RT to non-CNS sites with pazopanib, a selective multitargeted receptor tyrosine kinase inhibitor that blocks tumor growth and inhibits angiogenesis [82]. Three dose levels were evaluated (24 Gy/3 fractions, 30 Gy/3 fractions, and 36 Gy/3 fractions) in 13 patients, with one patient experiencing a dose-limiting grade 4 toxicity of hypoglycemia in the 36 Gy/3 fraction dose level. The investigators concluded that SBRT in combination with pazopanib is well tolerated with good local control and response rates outside the radiation field.

In 2023 Cem Onal et al. reported on 42 RCC patients with 5 or fewer lesions treated with TKI and SBRT. The 2-year OS and PFS rates were 58% and 51.3%. The 2-year LC was 94.1% per SBRT treated lesion. The authors concluded that SBRT in combination with TKIs is an effective and safe treatment option for RCC patients with five or fewer metastases. Distant metastasis was observed in 60% of the patients, indicating further improvement in systemic disease control is warranted [83].

Others are evaluating the efficacy of combined SBRT and anti-PD-1 antibody pembrolizumab to heighten the host immune system [84, 85] (see section “Immuno Radiotherapy”) through the abscopal effect. The abscopal effect refers to a rare phenomenon of tumor regression in lesions distant from the targeted site of radiotherapy, presumably through RT-induced activation of the host immune system. High-dose RT has been shown to preferentially enhance tumor-antigen presentation and later the tumor microenvironment when compared to conventionally fractionated RT [86].The Nives study recently reported results of a phase II single-arm multicenter trial in patients with metastatic RCC who progressed after antiangiogenic therapy, of whom at least one site was suitable for SBRT. A total of 69 patients received 30 Gy in three fractions to one metastatic site with concurrent Nivolumab. The authors concluded that Nivolumab in combination with SBRT does not provide evidence of improved outcomes in metastatic RCC over historical controls. However, they recommend that the approach be investigated in oligometastatic and oligoprogressive scenarios [87]. Prospective trials are currently underway to better understand the outcomes of combination targeted or immune therapies with SBRT in patients with RCC [84, 85, 88–90].

With regard to oligo progression there have been two prospective trials investigating progression directed MDT and maintenance on the current line systemic therapy. Cheung et al. reported on 38 patients receiving tyrosine kinase inhibitor monotherapy in a multicenter single-arm study [91]. They found that progression directed MDT prolonged the time until next systemic therapy by 12.6 months. Similarly, Hannan et al. reported on 20 patients receiving any systemic therapy [92]. This study found similar results, reporting time until new systemic therapy or death to be 11.1 months. In both studies MDT was associated with a low risk of grade 3 or higher toxicities (0 and 5%).

Immuno-Radiotherapy

Iodine-131 labeled tumor preferential monoclonal antibodies were shown to cause renal cell carcinoma xenograft regression and growth retardation in a nude mouse model [93]. The mice targeted with non-Iodine-131 labeled tumor preferential monoclonal antibodies failed to demonstrate variance from the control. Encouraging from a clinical standpoint, sequential computerized scintigraphy demonstrated that the radioisotopes were successfully targeted with high specificity for tumor tissue.

Radiation has also been postulated to enhance the antitumor response mediated by IL-2 in a murine metastatic renal adenocarcinoma model (Renca) [94]. Pulmonary metastases were induced by intravenous injection of Renca in Balb/c mice. Five days thereafter, a sublethal radiation dose (300 rads) was administered either to the whole body or the left lung alone. IL-2 (5000 Cetus units) was given intraperitoneally twice daily for 5 subsequent days. The mice were either sacrificed to assess tumor burden or followed for long-term survival. Pretreatment with irradiation significantly reduced pulmonary metastases and increased survival. Local irradiation of one lung was found to be equally as effective as whole-body irradiation. Metastases in the contralateral (nonirradiated) lung were found to be reduced following local irradiation, suggesting a systemic mechanism to increased antitumor response. The study's authors surmised this systemic mechanism was synergistic with IL-2 therapy. In a follow-up study at the same institution, investigators reported that immunohistochemistry demonstrated a macrophage influx following irradiation [95]. Meanwhile, IL-2 therapy induced T-cell infiltration into tumor nodules. The investigators concluded that macrophages, mobilized by radiation-induced tissue injury, phagocytosed apoptotic tumor cells and presented tumor antigens for a systemic immune response mediated by IL-2.

In a more recent study, cells of the human renal cancer cell line R11 were transfected by interferon-alpha gene and evaluated for radiation responses in vitro by clonogenic assays [96]. Investigators found that in addition to slowing cellular growth, transfection with the interferon-alpha gene increased radiosensitivity. Similar results have been reported for other cytokines, though not specifically in the context of renal cell carcinoma.

As previously discussed, clinical trials are underway to assess the role of a combination of immune modulators and radiation therapy in patients with RCC, where the immune system seems to play an important antitumor role. The University of Texas Southwestern is currently investigating the role of a combination of SBRT with IL-2 therapy in patients with metastatic RCC [88].

Conclusion

We have reached a far more expansive and nuanced understanding of the role of radiation therapy in the treatment of renal cell carcinoma over the course of the past decades. As radiotherapy evolves and as surgical, immunologic, and chemotherapeutic interventions evolve, this role will continue to be redefined. In addition to having an established role in palliation, the role of radiation to change the disease course in localized and metastatic RCC is emerging. If judiciously employed in this context, it is a safe, noninvasive, and efficacious treatment that bolsters the quality of life of patients afflicted with RCC. Further research is necessary to better understand the role radiation may play as an adjuvant therapy, a potential immune modulator, in the management of oligometastatic disease, and as a standard of care in the management of primary RCC.

References

1. Deschavanne PJ, Fertil B. A review of human cell radiosensitivity in vitro. Int J Radiat Oncol Biol Phys. 1996;34:251–66.
2. Michalski JM. Kidney, renal pelvis, and ureter. In: Perez C, Brady LW, Halperin EC, Schmidt-Ullrich RK, editors. Principles and practice of radiation oncology. 5th ed. Philadelphia, PA: Lippincott Williams and Wilkins; 2008.
3. Verma J, Mahajan A. The role of radiation therapy in renal cell carcinoma. In: Lara Jr PN, Jonasch E, editors. Kidney cancer. Berlin, Heidelberg: Springer-Verlag; 2012. p. 163–70.
4. Atkins MB, Avigan DE, Bukowski RM, Childs RW, Dutcher JP, Eisen TG, et al. Innovations and challenges in renal cancer. Clin Cancer Res. 2004;10(18):6277S–81S.
5. Lam JS, Shvarts O, Pantuck AJ. Changing concepts in the surgical management of renal cell carcinoma. Eur Urol. 2004;45:692–705.
6. Novick AC. Advances in the management of localized renal cell cancer. Can J Urol. 2000;7(2):960–6.
7. Haque W, Verma V, Lewis GD, Lo SS, Butler EB, Teh BS. Utilization of radiotherapy and stereotactic body radiation therapy for renal cell cancer in the USA. Future Oncol. 2018;14:819–27.
8. Otto U, Huland H, Baisch H, Klöppel G. Transplantation of human renal cell carcinoma into NMRI nu/nu mice. III. Effect of irradiation on tumor acceptance and tumor growth. J Urol. 1985;134:170–4.
9. Nias A. Radiobiological aspects of preoperative irradiation. Br J Radiol. 1967;40:166–9.
10. Riches E, Griffiths I, Thackray A. New growths of the kidney and ureter. Br J Urol. 1951;23:297–356.
11. Rost A, Brosig W. Preoperative irradiation of renal cell carcinoma. Urology. 1977;10:414–7.
12. Flocks R, Kadesky M. Malignant neoplasms of the kidney; an analysis of 353 patients followed five years or more. J Urol. 1958;79:196–201.
13. Riches E. The place of irradiation. JAMA. 1968;204(3):230–1.
14. Van der Werf-Messing B. Carcinoma of the kidney. Cancer. 1973;32:1056–61.
15. van der Werf-Messing B, van der Heul RO, Ledeboer RC. Renal cell carcinoma trial. Strahlentherapie [Sonderb]. 1981;76:169–75.
16. Juusela H, Malmio K, Alfthan O, Oravisto K. Preoperative irradiation in the treatment of renal adenocarcinoma. Scand J Urol Nephrol. 1977;11:277–81.
17. US National Library of Medicine. ClinicalTrials.gov. 2015. https://clinicaltrials.gov/ct2/show/NCT02473536. Accessed 1 Aug 2018.
18. Margulis V, Freifeld Y, Pop LM, Manna S, Kapur P, Pedrosa I, et al. Neoadjuvant SABR for renal cell carcinoma inferior vena cava tumor thrombus—safety lead-in results of a phase 2 trial. Int J Radiat Oncol Biol Phys. 2021;110(4):1135–42. PMID: 33549705.
19. Bratherton D III. The place of radiotherapy in the treatment of hypernephroma. Br J Radiol. 1964;37(434):141.
20. Rafla S. Renal cell carcinoma. Natural history and results of treatment. Cancer. 1970;25:26–40.
21. Finney R. The value of radiotherapy in the treatment of hypernephroma-a clinical trial. Br J Urol. 1973;45:258–69.
22. Kjaer M, Frederiksen PL, Engelholm S. Postoperative radiotherapy in stage II and III renal adenocarcinoma. A randomized trial by the Copenhagen Renal Cancer Study Group. Int J Radiat Oncol Biol Phys. 1987;13:665–72.

23. Rabinovitch RA, Zelefsky MJ, Gaynor JJ, Fuks Z. Patterns of failure following surgical resection of renal cell carcinoma: implications for adjuvant local and systemic therapy. J Clin Oncol. 1994;12:206–12.
24. Gez E, Libes M, Bar-Deroma R, Rubinov R, Stein M, Kuten A. Postoperative irradiation in localized renal cell carcinoma: the Rambam Medical Center experience. Tumori. 2002;88:500–2.
25. Kao GD, Malkowicz SB, Whittington R, D'Amico AV, Wein AJ. Locally advanced renal cell carcinoma: low complication rate and efficacy of postnephrectomy radiation therapy planned with CT. Radiology. 1994;193:725–30.
26. Makarewicz R, Zarzycka M, Kulińska G, Windorbska W. The value of postoperative radiotherapy in advanced renal cell cancer. Neoplasma. 1998;45:380.
27. Stein M, Kuten A, Halpern J, Coachman NM, Cohen Y, Robinson E. The value of postoperative irradiation in renal cell cancer. Radiother Oncol. 1992;24:41–4.
28. Tunio M, Hashmi A, Rafi M. Need for a new trial to evaluate postoperative radiotherapy in renal cell carcinoma: a meta-analysis of randomized controlled trials. Ann Oncol. 2010;21:1839–45.
29. Frydenberg M, Gunderson L, Hahn G, Fieck J, Zincke H. Preoperative external beam radiotherapy followed by cytoreductive surgery and intraoperative radiotherapy for locally advanced primary or recurrent renal malignancies. J Urol. 1994;152:15–21.
30. Krengli M, Calvo FA, Terrone C, Haddock MG, Hannoun-Levi JM, Thariat J, et al. Genitourinary cancer. In: Gunderson L, editor. Intraoperative irradiation: techniques and results. Totowa, NJ: Springer; 2011. p. 459–79.
31. Paly JJ, Hallemeier CL, Biggs PJ, et al. Outcomes in a multi-institutional cohort of patients treated with intraoperative radiation therapy for advanced or recurrent renal cell carcinoma. Int J Radiat Oncol Biol Phys. 2014;88:618–23.
32. Master VA, Gottschalk AR, Kane C, Carroll PR. Management of isolated renal fossa recurrence following radical nephrectomy. J Urol. 2005;174:473–7.
33. Choueiri TK, Tomczak P, Park SH, Venugopal B, Ferguson T, Symeonides SN, et al. Overall survival with adjuvant pembrolizumab in renal-cell carcinoma. N Engl J Med. 2024;390(15):1359–71. PMID: 38631003.
34. Choueiri TK, Tomczak P, Park SH, Venugopal B, Ferguson T, Chang Y-H, et al. Adjuvant pembrolizumab after nephrectomy in renal-cell carcinoma. N Engl J Med. 2021;385(8):683–94. PMID: 34407342.
35. Hui Z, Tretiakova M, Zhang Z, Li Y, Wang X, Zhu JX, Gao Y, Mai W, Furge K, Qian CN, Amato R, Butler EB, Teh BT, Teh BS. Radiosensitization by inhibiting STAT1 in renal cell carcinoma. Int J Radiat Oncol Biol Phys. 2009;73:288–95.
36. Siva S, Louie AV, Warner A, et al. Pooled analysis of stereotactic ablative radiotherapy for primary renal cell carcinoma: a report from the International Radiosurgery Oncology Consortium for Kidney (IROCK). Cancer. 2017;124:934–42.
37. Fuks Z, Kolesnick R. Engaging the vascular component of the tumor response. Cancer Cell. 2005;8:89–91.
38. Leith JT, Cook S, Chougule P, Calabresi P, Wahlberg L, Lindquist C, et al. Intrinsic and extrinsic characteristics of human tumors relevant to radiosurgery: comparative cellular radiosensitivity and hypoxic percentages. Acta Neurochir Suppl. 1994;62:18–27.
39. Walsh L, Stanfield JL, Cho LC, Chang C, Forster K, Kabbani W, et al. Efficacy of ablative high-dose-per-fraction radiation for implanted human renal cell cancer in a nude mouse model. Eur Urol. 2006;50:795–800.
40. Grant SR, Lei X, Hess KR, Smith GL, Matin SF, Wood CG, et al. Stereotactic body radiation therapy for the definitive treatment of early stage kidney cancer: a survival comparison with surgery, tumor ablation, and observation. Adv Radiat Oncol. 2020;5(3):495–502. PMID: 32529146.
41. Psutka SP, Master VA. Role of metastasis-directed treatment in kidney cancer. Cancer. 2018;124:3641. https://doi.org/10.1002/cncr.31341.
42. Beitler JJ, Makara D, Silverman P, Lederman G. Definitive, high-dose-per-fraction, conformal, stereotactic external radiation for renal cell carcinoma. Am J Clin Oncol. 2004;27:646–8.
43. Wersäll PJ, Blomgren H, Lax I, Kälkner KM, Linder C, Lundell G, et al. Extracranial stereotactic radiotherapy for primary and metastatic renal cell carcinoma. Radiother Oncol. 2005;77:88–95.
44. Siva S, Pham D, Gill S, Corcoran NM, Foroudi F. A systematic review of stereotactic radiotherapy ablation for primary renal cell carcinoma. BJU Int. 2012;110:E737. https://doi.org/10.1111/j.1464-410x.2012.11550.x.
45. Siva S, Jackson P, Kron T, et al. Impact of stereotactic radiotherapy on kidney function in primary renal cell carcinoma: establishing a dose–response relationship. Radiother Oncol. 2016;118:540–6.
46. Siva S, Pham D, Kron T, et al. Stereotactic ablative body radiotherapy for inoperable primary kidney cancer: a prospective clinical trial. BJU Int. 2017;120:623–30.
47. Siva S, et al. Stereotactic ablative body radiotherapy for primary kidney cancer (TROG 15.03 FASTRACK II): a non-randomized phase 2 trial. Lancet Oncol. 2024;3:308–16.
48. Gaudreault M, Hardcastle N, Jackson P, McIntosh L, Higgs B, Pryor D, et al. Dose-effect relationship of kidney function after SABR for primary renal cell carcinoma: TROG 15.03 FASTRACK II. Int J Radiat Oncol Biol Phys. 2024;120(3):648–54. PMID: 38679212.
49. Siva S, Ellis RJ, Ponsky L, et al. Consensus statement from the International Radiosurgery Oncology Consortium for Kidney for primary renal cell carcinoma. Future Oncol. 2016;12:637–45.
50. Siva S, et al. Stereotactic body radiotherapy for primary renal cell carcinoma: a systematic review and practice guideline from the International Society of

Stereotactic Radiosurgery (ISRS). Lancet Oncol. 2024;25(1):e18–28.
51. US National Library of Medicine. ClinicalTrials.gov. 2017. https://clinicaltrials.gov/ct2/show/NCT02613819. Accessed 1 Aug 2018.
52. US National Library of Medicine. ClinicalTrials.gov. 2017. https://clinicaltrials.gov/ct2/show/NCT03108703. Accessed 1 Aug 2018.
53. Wronski M, Arbit E, Russo P, Galicich JH. Surgical resection of brain metastases from renal cell carcinoma in 50 patients. Urology. 1996;47:187–93.
54. Wronski M, Maor MH, Davis BJ, Sawaya R, Levin VA. External radiation of brain metastases from renal carcinoma: a retrospective study of 119 patients from the MD Anderson Cancer Center. Int J Radiat Oncol Biol Phys. 1997;37:753–9.
55. Halperin EC, Harisiadis L. The role of radiation therapy in the management of metastatic renal cell carcinoma. Cancer. 1983;51:614–7.
56. Badalament RA, Kreutzer E, Cluck RW, Herr HW, Wong GY, Fair WR, et al. Surgical treatment of brain metastases from renal cell carcinoma. Urology. 1990;36(2):112–7.
57. Goyal LK, Suh JH, Reddy CA, Barnett GH. The role of whole brain radiotherapy and stereotactic radiosurgery on brain metastases from renal cell carcinoma. Int J Radiat Oncol Biol Phys. 2000;47:1007–12.
58. Amendola BE, Wolf AL, Coy SR, Amendola M, Bloch L. Brain metastases in renal cell carcinoma: management with gamma knife radiosurgery. Cancer J. 2000;6:372–6.
59. Ikushima H, Tokuuye K, Sumi M, Kagami Y, Murayama S, Ikeda H, et al. Fractionated stereotactic radiotherapy of brain metastases from renal cell carcinoma. Int J Radiat Oncol Biol Phys. 2000;48:1389–93.
60. Payne BR, Prasad D, Szeifert G, Steiner M, Steiner L. Gamma surgery for intracranial metastases from renal cell carcinoma. J Neurosurg. 2000;92:760–5.
61. Sheehan JP, Sun MH, Kondziolka D, Flickinger J, Lunsford LD. Radiosurgery in patients with renal cell carcinoma metastasis to the brain: long-term outcomes and prognostic factors influencing survival and local tumor control. J Neurosurg. 2003;98:342–9.
62. Kim WH, Kim DG, Han JH, Paek SH, Chung HT, Park CK, Kim CY, Kim YH, Kim JW, Jung HW. Early significant tumor volume reduction after radiosurgery in brain metastases from renal cell carcinoma results in long-term survival. Int J Radiat Oncol Biol Phys. 2012;82:1749–55.
63. Staehler M, Haseke N, Nuhn P, Tüllmann C, Karl A, Siebels M, et al. Simultaneous antiangiogenic therapy and single-fraction radiosurgery in clinically relevant metastases from renal cell carcinoma. BJU Int. 2011;108:673–8.
64. Gerszten PC, Burton SA, Ozhasoglu C, Vogel WJ, Welch WC, Baar J, et al. Stereotactic radiosurgery for spinal metastases from renal cell carcinoma. J Neurosurg Spine. 2005;3:288–95.
65. Onufrey V, Mohiuddin M. Radiation therapy in the treatment of metastatic renal cell carcinoma. Int J Radiat Oncol Biol Phys. 1985;11:2007–9.
66. Chang EL, Shiu AS, Mendel E, Mathews LA, Mahajan A, Allen PK, et al. Phase I/II study of stereotactic body radiotherapy for spinal metastasis and its pattern of failure. J Neurosurg Spine. 2007;7:151–60.
67. Yamada Y, Bilsky MH, Lovelock DM, Venkatraman ES, Toner S, Johnson J, et al. High-dose, single-fraction image-guided intensity-modulated radiotherapy for metastatic spinal lesions. Int J Radiat Oncol Biol Phys. 2008;71:484–90.
68. Zelefsky MJ, Greco C, Motzer R, Magsanoc JM, Pei X, Lovelock M, Mechalakos J, Zatcky J, Fuks Z, Yamada Y. Tumor control outcomes after hypofractionated and single-dose stereotactic image-guided intensity-modulated radiotherapy for extracranial metastases from renal cell carcinoma. Int J Radiat Oncol Biol Phys. 2012;82:1744–8.
69. Smith BW, Joseph JR, Saadeh YS, Marca FL, Szerlip NJ, Schermerhorn TC, Spratt DE, Younge KC, Park P. Radiosurgery for treatment of renal cell metastases to spine: a systematic review of the literature. World Neurosurg. 2018;109:e502. https://doi.org/10.1016/j.wneu.2017.10.011.
70. Freifeld Y, Pedrosa I, Mclaughlin M, Correa RM, Louie AV, Maldonado JA, et al. Stereotactic ablative radiation therapy for renal cell carcinoma with inferior vena cava tumor thrombus. Urol Oncol. 2022;40(4):166.e9–13. PMID: 35144866.
71. Shanker, et al. BJUI Compass. 2024 (in press).
72. Correa RJM, Ahmad B, Warner A, Johnson C, Mackenzie MJ, Pautler SE, Bauman GS, Rodrigues GB, Louie AV. A prospective phase I dose-escalation trial of stereotactic ablative radiotherapy (SABR) as an alternative to cytoreductive nephrectomy for inoperable patients with metastatic renal cell carcinoma. Radiat Oncol. 2018;13:47. https://doi.org/10.1186/s13014-018-0992-3.
73. Méjean A, Ravaud A, Thezenas S, Colas S, Beauval J-B, Bensalah K, et al. Sunitinib alone or after nephrectomy in metastatic renal-cell carcinoma. N Engl J Med. 2018;379(5):417–27. PMID: 29860937.
74. Tang C, Msaouel P. Charting the path to systemic therapy de-escalation-oligometastatic kidney cancer as a paradigm. JAMA Oncol. 2024;10(5):561–2. PMID: 38451536.
75. Tang C, Msaouel P, Hara K, Choi H, Le V, Shah AY, et al. Definitive radiotherapy in lieu of systemic therapy for oligometastatic renal cell carcinoma: a single-arm, single-centre, feasibility, phase 2 trial. Lancet Oncol. 2021;22(12):1732–9. PMID: 34717797.
76. Ranck MC, Golden DW, Corbin KS, Hasselle MD, Liauw SL, Stadler WM, Hahn OM, Weichselbaum RR, Salama JK. Stereotactic body radiotherapy for the treatment of oligometastatic renal cell carcinoma. Am J Clin Oncol. 2013;36:589–95.
77. Siva S, Kothari G, Muacevic A, Louie AV, Slotman BJ, Teh BS, Lo SS. Radiotherapy for renal cell carcinoma: renaissance of an overlooked approach. Nat Rev Urol. 2017;14:549–63.
78. Wang CJ, Christie A, Lin M-H, et al. Safety and efficacy of stereotactic ablative radiation therapy for

renal cell carcinoma extracranial metastases. Int J Radiat Oncol Biol Phys. 2017;98:91–100.
79. Hannan R, Christensen M, Christie A, Garant A, Pedrosa I, Robles L, et al. Stereotactic ablative radiation for systemic therapy-naïve oligometastatic kidney cancer. Eur Urol Oncol. 2022;5(6):695–703. PMID: 35985982.
80. Meyer E, Pasquier D, Bernadou G, et al. Stereotactic radiation therapy in the strategy of treatment of metastatic renal cell carcinoma: a study of the Getug group. Eur J Cancer. 2018;98:38–47.
81. Miller JA, Balagamwala EH, Angelov L, Suh JH, Rini B, Garcia JA, Ahluwalia M, Chao ST. Spine stereotactic radiosurgery with concurrent tyrosine kinase inhibitors for metastatic renal cell carcinoma. J Neurosurg Spine. 2016;25:766–74.
82. Wolf KD, Rottey S, Vermaelen K, et al. Combined high dose radiation and pazopanib in metastatic renal cell carcinoma: a phase I dose escalation trial. Radiat Oncol. 2017;12:157. https://doi.org/10.1186/s13014-017-0893-x.
83. Onal C, et al. Stereotactic body radiotherapy and tyrosine kinase inhibitors in patients with oligometastatic renal cell carcinoma: a multi-institutional study. Strahlentherapie und Onkologie. 2023;199:456–64.
84. US National Library of Medicine. ClinicalTrials.gov. 2016. https://clinicaltrials.gov/ct2/show/NCT02855203. Accessed 1 Aug 2018.
85. US National Library of Medicine. ClinicalTrials.gov. 2016. https://clinicaltrials.gov/ct2/show/NCT02599779. Accessed 1 Aug 2018.
86. Formenti SC, Demaria S. Systemic effects of local radiotherapy. Lancet Oncol. 2009;10:718–26.
87. Masini C, et al. Nivolumab in combination with stereotactic body radiotherapy in pretreated patients with metastatic renal cell carcinoma. Results of the phase II NIVES study. Eur Urol. 2022;81(3):274–82.
88. US National Library of Medicine. ClinicalTrials.gov. 2016. https://clinicaltrials.gov/ct2/show/NCT01896271. Accessed 1 Aug 2018.
89. US National Library of Medicine. ClinicalTrials.gov. 2017. https://clinicaltrials.gov/ct2/show/NCT02334709. Accessed 1 Aug 2018.
90. US National Library of Medicine. ClinicalTrials.gov. 2016. https://clinicaltrials.gov/ct2/show/NCT03065179. Accessed 1 Aug 2018.
91. Cheung P, Patel S, North SA, Sahgal A, Chu W, Soliman H, et al. Stereotactic radiotherapy for oligoprogression in metastatic renal cell cancer patients receiving tyrosine kinase inhibitor therapy: a phase 2 prospective multicenter study. Eur Urol. 2021;80(6):693–700. PMID: 34399998.
92. Hannan R, McLaughlin MF, Pop LM, Pedrosa I, Kapur P, Garant A, et al. Phase 2 trial of stereotactic ablative radiotherapy for patients with primary renal cancer. Eur Urol. 2023;84(3):275–86. PMID: 36898872.
93. Chiou RK, Vessella RL, Limas C, Shafer RB, Elson MK, Arfman EW, et al. Monoclonal antibody-targeted radiotherapy of renal cell carcinoma using a nude mouse model. Cancer. 1988;61(9):1766–75.
94. Chakrabarty A, Hillman GG, Maughan RL, Ali E, Pontes JE, Haas GP. Radiation therapy enhances the therapeutic effect of immunotherapy on pulmonary metastases in a murine renal adenocarcinoma model. In Vivo. 1994;8:25–31.
95. Dezso B, Haas GP, Hamzavi F, Kim S, Montecillo EJ, Benson PD, et al. The mechanism of local tumor irradiation combined with interleukin 2 therapy in murine renal carcinoma: histological evaluation of pulmonary metastases. Clin Cancer Res. 1996;2:1543–52.
96. Syljuåsen RG, Belldegrun A, Tso CL, Withers HR, McBride WH. Sensitization of renal carcinoma to radiation using alpha interferon (IFNA) gene transfection. Radiat Res. 1997;148:443–8.

Systemic Therapies for the Treatment of Renal Cell Carcinoma

22

Sonia Gowda and Paul Mathew

Introduction

In the United States, approximately 82,000 new cases with 14,000 deaths from metastatic kidney cancer are estimated in 2024 [1, 2]. Most kidney cancer deaths (90%) are secondary to metastatic CRCC. Only 10% of patients present with the classic triad of flank pain, hematuria, and a palpable mass on exam [3]. Synchronous metastases are present in about one-third of patients newly diagnosed with RCC, while approximately 30% will progress to distant metastasis after prior nephrectomy for localized disease [4]. The most common form of metastatic presentation of MRCC is lung metastases. Solitary metachronous lung metastases are particularly suitable for metastasectomy with curative intent and represent a first choice for consideration in the surgically fit patient [5, 6]. Low volume indolent metastases, such as may be observed in the lung or pancreas, can be monitored alone, particularly if the risk of systemic therapy is significant and resection is not practicable [7, 8]. Surgery and/or radiation therapy in MRCC may be required to control a dominant symptomatic metastasis, such as in the brain, with pathological fractures or cord compression from bone metastases, or to control a painful bleeding primary tumor in the kidney. These palliative imperatives may preclude the initiation of systemic therapy until surgical recovery and/or after the completion of radiation.

Systemic Therapy Options in Metastatic Disease

Translational Considerations Von-Hippel Lindau (*VHL*) disease is an autosomal dominant hereditary cancer syndrome at risk for CRCC, paragangliomas, phaeochromocytomas, and vascular tumors, including retinal, cerebellar, and spinal cord hemangioblastomas. Patients with VHL disease harbor a germline loss-of-function *VHL* allele, and tumors typically develop after the remaining wild-type allele is mutated or lost [9]. The majority of sporadic CRCC tumors (70–80%) have biallelic *VHL* mutation, less commonly hypermethylation, consistent with a Knudson two-hit tumor suppressor. Advances in the field of oxygen sensing have led to deep insights into the function of the VHL protein (pVHL) with translational implications [10]. Under normoxic conditions, HIF2α undergoes prolyl hydroxylation, which then marks it as a high-affinity substrate for binding to pVHL, which is a substrate recognition motif for an E3 ubiquitin ligase. This results in ubiquitination and proteosomal degradation of HIF2α. Either when pVHL is defective or under hypoxic conditions, HIF2α accumulates and can bind its partner HIF1β. The complex can now translocate to the nucleus to bind to hypoxia-

A correction to this chapter can be found at https://doi.org/10.1007/978-3-031-97599-8_25

S. Gowda · P. Mathew (✉)
Division of Hematology-Oncology, Tufts Medical Center, Boston, MA, USA
e-mail: Sonia.Gowda@tuftsmedicine.org; Paul.Mathew@tuftsmedicine.org

J. A. Libertino, J. R. Gee (eds.), *Renal Cancer*, https://doi.org/10.1007/978-3-031-97599-8_22

response elements (HREs) in promoter regions of multiple target genes, including *VEGFA* and *PDGFB*. VEGF plays a major role in both normal and tumor-associated angiogenesis. Among all epithelial tumors, CRCC tumors have the highest levels of VEGF expression [11, 12], supporting the rationale for targeting VEGF and its receptors, particularly VEGFR2 [13]. Allosteric inhibitors of HIF2α dimerization, such as belzutifan, represent an alternative strategy to target the molecular sequelae of VHL loss, central to the pathogenesis of CRCC [14] (Fig. 22.1).

The cytokine therapeutic era with interferon-alpha and interleukin-2 established the immune-responsiveness of CRCC, before it was eclipsed by VEGFR-TKI therapy, which demonstrated superior response rates, progression-free, and overall survival compared to this class of immunotherapeutics [15].

Immunotherapy forged a remarkable return to center-stage in CRCC with the advent of ICI therapy [16]. Although CRCCs are characterized as among the most highly inflamed solid tumors [17], they are associated with low mutation burdens as traditionally assessed by next-generation sequencing, which examines the presence of non-synonymous single-nucleotide variants in genomic hotspots associated with cancer, i.e., variants that result in a shift in the amino acid sequence of proteins. Whole-exome sequencing, however, demonstrated the highest proportion of frameshift insertion or deletions (indels) in CRCC, when compared to other solid tumors, projected as the principal mutagenic source of immunogenic neoantigens [18, 19]. Intriguingly, human endogenous retroviruses have also been proposed as drivers of immunogenicity in CRCC. Reactivation of evolutionary vestiges of these retroviruses is thought to trigger immune system recognition and contribute to immunogenicity [18, 20].

Taken together, this background sets the stage for the apparent synergy of VEGFR-TKIs and ICI therapy in CRCC that has yielded major survival advances in multiple Phase III trials over VEGFR-TKI monotherapy [21, 22]. VEGF has been identified as a major immunosuppressive cytokine in the tumor immune microenviron-

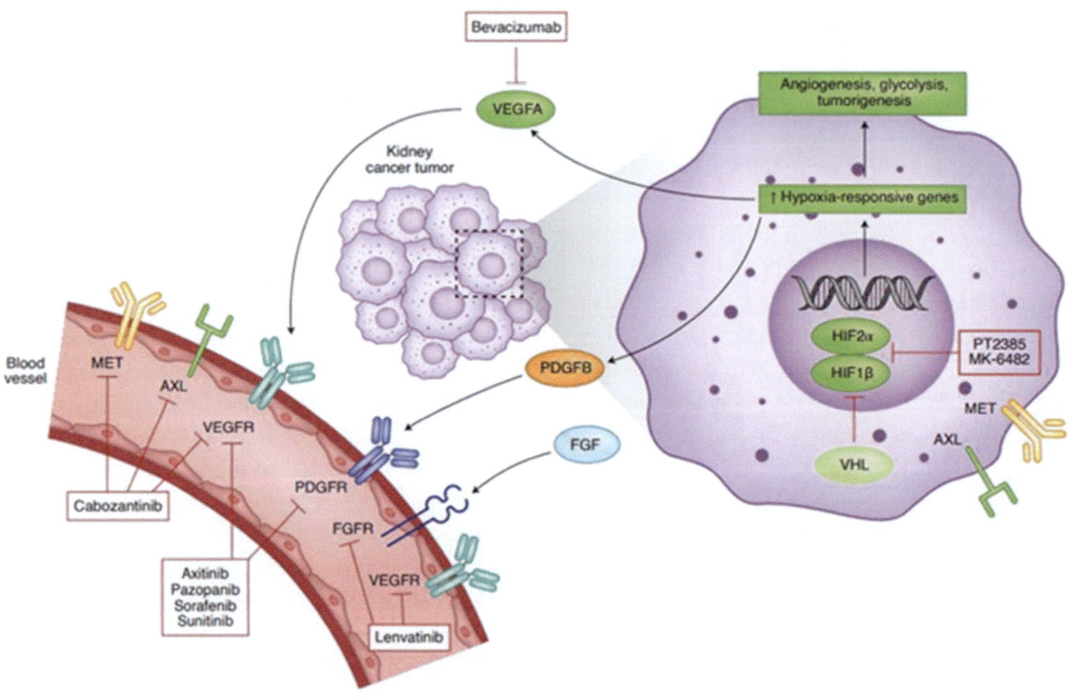

Fig. 22.1 Therapeutic targeting of pathological signaling secondary to VHL-inactivation [10]

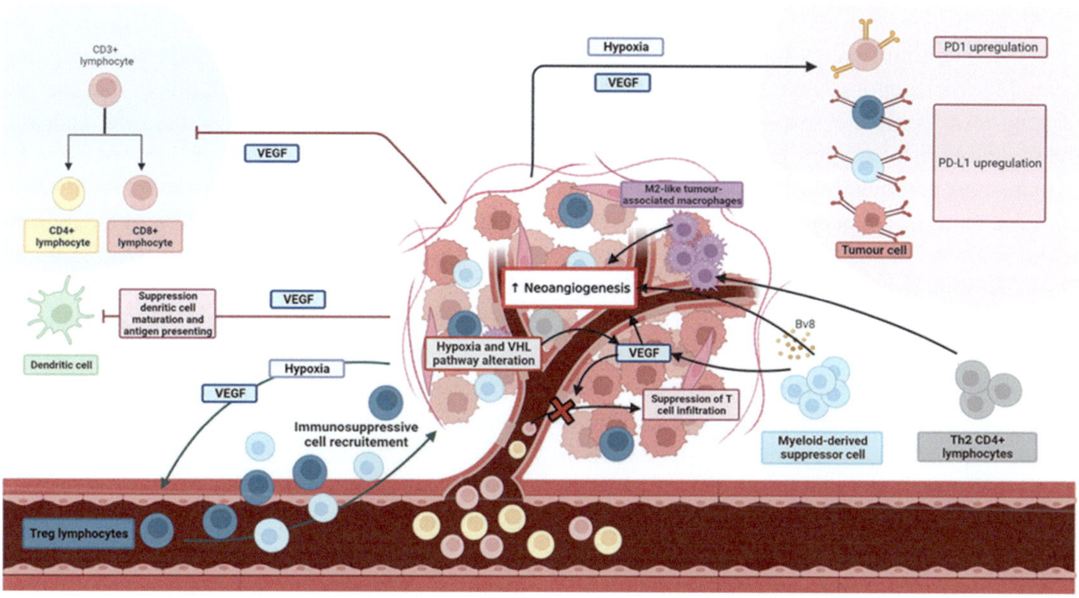

Fig. 22.2 VEGF regulates an immune-suppressed tumor microenvironment in renal cell carcinoma [22]

ment, impairing dendritic cell antigen presentation, natural killer and cytotoxic T cell function while upregulating inhibitory T-regulatory cells, M2 polarized macrophages, and myeloid-derived suppressor cells [22, 23] (Fig. 22.2). Control of VEGF signaling and/or blockade of diverse inhibitory immune checkpoint signaling can overcome the restraints imposed on the immune surveillance [24] in CRCC and generate high-quality and durable tumor responses.

Risk Stratification and Therapeutic Choices

The approach to treatment selection for patients with MRCC begins with the identification of risk status, which has evolved with time. The International Metastatic RCC Database Consortium (IMDC) Risk Model is currently the most widely utilized tool to inform front-line treatment for metastatic disease [25, 26]. The model incorporates time from diagnosis to initiation of therapy, Karnofsky performance score, hemoglobin, calcium level, with neutrophilia and thrombocytosis as independent factors of increased risk. Absence of any risk factors confers favorable risk, with a median survival of 43.2 months; one to two risk factors confer intermediate risk, with a median survival of 22.5 months, and three or more risk factors confer poor risk, with a median survival of 7.8 months. The model has been employed for clinical trial stratification, leading the way for interpretation of clinical trial outcomes and risk-adapted treatment selection.

In the front-line therapy of metastatic CRCC, four combination regimens—ipilimumab and nivolumab [27], axitinib and pembrolizumab [28], cabozantinib and nivolumab [29], and lenvatinib and pembrolizumab [30]—have demonstrated improved survival over sunitinib monotherapy and represent the current standard of care options in the field [31]. These represent either double ICI therapy or a combination of a VEGFR-TKI and a PD-1 antibody. Clinical trials that integrated PDL-1 antibody therapy, either avelumab or atezolizumab, have not yielded overall survival advantages in CRCC to date [32–35]. The long-term outcomes of the combination regimens that prolonged both PFS and overall survival, stratified by IMDC risk-category, are represented in Table I, with follow-up from 43 to 99 months [36–39]. Each of these regimens continues to demonstrate improved overall survival over sunitinib, except for patients within the favorable risk category. Nevertheless, the fraction of long-term complete responders (CR) within the favorable risk category is consistently higher with all four combinatorial regimens, up to 21% with lenvatinib and pembrolizumab versus 5% with sunitinib. This is also true for the combination of ipilimumab and nivolumab, approved for patients with intermediate and poor-risk disease, with a CR rate of 12.8% versus 6.5% with sunitinib. Although objective response and progression-free survival (PFS) rates in favorable-risk disease with ipilimumab and nivolumab is nearly half that compared to sunitinib, the durable complete response rates and duration of responses is nearly doubled. For the three VEGFR-TKI and PD-1 antibody combination regimens, tumor response rates, PFS, complete responses, and duration of response are superior across all IMDC risk groups compared to sunitinib, although overall survival failed to meet significance in the favorable-risk group. In all studies, the time to response favored combination therapy over sunitinib. The median duration of response in patients with intermediate and poor-risk disease receiving ipilimumab and nivolumab is nearly 7 years with CR rates of 12% compared to a 20 month median response duration and a 2.6% CR rate with sunitinib. It can be argued therefore that to achieve long-term CR outcomes in metastatic CRCC, combination therapy is superior to VEGFR-TKI monotherapy across all risk-groups. To date, the most favorable long-term response data are with the double ICI combination, although with further follow-up, the responses to VEGFR-TKI and PD-1 combinations may prove to be similarly durable.

There are no head-to-head comparisons of these combinations, and real-world comparisons may be required to assess community adoption of these regimens, their time on treatment with comparative survival and toxicity outcomes. Data suggest that axitinib and pembrolizumab may be the most commonly adopted regimen in community practice, with the most durable time on treatment and no difference in survival from ipililumab and nivolumab [40, 41]. Comparative toxicity outcomes may influence the choice of therapy. For example, systemic corticosteroids were required in 40% of patients treated with nivolumab and ipilimumab [27] which is higher than the approximately 15–20% of patients receiving VEGFR-TKI and ICI combinations. Treatment discontinuation rates for toxicity varied from 20% with cabozantinib and nivolumab to 37% with lenvatinib and pembrolizumab. In this regard, it is worth pointing out that it is unlikely that recommended starting VEGFR-TKI doses in these regimens represent the optimal biological dose for all patients, and dose-titration based on tolerance may be a reasonable option to consider for the frail (author's preference). There are no clear data to inform whether one combination regimen is superior to another in the presence of bone [42], liver [43] or brain metastases [44].

Triplet combination therapy with anti-CTLA-4/PD-1 blockade and VEGFR-TKI was investigated in the phase 3 COSMIC-313 study, in which patients with advanced clear cell RCC with IMDC intermediate- or poor-risk disease were randomized to receive first-line therapy with ipilimumab and nivolumab with either cabozantinib or placebo. The addition of cabozantinib was associated with an improvement in the primary endpoint, with a significantly prolonged PFS at 12 months, with a hazard ratio of 0.73, as well as a higher overall response rate of 43% in the triplet combination group versus 36% in the control group. However, the toxicity of the triplet regimen also appeared to be substantially higher, with grade 3 or 4 adverse events occurring in 79% of patients in the triplet therapy group and 56% of patients in the control group. The triplet regimen of ipilimumab, nivolumab, and cabozantinib is not currently approved, but overall survival follow-up is ongoing [45]. The PDIGREE Phase III study assesses the sequential integration of cabozantinib with nivolumab following induction with ipilimumab and nivolumab therapy alone and has completed accrual [46].

The frontline combination trials that have established superiority over sunitinib are limited by the absence of a single-agent PD-1 antibody control arm, and the role of ***ICI monotherapy in the front-line*** is undefined. Studies of first-line

PD-1/PD-L1 inhibitor monotherapy, followed by the addition of CTLA-4 blockade as salvage, only for those patients who have a suboptimal response to PD-1/PD-L1 monotherapy, demonstrate a modest response to salvage combination therapy, while other patients demonstrated progression too rapidly to receive this strategy [47, 48]. Therefore, PD-1 antibody monotherapy is only recommended in patients ineligible for integration of CTLA-4 inhibition or VEGFR-TKI therapy.

Front-line VEGFR-TKI monotherapy may be considered in metastatic disease for those who have absolute contraindications to immune checkpoint inhibitors including severe autoimmune disease or prior organ transplant, or in those with favorable risk and low burden of disease. The TKIs sunitinib, sorafenib, pazopanib, axitinib, lenvatinib, cabozantinib, and tivozanib have been approved by the FDA as monotherapy for advanced RCC. A randomized phase 3 inferiority trial compared pazopanib versus sunitinib as first-line therapy in patients with metastatic RCC [49]. The progression-free survival for patients treated with pazopanib was noninferior to the PFS for those treated with sunitinib, and the overall survival was similar. The safety profile favored pazopanib, although a higher incidence of hepatotoxicity was seen with pazopanib. Sunitinib-associated hypertension, defined as a maximum or mean systolic blood pressure greater than 140 mm Hg, was associated with an improvement in clinical outcome, suggesting that the development of hypertension during therapy may be a biomarker of response to VEGFR-TKIs [49]. The phase 2 CABOSUN trial demonstrated improvement in progression-free survival with cabozantinib compared to sunitinib in treatment-naïve intermediate or poor risk advanced RCC; however, the difference in overall survival was not statistically significant [50].

Active Surveillance in MRCC Patients who can be considered for active surveillance typically have low volume of metastatic disease with metastases in 1-2 organ systems at most, few or no symptoms related to disease, fall within IMDC favorable or intermediate risk categories, and display an absence of high risk pathologic features, e.g., low grade tumors with absence of sarcomatoid variant disease [51]. Those with a long interval between nephrectomy and the development of metastases, with an overall low burden of metastatic disease, may also be considered for active surveillance. Elderly patients, or those with significant comorbidities who have asymptomatic, slow-growing metastases may also be candidates for observation rather than immediate treatment.

Evolving Subsequent Lines of Therapy: Are They Effective?

Second-line therapy in the context of metastatic CRCC depends on prior treatment, e.g., VEGFR-TKI or ICI-only regimens. It is increasingly less common for patients to be PD-1-inhibitor-naïve or to have used an older-generation VEGFR-TKI in the front-line, such as sunitinib or sorafenib. There are no established standards of care for a VEGFR-TKI in the second-line setting for patients who have received a potent VEGFR-TKI such as cabozantinib, lenvatinib, or axitinib in the front-line. If an ICI and VEGFR-TKI combination was used as a first-line therapy, patients should be considered for a regimen that incorporates a different VEGFR-TKI such as cabozantinib, lenvatinib, or tivozanib. However, there are now two randomized trials that have demonstrated no advantage with an alternate VEGFR-TKI combined with PD-1 antibody retreatment; both cabozantinib and atezolizumab [52] and tivozanib and nivolumab [53] failed to demonstrate any advantage over the respective VEGF/R-inhibitor control arm. Older studies have demonstrated that patients with disease progression while undergoing older-generation VEGF-targeted therapy can experience a response to a more potent VEGF-targeted therapy, such as with axitinib [54] and cabozantinib [55], whereas the mTOR inhibitor everolimus was ineffective. Lenvatinib, which inhibits FGFR in addition to VEGF, has been shown to improve progression-free survival in combination with everolimus compared to everolimus alone in patients previously treated with antiangiogenic therapy [56].

This combination was FDA approved in 2016 for treatment of advanced renal cell carcinoma after one prior antiangiogenic therapy. In the third- or fourth-line setting, another VEGF-directed TKI, tivozanib, has demonstrated improved progression-free survival and less toxicity in comparison with sorafenib after two previous lines of therapy, including at least one VEGF-directed therapy, resulting in FDA approval for relapsed or refractory advanced renal cell carcinoma following two or more prior systemic therapies [57]. However, no improvement in overall survival was observed, and less than 30% of patients had received immunotherapy previously. In practice, clinicians may switch between VEGF inhibitors if other options are exhausted and clinical trials are not available. There may be a benefit in alternating between TKIs with broad-spectrum (cabozantinib, lenvatinib) and narrow-spectrum (axitinib, tivozanib) activity.

HIF2α Inhibitor Therapy The orally bioavailable HIF-2 inhibitor belzutifan was approved by the FDA in 2021 for patients with VHL syndrome and VHL-associated renal cell carcinoma, CNS hemangioblastomas, and pancreatic neuroendocrine tumors that do not require immediate surgery [58]. Belzutifan has also been shown to demonstrate efficacy in CRCC in those without VHL syndrome. The LITESPARK-005 trial compared belzutifan 120mg once daily versus everolimus 10mg once daily in 746 patients with unresectable locally advanced or metastatic clear-cell RCC with disease progression after 1 to 3 prior regimens, including at least one anti-PD-(L)1 monoclonal antibody and at least one VEGFR-TKI. Specifically, eligible patients had evidence of disease progression after treatment with both a PD1 or PD-L1 inhibitor and VEGFR-TKI, received in sequence or in combination. Approximately 50% of patients in the belzutifan arm had had one prior VEGFR-TKI, and the other 50% had had 2-3 prior VEGFR-TKIs. About 45% in the belzutifan arm had had three prior lines of therapy. Overall, 43% of participants had received two prior lines of treatment, and 42% had received three prior lines of treatment. The trial demonstrated an improvement in progression-free survival with belzutifan compared to everolimus (HR 0.74), with a median PFS of 5.6 in both arms. The estimated percentage of patients who were progression-free at 12 months was 33.4% in the belzutifan group and 17.1% in the everolimus group. The overall response rate was also higher with belzutifan, at 22.7%, versus 3.5% with everolimus. Difference in overall survival was not statistically different at the time of the final data report [59]. Based on the PFS benefit, the FDA approved belzutifan in December 2023 for advanced renal cell carcinoma patients following prior anti-PD-1/L1 and VEGFR-TKI [60]. Common adverse events with belzutifan include fatigue, anemia, hypoxia, dyspnea, and nausea. Anemia and hypoxia occurred at higher rates in the belzutifan arm; grade 3 to 5 anemia occurred at a rate of 32.5% with belzutifan compared with 18.1% in the everolimus arm, and grade 3 to 5 hypoxia occurred in 10.5% of patients in the belzutifan arm, compared with 1.1% of patients in the everolimus arm. While both were managed with blood transfusion and supportive oxygen, these adverse effects are important to note for a treatment population that may have these comorbidities at baseline due to advanced renal failure. More research is needed on the safety of belzutifan in this patient population, at the end stage of kidney disease, or in those who are dialysis dependent. Belzutifan has addressed the previously unmet need for therapies with novel targets in advanced RCC by targeting the HIF pathway. However, a major limitation of the trial is the choice of everolimus as the comparator drug, which has been shown in prior trials to be less efficacious as a monotherapy compared to cabozantinib, nivolumab, and combination lenvatinib and everolimus, and the lack of demonstrable survival benefit. Trials assessing the efficacy of combination VEGFR-TKIs and HIF inhibitors are in progress as a form of vertical combination therapy along the VHL-pathway, with and without ICI therapy as a novel triplet regimen.

In conclusion, given the major advances in front-line therapy of metastatic RCC, the second-line remains open to novel investigational approaches that address the biological heterogeneity of the disease and treatment resistance to potent front-line VEGFR-TKI therapy combined with ICI therapy, either PD-1 or combined CTLA-4 and PD-1 therapy. In this context, there are no survival advantages demonstrated to date.

Renal Cell Carcinoma with Sarcomatoid and Rhabdoid Differentiation RCC with sarcomatoid differentiation (sRCC) displays an aggressive phenotype characterized by epithelial–mesenchymal transition and tends to respond poorly to VEGFR-TKIs compared to epithelioid RCC. Front-line combination trials with ICI therapy have uniformly demonstrated better efficacy, potentially due to more prominent immune cell infiltration [61]. The long-term update of ipilimumab and nivolumab showed the best outcomes for sarcomatoid variant disease, with ORR of 61% versus 23.1%, and CR of 18.9% versus 3.1% versus sunitinib [62]. Tumors with elements of rhabdoid differentiation represent aggressive variants, but adequate data to assess the impact on ICI efficacy is lacking [61].

Considerations for Elderly Populations There are no readily established criteria for what is defined as an elderly patient and among the trials in CRCC, patients above the age of 75 years are significantly under-represented. Overall, there is little evidence of diminished evidence of activity of ICI therapy either alone or in combination with VEGFR-TKI therapy as a result of immune senescence. The PFS and overall survival advantage in patients between 65 and 75 years of age is more readily evaluable, and among these patients, there is little difference in outcomes compared to younger patients. Toxicity rates are not reported to be more frequent or serious in patients above 65 years of age [63].

Immunocompromised and Organ Transplant Immunocompromised patients also pose a challenge when considering optimal treatment for advanced disease. Trials routinely excluded patients with a previous history of transplant, who were diagnosed with active autoimmune disorders, or who were on significant dose levels of glucocorticoids at the time of enrollment; therefore, data regarding benefit and tolerance in this population are limited. In organ transplant patients, the risk of graft rejection with the use of immunotherapy is as high as 50%, and the most common oncologic outcome is progression. Rotation to the mTOR inhibitor sirolimus from calcineurin inhibitors and integration of a VEGFR-TKIs like lenvatinib would approximate the lenvatinib-everolimus combination regimen that is active in the second-line therapy of CRCC, but durable complete responses would not be anticipated. The use of pulse-dose steroids with mTOR inhibitors has been advanced as a potential strategy to maintain graft function without compromising efficacy of a concurrently administered PD-1 inhibitor in cutaneous squamous cell carcinoma, with sequential addition of CTLA-4 inhibitor therapy implemented for progression of disease [64]. It is not clear if such a strategy would have equivalent efficacy outcomes in other solid tumors [65]. A risk-adapted approach appears warranted. In the life-threatening evolution of metastatic CRCC in the organ transplant setting, combined ICI therapy may fully exploit the putative immunogenic credentials of a tumor that arose in a background of long-term immunosuppression. Transition to dialysis would need to be anticipated in such a scenario in which life-preservation is privileged over graft preservation. Informative biomarkers would guide therapy in such a scenario. The majority of RCCs will develop in the native kidney, however, these can occur in the allograft. [66] Allograft CRCC can either be transmitted by the donor or develop after transplant. As these patients are typically closely monitored, most CRCCs in this population are detected in the early stage, still amenable to surgical intervention such as partial or complete nephrectomy or radiofrequency ablation. A modification to the immunosuppressive regimen may be required; in this scenario, transition to mTOR inhibitors is an appropriate consideration. A multivariate analysis of posttransplant malignancies in 33,249 deceased donor primary solitary renal transplant recipients found that maintenance immunosuppression with mTOR inhibitor drugs, sirolimus and everolimus, is associated with a reduced risk of developing posttransplant de novo malignancy [67].

Adjuvant Systemic Therapy in Localized RCC

For patients with localized renal cancer, surgical excision via open or laparoscopic nephrectomy is the primary treatment, with either radical nephrectomy or nephron-sparing partial nephrectomy for smaller tumors. The role of lymphadenectomy is controversial and has not been proven to extend overall survival. Randomized studies conducted in the cytokine era failed to demonstrate an advantage for adjuvant interferon or interleukin-2 [68].

A large phase 3 randomized clinical study, KEYNOTE-564, evaluated the role of adjuvant pembrolizumab 200 mg intravenously every 3 weeks for 1 year versus placebo in patients with CRCC with intermediate-high or high risk of recurrence after prior nephrectomy, with or without metastasectomy. Eligible patients had no prior systemic therapy and had histologically confirmed locoregional renal cell carcinoma with a clear-cell component. They also met predefined criteria for high risk, including tumor stage 2 with nuclear grade 4 or sarcomatoid differentiation, tumor stage 3 or higher, regional lymph node metastasis, or stage M1 with no evidence of disease. Exclusion criteria included any major surgery other than nephrectomy/metastasectomy within 12 weeks prior to randomization, prior radiation therapy, prior immunotherapy, active autoimmune disease, infection, pneumonitis, or another active malignancy. Patients with M1 disease were excluded if bone or brain metastasis were the sites resected or the interval from resection was over 12 months. At prespecified interim analysis, the use of pembrolizumab had resulted in significant improvement in disease-free survival (HR 0.68; 24-month DFS 77.3% vs. 68.1%) [69]. Further follow-up showed an overall survival benefit with adjuvant pembrolizumab (HR 0.62) [70] with no adverse impact on quality of life among adjuvant therapy recipients [71]. Based on these results, pembrolizumab is FDA-approved as adjuvant therapy for renal cell carcinoma at intermediate high or high risk of recurrence following nephrectomy or following nephrectomy and resection of metastatic lesions.

Prior to KEYNOTE-564, there was no universally accepted standard adjuvant therapy. In the phase 3 S-TRAC study, 615 patients with high-risk clear cell–type renal cell carcinoma after nephrectomy received 1 year of adjuvant sunitinib or placebo. The median DFS was significantly longer in patients receiving sunitinib versus placebo at 6.8 versus 5.6 years, respectively [72]. S-TRAC resulted in FDA approval of sunitinib as adjuvant therapy. However, sunitinib is associated with several toxicities, and no data demonstrating OS benefit are available. Four additional phase 3 studies of adjuvant TKIs have all failed to meet their primary DFS endpoints, including studies with axitinib, pazopanib, sorafenib, as well as the ASSURE trial that included sunitinib [73]. TKIs are not preferred agents for adjuvant systemic therapy.

A lack of concordant benefit with adjuvant nivolumab [74] or adjuvant ipilimumab and nivolumab [75] in high-risk renal cell carcinoma may be seen to have conflicted with the results with pembrolizumab. However, there are no ready explanations for this variation based on patient population, mechanism of action, or duration of therapy. The data with adjuvant pembrolizumab are internally consistent, with progressively greater PFS benefit with increasing risk, such as patients with resected metastatic disease (PFS hazard ratio 0.4) [70] and may well reflect the unique activity of this PD-1 inhibitor. There are no randomized studies of adjuvant VEGFR-TKI in combination with ICI therapy. Neoadjuvant studies of VEGFR-TKI and/or ICI combinations require further exploration, as immunological control of distant microscopic disease may derive from optimal antigen priming in an intact primary tumor with a putatively large pool of immunogenic peptides [76]. This approach may be analogous to the improved outcomes with neoadjuvant pembrolizumab compared to adjuvant pembrolizumab in high-risk melanoma [77].

Predictive Biomarkers in CRCC Identifying biomarkers predictive of response and resistance would refine the therapeutic approach toward control of the disease. Genomic markers, including VHL status, transcriptional signatures, PDL-1 expression, tumor mutational burden, and T-lymphocytic infiltration, have all been probed for association with therapy outcomes [78–80], but none have proved impactful, particularly with the standardization of combinatorial VEGFR-TKI and PD-1 ICI regimens. Angiogenic, T-effector, and inflammatory myeloid signatures may be parsed from CRCC tumor tissue and predict for response to VEGFR-TKI or PDL-1 antibody therapy or the combination over monotherapy, respectively. [81] Since VEGFR-TKI or ICI monotherapy are uncommon therapy choices, and VEGFR-TKI and PDL-1 ICI combination therapy does not prolong survival, the value of this signature is hard to project and has not been prospectively validated. It nevertheless offers a glimpse into the biological heterogeneity of CRCC and a potential match of biology to therapeutic class that follow-on studies may refine and validate [82].

Research Directions There is an exciting range of investigative strategies in CRCC that seek to advance on the gains made with VEGFR-TKI and ICI therapies and to further refine their individualized application. Integration of HIF2α inhibitors in triplet combinations with VEGFR-TKI and ICI therapy is being studied in the frontline setting, while toxicity will be under particular scrutiny. Novel HIF2α inhibitors with increased potency and specificity are in clinical trials in the second line, seeking to improve on the results with belzutifan. Novel immune checkpoint inhibitors targeting LAG-3, TIGIT, and CD137, CAR-T cells, and personalized mRNA cancer vaccines are in the vanguard of immunotherapy research in CRCC. HIF2-independent pathways activated by VHL loss, tumor-stromal interactions, and angiogenic mechanisms of resistance to VEGFR-TKI therapy require additional scrutiny toward the identification of novel therapeutic targets. Personalization of systemic therapy in CRCC with molecular predictive tools remains a holy grail, as it did in the cytokine era [83].

References

1. Siegel RL, Giaquinto AN, Jemal A. Cancer statistics, 2024. CA Cancer J Clin. 2024;74(1):12–49. https://doi.org/10.3322/caac.21820.
2. Young M, Jackson-Spence F, Beltran L, et al. Renal cell carcinoma. Lancet (London, England). 2024;404(10451):476–91. https://doi.org/10.1016/s0140-6736(24)00917-6.
3. Padala SA, Barsouk A, Thandra KC, et al. Epidemiology of renal cell carcinoma. World J Oncol. 2020;11(3):79–87. https://doi.org/10.14740/wjon1279.
4. Ljungberg B, Alamdari FI, Rasmuson T, Roos G. Follow-up guidelines for nonmetastatic renal cell carcinoma based on the occurrence of metastases after radical nephrectomy. BJU Int. 1999;84(4):405–11. https://doi.org/10.1046/j.1464-410x.1999.00202.x.
5. Ouzaid I, Capitanio U, Staehler M, et al. Surgical metastasectomy in renal cell carcinoma: a systematic review. Eur Urol Oncol. 2019;2(2):141–9. https://doi.org/10.1016/j.euo.2018.08.028.
6. Zaid HB, Parker WP, Safdar NS, et al. Outcomes following complete surgical metastasectomy for patients with metastatic renal cell carcinoma: a systematic review and meta-analysis. J Urol. 2017;197(1):44–9. https://doi.org/10.1016/j.juro.2016.07.079.
7. Harrison MR, Costello BA, Bhavsar NA, et al. Active surveillance of metastatic renal cell carcinoma: results from a prospective observational study (MaRCC). Cancer. 2021;127(13):2204–12. https://doi.org/10.1002/cncr.33494.
8. Rini BI, Dorff TB, Elson P, et al. Active surveillance in metastatic renal-cell carcinoma: a prospective, phase 2 trial. Lancet Oncol. 2016;17(9):1317–24. https://doi.org/10.1016/s1470-2045(16)30196-6.
9. Kaelin WG Jr. Von Hippel-Lindau disease: insights into oxygen sensing, protein degradation, and cancer. J Clin Invest. 2022;132(18) https://doi.org/10.1172/jci162480.
10. Choueiri TK, Kaelin WG Jr. Targeting the HIF2-VEGF axis in renal cell carcinoma. Nat Med. 2020;26(10):1519–30. https://doi.org/10.1038/s41591-020-1093-z.
11. Takahashi A, Sasaki H, Kim SJ, et al. Markedly increased amounts of messenger RNAs for vascular endothelial growth factor and placenta growth factor in renal cell carcinoma associated with angiogenesis. Cancer Res. 1994;54(15):4233–7.
12. Berger DP, Herbstritt L, Dengler WA, Marmé D, Mertelsmann R, Fiebig HH. Vascular endothelial growth factor (VEGF) mRNA expression in human tumor models of different histologies. Ann Oncol. 1995;6(8):817–25. https://doi.org/10.1093/oxfordjournals.annonc.a059322.
13. Cébe-Suarez S, Zehnder-Fjällman A, Ballmer-Hofer K. The role of VEGF receptors in angiogenesis; complex partnerships. Cell Mol Life Sci. 2006;63(5):601–15. https://doi.org/10.1007/s00018-005-5426-3.
14. Chen W, Hill H, Christie A, et al. Targeting renal cell carcinoma with a HIF-2 antagonist. Nature. 2016;539(7627):112–7. https://doi.org/10.1038/nature19796.
15. Motzer RJ, Hutson TE, Tomczak P, et al. Overall survival and updated results for sunitinib compared with interferon alfa in patients with metastatic renal

cell carcinoma. J Clin Oncol. 2023;41(11):1965–71. https://doi.org/10.1200/jco.22.02623.
16. Motzer RJ, Escudier B, McDermott DF, et al. Nivolumab versus everolimus in advanced renal-cell carcinoma. N Engl J Med. 2015;373(19):1803–13. https://doi.org/10.1056/NEJMoa1510665.
17. Monjaras-Avila CU, Lorenzo-Leal AC, Luque-Badillo AC, D'Costa N, Chavez-Muñoz C, Bach H. The tumor immune microenvironment in clear cell renal cell carcinoma. Int J Mol Sci. 2023;24(9) https://doi.org/10.3390/ijms24097946.
18. Wolf MM, Rathmell WK, de Cubas AA. Immunogenicity in renal cell carcinoma: shifting focus to alternative sources of tumour-specific antigens. Nat Rev Nephrol. 2023;19(7):440–50. https://doi.org/10.1038/s41581-023-00700-5.
19. Yakirevich E, Patel NR. Tumor mutational burden and immune signatures interplay in renal cell carcinoma. Ann Transl Med. 2020;8(6):269. https://doi.org/10.21037/atm.2020.02.81.
20. Smith CC, Beckermann KE, Bortone DS, et al. Endogenous retroviral signatures predict immunotherapy response in clear cell renal cell carcinoma. J Clin Invest. 2019;128(11):4804–20. https://doi.org/10.1172/JCI121476.
21. Jonasch E, Atkins MB, Chowdhury S, Mainwaring P. Combination of anti-angiogenics and checkpoint inhibitors for renal cell carcinoma: is the whole greater than the sum of its parts? Cancer. 2022;14(3) https://doi.org/10.3390/cancers14030644.
22. Granet-Vaissiere E, Lefort F, Domblides C, et al. Combinations of anti-angiogenic agents and immune checkpoint inhibitors in renal cell carcinoma: best option? Cancer. 2023;15(4):1048.
23. Yang J, Yan J, Liu B. Targeting VEGF/VEGFR to modulate antitumor immunity. Front Immunol. 2018;9:978. https://doi.org/10.3389/fimmu.2018.00978.
24. Lee WS, Yang H, Chon HJ, Kim C. Combination of anti-angiogenic therapy and immune checkpoint blockade normalizes vascular-immune crosstalk to potentiate cancer immunity. Exp Mol Med. 2020;52(9):1475–85. https://doi.org/10.1038/s12276-020-00500-y.
25. Heng DYC, Xie W, Regan MM, et al. Prognostic factors for overall survival in patients with metastatic renal cell carcinoma treated with vascular endothelial growth factor–targeted agents: results from a large, multicenter study. J Clin Oncol. 2009;27(34):5794–9. https://doi.org/10.1200/jco.2008.21.4809.
26. Heng DY, Xie W, Regan MM, et al. External validation and comparison with other models of the International Metastatic Renal-Cell Carcinoma Database Consortium prognostic model: a population-based study. Lancet Oncol. 2013;14(2):141–8. https://doi.org/10.1016/s1470-2045(12)70559-4.
27. Motzer RJ, Tannir NM, McDermott DF, et al. Nivolumab plus Ipilimumab versus Sunitinib in advanced renal-cell carcinoma. N Engl J Med. 2018;378(14):1277–90. https://doi.org/10.1056/NEJMoa1712126.
28. Rini BI, Plimack ER, Stus V, et al. Pembrolizumab plus Axitinib versus Sunitinib for advanced renal-cell carcinoma. N Engl J Med. 2019;380(12):1116–27. https://doi.org/10.1056/NEJMoa1816714.
29. Choueiri TK, Powles T, Burotto M, et al. Nivolumab plus Cabozantinib versus Sunitinib for advanced renal-cell carcinoma. N Engl J Med. 2021;384(9):829–41. https://doi.org/10.1056/NEJMoa2026982.
30. Motzer R, Alekseev B, Rha SY, et al. Lenvatinib plus Pembrolizumab or Everolimus for advanced renal cell carcinoma. N Engl J Med. 2021;384(14):1289–300. https://doi.org/10.1056/NEJMoa2035716.
31. Navani V, Heng DYC. Treatment selection in first-line metastatic renal cell carcinoma—the contemporary treatment paradigm in the age of combination therapy: a review. JAMA Oncol. 2022;8(2):292–9. https://doi.org/10.1001/jamaoncol.2021.4337.
32. Motzer RJ, Penkov K, Haanen J, et al. Avelumab plus Axitinib versus Sunitinib for advanced renal-cell carcinoma. N Engl J Med. 2019;380(12):1103–15. https://doi.org/10.1056/NEJMoa1816047.
33. Motzer RJ, Penkov K, Uemura H, et al. Avelumab + axitinib vs sunitinib in patients (pts) with advanced renal cell carcinoma (aRCC): final overall survival (OS) analysis from the JAVELIN Renal 101 phase 3 trial. J Clin Oncol. 2024;42(16_suppl):4508. https://doi.org/10.1200/JCO.2024.42.16_suppl.4508.
34. Rini BI, Powles T, Atkins MB, et al. Atezolizumab plus bevacizumab versus sunitinib in patients with previously untreated metastatic renal cell carcinoma (IMmotion151): a multicentre, open-label, phase 3, randomised controlled trial. Lancet. 2019;393(10189):2404–15. https://doi.org/10.1016/S0140-6736(19)30723-8.
35. Motzer RJ, Powles T, Atkins MB, et al. Final over all survival and molecular analysis in IMmotion151, a phase 3 trial comparing atezolizumab plus bevacizumab vs sunitinib in patients with previously untreated metastatic renal cell carcinoma. JAMA Oncologia. 2022;8(2):275–80. https://doi.org/10.1001/jamaoncol.2021.5981.
36. Tannir NM, Albigès L, McDermott DF, et al. Nivolumab plus ipilimumab versus sunitinib for first-line treatment of advanced renal cell carcinoma: extended 8-year follow-up results of efficacy and safety from the phase III CheckMate 214 trial. Ann Oncol. 2024; https://doi.org/10.1016/j.annonc.2024.07.727.
37. Motzer RJ, Porta C, Eto M, et al. Lenvatinib plus pembrolizumab versus sunitinib in first-line treatment of advanced renal cell carcinoma: final prespecified overall survival analysis of clear, a phase III study. J Clin Oncol. 2024;42(11):1222–8. https://doi.org/10.1200/jco.23.01569.
38. Powles T, Burotto M, Escudier B, et al. Nivolumab plus cabozantinib versus sunitinib for first-line treatment of advanced renal cell carcinoma: extended follow-up from the phase III randomised CheckMate 9ER trial. ESMO Open. 2024;9(5):102994. https://doi.org/10.1016/j.esmoop.2024.102994.
39. Plimack ER, Powles T, Stus V, et al. Pembrolizumab plus axitinib versus sunitinib as first-line treat-

ment of advanced renal cell carcinoma: 43-month follow-up of the phase 3 KEYNOTE-426 study. Eur Urol. 2023;84(5):449–54. https://doi.org/10.1016/j.eururo.2023.06.006.
40. Shah NJ, Sura SD, Shinde R, et al. Real-world treatment patterns and clinical outcomes for metastatic renal cell carcinoma in the current treatment era. Eur Urol Open Sci. 2023;49:110–8. https://doi.org/10.1016/j.euros.2022.12.015.
41. Mori K, Mostafaei H, Miura N, et al. Systemic therapy for metastatic renal cell carcinoma in the first-line setting: a systematic review and network meta-analysis. Cancer Immunol Immunother. 2021;70(2):265–73. https://doi.org/10.1007/s00262-020-02684-8.
42. Brown J, Santini D, Charnley N, Ogareva A, Chisholm A, Jones R. Implications of bone metastasis on response to systemic therapy in patients with advanced renal cell carcinoma: a systematic literature review. Cancer Treat Rev. 2024:129. https://doi.org/10.1016/j.ctrv.2024.102792.
43. Grünwald V, Powles T, Eto M, et al. Phase 3 CLEAR study in patients with advanced renal cell carcinoma: outcomes in subgroups for the lenvatinib-plus-pembrolizumab and sunitinib arms. Front. Oncologia. 2023;13:1223282. https://doi.org/10.3389/fonc.2023.1223282.
44. Hasanov E, Yeboa DN, Tucker MD, et al. An interdisciplinary consensus on the management of brain metastases in patients with renal cell carcinoma. CA Cancer J Clin. 2022;72(5):454–89. https://doi.org/10.3322/caac.21729.
45. Choueiri Toni K, Powles T, Albiges L, et al. Cabozantinib plus Nivolumab and Ipilimumab in renal-cell carcinoma. N Engl J Med. 2023;388(19):1767–78. https://doi.org/10.1056/NEJMoa2212851.
46. Zhang T, Ballman KV, Choudhury AD, et al. PDIGREE: an adaptive phase III trial of PD-inhibitor nivolumab and ipilimumab (IPI-NIVO) with VEGF TKI cabozantinib (CABO) in metastatic untreated renal cell cancer (Alliance A031704). J Clin Oncol. 2021;39(6_suppl):TPS366. https://doi.org/10.1200/JCO.2021.39.6_suppl.TPS366.
47. McKay RR, McGregor BA, Xie W, et al. Optimized management of nivolumab and ipilimumab in advanced renal cell carcinoma: a response-based phase II study (OMNIVORE). J Clin Oncol. 2020;38(36):4240–8. https://doi.org/10.1200/jco.20.02295.
48. Atkins MB, Jegede OA, Haas NB, et al. Phase II study of nivolumab and salvage nivolumab/ipilimumab in treatment-naive patients with advanced clear cell renal cell carcinoma (HCRN GU16-260-Cohort A). J Clin Oncol. 2022;40(25):2913–23. https://doi.org/10.1200/jco.21.02938.
49. Motzer RJ, Hutson TE, Cella D, et al. Pazopanib versus sunitinib in metastatic renal-cell carcinoma. N Engl J Med. 2013;369(8):722–31. https://doi.org/10.1056/NEJMoa1303989.
50. Choueiri TK, Hessel C, Halabi S, et al. Cabozantinib versus sunitinib as initial therapy for metastatic renal cell carcinoma of intermediate or poor risk (Alliance A031203 CABOSUN randomised trial): Progression-free survival by independent review and overall survival update. Eur J Cancer. 2018;94:115–25. https://doi.org/10.1016/j.ejca.2018.02.012.
51. Beecroft N, Gauntner TD, Upadhyay R, et al. Active surveillance in metastatic renal cell carcinoma. J Kidney Cancer VHL. 2024;11(2):27–38. https://doi.org/10.15586/jkcvhl.v11i2.309.
52. Pal SK, Albiges L, Tomczak P, et al. Atezolizumab plus cabozantinib versus cabozantinib monotherapy for patients with renal cell carcinoma after progression with previous immune checkpoint inhibitor treatment (CONTACT-03): a multicentre, randomised, open-label, phase 3 trial. Lancet (London, England). 2023;402(10397):185–95. https://doi.org/10.1016/s0140-6736(23)00922-4.
53. Choueiri TK, Albiges L, Barthélémy P, et al. Tivozanib plus nivolumab versus tivozanib monotherapy in patients with renal cell carcinoma following an immune checkpoint inhibitor: results of the phase 3 TiNivo-2 study. Lancet (London, England). 2024; https://doi.org/10.1016/s0140-6736(24)01758-6.
54. Motzer RJ, Escudier B, Tomczak P, et al. Axitinib versus sorafenib as second-line treatment for advanced renal cell carcinoma: overall survival analysis and updated results from a randomised phase 3 trial. Lancet Oncol. 2013;14(6):552–62. https://doi.org/10.1016/s1470-2045(13)70093-7.
55. Choueiri TK, Escudier B, Powles T, et al. Cabozantinib versus everolimus in advanced renal-cell carcinoma. N Engl J Med. 2015;373(19):1814–23. https://doi.org/10.1056/NEJMoa1510016.
56. Motzer RJ, Hutson TE, Glen H, et al. Lenvatinib, everolimus, and the combination in patients with metastatic renal cell carcinoma: a randomised, phase 2, open-label, multicentre trial. Lancet Oncol. 2015;16(15):1473–82. https://doi.org/10.1016/s1470-2045(15)00290-9.
57. Rini BI, Pal SK, Escudier BJ, et al. Tivozanib versus sorafenib in patients with advanced renal cell carcinoma (TIVO-3): a phase 3, multicentre, randomised, controlled, open-label study. Lancet Oncol. 2020;21(1):95–104. https://doi.org/10.1016/S1470-2045(19)30735-1.
58. Jonasch E, Donskov F, Iliopoulos O, et al. Belzutifan for renal cell carcinoma in Von Hippel–Lindau disease. N Engl J Med. 2021;385(22):2036–46. https://doi.org/10.1056/NEJMoa2103425.
59. Choueiri TK, Powles T, Peltola K, et al. Belzutifan versus everolimus for advanced renal-cell carcinoma. N Engl J Med. 2024;391(8):710–21. https://doi.org/10.1056/NEJMoa2313906.
60. Albiges L, Rini BI, Peltola K, et al. LBA88 Belzutifan versus everolimus in participants (pts) with previously treated advanced clear cell renal cell carcinoma (ccRCC): randomized open-label phase III LITESPARK-005 study. Ann Oncol. 2023;34:S1329–30. https://doi.org/10.1016/j.annonc.2023.10.090.

61. Hahn AW, Lebenthal J, Genovese G, Sircar K, Tannir NM, Msaouel P. The significance of sarcomatoid and rhabdoid dedifferentiation in renal cell carcinoma. Cancer Treat Res Commun. 2022;33:100640. https://doi.org/10.1016/j.ctarc.2022.100640.
62. Tannir NM, Signoretti S, Choueiri TK, et al. Efficacy and safety of nivolumab plus ipilimumab versus sunitinib in first-line treatment of patients with advanced sarcomatoid renal cell carcinoma. Clin Cancer Res. 2021;27(1):78–86. https://doi.org/10.1158/1078-0432.Ccr-20-2063.
63. Lolli C, Altavilla A, Conteduca V, et al. A comprehensive review of the role of immune checkpoint inhibitors in elderly patients affected by renal cell carcinoma. Crit Rev Oncol Hematol. 2020;153:103036. https://doi.org/10.1016/j.critrevonc.2020.103036.
64. Koyfman SA, Geiger JL. Checkpoint inhibition for kidney transplant recipients with advanced cutaneous carcinomas: an emerging standard for select patients. J Clin Oncol. 2024;42(9):981–3. https://doi.org/10.1200/jco.23.02570.
65. Van Meerhaeghe T, Murakami N, Le Moine A, Brouard S, Sprangers B, Degauque N. Fine-tuning tumor- and allo-immunity: advances in the use of immune checkpoint inhibitors in kidney transplant recipients. Clin Kidney J. 2024;17(4) https://doi.org/10.1093/ckj/sfae061.
66. Yohannan B, Sridhar A, Kaur H, Golovine AD, Maithel N. Renal cell carcinoma in renal transplant recipients: is there a role for screening? J Clin Oncol. 2022;40(16_suppl):10528. https://doi.org/10.1200/JCO.2022.40.16_suppl.10528.
67. Kauffman HM, Cherikh WS, Cheng Y, Hanto DW, Kahan BD. Maintenance immunosuppression with target-of-rapamycin inhibitors is associated with a reduced incidence of de novo malignancies. Transplantation. 2005;80(7):883–9. https://doi.org/10.1097/01.tp.0000184006.43152.8d.
68. Massari F, Bria E, Maines F, et al. Adjuvant treatment for resected renal cell carcinoma: are all strategies equally negative? Potential implications for trial design with targeted agents. Clin Genitourin Cancer. 2013;11(4):471–6. https://doi.org/10.1016/j.clgc.2013.04.018.
69. Choueiri TK, Tomczak P, Park SH, et al. Adjuvant pembrolizumab after nephrectomy in renal-cell carcinoma. N Engl J Med. 2021;385(8):683–94. https://doi.org/10.1056/NEJMoa2106391.
70. Choueiri TK, Tomczak P, Park SH, et al. Overall survival with adjuvant pembrolizumab in renal-cell carcinoma. N Engl J Med. 2024;390(15):1359–71. https://doi.org/10.1056/NEJMoa2312695.
71. Choueiri TK, Tomczak P, Park SH, et al. Patient-reported outcomes in KEYNOTE-564: adjuvant pembrolizumab versus placebo for renal cell carcinoma. Oncologist. 2023;29(2):142–50. https://doi.org/10.1093/oncolo/oyad231.
72. Ravaud A, Motzer RJ, Pandha HS, et al. Adjuvant sunitinib in high-risk renal-cell carcinoma after nephrectomy. N Engl J Med. 2016;375(23):2246–54. https://doi.org/10.1056/NEJMoa1611406.
73. Haas NB, Manola J, Uzzo RG, et al. Adjuvant sunitinib or sorafenib for high-risk, non-metastatic renal-cell carcinoma (ECOG-ACRIN E2805): a double-blind, placebo-controlled, randomised, phase 3 trial. Lancet. 2016;387(10032):2008–16. https://doi.org/10.1016/s0140-6736(16)00559-6.
74. Motzer RJ, Bex A, Russo P, et al. Adjuvant nivolumab for localized renal cell carcinoma at high risk of recurrence after nephrectomy: part B of the randomized, placebo-controlled, phase III checkmate 914 trial. J Clin Oncol. 2024:Jco2400773. https://doi.org/10.1200/jco.24.00773.
75. Motzer RJ, Russo P, Grünwald V, et al. Adjuvant nivolumab plus ipilimumab versus placebo for localised renal cell carcinoma after nephrectomy (CheckMate 914): a double-blind, randomised, phase 3 trial. Lancet (London, England). 2023;401(10379):821–32. https://doi.org/10.1016/s0140-6736(22)02574-0.
76. Marandino L, Campi R, Amparore D, et al. Neoadjuvant and adjuvant immune-based approach for renal cell carcinoma: pros, cons, and future directions. Eur Urol Oncol. 2024; https://doi.org/10.1016/j.euo.2024.09.002.
77. Patel SP, Othus M, Chen Y, et al. Neoadjuvant–adjuvant or adjuvant-only pembrolizumab in advanced melanoma. N Engl J Med. 2023;388(9):813–23. https://doi.org/10.1056/NEJMoa2211437.
78. Cotta BH, Choueiri TK, Cieslik M, et al. Current landscape of genomic biomarkers in clear cell renal cell carcinoma. Eur Urol. 2023;84(2):166–75. https://doi.org/10.1016/j.eururo.2023.04.003.
79. Lyskjær I, Iisager L, Axelsen CT, Nielsen TK, Dyrskjøt L, Fristrup N. Management of renal cell carcinoma: promising biomarkers and the challenges to reach the clinic. Clin Cancer Res. 2024;30(4):663–72. https://doi.org/10.1158/1078-0432.Ccr-23-1892.
80. Labaki C, Saliby RM, Bakouny Z, et al. Emerging biomarkers of response to systemic therapies in metastatic clear cell renal cell carcinoma. Hematol Oncol Clin North Am. 2023;37(5):937–42. https://doi.org/10.1016/j.hoc.2023.05.021.
81. McDermott DF, Huseni MA, Atkins MB, et al. Clinical activity and molecular correlates of response to atezolizumab alone or in combination with bevacizumab versus sunitinib in renal cell carcinoma. Nat Med. 2018;24(6):749.
82. Motzer RJ, Banchereau R, Hamidi H, et al. Molecular subsets in renal cancer determine outcome to checkpoint and angiogenesis blockade. Cancer Cell. 2020;38(6):803–817.e4. https://doi.org/10.1016/j.ccell.2020.10.011.
83. Klapper JA, Downey SG, Smith FO, et al. High-dose interleukin-2 for the treatment of metastatic renal cell carcinoma : a retrospective analysis of response and survival in patients treated in the surgery branch at the National Cancer Institute between 1986 and 2006. Cancer. 2008;113(2):293–301. https://doi.org/10.1002/cncr.23552.

Unified Approaches to Surgery and Systemic Therapy for Renal Cell Carcinoma

23

Shayan Smani, Soum D. Lokeshwar, Alejandro Abello, and Patrick A. Kenney

Introduction

More than 80,000 people in the United States were diagnosed with kidney cancer in 2024, more than >14,000 died of the disease, accounting for an overall 5-year survival rate of 78.1% [1]. At diagnosis, 34% of patients have regionally advanced or metastatic disease, with an additional 10–28% developing recurrence or metastasis following surgery for previously localized disease [1]. This substantial percentage of patients may benefit from integrated surgical and systemic therapy. A multifaceted approach to the treatment of renal cell carcinoma (RCC) is increasingly undertaken to maximize clinical outcomes. This chapter will focus on the proper integration of surgery and systemic therapy with regard to adjuvant therapy for RCC, neoadjuvant therapy for locally advanced disease, and multimodal therapy for metastatic RCC (mRCC), including presurgical targeted therapy and cytoreductive nephrectomy.

S. Smani · S. D. Lokeshwar · P. A. Kenney (✉)
Department of Urology, Yale School of Medicine, Yale New Haven Hospital, New Haven, CT, USA
e-mail: patrick.kenney@yale.edu

A. Abello
Department of Urology, Beth Israel Deaconess Medical Center, Boston, MA, USA
e-mail: aabello1@bidmc.harvard.edu

Adjuvant Therapy

In this chapter, the phrase adjuvant therapy will define treatment that is administered after complete surgical resection with the goal of reducing the risk of recurrence [2]. Patients who develop distant metastatic disease have progressed to an incurable state, with 5-year survival rates of about 10% [1]. The ideal adjuvant therapy should have favorable toxicity, efficacy against the standard of care (observation or pembrolizumab) in phase 3 randomized trials and could be administered to the subset of patients who are most likely to benefit, ideally on an outpatient basis [3, 4].

Contemporary Approach to Quantifying the Risk of Recurrence

An important aspect of developing effective adjuvant therapy is to define the group of patients who are at elevated risk of recurrence and who are therefore most likely to benefit from adjuvant therapy. Identifying high-risk patients will address one of the recognized disadvantages of the adjuvant approach, namely that some patients are cured with surgery alone and will be treated with adjuvant therapy that offers the potential for harm but not benefit.

Existing predictive models are based solely on preoperative variables such as gender, symptoms, and imaging findings, including necrosis, lymphadenopathy, and tumor size [5–7]. These models

J. A. Libertino, J. R. Gee (eds.), *Renal Cancer*, https://doi.org/10.1007/978-3-031-97599-8_23

may help select intervention vs. active surveillance and may prove useful for identifying patients for neoadjuvant therapy [8, 9]. On the other hand, postoperative models that incorporate pathologic variables discriminate better than preoperative models and are therefore more appropriate for the selection of candidates for adjuvant therapy [9, 10].

Models Incorporating Clinical and Pathologic Data

Several models use clinical and pathologic variables to predict the risk of progression after surgery for localized RCC (Table 23.1) [11–14]. These models are useful but have shortcomings. Neither the modified UCLA Integrated Staging System (UISS) nor the MSKCC nomograms capture the nearly 20% rate of recurrence beyond 5 years [11, 14–18]. In addition, since there is a known association between nuclear grade and outcome, the exclusion of nuclear grade in the 2001 MSKCC nomogram may have limited its predictive capacity [11, 13, 16]. Finally, none of these models include molecular prognostic biomarkers.

The UISS, which has been externally validated and includes all RCC subtypes, groups patients in low-, medium-, or high-risk categories [14, 19]. Instead of tailoring risk to an individual patient like a nomogram, grouping risk into categories will limit the instrument's discriminatory ability since each group will encompass a range of outcomes [9, 14]. The 2001 MSKCC nomogram and the UISS were compared with a multicenter cohort of >2400 patients [10]. The concordance index were 0.71 and 0.68 for the MSKCC and UISS models, respectively. The varied outcomes in the UISS intermediate-risk category were able to be discriminated by the MSKCC nomogram [10].

Using Molecular Markers to Improve Prognostication

In addition to using clinical and pathologic data, molecular markers may improve our ability to predict the risk of recurrence or progression. Several early efforts demonstrated the feasibility of this approach. By incorporating expression of carbonic anhydrase IX, vimentin, and p53 with clinical variables (metastasis, T stage, performance status), investigators achieved slightly better ability to predict disease-specific survival compared to the UISS (C Index 0.79 vs. 0.75) [20]. The same group also used molecular data in a nomogram to predict disease-free survival (DFS) following nephrectomy for localized ccRCC (Fig. 23.1) [21]. In addition to clinical and pathologic variables, the molecular markers included Ki-67, p53, endothelial VEGFR-1, epithelial VEGFR-1, and epithelial VEGF-D. While the molecular markers alone exceeded the predictive ability of the UISS (C Index 0.84 vs. 0.78), the accuracy of the full nomogram which incorporated clinical, pathological, and molecular data was higher still (concordance index 0.90) (Fig. 23.2).

UISS (0.82 vs. 0.77) [22].

Additionally, Kidney Injury Molecule-1 (KIM-1) has emerged as a promising urinary and plasma biomarker for RCC, serving as both a diagnostic and prognostic indicator. KIM-1, a glycoprotein associated with acute proximal tubular injury, is primarily expressed in RCC subtypes originating from the proximal tubules, such as clear cell RCC [23]. Elevated KIM-1 concentrations have been shown to predict RCC up to 5 years before diagnosis and are linked to shorter survival durations [24]. Higher post-nephrectomy KIM-1 concentration has been associated with worse DFS and overall survival (OS) in RCC [25].

Over recent decades, research into liquid biopsies and circulating cancer biomarkers has gained momentum, driven by their potential for early disease detection and treatment monitoring. Among these, circulating tumor DNA (ctDNA), which originates from apoptotic or necrotic tumor cells, macrophage secretions, or circulating tumor cells, has shown strong correlations with advanced disease and progression in the treatment of various solid tumors [26, 27]. In RCC, studies by Jung et al., Lin et al., and Yamamoto et al. demonstrated that ctDNA detection was significantly associated with worse outcomes, including higher mortality risk and

Table 23.1 Models that use clinical and pathologic variables to predict oncologic outcomes after surgery for localized RCC [11–14]

Type	Study population (n)	TNM	Histology	Nephrectomy	Years	Symptoms	Performance status	Tumor size	pT	pN	Grade	Histology	Necrosis	Vascular invasion	Outcome	Time point (years)	Concordance index
Nomogram	601	T1–3c, N0/x, M0	Papillary, chromophobe, ccRCC	Partial, radical	1989–1998	✓		✓	✓ (1997)			✓			Recurrence-free survival	5	0.74
Algorithm (low, moderate, high risk)	468	T1–4, N0, M0	Any	Partial, radical	1989–2000		✓		✓ (1997)	✓	✓				Overall survival, disease-specific survival, local recurrence-free survival, and systemic recurrence-free survival	1, 2, 3, 4, 5	NA
Algorithm (score between 0 and 11)	1671	T1–4, Nx–N2, M0	ccRCC	Radical	1970–2000			✓	✓ (2002)	✓	✓	NA	✓		Metastasis-free survival	1, 3, 5, 7, 10	0.82
Nomogram	701	T1–3c, N0/x, M0	ccRCC	Partial, radical	1989–2002	✓		✓	✓ (2002)		✓	NA	✓	✓	Recurrence-free survival	5	0.82

Adapted from Kenney and Wood [15]

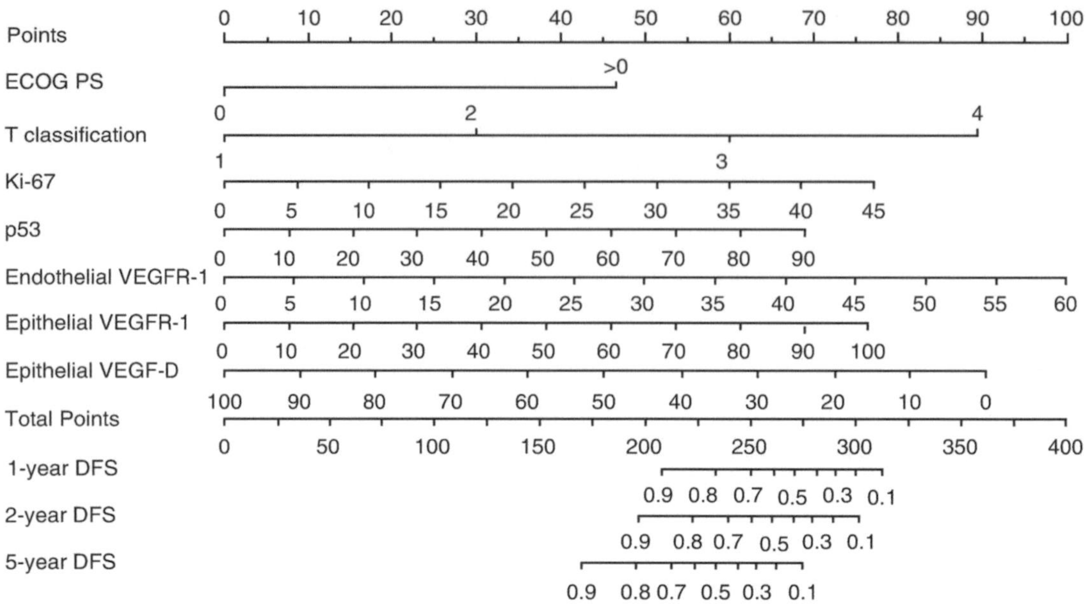

Fig. 23.1 This nomogram predicts disease-free survival using molecular data in addition to clinical and pathologic variables. The number of points assigned to each variable is determined by drawing a vertical line up to the points' axis. Total points correspond to predicted disease-free survival. (Reprinted with permission from Klatte et al. [21])

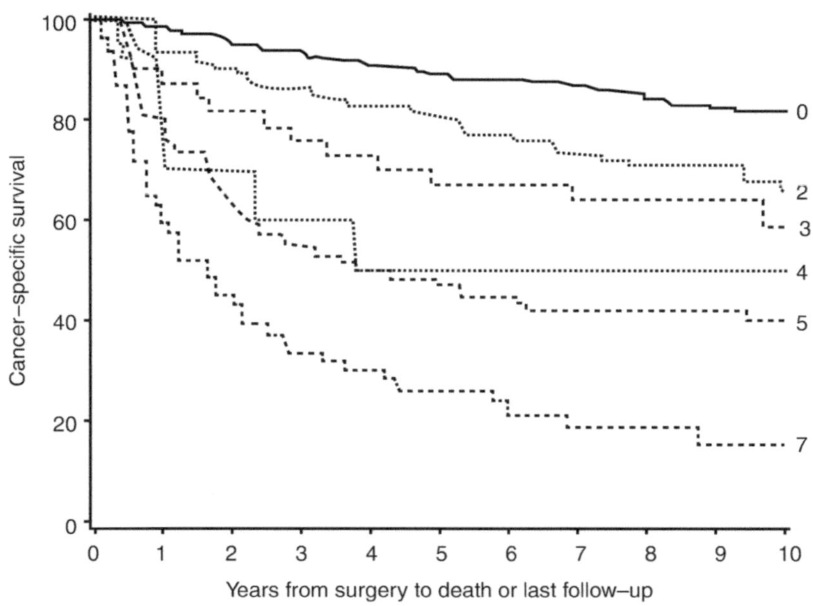

Fig. 23.2 BioScore is an algorithm that incorporates molecular markers to improve prognostication following nephrectomy for ccRCC. Total score is predictive of cancer-specific survival. (Reprinted with permission from Parker et al. [22])

shorter progression-free survival (PFS), cancer-specific survival, or OS [28–30]. While further prospective research is needed, these findings suggest that ctDNA holds promise as a prognostic biomarker in RCC, but overall ctDNA levels are low, requiring highly sensitive and expensive testing.

The great promise of biomarker models is that they may identify the molecular characteristics that drive tumor behavior and use them to predict clinical outcome. The molecular models mentioned above are promising but need independent validation and laboratory standardization [31].

The gains in prognostication thus far appear to be modest. The added cost of the assays must be weighed against the small incremental improvement over the user-friendly, readily available clinicopathologic models [16]. To date, there is little evidence supporting external validation of the value of molecular markers. They are not routinely used in clinical practice [32].

Adjuvant Trials

Radiotherapy

There are two reasons that one would expect little role for adjuvant therapy that is delivered locally. First, radical nephrectomy provides excellent local cancer control in most cases. Second, recurrence of RCC is typically distant from the primary [33]. Nonetheless, with a paucity of available systemic agents, the initial adjuvant studies in RCC used radiotherapy in an attempt to improve RCC control [4].

From 1961 to 1970, a prospective trial randomized patients with a completely resected primary tumor and no evidence of metastatic disease to adjuvant radiation to the renal bed, incision and para-aortic nodes (n = 51) or observation (n = 49) [34]. Radiotherapy was not associated with any improvement in recurrence or survival. Most notable among the substantial side effects that were attributed to the adjuvant radiation were four deaths from liver failure. Between 1979 and 1984, a similar multicenter trial randomized patients with stage II and III RCC to 50 Gy of external beam radiotherapy in 20 fractions to the kidney bed and nodes (n = 32) or observation (n = 33) [35]. Radiotherapy was associated with hepatic, gastric, and duodenal injuries, but no reduction in relapse. In nearly a fifth of patients, radiotherapy complications contributed to the patient's death. Based on these important trials, adjuvant radiotherapy is not employed for RCC.

Small retrospective studies in patients with advanced disease have shown a small benefit on 5-year survival rates after postoperative fractionated 40–50 Gy radiotherapy. However, due to the small sample size, high risk of bias from retrospective studies and absence of level 1 evidence, adjuvant radiotherapy is not currently recommended [36, 37].

Medical Therapy

Medroxyprogesterone acetate (MPA) can block glucocorticoid receptors that are expressed by some renal tumors [38]. MPA was investigated in a multicenter trial in which patients were randomized to 1 year of adjuvant MPA (n = 58) or observation (n = 62) following radical nephrectomy for non-metastatic RCC [39]. More than half of the patients had ≥T3 disease. After a median follow-up of 5 years, complications were common in the intervention arm, but rates of relapse were similar in the intervention and control groups (32.7% vs. 33.9%).

Another similar trial using adjuvant tegafur and uracil after radical nephrectomy did not show any significant differences in recurrence in comparison to the non-adjuvant group [40].

Immunotherapy

The primary tumor is thought to have an immunosuppressive effect [41–44]. It was proposed that once the "immune sink" was eliminated with nephrectomy, adjuvant immunotherapy could treat the remaining subclinical disease that leads to recurrence. Various adjuvant immune treatments have been evaluated, including vaccines, dendritic cell therapy, cytokines, and stem-cell transplant to engender a graft-versus-tumor effect [45–47].

The impact of immune surveillance on RCC is thought to be evidenced by the spontaneous regression of metastatic disease following tumor ablation or nephrectomy, as well as the infiltration of the tumor by immune cells that have antitumor activity [48–52]. In part, the immune system impact is thought to be mediated by interaction between CD8+ cytotoxic T lymphocytes and CD4+ helper T cells that secrete cytokines including Interleukin-2 (IL-2) and Interferon-α (IFN-α) [31]. Exogenous IL-2 and IFN-α are effective in metastatic disease, with response rates up to 20% and a 5% durable complete response for IL-2 [46, 53–55]. IL-2 and IFN-α do not appear to have activity in the adjuvant setting. Randomized trials have failed to show a survival benefit to adjuvant IL-2 or IFN-∝ [56–59]. Patients who received adjuvant chemoimmunotherapy in one trial had worse 5-year OS when compared to control (58% vs. 76%, $p = 0.028$) [60]. Another trial comparing adjuvant 5-Fluorouracil, IFN-∝, and IL-2 to placebo failed to show differences for the treatment arm in regard to DFS (61% vs. 50%, $p = 0.2$) or OS at 5 years (70% vs. 63%, $p = 0.4$) (Table 23.2) [61].

The Keynote-564 trial recently evaluated pembrolizumab, a programmed death receptor inhibitor (Keytruda), as adjuvant therapy for patients at high risk of recurrence following nephrectomy. This landmark study was the first to report a positive primary endpoint of DFS in this setting. The trial included 994 patients with intermediate- or high-risk localized RCC or M1 disease (no evidence of disease post-metastasectomy) and compared 17 cycles of pembrolizumab (administered every 3 weeks) to placebo. With a median follow-up of 24.1 months, pembrolizumab significantly improved DFS compared to placebo (HR: 0.68; 95% CI: 0.53–0.87; $P = 0.001$). A subsequent analysis, published in 2024, also demonstrated an improvement in OS, with a hazard ratio for death of 0.62 (95% CI: 0.44–0.87; $P = 0.005$) [62]. The findings from this trial introduced immune checkpoint inhibitor (ICI) therapy into the treatment landscape for localized RCC.

The IMmotion010 phase III trial assessed the efficacy of atezolizumab, a programmed death receptor ligand-1 inhibitor, as adjuvant therapy for patients at high risk of recurrence following surgery. A total of 778 patients with high-risk features were enrolled. Atezolizumab was administered at a dose of 1200 mg every 3 weeks for up to 16 cycles or 1 year, with outcomes compared to placebo over a median follow-up of 38.6 months. The trial did not meet its primary endpoint, as atezolizumab failed to significantly improve DFS compared to placebo. The HR for DFS was 0.93 (95% CI: 0.75–1.15; $P = 0.4950$), with a median DFS of 57.2 months (95% CI: 44.6, NE) for atezolizumab versus 49.5 months (95% CI: 47.4, NE) for placebo. Exploratory subgroup analyses also failed to show meaningful DFS benefits, including in the M1 NED subgroup, which constituted a larger proportion of patients (13.9%) compared to Keynote-564 (5.8%). The lack of DFS benefit across all subgroups, including those traditionally thought to derive the most benefit from immune checkpoint inhibition, underscores the need for further research to identify more effective adjuvant strategies [63].

Table 23.2 No randomized trial that investigated IL-2 and IFN-∝ as adjuvant therapy

Author	Year	Eligibility	Design	*N*	Median follow-up	Primary endpoint (intervention vs. control)	*P* value
Pizzocaro	2001	Robson II or III	IFN-alpha vs. observation	247	NA	5-year OS: 66.5% vs. 66.0%	0.861
Messing	2003	pT3–4a or N+	IFN-alpha vs. observation	283	10.4 years	Median OS: 5.1 vs. 7.4 years	0.09
Clark	2003	pT3b-4 or N+ or M1 (resected)	High-dose IL-2 vs. observation	69	22 months	2-year DFS: 48% vs. 55%	0.431
Atzpodien	2005	pT3b-4 or N+ or M1 (resected)	IFN-alpha + IL-2 + 5-FU vs. observation	203	4.3 years	5-year OS: 58% vs. 76%	0.028
Aitchison	2014	pT3b-4 or N+ or any pT + pN1 or pN2 or positive margins or positive microvascular invasion	IFN-alpha + IL-2 + 5-FU vs. observation	309	7 years	3-year DFS	0.23

Adapted from Kenney and Wood [15]

The CheckMate 914 phase III trial evaluated the combination of nivolumab, a programmed death receptor inhibitor, and ipilimumab, a cytotoxic T-lymphocyte-associated protein 4 (CTLA-4) inhibitor, in 816 patients at risk of recurrence following surgery. After a median follow-up of 37 months, the trial failed to meet its primary endpoint of DFS, with a HR of 0.92 (95% CI: 0.71–1.19; P = 0.5347). However, exploratory subgroup analyses suggested a potential benefit in patients with PD-L1 expression >1%, with a hazard ratio of 0.46 (95% CI: 0.23–0.94) favoring combination therapy. Notably, CheckMate 914 has been criticized for its high treatment discontinuation rate (33%) when compared to Keynote-564 (20%) [64].

Adjuvant active–specific immunotherapy using vaccines has also been employed with largely unfavorable results. In a trial reported in 1996, Galligioni et al. randomized patients to intradermal injection of irradiated tumor cells and BCG (n = 60) or observation (n = 60) [60]. The investigators were able to document that the vaccine induced a tumor-specific immune response by demonstrating a delayed-type cutaneous hypersensitivity reaction to autologous tumor cells in 70% of immunized patients a month after the end of therapy. This did not translate into improved outcomes with comparable 5-year DFS in the vaccine and control groups (63% vs. 72%, p = NS).

The first successful adjuvant trial in RCC was reported in 2004 by Jocham and colleagues [65]. In 1997 and 1998, the investigators enrolled 558 patients who were scheduled for radical nephrectomy at 55 German sites. Randomization took place prior to nephrectomy. An intervention consisting of six autologous tumor vaccinations at 4-week intervals was compared to observation. Following nephrectomy, only patients with pT2–3b, pN0–3, M0 RCC, and Eastern Cooperative Oncology Group (ECOG) performance status 0–2 were permitted to continue in the trial. It is important to note that patients with pT1 or pT4 disease were excluded, despite having already been randomized. The primary endpoint was tumor progression.

There was a large loss of patients from the trial. Five patients withdrew consent prior to surgery. After surgery, an additional 174 subjects were withdrawn for reasons including non-RCC histology, incorrect tumor stage, and inability to prepare the vaccine. More patients were lost from the vaccine arm than control (n = 99 vs. 75). Analyzing the remaining 379 patients, 5-year PFS was higher in the vaccine group (77.4% vs. 67.8%, p = 0.02). At 5 years, the hazard ratio for progression was 1.58 (95% CI: 1.05–2.37, p = 0.02) in favor of the intervention. In the group of patients with pT3 disease, the difference in PFS between intervention and control was larger (67.5% vs. 49.7%, p = 0.039).

The trial was criticized for the large loss of patients (32%), which was imbalanced between study arms [66]. Based on the study design, in which patients were randomized before pathologic diagnosis and staging, a loss of patients was assured. To address this criticism, an intention-to-treat analysis was later reported with larger vaccine (n = 233) and control (n = 244) groups [67], The vaccine was still associated with improved PFS (p = 0.048), though the magnitude of the benefit was not reported. There was no difference in OS (p = 0.12). The same vaccine protocol was recently evaluated with a retrospective matched-pair analysis in 495 patients [68]. At a median follow-up of 131 months, the vaccine was an independent predictor of OS (HR: 1.28, p = 0.030), as well as in the subset of pT3 patients (HR: 1.67, p = 0.011). Even with an improvement in PFS demonstrated in a randomized trial and similar retrospective findings, the adjuvant vaccine was not widely adopted and the manufacturer became insolvent [66].

In another adjuvant vaccine trial, patients were randomized to receive Vitespen (Oncophage, Antigenics, Inc., New York, NY) (n = 409) or observation (n = 409) following nephrectomy [69]. Vitespen is a heat shock protein (HSP) vaccine, which consists of HSP-peptide complexes that are isolated from a patient's tumor. HSPs are intracellular chaperones which play a role in the loading of antigenic peptides onto MHC class I molecules, eliciting an immune response [4, 38]. After a median follow-up of 1.9 years, the rate of recurrence was comparable in the Vitespen and control groups (37.7% vs. 39.8%, $p = 0.506$).

Despite the mixed results of adjuvant vaccine trials to date, there remains significant enthusiasm. It was previously speculated that the ideal adjuvant therapy should have proven efficacy in metastatic disease [3, 4]. This may not necessarily be the case. The mechanisms for survival, latency and subsequent activation of quiescent disseminated tumor cells are poorly understood, but immune escape is posited to play an important role. The promise of adjuvant tumor vaccines is to direct immune surveillance against quiescent disseminated tumor cells and thereby prevent future radiographic recurrence. There is emerging data to support the notion that personalized tumor vaccines can induce immune response and that activated T cells have antitumor activity. In a small single arm trial, none of the 9 patients who received a personalized peptide tumor vaccine experienced recurrence [70].

Based on these findings, there is growing interest in evaluating the role of adjuvant vaccine therapy in combination with ICIs across various oncologic domains. In KEYNOTE-942, a Phase 2b trial in patients with resected stage III/IV melanoma, the combination of mRNA-4157 (V940) and pembrolizumab demonstrated a significant improvement in recurrence-free survival (RFS) at 18 months compared to pembrolizumab monotherapymonths [71]. Building on this success, INTerpath-004 is a global, multicenter, randomized, double-blind Phase 2 study designed to assess the efficacy and safety of adjuvant pembrolizumab with mRNA-4157 or placebo in RCC [72]. The trial aims to enroll 272 patients, with primary completion expected in 2028. Beyond RFS, the study will also evaluate metastasis-free survival and OS, potentially broadening the applicability of this combination therapy in genitourinary malignancies.

Thalidomide is an antiangiogenic and immunomodulatory drug that was investigated as an adjuvant therapy in a single-institution trial [73]. Thalidomide has demonstrable activity in metastatic RCC [74]. High-risk patients (high-grade T2–T4 or node-positive disease) were randomized to 2 years of thalidomide ($n = 23$) or observation ($n = 23$). Following a scheduled interim analysis, the protocol was terminated early as adjuvant thalidomide was unlikely to demonstrate any benefit. There was no difference in cancer-specific survival at 2 or 3 years, but 3-year RFS was inferior in the thalidomide arm (28.7% vs. 69.3%, $p = 0.022$).

Targeted Agents

Four adjuvant trials have evaluated VEGF receptor tyrosine kinase inhibitors. The ASSURE trial randomized patients with high-grade pT1b or greater into sunitinib, sorafenib, or placebo groups. Approximately 44% of patients in the sunitinib group and 45% in the sorafenib group discontinued treatment because of drug-related toxicity. The trial was stopped early due to loss of power to achieve the primary endpoint, and no DFS differences were reported among the groups [75].

In contrast to ASSURE, the S-TRAC study comparing sunitinib to placebo in high-risk clear cell carcinoma did show a DFS advantage with sunitinib (6.8 years vs. 5.6 years, $p = 0.03$). There was no difference in OS. Furthermore, patients in the sunitinib group were more likely to have dose reductions (34.2% vs. 2%), dose interruptions (46.4% vs. 13.2%), and dose discontinuations (28.1% vs. 5.6%) for adverse events and toxicity [76]. The main difference with ASSURE was the selection criteria of the study population (Table 23.3).

Recently, the SORCE study assessed the efficacy of adjuvant sorafenib compared to placebo in 1711 patients with intermediate- and high-risk clear cell RCC. After 3 years, median DFS was not reached in either group, with no significant difference observed (HR 1.01; 95% CI: 0.83–1.23; $P = 0.95$). Notably, over half of the participants discontinued treatment within 12 months, primarily due to the severity of adverse effects [77]. Similarly, the ATLAS trial investigated axitinib, a potent VEGF inhibitor, as adjuvant therapy versus placebo in 721 patients who had undergone nephrectomy. The trial was terminated early during a pre-planned interim analysis due to futility, as it failed to demonstrate a significant improvement in DFS

Table 23.3 Comparison in inclusion criteria between ASSURE, S-TRAC, ATLAS, and SORCE trials

Trial	Intervention	Inclusion criteria
ASSURE	Sorafenib vs. sunitinib vs. placebo	Selection of patients using 2002 American Joint Committee on Cancer staging:pT1b/Grade 3–4/N0/M0pT2/any Grade/N0/M0pT3/any Grade/N0/M0pT4/any Grade/N0/M0Any T/any Grade/N+/M0
S-TRAC	Sunitinib vs. placebo	Selection of patients using modified UISS criteria: pT2/N0/M0pT3–4/N0/M0pTx/N1/M0
ATLAS	Axitinib vs placebo	Selection of patient with newly diagnosed RCC (≥pT2 and/or N+, any Fuhrman grade (FG), Eastern Cooperative Oncology Group performance status (ECOG PS) 0/1) and prior nephrectomy
SORCE	Sorafenib vs. placebo	Selection of patients with intermediate or high risk RCC per the Leibovich risk model

[78]. The combined findings of these four trials highlight the limitations of VEGF-targeted therapies in the adjuvant setting for RCC, perhaps highlighting the differences in disease state between metastatic disease and patients at risk of harboring microscopic disseminated disease, with targeting angiogenesis being of limited impact in the latter.

The PROTECT trial evaluated adjuvant pazopanib compared to placebo in patients with locally advanced RCC at high risk for relapse. In intention to treat analysis, the intervention group did not show significant differences in terms of DFS when compared to placebo (HR: 0.69, 95% CI: 0.70–1.06; $p = 0.1$) but exhibited higher rates of grade 3–4 adverse events (60% vs. 21%, respectively) [79]. Final analysis of the cohort was published in 2021, and similarly demonstrated no benefit to OS with the addition of pazopanib (HR 1.0, 95% CI 0.80–1.26, $p > 0.9$) [80].

The ARISER trial assessed weekly Girentuximab, a monoclonal antibody that binds CA IX, after nephrectomy in high-risk ccRCC. The trial enrolled 864 patients randomized into Girentuximab or placebo and showed no differences in DFS (HR: 0.97, 95% CI: 0.79–1.18) or OS (HR: 0.99, 95% CI: 0.74–1.32) with comparable adverse events between arms [81].

The EVEREST trial investigated the use of adjuvant everolimus, an mTOR complex 1 inhibitor approved in 2009 for metastatic RCC, in patients at intermediate, high, or very high risk of recurrence [82]. The trial compared daily everolimus for 54 weeks to placebo in 1545 patients. Although there was a trend toward improved RFS with everolimus, the difference was not statistically significant (HR: 0.85; 95% CI: 0.72–1.00; $P = 0.051$). However, the treatment was associated with a substantially higher rate of adverse events, with grade 3 adverse effects occurring nearly four times more frequently in the everolimus group compared to placebo [83].

Ongoing or Unreported Adjuvant Trials

Despite the demonstrated difficulty in identifying an effective adjuvant therapy, there are numerous ongoing adjuvant trials using targeted agents. Some of these trials compare immune checkpoint therapies with demonstrated activity among solid malignancies. For example, RAMPART aims to assess adjuvant durvalumab (PD-L1 inhibitor) and tremelimumab (CTLA-4 inhibitor) to placebo while LITESPARK-022 aims to investigate combination pembrolizumab and belzutifan to placebo. Similarly, INTerpath-004 is designed to evaluate the combination of pembrolizumab and the V940 vaccine compared to placebo (Table 23.4). All of the trials target patients with high risk of recurrence, some using the previously described predictive models.

Adjuvant Therapy: Current Status

For decades, there was no commonly accepted evidenced-based paradigm for adjuvant therapy following nephrectomy for clinically localized disease. Adjuvant radiotherapy, MPA, IL-2, IFN-α, and Thalidomide were evaluated in randomized con-

Table 23.4 Ongoing trials of adjuvant therapy for clinically localized RCC

Study name	Drug(s)	Study sponsor	Drug description	Clinicaltrials.gov	Design	Population	*n*	Adjuvant intervention	Primary outcome	Secondary outcome	Status
LITESPARK-022	Pembrolizumab and belzutifan	Merck Sharp & Dohme LLC	PD-L1 and HIF-2α inhibition	NCT05239728	Randomized, triple blind, placebo-controlled phase III	Intermediate-high risk, high risk, and M1		54 weeks of oral belzutifan and IV pembrolizumab or placebo	DFS	OS, adverse, events, RFS	Enrollment completed in 2023 and primary completion estimated in 2026
RAMPART	Durvalumab and tremelimumab	University College, London	PD-L1 and CTLA-4 inhibition	NCT03288532	Open-label, randomized, placebo-controlled phase III	Leibovich 3-11 risk	1750	1 year of durvalumab or 1 year of durvalumab and tremelimumab or active monitoring	DFS, OS	Metastasis-free survival, RCC specific survival	Recruitment began in July 2018 and is ongoing
TUOAD-RCC	Tremelimumab	Tianjin Medical University Second Hospital	CTLA-4 inhibitor	NCT06584435	Open-label, single arm, phase II clinical trial	High risk stage III/IV RCC		Tremelimumab every 3 weeks for one treatment cycle	PFS, OS	N/A	Recruitment began October 2022, expected completion March 2025
INTerpath-004	Pembrolizumab and mRNA-4157 (V940)	Merck Sharp & Dohme LLC	PD-L1 inhibition and individualized neoantigen therapy	NCT06307431	Randomized, triple blind, placebo-controlled phase II trial	Intermediate, high risk, or M1 disease	272	54 weeks of IV pembrolizumab and mRNA or 4154 or 54 weeks of IV pembrolizumab and placebo	DFS	OS, metastasis-free survival, adverse events	Recruitment began in April 2024 with completion estimated January 2028

(continued)

Table 23.4 (continued)

Study name	Drug(s)	Study sponsor	Drug description	Clinicaltrials.gov	Design	Population	*n*	Adjuvant intervention	Primary outcome	Secondary outcome	Status
IUNU-RC-102	Toripalimab and axitinib	Nanjing University Medical School	PD-L1 inhibition and VEGFR inhibition	NCT05768464	Single-arm, multicentre phase II clinical trial	Histologically confirmed non-clear cell RCC		240 mg toripalimab IV every 3 weeks and 5 mg axitinib oral twice daily	DFS	OS, localized disease recurrence-specific survival, adverse events	Recruitment began February 2023 with completion expected in 2026
MK-6482-022	Belzutifan and pembrolizumab	Merck Sharp & Dohme LLC	HIF-2α inhibition	NCT05239728	Randomized, double-blind, placebo-controlled phase III trial	Intermediate, high risk, or M1 disease		120 mg belzutifan for 54 weeks and pembrolizumab 400 mg IV every 6 weeks for 54 weeks	DFS	OS, adverse events, disease recurrence-specific survival, health-related QoL, FKSI-DRS survey of kidney cancer symptoms	Recruitment began in March 2022 and is expected to conclude in 2026

trolled trials, and neither improved disease progression or survival [34, 35, 39, 56–59, 73]. Although an adjuvant autologous tumor vaccination was associated with a PFS benefit in a randomized controlled trial, the study methodology has been criticized, and the intervention was not broadly adopted [65] No other adjuvant vaccine study had favorable results [60, 69] until 2025, when an adjuvant peptide neoantigen vaccine was shown to generate antitumor immunity in RCC. Sunitinib has not been shown to improve OS, had mixed results with regard to DFS, and nonetheless became the first US Food and Drug Administration (FDA)-approved agent for use in the adjuvant setting. Nonetheless, Sunitinib does not play an important role given mixed results, lack of OS benefit, and toxicity.

In 2021, the FDA approved the use of pembrolizumab as adjuvant treatment for patients at high risk of recurrence after nephrectomy, based on the results of the KEYNOTE-564 trial [84]. This multicenter, randomized, phase III trial evaluated the efficacy of pembrolizumab versus placebo in 994 participants. At a 57-month median follow-up, pembrolizumab demonstrated the first observed improvement in OS with adjuvant therapy in RCC (HR 0.62; 95% CI: 0.44–0.87; $P = 0.005$) [62]. While the addition of pembrolizumab was associated with an increase in grade 3 and 4 adverse events, no treatment-related deaths were reported.

By early 2022, both the National Comprehensive Cancer Network (NCCN) and the European Society for Medical Oncology (ESMO) updated their guidelines to include adjuvant pembrolizumab for patients with intermediate or high-risk RCC following nephrectomy. There are additional trials evaluating immune checkpoint inhibitors (e.g., nivolumab, avelumab) and combination approaches, aiming to further refine and expand adjuvant immunotherapy strategies in RCC.

Neoadjuvant Therapy for Locally Advanced RCC

In this chapter, we will use the term neoadjuvant therapy to designate therapy administered prior to surgical resection of clinically localized disease. The intent of neoadjuvant therapy for locally advanced RCC is not only to reduce the risk of recurrence but also to facilitate surgery by converting unresectable disease to resectable by making partial nephrectomy feasible or by simplifying resection of a venous tumor thrombus. Each of these goals continues to be theoretical, and there is little data to support the use of neoadjuvant systemic therapy in RCC.

Immunotherapy

A hallmark of immunotherapy for metastatic disease is that it appears to have little or no impact on the primary lesion. For instance, IL-2, IFN-α, and granulocyte-macrophage colony-stimulating factor were used to treat 16 patients with metastatic RCC with the primary in situ, and no response was seen in the primary tumors [85]. Applying this concept to the neoadjuvant setting, one would not expect cytokines to shrink the primary tumor [86].

On the other hand, there is some evidence that neoadjuvant renal artery embolization, which can be used to cut off the arterial inflow to locally advanced lesions prior to nephrectomy, might engender a beneficial immune response by releasing tumor-associated antigens. It is possible that angioinfarction augments the immune response to the renal tumor [87]. There are reports of regression of RCC metastases following RAE and nephrectomy [88, 89]. In addition, the common post-infarction syndrome may be cytokine-mediated. Several studies have shown that RAE is immunomodulatory with documented changes in natural killer cell activity, increased cell-mediated cytotoxicity, and alteration in lymphocyte proliferation [90–92]. A single case-control study of preoperative renal artery embolization demonstrated better OS at 5 years (62% vs. 35%, $p = 0.01$) and 10 years (47% vs. 23%, $p = 0.01$) [93]. Nonetheless, while it may be a helpful technical adjunct to surgery, no prospective clinical evidence supports the use of neoadjuvant renal artery embolization as a means of improving survival.

With the increasing recognition of the role of immune system evasion in the pathogenesis and progression of solid tumors, there has been growing interest in the use of immune checkpoint inhibitors as neoadjuvant therapy for locally advanced RCC. The PROSPER trial explored the perioperative use of nivolumab in patients with RCC. The study compared one cycle of neoadjuvant nivolumab followed by radical or partial nephrectomy and adjuvant nivolumab (480 mg IV every 4 weeks for nine doses) to surgery alone followed by surveillance, without a placebo control. Eligible patients included those with clinical stage >T2 or any T stage with N+ RCC, as well as individuals with selected oligometastatic disease, provided there was no evidence of disease within 12 weeks after surgery. The trial enrolled 819 patients, 87% of whom had clear cell RCC, with the remainder having non-clear cell subtypes. Biopsies were mandatory for patients in the nivolumab arm. The primary endpoint, RFS RFS, showed no significant difference between the nivolumab and control arms (HR: 0.97; 95% CI: 0.74–1.28; P = 0.43), prompting the Data and Safety Monitoring Committee to terminate the trial early. OS was also not statistically different between the groups (HR: 1.48; 95% CI: 0.89–2.48; P = 0.93), although OS data remained immature at the time of analysis. Grade III-IV adverse events were more frequent in the nivolumab arm (20%) compared to the control arm (6%). Mortality rates were similar, with 15 deaths (4%) in the nivolumab group and 18 deaths (4%) in the surgery-alone group [94].

Targeted Therapy

The advent of targeted therapy, which can have activity against the primary tumor, prompted a reevaluation of neoadjuvant systemic therapy prior to surgical resection. This section will review neoadjuvant targeted therapy for locally advanced disease. Much of the data is extrapolated from the presurgical (i.e., metastatic) literature. Presurgical therapy, which we use to denote therapy prior to planned cytoreductive surgery in mRCC, will be addressed later in the chapter.

Targeted Therapy Is Active Against the Primary Tumor

Response in the primary tumor is variable and depends on the individual tumor and the systemic agent employed. Profound responses to targeted agents have been reported, including complete histologic response, but these are the exception rather than the rule (Fig. 23.3a, b) [96]. The primary tumor typically has a more modest response to targeted agents.

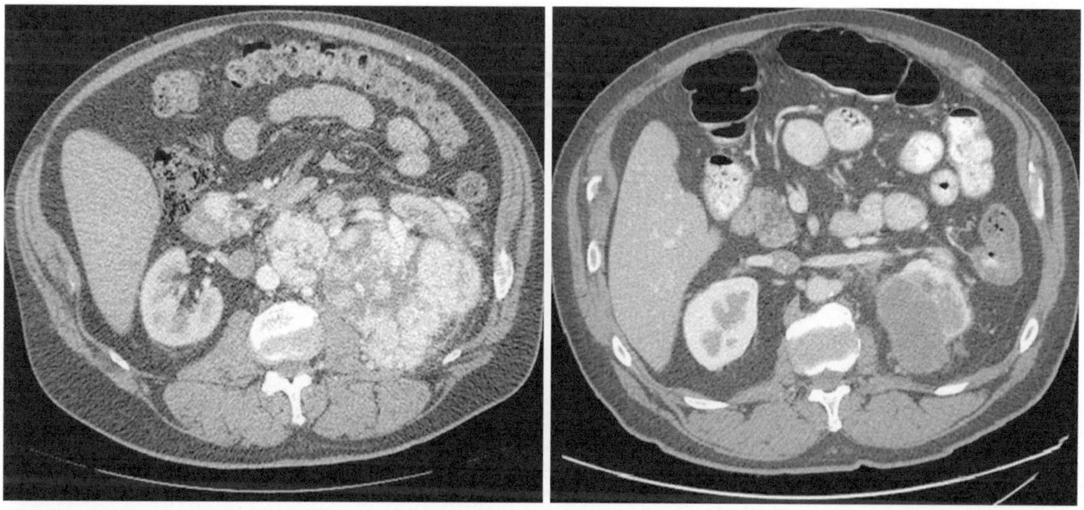

Fig. 23.3 Before therapy with Sunitinib (left), a CT scan demonstrates a large left-sided primary tumor with associated adenopathy. There was a significant decrease in both the primary tumor and nodes following treatment with Sunitinib (right). (Reprinted with permission from Abel et al. [95])

A number of retrospective analyses have described the impact of Sunitinib and other agents on the primary. Generally, Sunitinib has produced a more robust response in the primary tumor than any other targeted therapies [8]. Imaging for 17 patients who were treated with Sunitinib at two Dutch Centers from 2005 to 2007 was retrospectively analyzed [97]. The primary tumor was in place. Radiographic response in the primary was assessed using Response Evaluation Criteria in Solid Tumors (RECIST). It is important to note that RECIST, which is based on changes in tumor size, may underestimate the impact of targeted therapy whose impact may be better judged by assessing tumor necrosis and cavitation [98]. There were 4 partial responses, 1 progression, and 12 with stable disease by RECIST. Among the patients with partial response or stable disease, there was a 31% median reduction ($p = 0.001$) in tumor volume. There was a 39% concomitant increase ($p = 0.035$) in the median volume of necrosis.

Thomas et al. also reported a retrospective series of 19 patients with locally advanced or metastatic RCC who were treated with Sunitinib with the primary tumor in place [99]. By RECIST, there were three partial responses (16%), seven with stable disease (37%), and nine (47%) with progression. Of the eight (42%) patients who had tumor shrinkage, the mean decrease was 24% (range 2–46%) (Table 23.5).

A single-arm Phase II trial of presurgical Bevacizumab ($n = 23$) or Bevacizumab plus Erlotinib ($n = 27$) was undertaken in patients with metastatic RCC [100]. Most patients (58%) had stable disease, with some partial responses (10%) and a single complete response (2%). 52% of patients had regression of the primary tumor, although the size reductions were generally minor: 1–10% shrinkage (29%), 11–20% shrinkage (16%), and 20–30% shrinkage (7%).

Similarly, Cowey and colleagues performed a single-arm Phase II trial of neoadjuvant or presurgical Sorafenib in 30 patients with ≥ Stage II RCC [101]. Nephrectomy was planned in all patients. Median treatment duration was 33 days. The vast majority (93%) of patients had stable disease by RECIST criteria. The median change in tumor size was −9.6% (range from +16% to −40%).

In 2011, Abel and colleagues reported a single-institution retrospective review of patients with mRCC who received targeted therapy with the primary tumor in situ between 2004 and 2009 [95]. Adequate imaging was available for 168 patients with a median follow-up of 15 months. Two reviewers measured the diameter of primary and metastatic lesions on pre- and post-therapy imaging. Prior to therapy, the median diameter of the primary lesion was 9.6 cm. Patients received a variety of systemic targeted therapies (Table 23.3). The median maximum change in primary tumor diameter was −7.1% after a median 62 days of treatment. The median change in primary tumor diameter was −6.5 mm.

More recently, several single-arm phase II clinical trials have been conducted to assess the effectiveness of newer targeted therapies in

Table 23.5 In mRCC patients who were treated with systemic therapy with the primary tumor in situ, radiographic response in the primary tumor varied by drug

Agent	Number of patients	Median percentage change (IQR)	Median number days between imaging (IQR)
Sunitinib	75 (45%)	−10.2 (−21.1 to −2.8)	105 (76–201)
Bevacizumab	25 (15%)	0.1 (−4.2 to 4.6)	55 (54–56)
Bevacizumab plus erlotinib	26 (15%)	−10.1 (−17.1 to −6.0)	54.5 (54–56)
Sorafenib	16 (10%)	−6.0 (−12.3 to −0.4)	90 (61.5–124)
Temsirolimus	16 (10%)	−4.0 (−8.6 to −0.5)	56 (52–84)
Bevacizumab plus chemotherapy	7 (4%)	−6.1 (−11.9 to −0.7)	58 (43–118)
Erlotinib	2 (1%)	−5.1 (−9 to −1.3)	51.5 (41–62)
Pazopanib	1 (1%)	−11.1 (NA)	48 (NA)

Adapted from Abel et al. [95]

patients with localized RCC. Among these, the AXIPAN multicenter trial enrolled 18 patients to evaluate the efficacy of axitinib in reducing tumor size, thereby facilitating partial rather than radical nephrectomy [102]. Following axitinib therapy, 16 of 18 tumors decreased in diameter, with a mean reduction of 17%. Notably, among 12 patients with initial tumor sizes >7 cm, tumor shrinkage was sufficient to allow for partial nephrectomy. Similarly, De Velasco et al. reported a case series of four men with locally advanced RCC enrolled in the CABOPRE phase II trial, which investigated neoadjuvant cabozantinib [103]. The study concluded that cabozantinib induced a rapid and clinically significant response in intermediate-risk patients, making surgical resection more feasible. Lastly, the NeoAvAx trial, reported in 2022, was a single-arm phase II study that evaluated neoadjuvant avelumab and axitinib in 40 patients with localized RCC [104]. The trial, published in abstract form, found a 20% reduction in tumor size. Of the 12 patients who underwent post-treatment partial nephrectomy, 11 remained disease-free at a median follow-up of 23.5 months. In total, the findings from these small trials suggest that targeted therapies may be effective in reducing tumor size, promoting resectability in selected cases.

Permitting Resection

It has been proposed that neoadjuvant therapy may render initially unresectable lesions amenable to nephrectomy. It is clear that surgical resectability is a poorly defined, subjective characteristic that is dependent upon the surgeon and patient [86, 105]. Attributes that contribute to unresectability may include tumor size, extensive hilar involvement, considerable lymphadenopathy, or adjacent organ invasion [99]. In the series reported by Thomas and colleagues, there were four patients with locally advanced disease in whom the primary tumor was judged to be unresectable due to the proximity of adjacent structures ($n = 4$), vascular involvement ($n = 2$), and substantial adenopathy ($n = 2$) [99]. The average size of the primary tumor was 11.3 cm (range 6.4–20 cm). After being treated with neoadjuvant Sunitinib, three of the four patients had tumor shrinkage (range 11–24%) and subsequently had nephrectomy. The alterations in the primary that permitted transformation to "resectable" status were not described.

In 2012, Rini and colleagues reported the results of a Phase II trial of neoadjuvant or presurgical Sunitinib in 30 patients with a primary tumor that was deemed unresectable [106]. To be considered unresectable, patients had at least one of the following characteristics: large tumor, bulky adenopathy, tumor thrombus, or proximity to vital structures. The median change in the size of the primary tumor was a 22% decrease (median: 1.2 cm). Patients with non-clear cell histology had a median 1.4% increase (0.1 cm) in primary tumor size. Thirteen patients (45%) were able to go on to nephrectomy.

Although these findings are thought-provoking, it is estimated that <1% of RCC cases are characterized as unresectable [105]. In addition to being rare, unresectability is subjectively defined and may vary among surgeons. Moreover, existing drugs typically have at best a modest impact on the primary tumor. For these reasons, quantifying the impact of neoadjuvant therapy on unresectability in a reproducible manner will be a substantial challenge.

Enabling Nephron-Sparing Surgery

There is a growing body of evidence favoring nephron-sparing surgery over radical nephrectomy. There is a higher probability of renal insufficiency following radical nephrectomy compared to partial nephrectomy [107, 108]. It is presumed that the higher rate of chronic kidney disease following radical nephrectomy may place patients at higher risk of atherosclerotic disease and death. In a population-based analysis, radical nephrectomy was associated with a 1.4-fold higher number of cardiovascular events ($p < 0.05$) and a higher risk of overall mortality (HR: 1.38, $p < 0.01$) compared to partial nephrectomy [109]. Another population-based study that compared partial and radical nephrectomy for T1a RCC demonstrated comparable kidney cancer–specific survival (HR: 0.82; 95% CI: 0.19–3.49) but substantially lower risk of death with partial nephrectomy (HR: 0.54; 95% CI: 0.34–0.85) [110]. With partial nephrectomy, survival at 2, 5, and 8 years increased by 5.6%, 11.8%, and 15.5%, respectively ($p < 0.001$). It should be noted that these findings were not supported by a controversial and methodologically problematic prospective European Organization for the Research and Treatment of Cancer (EORTC) study that demonstrated improved OS with radical compared to partial nephrectomy [111].

Given the apparent benefits of partial nephrectomy, it has been proposed that one could employ neoadjuvant systemic therapy for large or locally advanced lesions to permit partial nephrectomy where it would otherwise not be feasible [86, 112]. There are reports of Sunitinib being utilized in the neoadjuvant setting to facilitate imperative partial nephrectomy, including a patient with two tumors in a solitary kidney after prior radical nephrectomy [113]. It was thought that partial nephrectomy of these centrally located lesions would not be possible. The patients were treated with neoadjuvant Sunitinib which resulted in a 20% decrease in size of the tumors. Subsequent partial nephrectomy was successful. Similarly, Thomas et al. described two cases of bilateral tumors in which neoadjuvant Sunitinib was followed by successful partial nephrectomy [114].

Sunitinib was also used in 12 patients, 5 of whom had metastatic disease, prior to partial nephrectomy as reported by Silberstein et al. in 2010 [115]. Each patient had an imperative indication for partial nephrectomy including chronic kidney disease ($n = 9$), solitary kidney ($n = 7$), or bilateral tumors ($n = 2$). In response to Sunitinib, all patients had measurable tumor shrinkage with the mean tumor diameter decreasing from 7.1 to 5.6 cm (21%). All patients underwent partial nephrectomy. There were three urine leaks. Follow-up was 23.9 months. Limitations of the study include lack of a control group and brief follow-up. In addition, the impact of Sunitinib on surgical complexity was not reported. It would have been valuable to quantify change in the surgical complexity of the tumor using anatomic or morphometric data (e.g., centrality index or nephrometry score) [116, 117]. A fundamental shortcoming of this study is that the indication for neoadjuvant or presurgical Sunitinib was not reported. It is unclear if Sunitinib had any impact on the feasibility, technical complexity, or oncologic outcome of partial nephrectomy.

A similar study was reported by Hellenthal et al., who performed a single-arm prospective study of neoadjuvant or presurgical Sunitinib in 20 patients with localized or metastatic ccRCC [112]. After 2 months of Sunitinib, 17 out of 20 (85%) patients had tumor shrinkage with a mean decrease of 11.8%. Eight patients had partial nephrectomy for pT1b–pT3a N0 M0 disease, and the remainder had radical nephrectomy. No complications were attributed to the upfront drug. These series provide evidence that partial nephrectomy following Sunitinib is feasible. Unfortunately, they do not provide efficacy data to support the use of systemic therapy prior to partial nephrectomy.

Downsizing Caval Tumor Thrombus

The data supporting the use of neoadjuvant targeted therapy to downsize caval tumor thrombus has similar problems. There are case reports in which neoadjuvant Sunitinib permitted a less morbid surgical approach for venous tumor thrombi. Karakiewicz and colleagues reported a patient who refused sternotomy for an 11 cm renal tumor with an atrial thrombus [118]. Following 12 weeks of neoadjuvant Sunitinib, the tumor thrombus had regressed to the infrahepatic IVC (Fig. 23.4a, b). In another report, presurgical Sunitinib was used to shrink a caval thrombus, which permitted laparoscopic rather than open cytoreductive nephrectomy [119].

These dramatic responses are not likely typical, and it is clear that not all caval tumor thrombi have gratifying responses to neoadjuvant therapy. Bex et al. described two patients with metastatic disease who were enrolled in a phase II trial of presurgical Sunitinib [120]. Despite treatment with Sunitinib, one patient developed a new caval tumor thrombus despite Sunitinib, and the second had growth of an existing infrahepatic thrombus up to the atrium.

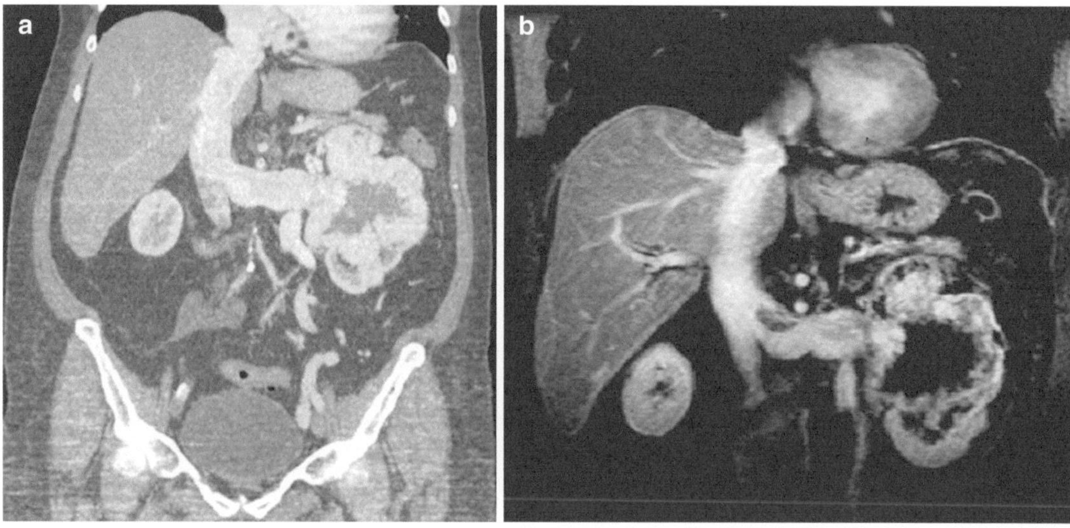

Fig. 23.4 CT scan demonstrating a left-sided RCC with an associated tumor thrombus extending into the right atrium (**a**). The thrombus substantially regressed in response to two cycles of Sunitinib. Following therapy, it is visible as a dark filling defect at the junction of the renal vein and cava (**b**). (Reprinted with permission from Karakiewicz et al. [118])

In a larger retrospective series, Cost et al. described 25 patients with an RCC tumor thrombus who were treated with targeted therapy [121]. The majority of the patients (76%) had ccRCC. Not all of the patients were considered surgical candidates. The tumor thrombus was level 2 ($n = 18$), level 3 ($n = 5$), or level 4 ($n = 2$). Systemic therapies were Sunitinib ($n = 12$), Bevacizumab ($n = 9$), Temsirolimus ($n = 3$), and Sorafenib ($n = 1$). In response to systemic therapy, the thrombus regressed in 44% of patients and expanded in 28%. In most patients, the thrombus level did not change. In one patient, the thrombus level increased (level 2–3). The thrombus level decreased in three patients, including one patient with a level 4 thrombus that became level 3. This was the only patient in whom the surgical approach would have been affected. A minority of the patients (36%) went on to radical nephrectomy and tumor thrombectomy. In addition to the retrospective design, other limitations are the heterogeneous patient population and drugs, and that not all patients were surgical candidates.

NAXIVA, a small phase II clinical trial assessed the use of neoadjuvant axitinib to reduce the extent of venous tumor thrombus among 20 patients with resectable RCC. Extensiveness of thrombus was defined by the Mayo Clinic venous tumor thrombus criteria. While statistical significance could not be assessed among this small sample size, 37.5% of patients with caval thrombus experienced a reduction in Mayo level. Overall, 41.2% of patients underwent less extensive surgery than was originally planned [122]. These findings suggest that neoadjuvant axitinib may have a role in minimizing surgical complexity in RCC patients with venous tumor thrombus, although larger studies are needed to confirm these preliminary results.

Two open-label phase II clinical trials are currently investigating the efficacy of combination immunotherapies for patients with RCC associated with IVC thrombus [123]. NEOPAX, conducted at the University of Colorado, Denver, aims to enroll 17 patients to receive neoadjuvant therapy with pembrolizumab and axitinib, with the primary endpoint being changes in IVC tumor thrombus extent based on Mayo classification. Similarly, a trial at the University of Texas Southwestern Medical Center seeks to evaluate tumor thrombus response in 30 patients treated with neoadjuvant pembrolizumab and lenvatinib. These small but important trials represent some of the first efforts to explore the expanded use of ICIs in patients with tumor thrombus, a novel treatment approach in this high-risk population.

Neoadjuvant Therapy: Current Status

In summary, rigorous research is needed to determine what role neoadjuvant approaches may have in the management of locally advanced RCC. While immunotherapies to date have had little impact on the primary tumor [85], their use in combination with targeted therapy may be reasonable [104]. Targeted therapies can affect the primary tumor, but overall, the impact with these agents is not robust. The impact of systemic therapy on resectability, feasibility of partial nephrectomy, and regression of tumor thrombus remains unclear, and this application is investigational, but can be a reasonable approach, especially in patients with solitary kidney or other imperative indications for nephron-sparing approaches.

Integrated Therapy for Metastatic Disease

While treatment of the primary tumor in other metastatic malignancies is usually limited to a palliative role, radical nephrectomy with therapeutic intent has been a core component of the treatment of metastatic RCC [4]. Cytoreductive nephrectomy was established as a treatment paradigm during the immunotherapy era. With the advent of targeted therapy, the ongoing role of cytoreductive nephrectomy remains to be elucidated and has been called into question by the results of CARMENA. In addition, the proper sequence of surgery and systemic therapy is not yet known. Advantages to presurgical systemic therapy in metastatic disease have been proposed and may significantly alter the existing integrated therapy archetype.

Cytoreductive Nephrectomy

During the first immunotherapy era, several findings prompted consideration of cytoreductive nephrectomy as a therapeutic adjunct to systemic therapy. First, immunotherapy appeared to have little or no impact on the primary tumor. Second, it was thought that the primary tumor inhibited immunosurveillance and could act as a source for further metastatic progression [124]. Further, nephrectomy was a favorable, independent prognostic factor in several retrospective immunotherapy series [125–129]. In particular, Motzer et al. created a multivariate model to predict survival by analyzing 670 patients with advanced RCC who were treated from 1975 to 1996. In addition to Karnofsky performance status <80%, lactate dehydrogenase (LDH) >1.5-fold normal, low hemoglobin, and corrected serum calcium >10 mg/dL, absence of nephrectomy was an independent predictor of shorter survival [129].

In 2001, two randomized trials from SWOG and the EORTC firmly established the role of cytoreductive nephrectomy prior to systemic treatment with IFN-α in patients with metastatic RCC [130, 131]. In both trials, patients were randomized to cytoreductive nephrectomy followed by IFN-α vs. IFN-α alone. In both trials, cytoreduction was associated with improved OS. In a combined analysis of the two similarly designed trials, cytoreductive nephrectomy followed by IFN-α was associated with longer median survival than IFN-α alone (13.6 months vs. 7.8 months, $p = 0.002$) [132]. Based on this considerable survival benefit, cytoreductive surgery followed by systemic therapy was confirmed as the principal treatment algorithm for mRCC.

In the combined analysis, there were 253 patients with measurable disease, and the objective response rates in the nephrectomy plus IFN and IFN alone groups were similarly low (6.9% vs. 5.7%, $p = 0.60$) [132]. Without a measurable improvement in metastatic disease, the mechanism of improved survival is unclear. Possibilities include tumoristasis induced by post-nephrectomy azotemia and metabolic acidosis, improved immune surveillance following removal of the immunologic sink, and elimination of a source of growth factors [2, 124].

The Importance of Proper Patient Selection

Cytoreductive nephrectomy is not without risks. Some patients may experience cancer progression during recovery from surgery. In addition, the morbidity of surgery may prevent a subset of patients from receiving the necessary systemic therapy. In addition, surgical convalescence may delay administration of systemic therapy.

Cytoreductive nephrectomy should clearly not be applied to all patients with metastatic RCC. It is essential to note the selection criteria of the SWOG and EORTC trials. In both trials, patients were excluded for ECOG performance status 2 or worse, prior systemic therapy, high-level tumor thrombus, or a primary tumor that was deemed unresectable. Patients with brain metastases were not eligible for the EORTC trial. The results of these trials should not be generalized to all patients with metastatic RCC, such as those with poor performance status.

Retrospective analyses identified clinical variables that were predictive of surgical benefit [4, 124, 133–137]. Good performance status, lack of central nervous system, liver or extensive bone metastases, absence of sarcomatoid or other poor prognosis histology, and debulking of a high fraction of disease were all associated with a favorable response to surgery [4].

In 2010, Culp et al. identified preoperative factors that were prognostic of a favorable response to cytoreductive nephrectomy [138]. In a retrospective analysis, the authors compared cytoreductive nephrectomy patients ($n = 566$) to those managed without cytoreduction ($n = 110$) from 1991 to 2007. The cohort of patients was similar to the ECOG and SWOG studies in that fewer than 3% had an ECOG performance status of 2, of and none had a performance status ≥3. There were brain metastases in 3.5%. The authors determined that cytoreductive nephrectomy patients who died within 8.5 months of surgery did not receive a survival benefit from surgery ($p < 0.05$). Independent predictors of inferior OS among cytoreductive nephrectomy patients included elevated LDH (HR: 1.66, $p < 0.001$), hypoalbuminemia (HR: 1.59, $p = 0.001$), symptomatic metastases (HR: 1.35, $p = 0.028$), liver metastases (HR: 1.47, $p = 0.039$), retroperitoneal adenopathy (HR: 1.29, $p = 0.040$), supradiaphragmatic adenopathy (HR: 1.48, $p = 0.001$), and clinical T3 (HR: 1.37, $p = 0.045$) or T4 (HR: 2.05, $p = 0.019$) disease. The survival curve of cytoreductive nephrectomy patients with ≥4 of these risk factors overlapped that of patients treated with medical therapy alone (Fig. 23.5). Even in a patient population that largely mirrored that of the SWOG and EORTC trials, not all candidates benefited from cytoreduction.

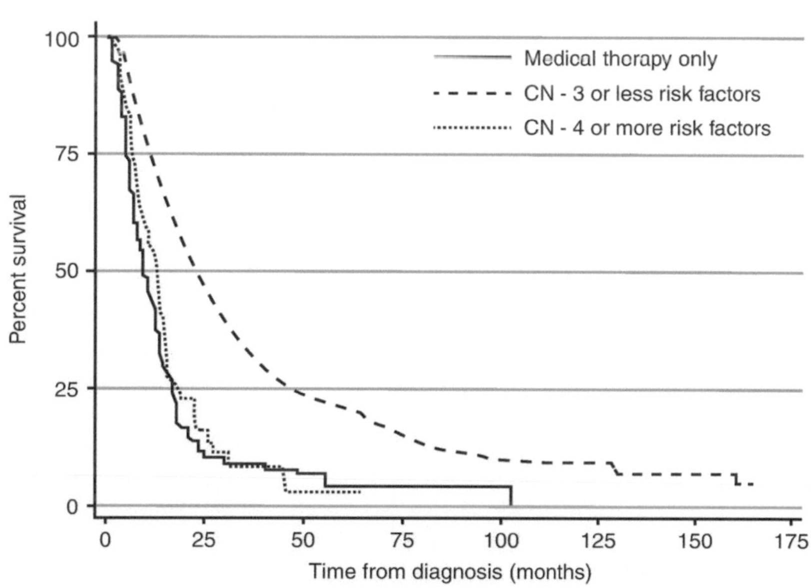

Fig. 23.5 In this Kaplan-Meier curve of overall survival after cytoreductive nephrectomy, survival of patients with four or more risk factors approximates that of patients treated with medical therapy alone. (Reprinted with permission from Culp et al. [138])

Targeted Therapy and Cytoreductive Nephrectomy

The benefit observed with cytoreductive nephrectomy may not be intrinsic to the operation but may be due to an interaction between the operation and the particular systemic agent employed thereafter. Cytoreductive surgery was established as a pillar of mRCC treatment in concert with early immunotherapy. It is not a foregone conclusion that there should continue to be a role for cytoreduction with targeted therapy or checkpoint inhibition.

Despite a paucity of data, cytoreduction retained its place in the treatment paradigm in the targeted therapy era. In the Phase III trials demonstrating progression-free or OS advantages for Sunitinib, Sorafenib, Temsirolimus, Everolimus, Bevacizumab/IFN-∝-2b, and Bevacizumab/IFN-∝-2a compared to control, the rates of prior nephrectomy in the intervention arms were 91%, 94%, 66%, 96%, 85%, and 100%, respectively [82, 139–143]. The lower rate of nephrectomy in the Temsirolimus trial is explained by the proportion of high-risk patients in that trial [139]. Although it was commonly employed, the uncertain benefit and potential adverse consequences of surgery prompted a reevaluation of the paradigm of integrated therapy.

Retrospective studies and subgroup analyses suggested that cytoreductive nephrectomy provided a survival advantage when followed by targeted therapy [144–146]. A multicenter collaboration reported a retrospective review of 645 patients who were treated with Sunitinib, Sorafenib, or Bevacizumab [145]. Patients who had a nephrectomy for clinically localized disease who later developed metastasis were excluded ($n = 331$). Patients who were treated with a cytoreductive nephrectomy ($n = 201$) were compared to those who were managed without nephrectomy ($n = 113$). Patients who had surgery were younger ($p < 0.01$), less often had poor performance status ($p < 0.01$), more often had >1 metastatic site ($p = 0.04$), less often received targeted therapy within a year of diagnosis ($p < 0.01$), and less often had hypercalcemia ($p < 0.01$). Cytoreductive nephrectomy was independently associated with better OS (HR: 0.68, $p = 0.04$), although the survival benefit was modest in patients with poor performance status and high-risk disease. These results support the continued use of cytoreduction in selected patients [147].

In summary, the Phase III trials that demonstrated the effectiveness of targeted therapeutics largely enrolled patients with prior cytoreductive nephrectomy. Second, retrospective data suggest that the addition of cytoreductive nephrectomy to targeted therapy is associated with improved survival.

The Clinical Trial to Assess the Importance of Nephrectomy (CARMENA) was a phase III non-inferiority trial comparing cytoreductive therapy and targeted therapy in intermediate to poor-risk patients with metastatic ccRCC and absence of brain metastases. The study randomized 450 patients to Sunitinib alone or cytoreductive nephrectomy followed by Sunitinib. The primary endpoint was OS, with secondary endpoints including objective response, PFS, and postoperative morbidity [148].

After a median follow-up of approximately 50.9 months, sunitinib alone was non-inferior to sunitinib + cytoreductive nephrectomy in regard to OS, response rate, or PFS [148]. CARMENA was criticized for alterations in the study protocol and differences between the study groups. For example, the initial recruitment goal was 576 patients, and the study closed after only 450 participants had been included over a period of 8 years for poor accrual. Moreover, 70.1% of the patients in the cytoreductive nephrectomy + sunitinib group had T3 and T4 tumors in comparison to 51% in the sunitinib alone cohort, possibly creating imbalances between the groups.

Similarly, SURTIME evaluated immediate vs. deferred cytoreductive nephrectomy in metastatic ccRCC patients receiving sunitinib. The study intended to recruit 458 patients to have adequate power for PFS estimation. However, due to poor accrual, ITT 28-week progression-free rate was assessed for 99 recruited patients showing no difference in immediate vs. deferred cytoreductive nephrectomy (42% vs. 43%, respectively, $p = 0.61$). Considering secondary endpoints in exploratory analysis, deferred cytoreductive nephrectomy group showed an advantage of approximately 17 months in OS when compared to immediate surgery (32.4 months for the deferred arm vs. 15 months for the immediate arm). Of note, 98% of the patients in the deferred arm received sunitinib while only 80% received this medication in the deferred arm. Moreover, 29% of the patients in the deferred arm did not undergo cytoreductive nephrectomy due to disease progression, indicating a possible role for presurgical therapy to select the right patients who could benefit from the surgical procedure after sunitinib therapy [149].

Treatment Chronology: Upfront Nephrectomy Versus Presurgical Targeted Therapy

The Argument for Presurgical Targeted Therapy

While surgery prior to immunotherapy was accepted as the proper order of therapy, it is not clear that upfront surgery followed by targeted therapy is the best sequence [4, 150].Investigators have proposed several reasons that presurgical targeted therapy might be beneficial. First, pre surgical therapy may decrease RCC-related morbidity prior to surgery [150]. Second, molecular evaluations of post-treatment nephrectomy specimens may elucidate markers of response and resistance [2, 4].

Third, the primary tumor may be more amenable to excision following presurgical targeted therapy. In a retrospective review by van der Veldt et al., three patients with mRCC had unresectable primaries due to suspected liver invasion [97]. Presurgical Sunitinib reduced primary tumor volume by 30–46%, and all were able to have subsequent cytoreductive surgery. Another retrospective analysis included ten patients with mRCC who received Sunitinib with the primary tumor in situ due to uncertain resectability, which was defined as adjacent organ invasion or involvement of essential vascular structures such as the great vessels, celiac axis, or superior mesenteric artery [151]. There were two partial responses by RECIST. The median change in primary tumor size was −10% (range from −20% to +11%). The tumor site that prohibited surgery shrank in six patients. This happened after 2–4 months of therapy and permitted cytoreductive nephrectomy in three patients. The ability of current agents to downsize complex primary tumors in mRCC patients is limited [2]. Barring the emergence of future therapies that are substantially more effective at downsizing the primary, other benefits will have to be recognized for presurgical therapy to be embraced.

Fourth, presurgical targeted therapy may have a role as a "litmus test" to identify a subset of patients with stable or responsive disease who will most benefit from cytoreductive nephrectomy [4]. Patients with rapidly progressive disease in the face of targeted therapy may not benefit from surgery. Rather than surgery, these patients with an aggressive phenotype would be selected for another systemic therapy [4]. At present, there is only limited data to support the "litmus test" concept. The long-term SWOG trial results demonstrate that disease progression within 90 days independently predicts worse OS (HR: 2.1, $p < 0.0001$) [152]. Additionally, there were six patients (12%) in the presurgical Bevacizumab trial who had progressive disease despite presurgical systemic therapy and did not go onto nephrectomy [100]. Despite being switched to alternative systemic therapies, none achieved disease stabilization or response, and it appears that they were spared unnecessary surgery.

The Supporting Evidence

The feasibility of presurgical targeted therapy has been demonstrated in case reports and retrospective series [99, 114, 119, 151, 153–157]. Additionally, the safety and efficacy of presurgical targeted agents have been addressed in several prospective single-arm studies [100, 101, 151, 158].

In the single-arm Phase II presurgical Bevacizumab (with or without Erlotinib) trial, outcomes appeared similar to postsurgical treatment with median PFS of 11.0 months and with median OS of 25.4 months. In 2011, results from two single-arm Phase II trials of presurgical Sunitinib in metastatic ccRCC were published by Powles et al., a total of 17 patients (33%) had MSKCC poor-risk disease [158]. The rest had intermediate-risk disease. Patients received two or three cycles of Sunitinib prior to nephrectomy. Median decrease in the primary was 12%. Cytoreductive nephrectomy was undertaken in 37 out of 53 (70%) patients. Patients with disease progression ($n = 9$) did not have surgery. In addition, surgery was not employed in some due to patient preference ($n = 3$) or being unfit for surgery ($n = 2$). It is important to note that no patients became ineligible for surgery due to local progression. At a median of 21 days after surgery, Sunitinib was resumed. Among the 27% rate of complications was a case of postoperative respiratory failure leading to death. The median PFS was 8 months (95% CI: 5–15).

The Southwest Oncology Group is currently conducting PROBE (SWOG 1931), a phase III study evaluating the role of combination immune checkpoint therapy prior to cytoreductive nephrectomy in metastatic RCC [159]. The trial began accrual in 2021 and is expected to be completed by 2033, with an estimated enrollment of 364 patients. Participants will be randomized 1:1 to receive either standard-of-care immunotherapy alone or immunotherapy combined with surgery. The study aims to assess OS, PFS, objective response, and changes in tumor diameter. The authors hypothesize that adding cytoreductive nephrectomy to immunotherapy will improve OS by reducing antigen spread and neoantigen load from the primary tumor, thereby enhancing the efficacy of immunotherapy. Beyond clinical outcomes, the trial will also investigate quality of life, tumor genomic testing, microbiome composition, radiomics, and ctDNA as potential predictive biomarkers.

Is Pre Surgical Therapy Safe?

One argument against pre surgical therapy is that it might adversely affect disease biology by increasing invasion, metastasis, and resistance [160–162]. Another concern is that wound healing could be impaired by presurgical therapy, leading a higher complication rate after cytoreductive nephrectomy [2]. Chapin et al. retrospectively evaluated cytoreductive nephrectomy patients at a single center from 2004 to 2010 [163]. Patients had received a variety of presurgical targeted agents such as bevacizumab, bevacizumab plus erlotinib, sunitinib, sorafenib, erlotinib, and temsirolimus. Clavien-Dindo complications within 1 year of surgery were assessed for patients who received presurgical systemic therapy ($n = 70$) and those who had immediate cytoreductive nephrectomy ($n = 103$). A total of 99 out of 173 (57%) patients had 232 complications. No increased risk of overall or severe complications (Grade 3 or higher) was noted on multivariable analysis. On the other hand, presurgical targeted therapy was associated with a higher rate of wound complications such as superficial wound dehiscence or infection (HR: 4.14, $p = 0.003$).

Determining the Proper Duration of Presurgical Therapy

The correct duration of presurgical therapy will likely be determined by factors including the particular drug and demonstrated response to therapy. Abel and colleagues retrospectively reviewed a single institution's experience with treating mRCC patients with Sunitinib without prior nephrectomy from 2004 to 2009 [95]. The median maximum change in the size of the primary tumor was −10.2%. The maximum size change was noted after a median of 120 days of therapy. Early tumor response was defined as a ≥10% decrease in size within 60 days. This independently predicted improved overall survival (HR: 0.26, $p = 0.031$). Since the maximal response in the primary tumor occurs in the first 2–4 months, some have logically concluded that three cycles of presurgical Sunitinib would be adequate [2, 97]. It is nevertheless important to consider that the correct duration of presurgical therapy ultimately may not be dictated by the radiographic response in the primary tumor.

Integration of Cytoreductive Nephrectomy and Systemic Therapy: Current Status

Clinical data should be used to select the patients most likely to benefit from extirpative surgery. Despite the fact that we have not prospectively demonstrated a survival benefit for cytoreductive nephrectomy in the modern era, it is likely to remain a component of the treatment paradigm for select patients, especially for those without poor-risk disease, pending the results of ongoing studies [82, 141, 142].

Conclusion

It will be essential to rationally integrate surgery and systemic therapy to improve outcomes in RCC. Adjuvant pembrolizumab has been demonstrated to improve DFS and OS in ccRCC at high risk of recurrence. Adjuvant tumor vaccines are a promising area of investigation. In selected cases of locally advanced disease, neoadjuvant therapy may make unresectable disease resectable, enable partial nephrectomy, or shrink venous tumor thrombus. For patients with metastatic RCC, the correct paradigm remains to be elucidated, but the role of cytoreductive nephrectomy in the immune checkpoint era is an area of active investigation. It is not a therapy that should be employed for all.

References

1. Kosary C. SEER cancer stat facts: kidney and renal pelvis cancer. Bethesda: National Cancer Institute; 2024.
2. Bex A, Jonasch E, Kirkali Z, et al. Integrating surgery with targeted therapies for renal cell carcinoma: current evidence and ongoing trials. Eur Urol. 2010;58:819.
3. Jacobsohn KM, Wood CG. Adjuvant therapy for renal cell carcinoma. Semin Oncol. 2006;33(5):576–82.
4. Wood CG. Multimodal approaches in the management of locally advanced and metastatic renal cell carcinoma: combining surgery and systemic therapies to improve patient outcome. Clin Cancer Res. 2007;13:697s.
5. Raj GV, Thompson RH, Leibovich BC, et al. Preoperative nomogram predicting 12-year probability of metastatic renal cancer. J Urol. 2008;179:2146.
6. Yaycioglu O, Roberts WW, Chan T, et al. Prognostic assessment of nonmetastatic renal cell carcinoma: a clinically based model. Urology. 2001;58:141.
7. Cindolo L, De La Taille A, Messina G, et al. A preoperative clinical prognostic model for non-metastatic renal cell carcinoma. BJU Int. 2003;92:901.
8. Smaldone MC, Fung C, Uzzo RG, et al. Adjuvant and neoadjuvant therapies in high-risk renal cell carcinoma. Hematol Oncol Clin North Am. 2011;25:765.
9. Lane BR, Kattan MW. Prognostic models and algorithms in renal cell carcinoma. Urol Clin N Am. 2008;35:613.
10. Cindolo L, Patard JJ, Chiodini P, et al. Comparison of predictive accuracy of four prognostic models for nonmetastatic renal cell carcinoma after nephrectomy: a multicenter European study. Cancer. 2005;104:1362.
11. Kattan MW, Reuter V, Motzer RJ, et al. A postoperative prognostic nomogram for renal cell carcinoma. J Urol. 2001;166:63.
12. Sorbellini M, Kattan MW, Snyder ME, et al. A postoperative prognostic nomogram predicting recurrence for patients with conventional clear cell renal cell carcinoma. J Urol. 2005;173:48.
13. Leibovich BC, Blute ML, Cheville JC, et al. Prediction of progression after radical nephrectomy for patients with clear cell renal cell carcinoma: a stratification tool for prospective clinical trials. Cancer. 2003;97:1663.
14. Zisman A, Pantuck AJ, Wieder J, et al. Risk group assessment and clinical outcome algorithm to predict the natural history of patients with surgically resected renal cell carcinoma. J Clin Oncol. 2002;20:4559.
15. Kenney PA, Wood CG. Integration of surgery and systemic therapy for renal cell carcinoma. Urol Clin. 2012;39:211.
16. Crispen PL, Boorjian SA, Lohse CM, et al. Predicting disease progression after nephrectomy for localized renal cell carcinoma: the utility of prognostic models and molecular biomarkers. Cancer. 2008;113:450.
17. Levy DA, Slaton JW, Swanson DA, et al. Stage specific guidelines for surveillance after radical nephrectomy for local renal cell carcinoma. J Urol. 1998;159:1163.
18. Klatte T, Lam JS, Shuch B, et al. Surveillance for renal cell carcinoma: why and how? When and how often? Urol Oncol. 2008;26(5):550–4.
19. Patard J-J, Kim HL, Lam JS, et al. Use of the University of California Los Angeles integrated staging system to predict survival in renal cell carcinoma: an international multicenter study. J Clin Oncol. 2004;22:3316.
20. Kim HL, Seligson D, Liu X, et al. Using protein expressions to predict survival in clear cell renal carcinoma. Clin Cancer Res. 2004;10:5464.
21. Klatte T, Seligson DB, LaRochelle J, et al. Molecular signatures of localized clear cell renal cell carcinoma to predict disease-free survival after nephrectomy. Cancer Epidemiol Biomarkers Prev. 2009;18:894.
22. Parker AS, Leibovich BC, Lohse CM, et al. Development and evaluation of BioScore: a biomarker panel to enhance prognostic algorithms for clear cell renal cell carcinoma. Cancer. 2009;115:2092.

23. Zhang KJ, Wilson GD, Kara S, et al. Diagnostic role of kidney injury molecule-1 in renal cell carcinoma. Int Urol Nephrol. 2019;51:1893.
24. Scelo G, Muller DC, Riboli E, et al. KIM-1 as a blood-based marker for early detection of kidney cancer: a prospective nested case-control study. Clin Cancer Res. 2018;24:5594.
25. Xu W, Puligandla M, Halbert B, et al. Plasma KIM-1 is associated with recurrence risk after nephrectomy for localized renal cell carcinoma: a trial of the ECOG-ACRIN Research Group (E2805). Clin Cancer Res. 2021;27:3397.
26. Kidess E, Jeffrey SS. Circulating tumor cells versus tumor-derived cell-free DNA: rivals or partners in cancer care in the era of single-cell analysis? Genome Med. 2013;5:70.
27. Esposito A, Bardelli A, Criscitiello C, et al. Monitoring tumor-derived cell-free DNA in patients with solid tumors: clinical perspectives and research opportunities. Cancer Treat Rev. 2014;40:648.
28. Jung M, Ellinger J, Gevensleben H, et al. Cell-free SHOX2 DNA methylation in blood as a molecular staging parameter for risk stratification in renal cell carcinoma patients: a prospective observational cohort study. Clin Chem. 2019;65:559.
29. Yamamoto Y, Uemura M, Fujita M, et al. Clinical significance of the mutational landscape and fragmentation of circulating tumor DNA in renal cell carcinoma. Cancer Sci. 2019;110:617.
30. Lin YL, Wang YP, Li HZ, et al. Aberrant promoter methylation of PCDH17 (Protocadherin 17) in serum and its clinical significance in renal cell carcinoma. Med Sci Monit. 2017;23:3318.
31. Choueiri M, Tannir N, Jonasch E. Adjuvant and neoadjuvant therapy in renal cell carcinoma. Curr Clin Pharmacol. 2011;6:144.
32. EAU Guidelines. Edn. Presented at the EAU Annual Congress Paris 2024. ISBN 978-94-92671-23-3.
33. Aref I, Bociek RG, Salhani D. Is postoperative radiation for renal cell carcinoma justified? Radiother Oncol. 1997;43:155.
34. Finney R. The value of radiotherapy in the treatment of hypernephroma – a clinical trial. Br J Urol. 1973;45:258.
35. Kjaer M, Iversen P, Hvidt V, et al. A randomized trial of postoperative radiotherapy versus observation in stage II and III renal adenocarcinoma: a study by the Copenhagen Renal Cancer Study Group. Scand J Urol Nephrol. 1987;21:285.
36. Hallemeier CL, Choo R, Davis BJ, et al. Long-term outcomes after maximal surgical resection and intraoperative electron radiotherapy for locoregionally recurrent or locoregionally advanced primary renal cell carcinoma. Int J Radiat Oncol Biol Phys. 2012;82:1938.
37. Ulutin HC, Aksu G, Fayda M, et al. The value of postoperative radiotherapy in renal cell carcinoma: a single-institution experience. Tumori J. 2006;92:202.
38. Lam JS, Belldegrun AS, Figlin RA. Adjuvant treatment for renal cell carcinoma. Expert Opin Pharmacother. 2006;7:705.
39. Pizzocaro G, Piva L, Di Fronzo G, et al. Adjuvant medroxyprogesterone acetate to radical nephrectomy in renal cancer: 5-year results of a prospective randomized study. J Urol. 1987;138:1379.
40. Naito S, Kumazawa J, Omoto T, et al. Postoperative UFT adjuvant and the risk factors for recurrence in renal cell carcinoma: A long-term follow-up study. Int J Urol. 1997;4:8.
41. Fujikawa K, Matsui Y, Miura K, et al. Serum immunosuppressive acidic protein and natural killer cell activity in patients with metastatic renal cell carcinoma before and after nephrectomy. J Urol. 2000;164:673.
42. Dadian G, Riches P, Henderson D, et al. Immunological parameters in peripheral blood of patients with renal cell carcinoma before and after nephrectomy. Br J Urol. 1994;74:15.
43. Montie JE, Straffon RA, Deodhar SD, et al. In vitro assessment of cell-mediated immunity in patients with renal cell carcinoma. J Urol. 1976;115:239.
44. Rayman P, Wesa AK, Richmond AL, et al. Effect of renal cell carcinomas on the development of type 1 T-cell responses. Clin Cancer Res. 2004;10:6360S.
45. Arya M, Chao D, Patel HR. Allogeneic hematopoietic stem-cell transplantation: the next generation of therapy for metastatic renal cell cancer. Nat Clin Pract Oncol. 2004;1:32.
46. McDermott DF, Regan MM, Clark JI, et al. Randomized phase III trial of high-dose interleukin-2 versus subcutaneous interleukin-2 and interferon in patients with metastatic renal cell carcinoma. J Clin Oncol. 2005;23:133.
47. Lam JS, Leppert JT, Belldegrun AS, et al. Novel approaches in the therapy of metastatic renal cell carcinoma. World J Urol. 2005;23:202.
48. Shimabukuro T, Naito K. Tumor-infiltrating lymphocytes derived from human renal cell carcinoma: clonal analysis of its characteristics. Int J Urol. 2008;15:241.
49. Kradin R, Lazarus D, Dubinett S, et al. Tumour-infiltrating lymphocytes and interleukin-2 in treatment of advanced cancer. Lancet. 1989;333:577.
50. Finke J, Tubbs R, Connelly B, et al. Tumor-infiltrating lymphocytes in patients with renal-cell carcinoma. Ann N Y Acad Sci. 1988;532:387.
51. Vogelzang NJ, Priest ER, Borden L. Spontaneous regression of histologically proved pulmonary metastases from renal cell carcinoma: a case with 5-year followup. J Urol. 1992;148:1247.
52. Sanchez-Ortiz RF, Tannir N, Ahrar K, et al. Spontaneous regression of pulmonary metastases from renal cell carcinoma after radio frequency ablation of primary tumor: in situ tumor vaccine? J Urol. 2003;170:178.
53. Collaborators MRCRC. Interferon-α and survival in metastatic renal carcinoma: early results of a randomised controlled trial. Lancet. 1999;353:14.

54. Pyrhönen S, Salminen E, Ruutu M, et al. Prospective randomized trial of interferon alfa-2a plus vinblastine versus vinblastine alone in patients with advanced renal cell cancer. J Clin Oncol. 1999;17:2859.
55. Fyfe G, Fisher RI, Rosenberg SA, et al. Results of treatment of 255 patients with metastatic renal cell carcinoma who received high-dose recombinant interleukin-2 therapy. J Clin Oncol. 1995;13:688.
56. Messing EM, Manola J, Wilding G, et al. Phase III study of interferon alfa-NL as adjuvant treatment for resectable renal cell carcinoma: an Eastern Cooperative Oncology Group/Intergroup trial. J Clin Oncol. 2003;21:1214.
57. Pizzocaro G, Piva L, Colavita M, et al. Interferon adjuvant to radical nephrectomy in Robson stages II and III renal cell carcinoma: a multicentric randomized study. J Clin Oncol. 2001;19:425.
58. Clark JI, Atkins MB, Urba WJ, et al. Adjuvant high-dose bolus interleukin-2 for patients with high-risk renal cell carcinoma: a cytokine working group randomized trial. J Clin Oncol. 2003;21:3133.
59. Atzpodien J, Schmitt E, Gertenbach U, et al. Adjuvant treatment with interleukin-2-and interferon-alpha 2a-based chemoimmunotherapy in renal cell carcinoma post tumour nephrectomy: results of a prospectively randomised trial of the German Cooperative Renal Carcinoma Chemoimmunotherapy Group (DGCIN). Br J Cancer. 2005;92:843.
60. Galligioni E, Quaia M, Merlo A, et al. Adjuvant immunotherapy treatment of renal carcinoma patients with autologous tumor cells and bacillus Calmette-Guerin: five-year results of a prospective randomized study. Cancer. 1996;77:2560.
61. Aitchison M, Bray C, Van Poppel H, et al. Adjuvant 5-fluorouracil, alpha-interferon and interleukin-2 versus observation in patients at high risk of recurrence after nephrectomy for renal cell carcinoma: results of a phase III randomised European Organisation for Research and Treatment of Cancer (Genito-Urinary Cancers Group)/National Cancer Research Institute trial. Eur J Cancer. 2014;50:70.
62. Choueiri TK, Tomczak P, Park SH, et al. Overall survival with adjuvant pembrolizumab in renal-cell carcinoma. N Engl J Med. 2024;390:1359.
63. Pal SK, Uzzo R, Karam JA, et al. Adjuvant atezolizumab versus placebo for patients with renal cell carcinoma at increased risk of recurrence following resection (IMmotion010): a multicentre, randomised, double-blind, phase 3 trial. Lancet. 2022;400:1103.
64. Motzer RJ, Russo P, Grünwald V, et al. Adjuvant nivolumab plus ipilimumab versus placebo for localised renal cell carcinoma after nephrectomy (CheckMate 914): a double-blind, randomised, phase 3 trial. Lancet. 2023;401:821.
65. Jocham D, Richter A, Hoffmann L, et al. Adjuvant autologous renal tumour cell vaccine and risk of tumour progression in patients with renal-cell carcinoma after radical nephrectomy: phase III, randomised controlled trial. Lancet. 2004;363:594.
66. Rassweiler J. Re: ten-year survival analysis for renal carcinoma patients treated with an autologous tumour lysate vaccine in an adjuvant setting. Eur Urol. 2012;61:219.
67. Doehn C, Richter A, Theodor R, et al. An adjuvant vaccination with Reniale® prolongs survival in patients with renal cell carcinoma following radical nephrectomy: secondary analysis of a multicentre phase-III trial. Eur Urol Suppl. 2006;2:286.
68. May M, Brookman-May S, Hoschke B, et al. Ten-year survival analysis for renal carcinoma patients treated with an autologous tumour lysate vaccine in an adjuvant setting. Cancer Immunol Immunother. 2010;59:687.
69. Wood C, Srivastava P, Bukowski R, et al. An adjuvant autologous therapeutic vaccine (HSPPC-96; vitespen) versus observation alone for patients at high risk of recurrence after nephrectomy for renal cell carcinoma: a multicentre, open-label, randomised phase III trial. Lancet. 2008;372:145.
70. Braun DA, Moranzoni G, Chea V, et al. A neoantigen vaccine generates antitumour immunity in renal cell carcinoma. Nature. 2025;639(8054):474–82.
71. Weber JS, Carlino MS, Khattak A, et al. Individualised neoantigen therapy mRNA-4157 (V940) plus pembrolizumab versus pembrolizumab monotherapy in resected melanoma (KEYNOTE-942): a randomised, phase 2b study. Lancet. 2024;403:632.
72. Choueiri TK, Powles T, Braun D, et al. 45 INTerpath-004: A phase 2, randomized, double-blind study of pembrolizumab with V940 (mRNA-4157) or placebo in the adjuvant treatment of renal cell carcinoma. Oncologist. 2024;29:S15.
73. Margulis V, Matin SF, Tannir N, et al. Randomized trial of adjuvant thalidomide versus observation in patients with completely resected high-risk renal cell carcinoma. Urology. 2009;73:337.
74. Daliani DD, Papandreou CN, Thall PF, et al. A pilot study of thalidomide in patients with progressive metastatic renal cell carcinoma. Cancer. 2002;95:758.
75. Belldegrun AS, Chamie K, Kloepfer P, et al. ARISER: A randomized double blind phase III study to evaluate adjuvant cG250 treatment versus placebo in patients with high-risk ccRCC—results and implications for adjuvant clinical trials. J Clin Oncol. 2013;31(15)
76. Ravaud A, Motzer RJ, Pandha HS, et al. Adjuvant sunitinib in high-risk renal-cell carcinoma after nephrectomy. N Engl J Med. 2016;375:2246.
77. Eisen T, Frangou E, Oza B, et al. Adjuvant sorafenib for renal cell carcinoma at intermediate or high risk of relapse: results from the SORCE randomized phase III intergroup trial. J Clin Oncol. 2020;38:4064.
78. Gross-Goupil M, Kwon TG, Eto M, et al. Axitinib versus placebo as an adjuvant treatment of renal cell carcinoma: results from the phase III, randomized ATLAS trial. Ann Oncol. 2018;29:2371.
79. Motzer RJ, Haas NB, Donskov F, et al. Randomized phase III trial of adjuvant pazopanib versus pla-

cebo after nephrectomy in patients with localized or locally advanced renal cell carcinoma. J Clin Oncol. 2017;35:3916.
80. Motzer RJ, Russo P, Haas N, et al. Adjuvant pazopanib versus placebo after nephrectomy in patients with localized or locally advanced renal cell carcinoma: final overall survival analysis of the phase 3 PROTECT trial. Eur Urol. 2021;79:334.
81. Chamie K, Donin NM, Klöpfer P, et al. Adjuvant weekly girentuximab following nephrectomy for high-risk renal cell carcinoma: the ARISER randomized clinical trial. JAMA Oncol. 2017;3:913.
82. Motzer RJ, Escudier B, Oudard S, et al. Efficacy of everolimus in advanced renal cell carcinoma: a double-blind, randomised, placebo-controlled phase III trial. Lancet. 2008;372:449.
83. Ryan CW, Tangen CM, Heath EI, et al. Adjuvant everolimus after surgery for renal cell carcinoma (EVEREST): a double-blind, placebo-controlled, randomised, phase 3 trial. Lancet. 2023;402:1043.
84. Brown JT. Adjuvant therapy for non–clear cell renal cell carcinoma—the ascent continues. JAMA Netw Open. 2024;7:e2425251.
85. Bex A, Horenblas S, Meinhardt W, et al. The role of initial immunotherapy as selection for nephrectomy in patients with metastatic renal cell carcinoma and the primary tumor in situ. Eur Urol. 2002;42:570.
86. Jonasch E, Tannir NM. Targeted therapy for locally advanced renal cell carcinoma. Target Oncol. 2010;5:113.
87. Kalman D, Varenhorst E. The role of arterial embolization in renal cell carcinoma. Scand J Urol Nephrol. 1999;33:162.
88. Mohr SJ, Whitesel JA. Spontaneous regression of renal cell carcinoma metastases after preoperative embolization of primary tumor and subsequent nephrectomy. Urology. 1979;14:5.
89. Swanson DA, Johnson DE, von Eschenbach AC, et al. Angio Infarction plus nephrectomy for metastatic renal cell carcinoma—an update. J Urol. 1983;130:449.
90. Bakke A, Göthlin JH, Haukaas SA, et al. Augmentation of natural killer cell activity after arterial embolization of renal carcinomas. Cancer Res. 1982;42:3880.
91. Nakano H, Nihira H, Toge T. Treatment of renal cancer patients by transcatheter embolization and its effects on lymphocyte proliferative responses. J Urol. 1983;130:24.
92. Johnson G, Kalland T. Enhancement of mouse natural killer cell activity after dearterialization of experimental renal tumors. J Urol. 1984;132:1250.
93. Zielinski H, Szmigielski S, Petrovich Z. Comparison of preoperative embolization followed by radical nephrectomy with radical nephrectomy alone for renal cell carcinoma. Am J Clin Oncol. 2000;23:6.
94. Allaf M, Kim S, Harshman L, et al. LBA67 phase III randomized study comparing perioperative nivolumab (nivo) versus observation in patients (pts) with renal cell carcinoma (RCC) undergoing nephrectomy (PROSPER, ECOG-ACRIN EA8143), a National Clinical Trials Network trial. Ann Oncol. 2022;33:S1432.
95. Abel EJ, Culp SH, Tannir NM, et al. Primary tumor response to targeted agents in patients with metastatic renal cell carcinoma. Eur Urol. 2011;59:10.
96. Robert G, Gabbay G, Bram R, et al. Complete histologic remission after sunitinib neoadjuvant therapy in T3b renal cell carcinoma. Eur Urol. 2009;55:1477.
97. Van der Veldt AA, Meijerink MR, van den Eertwegh AJ, et al. Sunitinib for treatment of advanced renal cell cancer: primary tumor response. Clin Cancer Res. 2008;14:2431.
98. Desar I, Van Herpen C, Van Laarhoven H, et al. Beyond RECIST: molecular and functional imaging techniques for evaluation of response to targeted therapy. Cancer Treat Rev. 2009;35:309.
99. Thomas AA, Rini BI, Lane BR, et al. Response of the primary tumor to neoadjuvant sunitinib in patients with advanced renal cell carcinoma. J Urol. 2009;181:518.
100. Jonasch E, Wood CG, Matin SF, et al. Phase II presurgical feasibility study of bevacizumab in untreated patients with metastatic renal cell carcinoma. J Clin Oncol. 2009;27:4076.
101. Cowey CL, Amin C, Pruthi RS, et al. Neoadjuvant clinical trial with sorafenib for patients with stage II or higher renal cell carcinoma. J Clin Oncol. 2010;28:1502.
102. Lebacle C, Bensalah K, Bernhard J-C, et al. Evaluation of axitinib to downstage cT2a renal tumours and allow partial nephrectomy: a phase II study. BJU Int. 2019;123:804.
103. de Velasco G, Carril-Ajuria L, Guerrero-Ramos F, et al. A case series of advanced renal cell carcinoma patients treated with neoadjuvant cabozantinib prior to cytoreductive nephrectomy within the phase 2 CABOPRE trial. Oncotarget. 2020;11:4457.
104. Bex A, Abu-Ghanem Y, Thienen JVV, et al. Efficacy, safety, and biomarker analysis of neoadjuvant avelumab/axitinib in patients (pts) with localized renal cell carcinoma (RCC) who are at high risk of relapse after nephrectomy (NeoAvAx). J Clin Oncol. 2022;40:289.
105. Ficarra V, Novara G. Neoadjuvant targeted therapies in renal cell carcinoma. Nat Rev Urol. 2010;7:63.
106. Rini BI, Garcia J, Elson P, et al. The effect of sunitinib on primary renal cell carcinoma and facilitation of subsequent surgery. J Urol. 2012;187:1548.
107. Lau WK, Blute ML, Weaver AL, et al. Matched comparison of radical nephrectomy vs nephron-sparing surgery in patients with unilateral renal cell carcinoma and a normal contralateral kidney. Mayo Clin Proc. 2000;75(12):1236–42.
108. McKiernan J, Simmons R, Katz J, et al. Natural history of chronic renal insufficiency after partial and radical nephrectomy. Urology. 2002;59:816.
109. Huang WC, Elkin EB, Levey AS, et al. Partial nephrectomy versus radical nephrectomy in patients with small renal tumors—is there a difference in

mortality and cardiovascular outcomes? J Urol. 2009;181:55.
110. Tan H-J, Norton EC, Ye Z, et al. Long-term survival following partial vs radical nephrectomy among older patients with early-stage kidney cancer. JAMA. 2012;307:1629.
111. Van Poppel H, Da Pozzo L, Albrecht W, et al. A prospective, randomised EORTC intergroup phase 3 study comparing the oncologic outcome of elective nephron-sparing surgery and radical nephrectomy for low-stage renal cell carcinoma. Eur Urol. 2011;59:543.
112. Hellenthal NJ, Underwood W, Penetrante R, et al. Prospective clinical trial of preoperative sunitinib in patients with renal cell carcinoma. J Urol. 2010;184:859.
113. Ansari J, Doherty A, McCafferty I, et al. Neoadjuvant sunitinib facilitates nephron-sparing surgery and avoids long-term dialysis in a patient with metachronous contralateral renal cell carcinoma. Clin Genitourin Cancer. 2009;7:E39.
114. Thomas AA, Rini BI, Stephenson AJ, et al. Surgical resection of renal cell carcinoma after targeted therapy. J Urol. 2009;182:881.
115. Silberstein JL, Millard F, Mehrazin R, et al. Feasibility and efficacy of neoadjuvant sunitinib before nephron-sparing surgery. BJU Int. 2010;106:1270.
116. Simmons MN, Ching CB, Samplaski MK, et al. Kidney tumor location measurement using the C index method. J Urol. 2010;183:1708.
117. Kutikov A, Uzzo RG. The RENAL nephrometry score: a comprehensive standardized system for quantitating renal tumor size, location and depth. J Urol. 2009;182:844.
118. Karakiewicz PI, Suardi N, Jeldres C, et al. Neoadjuvant sutent induction therapy may effectively down-stage renal cell carcinoma atrial thrombi. Eur Urol. 2008;53:845.
119. Harshman LC, Srinivas S, Kamaya A, et al. Laparoscopic radical nephrectomy after shrinkage of a caval tumor thrombus with sunitinib. Nat Rev Urol. 2009;6:338.
120. Bex A, Van der Veldt AA, Blank C, et al. Progression of a caval vein thrombus in two patients with primary renal cell carcinoma on pretreatment with sunitinib. Acta Oncol. 2010;49:520.
121. Cost NG, Delacroix SE Jr, Sleeper JP, et al. The impact of targeted molecular therapies on the level of renal cell carcinoma vena caval tumor thrombus. Eur Urol. 2011;59:912.
122. Stewart GD, Welsh SJ, Ursprung S, et al. A phase II study of neoadjuvant axitinib for reducing the extent of venous tumour thrombus in clear cell renal cell cancer with venous invasion (NAXIVA). Br J Cancer. 2022;127:1051.
123. Parikh M. Clinical trials corner: the dreaded IVC thrombus - optimizing management. Kidney Cancer. 2024;8:27.
124. Flanigan RC. Debulking nephrectomy in metastatic renal cancer. Clin Cancer Res. 2004;10:6335S.
125. Mani S, Todd MB, Katz K, et al. Prognostic factors for survival in patients with metastatic renal cancer treated with biological response modifiers. J Urol. 1995;154:35.
126. Fisher RI, Coltman CA Jr, Doroshow JH, et al. Metastatic renal cancer treated with interleukin-2 and lymphokine-activated killer cells: a phase II clinical trial. Ann Intern Med. 1988;108:518.
127. Muss HB, Costanzi J, Leavitt R, et al. Recombinant alfa interferon in renal cell carcinoma: a randomized trial of two routes of administration. J Clin Oncol. 1987;5:286.
128. Motzer RJ, Russo P. Systemic therapy for renal cell carcinoma. J Urol. 2000;163:408.
129. Motzer RJ, Mazumdar M, Bacik J, et al. Survival and prognostic stratification of 670 patients with advanced renal cell carcinoma. J Clin Oncol. 1999;17:2530.
130. Flanigan RC, Salmon SE, Blumenstein BA, et al. Nephrectomy followed by interferon alfa-2b compared with interferon alfa-2b alone for metastatic renal-cell cancer. N Engl J Med. 2001;345:1655.
131. Mickisch G, Garin A, van Poppel H, et al. Radical nephrectomy plus interferon-alfa-based immunotherapy compared with interferon alfa alone in metastatic renal-cell carcinoma: a randomised trial. Lancet. 2001;358:966.
132. Flanigan RC, Mickisch G, Sylvester R, et al. Cytoreductive nephrectomy in patients with metastatic renal cancer: a combined analysis. J Urol. 2004;171:1071.
133. Pantuck AJ, Zisman A, Dorey F, et al. Renal cell carcinoma with retroperitoneal lymph nodes: impact on survival and benefits of immunotherapy. Cancer. 2003;97:2995.
134. Vasselli JR, Yang JC, Linehan WM, et al. Lack of retroperitoneal lymphadenopathy predicts survival of patients with metastatic renal cell carcinoma. J Urol. 2001;166:68.
135. Han K-R, Pantuck AJ, Bui MH, et al. Number of metastatic sites rather than location dictates overall survival of patients with node-negative metastatic renal cell carcinoma. Urology. 2003;61:314.
136. Motzer RJ, Russo P. Cytoreductive nephrectomy—patient selection is key. N Engl J Med. 2018;379:481–2.
137. Manley BJ, Tennenbaum DM, Vertosick EA, et al. The difficulty in selecting patients for cytoreductive nephrectomy: an evaluation of previously described predictive models. Urol Oncol. 2017;35(1):35.e1–5.
138. Culp SH, Tannir NM, Abel EJ, et al. Can we better select patients with metastatic renal cell carcinoma for cytoreductive nephrectomy? Cancer. 2010;116:3378.
139. Hudes G, Carducci M, Tomczak P, et al. Temsirolimus, interferon alfa, or both for advanced renal-cell carcinoma. N Engl J Med. 2007;356:2271.

140. Motzer RJ, Hutson TE, Tomczak P, et al. Sunitinib versus interferon alfa in metastatic renal-cell carcinoma. N Engl J Med. 2007;356:115.
141. Escudier B, Eisen T, Stadler WM, et al. Sorafenib in advanced clear-cell renal-cell carcinoma. N Engl J Med. 2007;356:125.
142. Rini BI, Halabi S, Rosenberg JE, et al. Bevacizumab plus interferon alfa compared with interferon alfa monotherapy in patients with metastatic renal cell carcinoma: CALGB 90206. J Clin Oncol. 2008;26:5422.
143. Escudier B, Pluzanska A, Koralewski P, et al. Bevacizumab plus interferon alfa-2a for treatment of metastatic renal cell carcinoma: a randomised, double-blind phase III trial. Lancet. 2007;370:2103.
144. Szczylik C, Porta C, Bracarda S, et al. Sunitinib in patients with or without prior nephrectomy (Nx) in an expanded access trial of metastatic renal cell carcinoma (mRCC). J Clin Oncol. 2008;26:5124.
145. Choueiri TK, Xie W, Kollmannsberger C, et al. The impact of cytoreductive nephrectomy on survival of patients with metastatic renal cell carcinoma receiving vascular endothelial growth factor targeted therapy. J Urol. 2011;185:60.
146. Warren M, Venner PM, North S, et al. A population-based study examining the effect of tyrosine kinase inhibitors on survival in metastatic renal cell carcinoma in Alberta and the role of nephrectomy prior to treatment. Can Urol Assoc J. 2009;3:281.
147. Singer EA, Srinivasan R, Bratslavsky G. Editorial comment. The impact of cytoreductive nephrectomy on survival of patients with metastatic renal cell carcinoma receiving vascular endothelial growth factor targeted therapy. J Urol. 2011;185:66.
148. Méjean A, Ravaud A, Thezenas S, et al. Sunitinib alone or after nephrectomy in metastatic renal-cell carcinoma. N Engl J Med. 2018;379:417.
149. Bex A, Mulders P, Jewett M, et al. Comparison of immediate vs deferred cytoreductive nephrectomy in patients with synchronous metastatic renal cell carcinoma receiving sunitinib: the SURTIME randomized clinical trial. JAMA Oncol. 2019;5:164.
150. Margulis V, Wood CG. Cytoreductive nephrectomy in the era of targeted molecular agents: is it time to consider presurgical systemic therapy? Eur Urol. 2008;54:489.
151. Bex A, van der Veldt AA, Blank C, et al. Neoadjuvant sunitinib for surgically complex advanced renal cell cancer of doubtful resectability: initial experience with downsizing to reconsider cytoreductive surgery. World J Urol. 2009;27:533.
152. Lara PN Jr, Tangen CM, Conlon SJ, et al. Predictors of survival of advanced renal cell carcinoma: long-term results from Southwest Oncology Group Trial S8949. J Urol. 2009;181:512.
153. Faba OR, Breda A, Rosales A, et al. Neoadjuvant temsirolimus effectiveness in downstaging advanced non–clear cell renal cell carcinoma. Eur Urol. 2010;58:307.
154. Shuch B, Riggs SB, LaRochelle JC, et al. Neoadjuvant targeted therapy and advanced kidney cancer: observations and implications for a new treatment paradigm. BJU Int. 2008;102:692.
155. Amin C, Wallen E, Pruthi RS, et al. Preoperative tyrosine kinase inhibition as an adjunct to debulking nephrectomy. Urology. 2008;72:864.
156. Wood CG, Margulis V. Neoadjuvant (presurgical) therapy for renal cell carcinoma: a new treatment paradigm for locally advanced and metastatic disease. Cancer. 2009;115:2355.
157. Patard J-J, Thuret R, Raffi A, et al. Treatment with sunitinib enabled complete resection of massive lymphadenopathy not previously amenable to excision in a patient with renal cell carcinoma. Eur Urol. 2009;55:237.
158. Powles T, Kayani I, Blank C, et al. The safety and efficacy of sunitinib before planned nephrectomy in metastatic clear cell renal cancer. Ann Oncol. 2011;22:1041.
159. Bell H, Cotta BH, Salami SS, et al. "PROBE"ing the role of cytoreductive nephrectomy in advanced renal cancer. Kidney Cancer J. 2022;6:3.
160. Plimack ER, Tannir N, Lin E, et al. Patterns of disease progression in metastatic renal cell carcinoma patients treated with antivascular agents and interferon: impact of therapy on recurrence patterns and outcome measures. Cancer. 2009;115:1859.
161. Ebos JM, Lee CR, Cruz-Munoz W, et al. Accelerated metastasis after short-term treatment with a potent inhibitor of tumor angiogenesis. Cancer Cell. 2009;15:232.
162. Pàez-Ribes M, Allen E, Hudock J, et al. Antiangiogenic therapy elicits malignant progression of tumors to increased local invasion and distant metastasis. Cancer Cell. 2009;15:220.
163. Chapin BF, Delacroix SE Jr, Culp SH, et al. Safety of presurgical targeted therapy in the setting of metastatic renal cell carcinoma. Eur Urol. 2011;60:964.

CAR-T Therapy for Kidney Cancer

24

Jonathan Yeshwanth Daniel, Sheron Raja, S. Iswarya, V. Yohitha, Meenu Soorajj, Zulfiqur Ali, Alex Khariton, Merrel Holley, and Vinoth-Kumar Lakshmanan

Introduction

Kidney cancer is a relatively common rating itself among the top fourteen types of cancers. It is age-related, rare in younger individuals, typically presenting itself in the sixth and seventh decades of life, with a male predominance. Men are diagnosed with the disease with a lifetime risk of about 1 in 43 whereas the same for women being 1 in 73. The incidence increases with age, and several modifiable risk factors have been identified. The substantial variation in geographical distribution underscores the fact that kidney cancer remains a significant public health concern globally [1]. Kidney cancer includes several histological subtypes of which renal cell carcinoma (RCC) is attributed to over 90% of the observed cases [2]. The number of cases of RCC has shown steady increase, which can be presumably attributed to the exhaustive utilization of modern imaging techniques, namely ultrasound and computed tomography (CT), leading to earlier detection, which has also helped to decrease mortality [3]. In 2022, the global mortality rate from renal cell carcinoma (RCC) reached 179,368 deaths, with the ratio of men to women being 1.8:1, with an age-adjusted rate of nearly 2 per 100,000 individuals [4]. Risk factors include smoking, obesity, hypertension, and certain genetic predispositions such as mutations or loss of function in the VHL (Von Hippel-Lindau) gene, which is often implicated in sporadic and hereditary forms of clear cell RCC [2]. Evidence also suggests that chronic kidney disease (CKD) can lead to cancer. A reduced GFR despite age-related reduction clearly indicates the influence of CKD on cancer worsening the prognosis up to 27% [5]. The interplay of lifestyle choices, genetic predispositions, and environmental exposures continues to be investigated vigorously, highlighting the need for further studies to understand their causal relationships fully [6]. However, certain correlations can be made: for example, kidney cancer stands seventh in the USA, making its occurrence twice as that of the world average; a sizeable number of the patients diagnosed are Black Americans. This data can possibly be correlated with the increasing smoking habits and

J. Y. Daniel · S. Raja · S. Iswarya · V. Yohitha · M. Soorajj · V.-K. Lakshmanan (✉)
Prostate Cancer Biomarker Laboratory, Faculty of Clinical Research, Sri Ramachandra Institute of Higher Education & Research, Chennai, India
e-mail: u022401025@sriramachandra.edu.in; C2223003@sriher.edu.in; C2223004@sriher.edu.in; meenusfcr@sriramachandra.edu.in; vinoth.lakshmanan@sriramachandra.edu.in

Z. Ali
Teesside University, Middlesbrough, England, UK
e-mail: z.ali@tees.ac.uk

A. Khariton
Sidney Kimmel Comprehensive Cancer Center, Philadelphia, PA, USA
e-mail: alex.khariton@jefferson.edu

M. Holley
International Hyperbaric Medical Foundation, Morgan City, LA, USA

J. A. Libertino, J. R. Gee (eds.), *Renal Cancer*, https://doi.org/10.1007/978-3-031-97599-8_24

obesity within the country. Interestingly, recent study of multi-ancestry GWAS meta-analysis represents an important avenue in understanding the genetic underpinnings of kidney cancer, particularly RCC subtypes, and lays the groundwork for future functional studies and potential clinical applications [7].

Renal Cell Carcinoma

Renal cell carcinoma is a series of malignancies that originate from the tubular epithelial cells. Renal cancer predominantly affects people in Europe and North America, with the lowest rates seen in Asia. The geographic differences in prevalence and mortality rates highlight the influence of genetic, environmental, and social factors on incidence progression and prognosis. Understanding these local differences is key to tailoring preventive and therapeutic strategies to effectively combat renal cancer worldwide. This heterogeneity in RCC reflects different genetic and molecular mechanisms involved in its development and progression. As these cancers originate from the tubular epithelium of the kidney, they present with a wide range of clinical behaviors, making diagnosis and treatment difficult. Understanding the diverse characteristics of RCC is critical for developing targeted therapies and improving patient outcomes [2]. The most important risk factors for renal cell carcinoma (RCC) are age and sex. Other notable predisposing factors are location, race, smoking history, tobacco use, hypertension, and obesity. Interestingly, recent research suggests that obese patients with RCC may have better chances of improvement, challenging the conventional view that obesity is a risk factor for RCC constitutes necessity highlighting the need for further research. Other less prominent risk factors that may be associated with RCC include chronic kidney disease, acquisition of renal cystic disease, end-stage renal disease, long-term use of palliative medications, conditions such as cadmium and trichlorethylene exposure, red and processed meat consumption, viral hepatitis, vitamin D levels, type 2 diabetes, elevated triglycerides, lack of physical activity, and

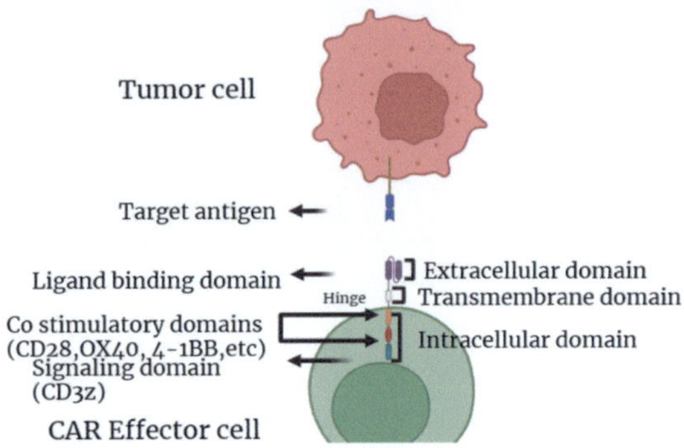

Fig. 24.1 Evolution of CAR-T therapy for renal cell carcinoma

genetics certain diseases. Mutations or epigenetic silencing of the Von-Hippel Landau (VHL) gene, a critical tumor suppressor, is associated with the most common subtype of RCC, which is clear cell renal cell carcinoma (ccRCC). Loss of heterozygosity caused by somatic mutations accounts for ~50–60% of cases of sporadic RCC, with ~20% of cases attributed to gene silencing caused by VHL promoter hypermethylation caused by exogenous chemical exposures. Biallelic VHL inactivation accounts for ~90% of sporadic cases of ccRCC, driving aggressive tumor development by runaway activation of Hypoxia-Inducible Factor (HIF). Understanding the complex interplay of these factors is critical to improving RCC prevention, diagnosis, and therapeutic strategies [8, 9]. Localized RCC is usually treated with surgery, comprising partial or radical nephrectomy, depending on the size and location of the tumor. Systemic therapies, especially checkpoint blockade therapies (such as nivolumab and pembrolizumab) and tyrosine kinase inhibitors (like sunitinib or pazopanib), that target critical signaling pathways in tumor growth and angiogenesis would be used against metastatic RCC [10] (Fig. 24.1).

The CAR consists of an extracellular hinge region linked to a transmembrane region and the intracellular co-stimulatory domain [e.g., CD28] and stimulatory domains [CD3Z]. The CAR can be expressed in different immune cells [e.g., T cells, NK cells] and recognize specific tumor antigens independently to MHC presentation. The above figure was created with the Biorender app.

Chimeric Antigen Receptor

Chimeric antigen receptors (CARs) are bioengineering marvels that are articulated to redirect the specificity of immune cells, particularly T lymphocytes, in the direction of target cells, often utilized in cancer immunotherapy [11]. CARs are fusion molecules generally composed of numerous elements: an extracellular single chain variable fragment (scFv) derived from a monoclonal antibody (mAb) targeting a surface molecule on the tumor cell, a spacer domain for flexibility and improving interplay between T cells and target cells, a transmembrane area, and signaling modules that prompt T cellular features [12]. The modular structure of CARs make it possible to improvise on its efficiency, making way for its evolution over several generations. The first generation CAR simply consisted of the scFv bound to CD3ζ intracellular domain which lacked persistence and proliferation [13]. This model failed to raise sufficient cytokine response ergo resulting in poor treatment outcomes. In order to successfully activate CAR-T cells, the participation of three receptors namely, T-cell antigen receptor, cytokine receptor and co-stimulatory receptor are essential. An antigen presenting cell interacting with a T-cell triggers an initial signal followed by a secondary signal, promoting IL-2. Only under the condition of this secondary co-stimulatory signal would the activation be complete. Thus, a second generation of CARs were introduced, incorporating a co-stimulatory component such as CD-28 [14]. Third gen CARs included more such domains but have not shown much promise in comparison to the second [15]. The latest generation of CARs are the "T cell redirected for universal cytokine-mediated killing (TRUCKs)." They are engineered to deploy the transgenic product to the tumor region. The inclusion of a nuclear factor of activated T cells (NFAT)-responsive expression cassette, enabling the inducible expression of a transgenic cytokine like interleukin-12, makes this achievable. CD3ζ signaling upon activation orders the induction of the NFAT, which in turn leads to the production of IL-12. This mass-recruits immune cells, which might help eliminate cancerous cells that may have not been recognized by the CAR-T cells as well [16]. Researchers have investigated various methods of gene switch and one-of-a-kind forms of effector cells for CAR remedy. While a few CAR options have shown clear benefits in sure cases, figuring out the suitable CAR design stays an assignment. There's no set guiding principle for making those selections, as the ultimate parameters vary depending on the specific case. CAR layout studies have performed an essential function in advancing CAR treatment options into clinical trials globally, however the journey towards optimization is ongoing [17]. Chimeric antigen receptors (CARs) have shown noticeable outcomes in scientific trials, highlighting the promise of novel immune-priming based approaches to the remedy of most cancers [18]. The US Food and Drug Administration has permitted chimeric antigen receptor (CAR) T-cell cures. To maintain development in this field, it is important to broaden new CAR designs. These designs may additionally include extraordinary antigen-binding domains, together with antigen-ligand binding companions and variable lymphocyte receptors. Another latest innovation in CAR layout includes integrating Boolean logic gates, which can potentially reduce the dangers of on-target, off-tumor toxicities. Recent research specializing in optimizing costimulatory signaling has additionally found out how CAR layout affects capability. By utilizing particular signaling pathways and transcription factors, CARs can have an impact on T-cell gene expression to enhance their effectiveness. Employing those techniques holds the promise of absolutely understanding the utility of CAR-T cellular treatment options for treating strong tumors [19] (Fig. 24.2).

Blood is collected from the patient diagnosed with renal cell carcinoma (1). The T cells that protect against infections are separated. The blood is directed into an apheresis machine, which removes T lymphocytes (2). Reprogramming the collected cells into CAR-T cells in the laboratory (3). Engineering and genetic alteration of T cells to have a chimeric antigen receptor (4). Numerous CAR-T cells

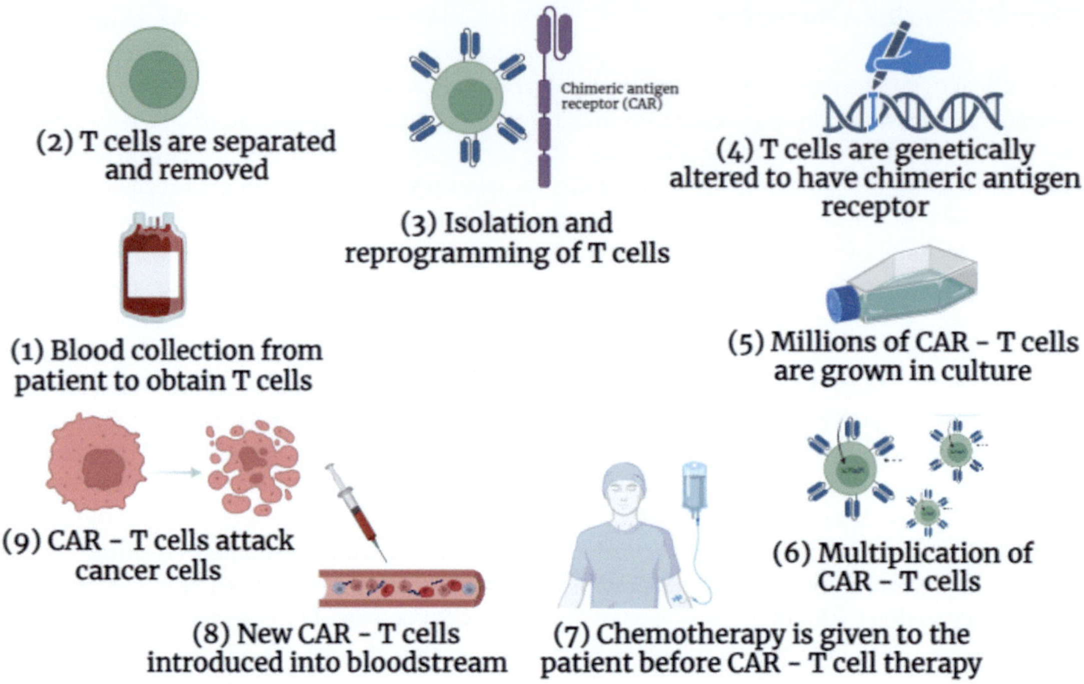

Fig. 24.2 CAR-T cell therapy

are grown in culture (5). The CAR-T cells grow and multiply until there are enough cells to target the cancer cells effectively (6). The patient must undergo chemotherapy prior to the introduction of CAR-T cells (7). Introducing the CAR-T cells into the bloodstream of the patient (8). Once in the bloodstream, these cells will be capable of detecting and destroying cancerous cells (9). The above figure was created with the Biorender app.

CAR-T Cell

The technology revolving around chimeric antigen receptors (CARs) empowers us to create T-cells which are able to target a wide range of protein structures located on numerous cells. By genetically editing T-cells to a specific CAR, we equip them with the potential to understand precise antigens on most cancer cells. Subsequently, these CAR-T cells can discern cancerous cells and proceed to get rid of them from the body. It's vital that the target antigen on tumors are particularly specific, as their presence in healthy tissues ought to trigger intense detrimental reactions, doubtlessly resulting in undesirable cell death. Therefore, meticulous attention is given to deciding on antigens for CAR-T-cellular remedy to decrease off-target. Outcomes and making sure of the safeness and efficacy of the treatment [20]. CAR-T cells are sourced from the affected person's own cells, ensuring that they are autologous and thereby keeping off complications related to allogeneic rejection or graft-as opposed to-host disease (GvHD). However, this personalized method necessitates tailor-made manufacturing for each patient, which can be difficult and useful resource-in depth. It is worth noting that CARs incorporate overseas sequences that can probably cause rejection by the patient's immune machinery. To deal with this issue, fludarabine, an antimetabolite, is blanketed within the preparative chemotherapy regimen. This serves to induce lymphodepletion, creating an environment conducive for the CAR-T cells to proliferate and function optimally. Thus, while there remains a risk of rejection, using fludarabine helps to mitigate this possibility to some extent [21]. However, determining the ideal CAR-T cell remains a subject of debate within the area. A complicating component in clinical trial is the variety among CAR-T-cell products, as each is customized from the T cells of a patient. Analysis of medical facts has revealed that fine responses are associated with the proliferation, sturdiness, and reminiscence-like traits of CAR-T cells. Therefore, the number one goal is to save or put off the exhaustion of T cells, which is taken into consideration as essential for reaching healing efficacy. This involves techniques designed to preserve the activity and characteristics of CAR-T cells through the years, relentlessly improving their effectiveness in treating the focused circumstance [22]. In 2011, a pivotal medical trial performed by Carl June's research group marked a large milestone in CAR-T cell remedy. They focused on treating chronic lymphocytic leukemia (CLL) by using a CAR specially designed in opposition to the B-cellular antigen CD19. Remarkably, in three patients, the infused CAR-T-cells underwent an exceptional enlargement of 1000-fold post-transfusion. This robust enlargement facilitated the eradication of lymphoma cells, leading to complete and sustained remission of the disorder. Since then, CAR-T-cellular-based technology have made superb strides, with the primary therapeutic merchandise making their way into clinical exercise. Among these, Kymriah (evolved by way of Novartis) and Yescarta (advanced by means of Gilead-Kite Pharma) have garnered approval from the FDA for the remedy of B-cell-related malignancies. Notably, each Kymriah and Yescarta target CD19, underscoring the efficacy of this approach in fighting B-cell malignancies. While CAR-T cell therapy has verified outstanding achievement in treating hematological oncogenic illnesses, specifically B-cellular malignancies, it is critical to acknowledge undesired outcomes in parallel. Notably, the remedy may set off B-cellular aplasia because of the focus on the healthy B-cells along with the malignant ones. However, this situation is clinically practicable, highlighting the overall therapeutic promise of remedy in combating most cancers [23, 24].

CAR-T and Cancer

Currently, the adoption of immune cells is a very assuring strategy for the treatment of cancer and the results in clinical trials have motivated the pharmaceutical industry to invest in cancer treatment. Because modified CAR-T is derived from the immune system, it is highly effective against hematologic malignancies. It achieved success in the treatment of some blood cancers, namely acute lymphoblastic leukemia (ALL), chronic lymphocytic leukemia (CLL), and non-Hodgkin lymphoma (NHL). In this therapy, T cells isolated from patients are genetically manipulated to express chimeric antigen receptors (CARs), which are designed to specifically target cancer proteins like CD19 or CD20. These modified T cells are then reintroduced into the patient's body, where they recognize and destroy the cancer cells [25]. However, alongside its curative potential, the therapy frequently brings about substantial toxic effects. These unfavorable reactions can consist of cytokine release syndrome, neurotoxicity, tumor lysis syndrome, and numerous other toxicities. Unfortunately, these toxicities have grown to be a barrier to the improvement of CAR-T cell therapy. Moreover, no matter its promising effects, the overall healing effectiveness of CAR-T cell remedy is restricted by way of high rates of relapse. Additionally, the implementation of this treatment is obstructed by arduous production process and its high cost. These factors contribute to the challenges in realizing the full potential of CAR-T cell therapy in clinical settings. In precise, while CAR-T cell therapy gives sizeable advantages in treating hematological malignancies, its efficacy is regularly offset by using the occurrence of toxic secondary effects and high fees of relapse. Further progress in this field is hampered by way of the complexities of manufacturing and the associated financial burden, restricting its broader adoption and effect in scientific practice [26].

Solid Tumors

Immunotherapy with CAR-T cells has achieved tremendous successes in the treatment of hematological malignancies. However, due to intricacies of solid tumors and their sites of occurrence, treatment of non-hematologic malignant masses with CAR-T cells is facing multiple obstacles, such as the hostile tumor microenvironment, on-tumor/off-tumor toxicities, and undesired antigen specificity. Many approaches have been attempted to triumph over these obstacles, including arming CAR-T cells with knock-out of PD-1 expression or secretion of cytokines/chemokines and using CAR-T cells in combination with other treatments. CAR-T therapy, famous for its victories against blood cancers, faces formidable obstacles when applied to solid tumors. These tumors exhibit a complexity not present in blood cancers, presenting challenges at every step of the treatment process. One of the main obstacles is the heterogeneity of solid tumors, which contain cell populations with different characteristics. Identifying a uniform target antigen expressed in all tumor cells has proven difficult. Furthermore, the hostile microenvironment surrounding solid tumors promotes immunosuppression, inhibiting CAR-T cell activity, promoting tumor growth. Factors such as hypoxia and immune checkpoint molecules contribute to this inhibition. In addition, solid tumors often lack sufficient T cell infiltration, which is essential for CAR-T action. Strategies aimed at enhancing T cell infiltration are under intense investigation to strengthen therapeutic outcomes. Despite advances, extra-tumor toxicity remains a concern, as healthy tissues carrying the same antigens may become unintentional targets of CAR-T cells, leading to unintended consequences. Nevertheless, researchers are exploring different strategies to overcome these barriers. Novel antigen discovery, combination therapies with conventional treatments or checkpoint blockade therapies, and engineering CAR-T cells with augmented functionalities are among the avenues being explored. Furthermore, local delivery methods hold promise for improving CAR-T accumulation within tumors while minimizing systemic toxicity. While the road ahead is challenging, ongoing research efforts offer hope for harnessing its full potential in fighting solid tumors [27]. CAR-T cells function by recognizing specific cell surface epitopes through single-chain variable fragment (scFv) systems, which typically consist of both light-chain and heavy-chain. This knowledge occurs in a non-MHC (major histocompatibility complex) limited manner. For example, CD19 (a membrane protein) is well expressed on nearly all B cells, making it an important target for CAR-T therapy in B-cell hematologic malignancies, which generally share the same structural characteristics. As a result, many patients with B-cell malignancies have experienced dramatic clinical outcomes following CD19 CAR-T cell therapy. However, its employment in the treatment of solid tumors faces severe limitations due to the heterogeneity of these tumors, the rarity of tumor-specific antibodies, and low immunogenicity because of its resistance to disease. In the case of solid tumors, several factors hamper the impact of CAR-T cell therapy. First of all, solid tumors exhibit a high degree of heterogeneity, composed of diverse cell types with different molecular compositions. These differences make it difficult to identify appropriate tumor antigens that are consistently expressed in all aberrant cells, hindering effectiveness of CAR-T cell therapy. In addition, solid tumors often lack specific antigens that these cells can identify, limiting the therapeutic potential of this approach. Furthermore, the immunosuppressive microenvironment surrounding solid tumors creates a hostile environment that inhibits CAR-T function, leading to tumor immune evasion and migration. Despite these challenges, efforts are being made to overcome the limitations of CAR-T cell therapy in the treatment of solid tumors. Various strategies aimed at narrowing specificity thereby enhancing potency of CAR-T cells are being ventured, such as the discovery of novel target antigens unique to solid tumors and engineering CAR-T cells with the advanced function. In addition, strategies to combine CAR-T therapy with other therapeutic strategies, such as immunosuppressive agents or targeted therapies, hold promise for improving treatment efficacy. By addressing these limiting factors and implementing novel resistance strategies, researchers aim to unlock the potential of CAR-T cell therapy in the fight against solid tumors [28, 29].

CART in RCC

Chimeric antigen receptor (CAR) T-cells show striking advances in immunotherapy for RCC and may lead to higher survival rates of long-term disease. For successful use of this therapy, it is important to identify the most appropriate tumor antigens and optimize T cell manipulation. Success will also depend on achieving remission while maintaining acceptable toxicity profiles, and ensuring overall efficacy and safety in patients. Despite the high levels of carbonic anhydrase IX (CA IX) in malignant RCC tissues, targeting this antigen resulted in significant toxicity to the hepatobiliary system at the target, non-tumor, and led to early termination of the clinical trials. Another attempted target is the vascular endothelial growth factor (VEGF) receptor.

Many RCC tumors exhibit mutations in the Von Hippel-Lindau gene, producing VEGF, a pathway essential for RCC survival is more than obvious. The success of small molecule inhibitors targeting this pathway provides a rationale for CAR-T-cell therapy against VEGFR2. However, this particular clinical trial (NCT01218867) was discontinued due to a lack of objective treatment response in patients [30, 31]. The underlying causes of early failure in CAR-T-cell therapy for renal cell carcinoma (RCC) remain unclear. Insights from studies of hematologic malignancies and other solid tumors suggest possible mechanisms. One such mechanism involves loss or downregulation of the target tumor antigen, known as "antigen escape." For example, in patients with refractory acute lymphoblastic leukemia (ALL) treated with CD19-targeting CAR-T cells, 70–90% initially showed durable responses. However, approximately 30–70% subsequently experienced disease relapse due to CD19 depletion or loss, suggesting antigen escape. This phenomenon has also been observed in multiple myeloma and glioblastoma [32–35]. Another factor limiting the efficacy of CAR-T-cell therapy for RCC is the immunosuppressive tumor microenvironment (TME). Unlike malignant hematologic malignancies, solid tumors typically have a limited endothelial T-cell infiltrate and an immunosuppressive environment in which T (Treg) cells contain regulators, myeloid-derived suppressor cells (MDSCs), and an immunomodulatory ligand such as PD-L1. Studies have shown that RCC tumors tend to have high numbers of Treg cells and MDSCs, which may suppress CAR-T-cell function. Physical and stromal barriers also play a role in limiting the efficacy of CAR-T-cell therapy. One such barrier is heparan sulfate proteoglycan (HSPG), which prevents trafficking of cells to the tumor. CAR-T cells engineered to express heparinase can disrupt the HSPG barrier, allowing tumor invasion and antitumor activity. Furthermore, many solid tumors, including RCC, have a hypoxic TME that negatively affects the survival of effector T-cells and immune cells. Hypoxia promotes ATP degradation, leading to adenosine accumulation, and interferes with TCR signaling by targeting A2AR and A2BR receptors on T cells, thus inhibiting their antitumor activity. In conclusion, the initial barriers to CAR-T-cell therapy for RCC can be attributed to several factors, including antigen escape, TME immunosuppression, and physiology of the tumor barriers. Overcoming these challenges requires novel strategies, such as the development of CAR-T-cells to disrupt stromal barriers and counteract immunosuppressive signals, to activate CAR-T-cell therapy effective in the treatment of RCC and other solid tumors [36, 37] (Fig. 24.3).

Collection of Blood from the patient diagnosed with renal cell carcinoma (1). Leukapheresis is a procedure to remove white blood cells from the blood sample (2). Insertion of CAR T gene through viral vectors such as Gamma-retroviruses and Lentiviruses (3). Amplification of cells with the incorporated CAR-T gene in culture (4). Administering the modified T cells expressing CARs into the bloodstream of the patient (5). Once in bloodstream, CAR-T receptor detects

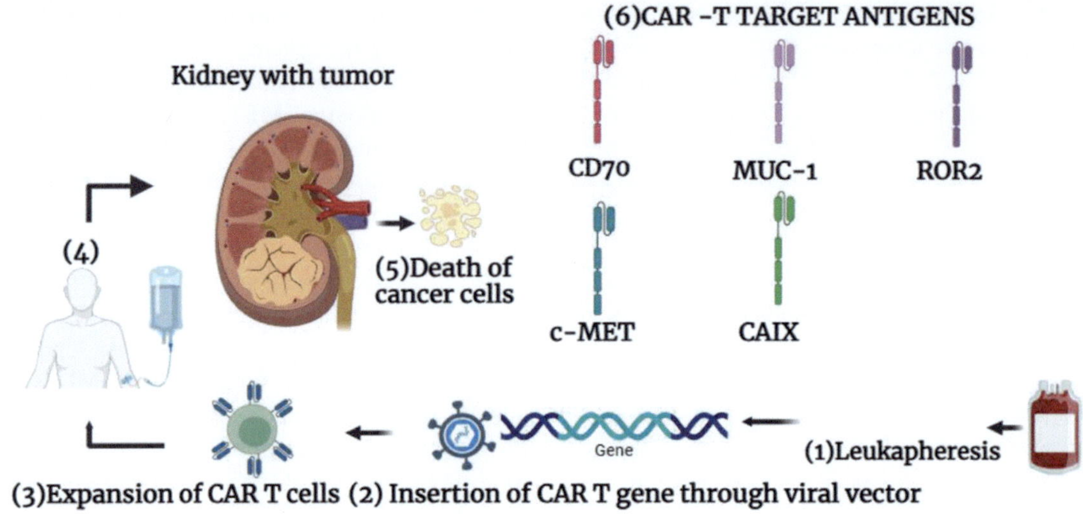

Fig. 24.3 CAR-T cell therapy for renal cell carcinoma

and destroys the tumor cells in the kidney (6). Target antigens: CD70—Cluster of differentiation 70, MUC-1—Mucin 1, ROR2—receptor tyrosine kinase-like orphan receptor 2, C-MET—mesenchymal epithelial transition factor, CAIX—carbonic anhydrase IX. The above figure was created with the Biorender app.

The Synergistic Potential of CAR-T with Radiotherapy

The search for a combination of chemo and radiation therapies has long been the focus of specialized research, with several studies suggesting its potential efficacy in a variety of cancers, including renal cell carcinoma (RCC) [38, 39]. This combined approach uses the strengths of both treatments to maximize overall treatment effects. The reason behind this combination is based on the overlapping mechanisms by which the immune system can improve the body's innate responses against cancer cells, and radiation therapy may directly contribute to tumor volume reduction and alter tumor microenvironment to be more flexible to immune penetration. Recently, the advancement of CAR-T therapy in solid tumors has boosted interest in its addition in radiation therapy. It is suggested that radiation therapy enhances CAR-T cell therapy by inducing cancer cell immunosuppression, thereby inducing CAR-T cell chemotaxis towards the tumor. This collaboration is believed to occur when radiation therapy can expose tumor antigens to the surface of cancer cells, resulting in increased recognition and targeting by CAR-T cells. Furthermore, γ-radiation, which is a specific form of radiation therapy, has been shown to increase CAR-T cell susceptibility by stimulating interferon-gamma (IFN-γ) from cancer cells. The secretion of IFN-γ is critical because it allows immune cells to penetrate the tumor microenvironment and modulate the tumor histology, thereby improving lymphocyte infiltration. Despite a promising theoretical framework, empirical data on the specificity of combining radiotherapy with CAR-T cell therapy in RCC are scarce. Initial results are encouraging, providing a strong rationale for this combined approach. The ability of radiation therapy to alter the tumor microenvironment and activate the immune system is a challenging issue that requires further investigation [40–42]. Consequently, more research is required to comprehend the overall potential and optimize the strategies of this combination therapy in RCC, aiming to move patient outcomes effective with a combination of new therapeutic strategies.

CAR-T Cell Therapy: Current Trials in RCC

Several active clinical trials are exploring the safety, tolerability, and efficacy of CAR-T cell therapy in individuals diagnosed with advanced and metastatic renal cell carcinoma (RCC). These studies investigate combinations of molecular targets and therapies to enhance outcomes for patients with relapsed or refractory stage IV mRCC. One separate phase II, two-arm, open-label clinical trial (NCT03393936) is investigating autologous CAR-T cells, specifically CCT 301-38 and CCT 301-59, in patients with relapse or stage failure IV in mRCC patients. This study targets receptor tyrosine kinase-like orphan receptor 2 (ROR2) with CCT301-59 and AXL-positive biopsies with CCT301-38 [43, 44]. Radiation therapy is used to induce cancer antigenicity, enhancing CAR-T cell chemotaxis, and making the tumor microenvironment more sensitive to immune function. Other trials included a randomized phase I/II study (NCT01218867) that evaluated a retrovirus engineered to target anti-VEGF receptor 2 in mRCC patients, but was discontinued due to no observed response. Another phase I/II trial (NCT02830724) is evaluating CAR-T cells treated with anti-hCD70, targeting CD70 expression, which is associated with poor survival in RCC patients [45–47] (Table 24.1). In addition, a single-arm, open-label phase I study (NCT04438083) is investigating CRISPR-Cas9 engineered CAR-T cells (CTX 130) targeting CD70 in advanced, relapsed ccRCC patients who have not been, or cannot be saved. Similarly, another phase I/II trial (NCT03638206) is testing

Table 24.1 Notable clinical trials in treatment of renal cell carcinoma with CAR-T Therapy

Serial number	NCI TRIAL ID	STUDY TITLE	Clinical phase	RCC stage	Type of CAR-T cell	Study start
1.	NCT03393936 [52]	Safety and efficacy of CCT301 CART in adult subjects with recurrent or refractory stage IV RCC	I/II	Recurrent or refractory stage IV RCC	CCT301-59 CCT301-28	26-03-2018
2.	NCT01218867 [53]	CAR-T cell receptor immunotherapy targeting VEGFR2 for patients with metastatic cancer	I/II	Metastatic RCC	Anti-VEGFR2 CAR-T cell	10-11-2010
3.	NCT02830724 [54]	Administering peripheral blood lymphocytes transduced with a CD70 binding chimeric antigen receptor to people with CD70 expressing cancers	I/II	RCC	Anti-HCD70CAR-T CELL	06-04-2017
4.	NCT04438083 [55]	COBALT-RCC	I	Relapsed or refractory RCC	CTX130	16-06-2020
5.	NCT03638206 [56]	Autologous CAR-T/TCR-T cell immunotherapy for malignancies	I/II	RCC	CAR-T cell/ TCR-T cell	01-03-2018
6.	NCT04969354 [57]	The clinical study of CAIX-targeted CAR-T cells in the treatment of advanced renal cell carcinoma	I	Advanced RCC	Allogenic CAR-T cell	01-10-2021
7.	NCT06010875 [58]	A clinical research about CD-70 targeted CAR-T in the treatment of CD70-positive advanced/ metastatic solid tumors	I	Metastatic RCC	CD70 CAR-T cells	30-11-2023
8.	NCT05420519 [59]	Clinical study of CD70-targeted CAR-T therapy for advanced/ advanced renal cancer	I	Advanced RCC	CD70 CAR-T cells	31-12-2021

(continued)

Table 24.1 (continued)

Serial number	NCI TRIAL ID	STUDY TITLE	Clinical phase	RCC stage	Type of CAR-T cell	Study start
9.	NCT05239143 [60]	P-MUC1C-ALLO1 allogeneic CAR-T cells in the treatment of subjects with advanced or metastatic solid tumors	I	Metastatic RCC	P-MUC1C-ALLO1 CAR-T cells	15-02-2022
10.	NCT04696731 [61]	Safety and efficacy of ALLO-316 in subjects with advanced or metastatic clear cell renal cell carcinoma (TRAVERSE)	I	Advanced RCC	ALLO-316	24-02-2021
11.	NCT06480565 [62]	A phase 1/2 trial of ADI-270 in ccRCC	I/II	Relapsed or refractory RCC	ADI-270	09-2024
12.	NCT05518253 [63]	A clinical study of CD70-targeted CAR-T in the treatment of CD70-positive advanced/ metastatic solid tumors	I	Advanced RCC	CD70 CAR-T cells	30-05-2022
13.	NCT05420545 [64]	A clinical study of CD70-targeted CAR-T in the treatment of CD70-positive advanced/ metastatic solid tumors	I	Advanced RCC	CD70 CAR-T cells	31-12-2021

1. NCT03393936: This clinical study is a two-arm, open-label, dose escalation and dose expansion trial designed to evaluate the safety and efficacy of autologous CAR-T cell therapies, specifically CCT301–38 and CCT301–59, in adult patients with relapsed and refractory stage IV metastatic renal cell carcinoma (m RCC). **2. NCT01218867:** In this clinical study, patient's white blood cells were modified with a retrovirus that has the gene for anti-vascular endothelial growth factor receptor (VEGFR2) incorporated in the retrovirus. **3. NCT02830724:** Researchers are exploring a new cancer therapy that involves gene transfer using anti-CD70-modified white blood cells. This approach aims to harness the body's immune system to target and shrink tumors safely. **4. NCT04438083:** The Phase 1 study evaluating CTX130, an allogeneic CAR-T-cell therapy targeting CD70, in patients with relapsed or refractory clear cell renal cell carcinoma (ccRCC) has shown promising results regarding safety and efficacy. This multicenter, open-label trial, known as COBALT-RCC, included patients who had previously undergone treatment with checkpoint inhibitors (CPIs) and tyrosine kinase inhibitors (TKIs). **5. NCT03638206:** This study is designed to assess the safety and effectiveness of chimeric antigen receptor T-cell (CAR-T) and T-cell receptor T-cell (TCR-T) immunotherapy in patients with various malignancies. As a single-arm, open-label, uni-center, phase I-II trial, it aims to provide crucial insights into how these innovative therapies can be utilized in the treatment of cancer. **6. NCT04969354:** This is an experimental study to evaluate the safety and efficacy of CAR-T cells targeting CAIX in the treatment of advanced renal cancer. **7. NCT06010875:** The study describes a single-center, double-arm, open-label trial aimed at evaluating the safety and efficacy of CD70-targeting CAR-T cells in patients with CD70-positive advanced or metastatic solid tumors. The primary objectives of this study include identifying the recommended doses and infusion patterns for the CAR-T cell therapy. **8. NCT05420519:** This is a phase I clinical study to evaluate the safety and tolerability of CAR-T in patients with advanced/ metastatic renal cell carcinoma, and to obtain the maximum tolerated dose of CAR-T and phase II Recommended dose. **9. NCT05239143:** The study titled "A Phase 1, Open Label, Dose Escalation and Expanded Cohort Study of P-MUC1C-ALLO1 in Adult Subjects with Advanced or Metastatic Epithelial Derived Solid Tumors is a multicenter clinical trial designed to evaluate the safety, tolerability, and preliminary efficacy of P-MUC1C-ALLO1, an allogeneic CAR-T-cell therapy targeting the MUC1-C antigen expressed on various epithelial tumors. **10. NCT04696731:** This is a Phase 1 dose escalation study following a 3 + 3 study design. The purpose of the TRAVERSE study is to assess the safety, efficacy, and cell kinetics of ALLO-316 in adults with advanced or metastatic clear cell renal cell carcinoma after a lymphodepletion regimen comprising fludarabine, cyclophosphamide, and ALLO-647 to define a Phase 2 dose. **11. NCT06480565**: This study is a Phase 1/2 multicenter, open-label trial designed to evaluate ADI-270, an engineered gamma-delta chimeric antigen receptor (CAR) Vδ1 T Cell product targeting CD70, in patients with relapsed or refractory clear cell renal cell carcinoma (ccRCC). The trial aims to assess the safety, tolerability, and preliminary anti-tumor activity of ADI-270, particularly in patients who have previously been treated with immune checkpoint inhibitors and vascular endothelial growth factor (VEGF) inhibitors. **12. NCT05518253:** Phase I clinical studies for chimeric antigen receptor T-cell (CAR-T) therapy are crucial for evaluating the safety and tolerability of these innovative treatments, particularly in patients with advanced or metastatic solid tumors that express specific antigens, such as CD70. The primary objectives of these trials include determining the maximum tolerated dose (MTD) and establishing a recommended phase II dose (RP2D). **13. NCT05420545:** This is a phase I clinical study to evaluate the safety and tolerability of CAR-T in patients with CD70-positive advanced/metastatic solid tumor, and to obtain the maximum tolerated dose of CAR-T and phase II Recommended dose the targeting of tyrosine-protein kinase MET (c-MET), with a focus on prognosis. The TRAVERSE trial (NCT04696731) has received FDA emergency designation and is evaluating ALLO-316, an allogeneic CAR-T cell therapy that targets CD70. Another study (NCT04969354) is investigating CAR-T cells targeting CAIX in advanced RCC, involving a two-step approach to determine safety and efficacy. Recently, a phase I study (NCT05239143) was initiated to evaluate P-MUC1C-ALLO1, an allogeneic CAR-T cell therapy targeting the Mucin 1 cell surface associated C-terminal antigen in tumor form advanced or metastatic hardness, including RCC. These studies clearly project the ongoing research and potential of CAR-T cell therapies for the treatment of advanced and metastatic RCC [48–51].

Conclusion

The development of CAR-T cells signifies a revolutionary transformation in cancer immunotherapy, offering unprecedented potential to identify and annihilate cancer cells. The technology of genetic manipulation of T cells to express CARs that target characteristic antigens on tumor cells has shown efficacy in hematologic malignancies. Despite the tremendous success in leukemia, challenges persist in improving CAR design, improving manufacturing processes, and addressing undesired effects such as cytokine release syndrome and neurotoxicity.

In solid tumors, including renal cell carcinoma (RCC), challenges such as tumor heterogeneity, immune microenvironment, and physical barriers to CAR-T cell entry and activation need to be addressed. While initial attempts to target RCC with CAR-T cells, such as those for carbonic anhydrase IX (CA IX) and vascular endothelial growth factor receptor 2 (VEGFR2), faced setbacks due to extra-tumor toxicity and due to its limited efficacy, ongoing research is exploring alternative ways to overcome these obstacles. Promising strategies include chemo-radiotherapy, which can enhance tumor immunogenicity and improve infiltration and action. Furthermore, the integration of Boolean logic gates and adaptation to counteract immune signals holds the potential to enable CAR-T therapies an improved efficacy and safety in solid tumors. Several clinical trials are presently involved in exploring the use of CAR-T cell therapy in RCC, targeting antigens such as CD70, c-MET, and ROR2. These studies aim to refine CAR-T cell architecture and clinical strategies to achieve optimal outcomes for patients with recurrent or refractory RCC. Despite the challenges, ongoing research and clinical trials underscore the dynamic and evolving landscape of this therapy, noting its potential to revolutionize cancer treatment and improve patient survival. In summary, while CAR-T cell therapy has already made significant progress in the treatment of leukemia, its application in solid tumors such as RCC is still in experimental stages. The journey toward optimizing CAR-T cell therapies for widespread use continues, with ongoing research focused on overcoming the unique challenges posed by solid tumors. The outlook of CAR-T cell therapy is bright, with the potential for significant breakthroughs in cancer therapy, raising hopes for effective and personalized cancer therapies.

References

1. Mousavi SE, Najafi M, Aslani A, Fazlollahi A, Yekta Z, Sadri M, et al. A population-based study on incidence trends of kidney and renal pelvis cancers in the United States over 2000–2020. Sci Rep. 2024;14(1):11294.
2. Hsieh JJ, Purdue MP, Signoretti S, Swanton C, Albiges L, Schmidinger M, et al. Renal Cell Carcinoma. Nat Rev Dis Primers. 2017;3(1):17009.
3. Capitanio U, Montorsi F. Renal Cancer. Lancet. 2016;387(10021):894–906.
4. Bukavina L, Bensalah K, Bray F, Carlo M, Challacombe B, Karam JA, et al. Epidemiology of renal cell carcinoma: 2022 update. Eur Urol. 2022;82(5):529–42.
5. Rosner MH, Jhaveri KD, McMahon BA, Perazella MA. Onconephrology: the intersections between the kidney and cancer. CA Cancer J Clin. 2020;71(1):47–77.
6. Chow WH, Dong LM, Devesa SS. Epidemiology and risk factors for kidney cancer. Nat Rev Urol. 2010;7(5):245–57.
7. Purdue MP, Dutta D, Machiela MJ, Gorman BR, Winter T, Okuhara D, et al. Multi-ancestry genome-

wide association study of kidney cancer identifies 63 susceptibility regions. Nat Genet. 2024;56:809–18.
8. Kim CS, Han KD, Choi HS, Bae EH, Ma SK, Kim SW. Association of hypertension and blood pressure with kidney cancer risk. Hypertension. 2020;75(6):1439–46.
9. Johansson M, Carreras-Torres R, Scelo G, Purdue MP, Mariosa D, Muller DC, et al. The influence of obesity-related factors in the etiology of renal cell carcinoma—a mendelian randomization study. PLoS Med. 2019;16(1):e1002724.
10. Motzer RJ, Jonasch E, Agarwal N, Alva A, Baine M, Beckermann K, et al. Kidney cancer, version 3.2022, NCCN clinical practice guidelines in oncology. J Natl Compr Cancer Netw. 2022 Jan;20(1):71–90.
11. Sadelain M, Brentjens R, Rivière I. The basic principles of chimeric antigen receptor design. Cancer Discov. 2013;3(4):388–98.
12. Jensen MC, Riddell SR. Designing chimeric antigen receptors to effectively and safely target tumors. Curr Opin Immunol. 2015;33:9–15.
13. Jayaraman J, Mellody MP, Hou AJ, Desai RP, Fung AW, Pham AHT, Chen YY, Zhao W. CAR-T design: elements and their synergistic function. EBioMedicine. 2020;58:102931.
14. Finney HM, Lawson ADG, Bebbington CR, Weir ANC. Chimeric receptors providing both primary and costimulatory signaling in T cells from a single gene product. J Immunol. 1998;161(6):2791–7.
15. Zhang C, Liu J, Zhong JF, Zhang X. Engineering CAR-T cells. Biomarker. Research. 2017;5:22.
16. Chmielewski M, Abken H. TRUCKs: the fourth generation of CARs. Expert Opin Biol Ther. 2015;15(8):1145–54.
17. Oldham RAA, Medin JA. Practical considerations for chimeric antigen receptor design and delivery. Expert Opin Biol Ther. 2017;17(8):961–78.
18. Walsh Z, Yang Y, Kohler ME. Immunobiology of chimeric antigen receptor T cells and novel designs. Immunol Rev. 2019;290(1):100–13.
19. Boucher JC, Davila ML. Chimeric antigen receptor design today and tomorrow. Cancer J. 2021;27(2):92–7.
20. Lukjanov V, Koutná I, Šimara P. CAR T-cell production using nonviral approaches. J Immunol Res. 2021;2021:6644685.
21. Larson RC, Maus MV. Recent advances and discoveries in the mechanisms and functions of CAR T cells. Nat Rev Cancer. 2021;21(3):145–61.
22. Fraietta JA, Lacey SF, Orlando EJ, Pruteanu-Malinici I, Gohil M, Lundh S, et al. Determinants of response and resistance to CD19 chimeric antigen receptor (CAR) T cell therapy of chronic lymphocytic leukemia. Nat Med. 2018;24(5):563–71.
23. Porter DL, Levine BL, Kalos M, et al. Chimeric antigen receptor–modified T cells in chronic lymphoid leukemia. N Engl J Med. 2011;365(8):725–33.
24. Kalos M, Levine BL, Porter DL, Katz S, Grupp SA, Bagg A, et al. T cells with chimeric antigen receptors have potent antitumor effects and can establish memory in patients with advanced leukemia. Sci Transl Med. 2011;3(95):95ra73–3.
25. Skorka K, Ostapinska K, Malesa A, Giannopoulos K. The application of CAR-T cells in haematological malignancies. Arch Immunol Ther Exp. 2020;68(6)
26. Han D, Xu Z, Zhuang Y, Ye Z, Qian Q. Current progress in CAR-T cell therapy for hematological malignancies. J Cancer. 2021;12(2):326–34.
27. Ma S, Li X, Wang X, et al. Current progress in CAR-T cell therapy for solid tumors. Int J Biol Sci. 2019;15(12):2548.
28. Sadelain M. T-cell engineering for cancer immunotherapy. Cancer J. 2009;15(6):451–5.
29. Gill S, Porter DL. CAR-modified anti-CD19 T cells for the treatment of B-cell malignancies: rules of the road. Expert Opin Biol Ther. 2013;14(1):37–49.
30. Lyou Y, Dorff TB. Chimeric antigen receptor (CAR) T-cell treatment in renal cell carcinoma: current clinical trials and future directions. Kidney Cancer. 2022;6(3):159–68.
31. Lamers CH, Sleijfer S, van Steenbergen S, van Elzakker P, van Krimpen B, Groot C, et al. Treatment of metastatic renal cell carcinoma with CAIX CAR-engineered T cells: clinical evaluation and management of on-target toxicity. Mol Ther. 2013;21(4):904–12.
32. Majzner RG, Mackall CL. Tumor antigen escape from CAR T-cell therapy. Cancer Discov. 2018;8(10):1219–26.
33. Cohen AD, Garfall AL, Stadtmauer EA, Melenhorst JJ, Lacey SF, Lancaster E, et al. B cell maturation antigen–specific CAR T cells are clinically active in multiple myeloma. J Clin Invest. 2019;129(6):2210–21.
34. Montironi C, Muñoz-Pinedo C, Eldering E. Hematopoietic versus solid cancers and T cell dysfunction: looking for similarities and distinctions. Cancers. 2021;13(2):284.
35. Najjar YG, Rayman P, Jia X, Pavicic PG, Rini BI, Tannenbaum CS, et al. Myeloid-derived suppressor cell subset accumulation in renal cell carcinoma parenchyma is associated with intratumoral expression of IL1β, IL8, CXCL5, and Mip-1α. Clin Cancer Res. 2017;23(9):2346–55.
36. Zhang BL, Qin DY, Mo ZM, Li Y, Wei W, Wang YS, et al. Hurdles of CAR-T cell-based cancer immunotherapy directed against solid tumors. Sci China Life Sci. 2016;59(4):340–8.
37. Marofi F, Achmad H, Bokov D, Abdelbasset WK, Alsadoon Z, Chupradit S, et al. Hurdles to breakthrough in CAR T cell therapy of solid tumors. Stem Cell Res Ther. 2022;13(1):140.
38. Seyedin SN, Schoenhals JE, Lee DA, Cortez MA, Wang X, Niknam S, et al. Strategies for combining immunotherapy with radiation for anticancer therapy. Immunotherapy. 2015;7(9):967–80.
39. Ngiow S, McArthur Grant A, Smyth MJ. Radiotherapy complements immune checkpoint blockade. Cancer Cell. 2015;27(4):437–8.
40. Tang C, Welsh JW, Patricia ME, Chang JY, Hess KR, et al. Ipilimumab with stereotactic ablative radia-

tion therapy: phase I results and immunologic correlates from peripheral T cells. Clin Cancer Res. 2017;23(6):1388–96.
41. Formenti SC, Rudqvist NP, Golden E, Cooper B, Wennerberg E, Lhuillier C, et al. Radiotherapy induces responses of lung cancer to CTLA-4 blockade. Nat Med. 2018;24(12):1845–51.
42. Santoni M, Heng DYC, Aurilio G, Iozzelli A, Servi L, Fabiani A, et al. Combining radiotherapy with immunocheckpoint inhibitors or CAR-T in renal cell carcinoma. Curr Drug Targets. 2020;21(4):416–23.
43. Yang C, Ji S, Li Y, Fu L, Jiang T, Meng F. Ror2, a developmentally regulated kinase, is associated with tumor growth, apoptosis, migration, and invasion in renal cell carcinoma. Oncol Res. 2017;25(2):195–205.
44. Dai H, Wang Y, Lu X, Han W. Chimeric antigen receptors modified T-cells for cancer therapy. JNCI J Natl Cancer Inst. 2016;108(7)
45. Zhu C, Wei Y, Wei X. AXL receptor tyrosine kinase as a promising anti-cancer approach: functions, molecular mechanisms and clinical applications. Mol Cancer. 2019;18(1):153.
46. Hou B, Tang Y, Li W, Zeng Q, Chang D. Efficiency of CAR-T therapy for treatment of solid tumor in clinical trials: a meta-analysis. Dis Markers. 2019;2019:3425291.
47. Yang DC, Chen CH. Potential new therapeutic approaches for renal cell carcinoma. Semin Nephrol. 2020;40(1):86–97.
48. Albinger N, Hartmann J, Ullrich E. Current status and perspective of CAR-T and CAR-NK cell therapy trials in Germany. Gene Ther. 2021;28(9):513–27.
49. Xu Y, Miller CP, Warren EH, Tykodi SS. Current status of antigen-specific T-cell immunotherapy for advanced renal-cell carcinoma. Hum Vaccin Immunother. 2021;17(7):1882–96.
50. Kim I, Lee HJ. The frontline immunotherapy-based treatment of advanced clear cell renal cell carcinoma: current evidence and clinical perspective. Biomedicines. 2022;10(2):251.
51. Kyte JA. Strategies for improving the efficacy of CAR T cells in solid cancers. Cancers. 2022;14(3):571.
52. NCT03393936: https://clinicaltrials.gov/study/NCT03393936?cond=NCT03393936&rank=1
53. NCT01218867: https://clinicaltrials.gov/study/NCT01218867?cond=NCT01218867&rank=1
54. NCT02830724: https://clinicaltrials.gov/study/NCT02830724?cond=NCT02830724&rank=1
55. NCT04438083: https://clinicaltrials.gov/study/NCT04438083?cond=NCT04438083&rank=1
56. NCT03638206: https://clinicaltrials.gov/study/NCT03638206?cond=NCT03638206&rank=1
57. NCT04969354: https://clinicaltrials.gov/study/NCT04969354?cond=NCT04969354&rank=1
58. NCT06010875: https://clinicaltrials.gov/study/NCT06010875?cond=NCT06010875&rank=1
59. NCT05420519: https://clinicaltrials.gov/study/NCT05420519?cond=NCT05420519&rank=1
60. NCT05239143: https://clinicaltrials.gov/study/NCT05239143?cond=NCT05239143&rank=1
61. NCT04696731: https://clinicaltrials.gov/study/NCT04696731?cond=NCT04696731&rank=1
62. NCT06480565: https://clinicaltrials.gov/study/NCT06480565?cond=NCT06480565&rank=1
63. NCT05518253: https://clinicaltrials.gov/study/NCT05518253?cond=NCT05518253&rank=1
64. NCT05420545: https://clinicaltrials.gov/study/NCT05420545?cond=NCT05420545&rank=1

Correction to: Systemic Therapies for the Treatment of Renal Cell Carcinoma

Sonia Gowda and Paul Mathew

Correction to:
Chapter 22 in: J. A. Libertino, J. R. Gee (eds.), *Renal Cancer*, https://doi.org/10.1007/978-3-031-97599-8_22

The book was inadvertently published without Table 22.1 in chapter 22. This correction chapter includes the missing table as follows:

The original chapter can be found at
https://doi.org/10.1007/978-3-031-97599-8_22

J. A. Libertino, J. R. Gee (eds.), *Renal Cancer*, https://doi.org/10.1007/978-3-031-97599-8_25

Table 22.1 Long-term follow-up of combination regimens that improve overall survival in MRCC, compared to sunitinib

Combination	Follow-up (months)	IMDC category	(%)	ORR (%)	Time to response (months)	CR (%)	Response duration (months)	PFS % or HR	OS (HR)
Ipilimumab and nivolumab	**99**	**Total**	**1096**	**39.5 vs 33**	**2.8 vs 4.0**	**12 vs 3.5**	**76.2 vs 25**	**22.8% vs 10.8%**	**0.72**
		Good	23%	29.6 vs 51.6	2.8 vs 4.2	12.8 vs 6.5	61.5 vs 33.2	12.7% vs 17%	0.82*
		Intermediate	61%	42.4 vs 27.5	2.8 vs 3.1	11.8 vs 2.6	82.8 vs 19.8	25.4% vs 8.5%	0.69
		Poor	17%						
Axitinib and pembrolizumab	**43**	**Total**	**861**	**60 vs 40**	**N/A**	**10 vs 3.5**	**24 vs 15**	**0.67**	**0.73**
		Good	32%	69 vs 50		–	–	0.76	1.2*
		Intermediate	55%	61 vs 40		–	–	0.69	0.67
		Poor	13%	39 vs 12		–	–	0.53	0.51
Cabozantinib and nivolumab	**44**	**Total**	**651**	**56 vs 28**	**2.8 vs 4.3**	**13 vs 5**	**22.1 vs 16.1**	**0.59**	**0.7**
		Good	23%	67.6 vs 45.8	2.8 vs 4.2	16.2 vs 9.7	19.8 vs 17.8	0.72*	1.07*
		Intermediate	58%	56.4 vs 27.7	2.8 vs 5.4	28 vs 8	22.9 vs 19.3	0.63	0.75
		Poor	19%	41 vs 10.3	3.3 vs 3.1	3 vs 1	35.9 vs 4.9	0.37	0.46
Lenvatinib and pembrolizumab	**50**	**Total**	**712**	**71.3 vs 36.7**	**1.9 vs 2.0**	**18.3 vs 4.8**	**26.7 vs 14.7**	**0.47**	**0.79**
		Good	31%	68.2 vs 50.8	–	20.9 vs 4.8	26.3 vs 14.7	0.50	0.94*
		Intermediate	59%	72.9 vs 31.8	–	15.2 vs 4.7	25.9 vs 12.9	0.43	0.74
		Poor	9%	69.7 vs 13.5	–	6.1 vs 0	20.4 vs NR		

ORR overall response rate, *CR* complete response, *PFS* progression-free survival, *OS* overall survival, *HR* hazard ratio, *NR* not reached, *N/A* not available; * Confidence interval includes 1.0

Index

A
Ablative techniques, 263
Abscopal effect, 429
Acquired cystic kidney disease (ACKD), 6
Acrylic polymer microspheres, 129
Active surveillance (AS), 141
    indications for, 153–156
    outcomes, 157–160
        cost-effectiveness, 160
        delayed intervention, 157
        growth rate, 157
        quality of life, 160
        renal function, 158–160
        risk of metastasis, 158
        survival and mortality, 158
    protocols, 155–157
    rationale for, 153
    shared decision-making model, 156
    short-term stability, 157
Acute lymphoblastic leukemia (ALL), 481
Adaptive statistical iterative reconstruction (ASIR) algorithms, 89
Adjuvant chemotherapy, 380, 381
Adjuvant therapy
    ARISER trial, 455
    ASSURE, S-TRAC, ATLAS, and SORCE trials, 454, 455
    clinical and pathologic data, 448, 449
    definition, 447
    EVEREST trial, 455
    immunotherapy, 451
        CheckMate 914 phase III trial, 453
        IL-2 and IFN-∝, 451, 452
        IMmotion010 phase III trial, 452
        Keynote-564 trial, 452
        RFS, 454
        surveillance, 451
        thalidomide, 454
        vaccines, 453, 454
        Vitespen, 453
    medical therapy, 451
    ongoing/unreported trials, 455–457
    pembrolizumab, 458
    prognostication, 448, 450, 451
    PROTECT trial, 455
    radiotherapy, 451
    risk of recurrence, 447, 448
Adult renal cancers, 86
ALARA, 89
American Joint Committee on Cancer (AJCC), 11, 282–284
American Society of Anesthesiologists (ASA), 250
American Urological Association (AUA), 11, 263, 274, 338
Angioinfarction, 127, 131, 137
Angiomyolipoma (AML), 68, 69, 94–97, 106, 137
    of kidney, 107
AngioVac procedure, 302, 303, 305
ANGPTL4, 28
Anterior surgical approach, 250
Anti-inflammatory cytokine inhibitors, 181
Anti-VEGF agents, 350
Anti-VEGF targeted therapies, 355
Aortic calcium volume scores (ACS), 181
APOBEC3B expression, 29
Apoptosis, 224
Apparent diffusion coefficient (ADC) values, 95–97
Aquaporin-1 (AQP1), 8
Area under receiver operating curve (AUROC), 8
Aristolochic acid (AA), 7, 368, 369
Arterial-based complexity (ABC) system, 210
Arteriovenous fistula (AVF), 272
Artery-only clamping, 267
Artificial intelligence (AI), 99
ASPEN trial, 351
ASSURE trial, 337
Asymptomatic recurrences, 392
Atezolizumab, 452
Atriotomy, 297, 299
Augmented reality (AR), 263, 276
Autosomal dominant disorders, 10
Autotransplantation, 378–379
Axitinib, 31, 115

J. A. Libertino, J. R. Gee (eds.), *Renal Cancer*, https://doi.org/10.1007/978-3-031-97599-8

B
Balloon or stent-assisted coiling, 128
BAP1-associated RCC, 41
BAP1 tumor suppressor gene, 10
Belzutifan, 436
Benign renal tumors, 104
Bevacizumab, 467
BHD-associated lesions, 39
Bilateral, multifocal (BMF), 43
Biomarkers, 327
Birt-Hogg-Dubé (BHD) syndrome, 30, 39, 56, 67
Bladder cancer recurrence (BCR), 366, 375
Blake or Jackson-Pratt drain, 269
Blood cancers, 479, 480
Bone
  distant recurrence, 392–393
  metastasis, 112, 113
BONSAI study, 356
Bookwalter retractors, 288
Bosniak renal cyst classification, 88
Bowel injury, 272
Brain
  distant recurrence, 393
  metastases, local therapy, 341
BRCA1-associated protein-1 (BAP1), 27, 41
Budd-Chiari syndrome, 426

C
Cabozantinib, 352, 356
Cancer dissemination, 45–46
Cancer-specific survival (CSS), 314
Cancer symptom questionnaire, 160
Capillary occlusion, 130–133
Carbonic anhydrase IX (CA IX), 28, 119, 120, 321, 322
Carcinogenesis, 368–369
Cardiopulmonary bypass (CPB), 288, 291, 297, 299, 300
Caval–atrial shunt, 292, 293
Caval interruption, 301
Caval tumor thrombus, 462, 463
Caval wall resection, 301
Cavotomy, 291–293, 295, 299
CDK4/6 inhibitors, 356
Cell death, 224
Centers for Disease Control and Prevention, 5
Centrality Index (C-Index), 205–207, 247, 249
Centrally located tumors, 255
Central necrosis, 92
Central occlusion, 127–129
Cephalad level of the tumor thrombus, 287
CheckMate 914 phase III trial, 453
Chemical shift imaging, 92
Chimeric antigen receptor (CAR) T-cell therapy
  B-cellular malignancies, 479
  blood, 477, 478
  cancer treatment, 479
  clinical trials, 479
  co-stimulatory component, 477
  definition, 477
  GvHD, 478
  incidence, 475
  lymphoma cells, 479
  modular structure, 477
  occurrence, 475
  protein structures, 478
  radiotherapy, 482
  RCC
    ALL, 481
    clinical trials, 483, 485
    development, 481
    evolution of, 476
    hypoxia, 481
    immunotherapy, 481
    incidence, 476
    leukapheresis, 481
    MDSCs, 481
    progression, 476
    risk factors, 476
    target antigens, 482
    VHL, 481
  risk factors, 475
  signalling pathways and transcription factors, 477
  solid tumours, 480, 481
  treatment options, 477, 478
  TRUCKs, 477
Chimeric-G250 (girentuximab), 149
Chromophobe renal cell carcinoma (ChRCC), 30, 94, 350, 353, 354
  clinical features, 56
  molecular genetics, 56
  pathology, 56
  prognosis, 57
Chromosome 3 translocation, 43
Chromosome 7q31, 29
Chronic hypertension, 5
Chronic kidney disease (CKD), 221–227, 232, 239, 397
  ACS, 181
  cardiovascular events, 180
  finerenone, 181
  hypertension and left ventricular dysfunction, 181
  KDIGO guidelines, 180
  prevalence and incidence, 178, 179
  renal dysfunction, 181
  risk factor, 181
  serum abnormalities, 181
  SGLT2 inhibitors, 181
Chronic lymphocytic leukemia (CLL), 479
Chronic obstructive pulmonary disease (COPD), 4
Chronic renal disease, 6
Chronic renal insufficiency, 177
Circulating tumor DNA (ctDNA), 31
Clear cell histology, 25, 351
Clear cell renal cell carcinoma (ccRCC), 4, 39, 103–105, 107, 111–113, 115, 116, 118–120
  clinical features, 52
  definition, 27
  hypoxia-induced genes, 27, 28
  molecular genetics, 53, 54
  pathology, 52, 53
  prognosis, 54

Collecting duct carcinoma, 355, 356
Collecting system, 268
Combined central and peripheral occlusion, 129–130
Complete metastasectomy, 342
Comprehensive metabolic panel (CMP), 396
Computed tomography (CT) scanning, 8
Contemporary classification systems
  C-index model, 205
  PADUA, 205
  renal nephrometry score
    components, 203
    and nephrometry sum, 204
    polar lines, 204
    radiographic measures, 203
    tumor size, 203
    web-based tool, 205
Contrast-enhanced ultrasound (CEUS), 81, 148–149, 161, 397, 412
  small renal masses, 148
Conventional imaging methods, 318
Conventional renal cell carcinoma (CRCC)
  incidence, 435
  localized renal cancer
    biomarkers, 442, 443
    KEYNOTE-564, 442
    lymphadenectomy, 442
    nivolumab/ipilimumab, 442
    pembrolizumab, 442
    research directions, 443
  metastatic disease
    elderly populations, 441
    immunocompromised and organ transplant, 441
    risk stratification, 437–439
    sarcomatoid and rhabdoid differentiation, 441
    second-line therapy, 439–441
    translational considerations, 435–437
Copenhagen Renal Cancer Study, 421
Cost-effective techniques, 8
Cowden syndrome, 10
Cryoablation (CA), 82, 90, 91, 274, 410–412
Curaspon, 130
Cylindrical volume ratio method, 229
Cytoreduction, 325–327
Cytoreductive nephrectomy, 313, 325, 326, 358
  clinical evidence, 467, 468
  definition, 464
  multivariate model, 464
  patient selection, 464, 465
  presurgical targeted therapy
    argument for, 467
    duration, 468
    safety, 468
  SWOG and the EORTC trials, 464
  targeted therapy, 466, 467
Cytotoxic chemotherapy, 356

D

da Vinci Xi robotic system, 269, 270
Debakey vascular clamp, 288, 289, 291
Decision analytic models, 160
Deep hypothermic circulatory arrest (DHCA), 299, 301
Deep vein thrombosis (DVT) prophylaxis, 273
Detachable balloons, 128
Diagnostic ureteroscopy, 371–372
Diameter-axial-polar (DAP) nephrometry scoring system, 210
Diaphragmatic injury, 272
Disease-free survival (DFS), 448, 452
Distant metastasis, 110, 325–327
Distant recurrence
  bone, 392–393
  brain, 393
  liver, 393
  lung, 392
  lymph node, 393–394
DNA methylation, 28
Doyen clamps, 306
Dual energy CT (DECT), 98

E

EGLN3, 27
18F-labeled acetate, 121
18F-labeled choline, 121
18F-labeled thymidine (FLT), 120
11C-acetate, 121
Embolization procedures, 127
Endovascular downstaging, 288, 302–305
Endovascular procedures, 127
End-stage renal disease (ESRD), 6
Eosinophilic vacuolated tumors (EVTs), 57
Epithelial-to-mesenchymal transition (EMT), 71, 368
ESPN trial, 351
Estimated glomerular filtration rate (eGFR), 6, 177, 397
European Association of Urology (EAU) guidelines, 144, 150, 155, 338, 340
Evarrest fibrin sealant patch, 289
EVEREST study, 359
Evidence-based approach, 327
Excretory urography, 78, 369, 371
EXIST-2 trial in TSC, 45
Extended LND (eLND), 313, 315, 316, 322
Extracorporeal oxygen membrane (ECMO) device, 302

F

Facultative LND, 314
Familial and hereditary syndromes
  cancer-specific survival, 43
  de novo mutation, 36
  forms of RCC, 35
  genetic counseling, 35
  genetic testing, 37
  multifocality, 43
  resection of multiple lesions, 44
  surveillance of small renal masses, 43
  tumor removal without ischemia, 44
  wide surgical excision, 45
FASTRACK study, 424

Finerenone, 181
FLCN inactivation in sporadic renal cancers, 354
Follicular renal cell carcinoma, 357
Folliculin (FLCN) gene, 30
Fuhrman grade, 406
Fumarate hydratase-deficient RCC, 358
Fumarate hydratase (FH) gene, 10, 29, 65, 358
Fumarate hydrogenase tumor predisposition syndrome, 10

G
Gelfoam, 130
Gelitaspon, 130
Genetic testing, 45
Genomic alterations (GA), 11, 71, 367
 UTUC, 367
Genomic biomarkers, 322
Germline chromosome 3 translocations, 42
Gerota's fascia, 269
Girentuximab, 120, 149, 172, 275, 318, 321, 322, 455
Glomerular filtration rate (GFR), 176
Goblet sign, 369
Growth kinetics, 154, 157, 158, 161

H
Hand-assisted laparoscopic nephrectomy, 377
Hand-assisted laparoscopic partial nephrectomy, 265, 266
Health record systems, 2
Heat shock protein (HSP), 453
Hemorrhage, 188
Hemostasis, 253
 resected bed of kidney, 268, 269
Heparan sulfate proteoglycan (HSPG), 481
Hepatic venous bleeding, 293
Hereditary kidney cancer, 35, 36
 syndromes, 36, 43, 45
Hereditary leiomyomatosis and renal cell carcinoma (HLRCC), 39, 40, 64, 65
Hereditary papillary renal carcinoma (HPRC/HPRCC), 36, 38–40, 43, 44, 54, 64
Hereditary pheochromocytoma paraganglioma syndrome, 65, 66
Hereditary renal cancer syndrome, 10
HIF2α dimerization, 435, 436
HIF2α inhibitor therapy, 440, 441
High-intensity focused ultrasound (HIFU), 77, 82, 276
Hilar clamping, 267
Hockey-stick or cobra configuration, 127
Hounsfield units (HU), 86
Human epidermal growth factor receptor 2 (HER2), 368
Hybrid oncocytic/chromophobe tumors (HOCTs), 149, 152
Hypertension, 5, 6
Hypervascular angiomyolipoma, 137
Hypervascular tumor, 92
Hypovascular left renal mass, 287
Hypoxia, 120, 481
Hypoxia-induced genes, 27, 28
Hypoxia-inducible factor 1 (HIF-1), 10
Hypoxia-response elements (HREs), 435–436

I
IMmotion010 phase III trial, 452
Immune checkpoint inhibitors (ICIs), 31, 115, 381
Immune-oncologic (IO) therapies, 339
Immunotherapy, 115
Imperative partial nephrectomy (IPN), 305
Incidental renal masses, 338
Inferior vena cava (IVC), 15, 288, 426
 filter, 287
Inflammatory lymphadenopathies, 318
Infrahepatic IVC, 294
Infrahepatic thrombus, 282
Infrahepatic tumor thrombus level II, 288, 290, 291
Initial nephrometry classification systems, 209
Insulin-like growth factor 1 (IGF-1), 10
Integrated system, 17
Interaortocaval lymph nodes, 313
Interferon-alpha, 429, 436
Interferon-gamma (IFN-γ), 482
Interferon-∝ (IFN-∝), 452
Interleukin-2 (IL-2), 429, 436, 451
International Agency for Research on Cancer (IARC), 4
International Renal Cell Carcinoma–Venous Thrombus Consortium (IRCC-VTC), 307, 309, 323
International Society of Stereotactic Radiosurgery (ISRS), 424
Internist's tumor, 284
Intraperitoneal access, 265
Intratumoral hemorrhage, 92
Intravenous pyelogram (IVP), 78–79
Intussusception, 377, 378
Ischemia, 6, 44, 71, 202, 207, 209, 211, 218, 221–233, 239, 249, 250, 252, 255, 267–269, 273, 276, 337
 adverse impact of, 255, 256

K
Kaplan-Meier curve, 465
KEYNOTE-427 trial, 352
KEYNOTE-564 trial, 334, 342, 452
Ki-67, 368
Kidney cancer, 1
 cancer specific survival (CSS), 334
 laparoscopic approaches, 334
 localized stage, 334
 long-term survival, 334
 open surgical excision, 334 (*see* Renal cell carcinoma (RCC))
 standardized treatment protocol, 334
Kidney Disease Outcomes Quality Initiative (KDOQI), 179
Kidney Injury Molecule-1 (KIM-1), 448
Kocher maneuver, 294

L

Langenbeck, 295
Laparoscopic partial nephrectomy (LPN), 188, 263, 264
Large renal vein thrombus, 289
Lazarus effect, 306
Leukapheresis, 481
Litmus test, 467
Liver
  distant recurrence, 393
  metastasis, 113, 114, 117
  mobilization, 293, 294
Locoregional metastasis, 108–110
Lower extremity sequential compression devices, 264
Low-grade oncocytic tumor (LOT), 57
Lung
  distant recurrence, 392
  metastasis, 110–111
Lung metastases from RCC (LM-RCC), 340
Lymphadenectomy, 311, 314, 379–380
Lymph node dissection (LND), in RCC management, 311
  lymph node metastasis, prevalence of, 318, 319
  morbidity, 316
  and oncological outcomes, 313–315
  perform
    clinical node-positive (cT1-4, N+M0) RCC, 324, 325
    distant metastasis and cytoreduction (cTanyNanyM1), 325–327
    larger tumors (cT2abN0M0), 323
    localized disease (cT1abN0M0), 322, 323
    locally advanced disease (cT3-T4N0M0), 323, 324
  predicting lymph node involvement, 319
    intraoperative lymph node assessment, 320, 321
    molecular and genomic biomarkers, 322
    protocols and nomograms, 319, 320
    sentinel lymph node biopsy, 321
  scope of, 313–315
  survival benefit, 312
  templates and techniques, 327
  therapeutic benefit, 311
Lymph node, distant recurrence, 393–394
Lymph node invasion (LNI), 72, 312, 313, 316–318
  imaging for detection, 316–318
Lymph node metastasis, 283
  prevalence of, 318, 319
Lymphovascular invasion (LVI), 314, 368, 380
Lynch syndrome (LS), 365, 366

M

Magnetic resonance imaging (MRI), 10
Massive pulmonary embolism, 302
Matrixmetalloproteinase (MMP)-9, 368
Mayo classification, 463
Mayo Staging System, 282
Median sternotomy (MS), 294, 295, 297–301
Medroxyprogesterone acetate (MPA), 451
Memorial Sloan Kettering Cancer Center (MSKCC), 176, 177, 337, 341, 448
Mesenchymal–epithelial transition (MET)
  inhibitors, 64
  mutations, 352
  mutations or activation in pRCC proliferation, 352
  pathway, 351
  proto-oncogene, 10
Metabolic tumor burden (MTB), 115
Metastasectomy, 340, 341
  solitary or multiple metastases, 340
Metastases-directed therapy (MDT), 428, 429
Metastasis, 16, 17, 137
Metastasis-associated lung adenocarcinoma transcript 1 (MALAT1), 322
Metastatic renal cell carcinoma (mRCC), 104, 110, 115–118, 121, 333, 339, 340, 342, 447, 460, 464, 466–468, 483
  management, 333
Metastectomy, 306
Methotrexate, vinblastine, doxorubicin, and cisplatin (MVAC), 356
Microphthalmia-associated transcription factor (MiTF) family of genes, 41, 42
  translocation renal cancer, 356
Microsatellite alterations, 367
  UTUC, 367
Microvascular invasion (MVI), 72
Microwave therapy, 274, 275
Minimally access approach, 297, 299–301
Minimally invasive partial nephrectomy (MIPN)
  cardiac performance, 264
  complication rates, 271
  cross-sectional imaging, 264
  factors, 263
  improved technology, 263
  invasive surgical techniques of laparoscopy, 263
  magnesium citrate bowel preparation, 264
  medical comorbidities, 264
  nephrometry score, 209
  patient positioning, 264
  peritoneal insufflation, 264
  pneumoperitoneum, 264
  preoperative bowel preparation, 264
  radiologic imaging, 263
  surgical skill set, 263
  technique and histological assessment, 263
  venous injuries, 272
Minimally invasive surgery (MIS), 174, 246, 337
  in treatment of renal malignancies, 337
Minimally invasive techniques, 246, 247, 301, 316
  nephrectomy, 217
Minimally invasive thermal ablative (TA) therapies for renal tumors, 274
Minor thermal injury, 272
MiR-26a-5p expression, 368
MiRNA-151b, 368
Mitomycin C, 374
Model-based iterative reconstruction (MIR) algorithms, 89

Modification of Diet in Renal Disease (MDRD) equation, 177, 245, 251
Molecular imaging
bone metastasis, 111–113
CA IX, 119, 120
distant metastases, 110
18F-DCFPyl, 119
18F-FMISO, 120
18F-labeled acetate, 121
18F-labeled choline, 121
18F-labeled thymidine (FLT), 120
11C-acetate, 121
hypoxia, 120
liver metastasis, 113–114
locoregional metastasis, 108–110
lung metastasis, 110–111
management of, 118–119
monitoring therapeutic response, 115–118
primary RCC diagnosis, 104–108
prognostic values of FDG PET, 114, 115
surveillance, 114
Mortality rates, 3
mRNA editing, 29
mTOR inhibitors, 45, 350, 355
Mucinous tubular and spindle cell carcinoma (MTSCC), 356, 357
Myeloid-derived suppressor cells (MDSCs), 481

N
N-acetyl-p-benzoquinone imine (NAPQI), 7
National Cancer Institute, 41
National Comprehensive Cancer Network (NCCN) guidelines, 155, 340
National Kidney Foundation Disease Outcomes Quality Initiative CKD classification, 244, 245
Neoadjuvant chemotherapy, 306, 380
Neoadjuvant therapy
downsizing caval tumor thrombus, 462, 463
immunotherapy, 458, 459
nephron-sparing surgery, 461, 462
recurrence, 458
resection, 461
targeted therapy, 459–461
Nephrectomy, 3, 319, 325, 359
Nephrometry scoring systems, 210, 211
Nephrons atrophy, 176
Nephron-sparing partial nephrectomy, 82
Nephron-sparing surgery (NSS), 189, 190, 216, 217, 239, 240, 256, 263, 461, 462
Nephroureterectomy, 375–377
bladder cuff removal
pluck technique, 378
intussusception, 377–378
open technique, 377
transvesical approach, 378
unroofing technique, 378
Neuropathies, 264
New baseline glomerular filtration rate (NBGFR), 229
Next-generation 3D display and image processing, 275
Nivolumab, 31, 429
Non-clamping partial nephrectomy technique, 202, 207, 218, 222, 225
Non-clamping technique, 252, 254, 267
Non-clear cell renal cell carcinoma, 352
Non-functioning renal graft, 137
Non-ischemic partial nephrectomy, 222, 225, 267
Nonsteroidal anti-inflammatory drugs (NSAIDs), 7
NRF2-ARE pathway, 29
Nuclear factor of activated T cells (NFAT), 477

O
Obesity, 5
Occluded vasculature management, 301
Occult multifocal renal tumors, 217
Oligometastatic disease, 428, 429
Oncocytomas, 104–106, 142–145, 149, 150
Open non-clamping technique, 252
Open partial nephrectomy (OPN)
advantages, 239
assessment of renal function, 251
cardiopulmonary complications, 250
excision of tumor, 254, 255
history, 240
imaging, 251
ischemia, adverse impact of, 255, 256
minimally invasive techniques, 246, 247
mobilizing the kidney, 252
oncologic efficacy of, 241, 242
oncologic outcomes, 244
outcomes, 243
preoperative evaluation, 250
prophylaxis, 251
renal preservation, 244–246
renorrhaphy, 255
risks and benefits of treatment options, 244
small renal masses, epidemiology of, 240, 241
stages of CKD, 244, 245
surgical approaches, 251, 252
TNM staging of renal cancer, 242
T1 tumors, 243, 244
T1a tumors, 243
T1b tumors, 243
tumor complexity, 247–250
underutilization of, 246
vascular clamping, 252–254
vascular control, 252
Open surgical technology, advancements, 218
Open technique, 377

P
p53, 368, 369
Palliative embolization
angiomyolipoma, 137
nonfunctioning renal graft, 137
primary renal mass, 137
renal cell carcinoma, 137
Pancreatic and splenic injuries, 272

Papillary adenomas, 67
Papillary renal cell carcinoma (PRCC), 4, 29, 30, 351–353
clinical features, 54
molecular genetics, 55
pathology, 54, 55
prognosis, 55
PAPMET trial, 352
Partial nephrectomy (PN), 216, 221–236, 263, 266, 312, 335–337, 342
and ablative therapies, 274
oncological outcomes, 274
candidate selection, 191, 192
CKD
ACS, 181
cardiovascular events, 180
finerenone, 181
hypertension and left ventricular dysfunction, 181
KDIGO guidelines, 180
prevalence and incidence, 178, 179
renal dysfunction, 181
risk factor, 181
serum abnormalities, 181
SGLT2 inhibitors, 181
complications of, 187–189
cross-sectional imaging, 170
epidemiology, 170–172
history of, 169, 172–174
long-term follow-up, 170
nephrometry score, 208
oncologic outcomes, 174–176
open partial nephrectomy (*see* Open partial nephrectomy (OPN))
RCTs, 172
recurrence after, 394–395
renal functional outcomes, 176–178
renal surgery
cardiovascular events, 182, 183
cardiovascular mortality, 185–187
CKD, 182, 184–186
clinical trial, 183
eGFR, 182
overall survival rate, 183, 184
randomized trial, 184
retrospective data, 184
risk factor, 182
SEER data, 182
small renal masses, 192, 193
surveillance
abdominal imaging modalities, 397
components, 396–397
prognostic factor, 397–399
rationale, 395–396
with sporadic RCC, 399–407
utilization of, 189–191
Pazopanib, 342, 428
Peak early enhancement ratio (PEER), 145
Pembrolizumab, 31, 334, 335, 442, 458
Percutaneous biopsy, 160
Perilipin-2 (PLIN2), 8
Perinephric fat, 173
Perioperative chemotherapy, 380, 381
Perivascular epithelioid tumor (PEComa), 69
Persistent urinary tract infection, 215
Personalized treatment approaches, 326
PET with fluorine-18 fluorodeoxyglucose (FDG), 321
Pluck technique, 378
Pneumoperitoneum, 265
Polar nephrectomy, 254
Polybromo 1 (PBRM1), 27
Polymer-coated particles with a hydrogel core, 129
Polyvinyl alcohol, 129
microspheres, 129
Positive surgical margins (PSMs), 395
Post-embolization syndrome, 133, 137
Post-infarction syndrome, 287
Postoperative renal function
chronic kidney disease, 226, 227
clamping versus non-clamping partial nephrectomy, 225, 226, 229
clinical cases, 233–236
combined ischemia and volume, 231, 232
long-term follow-up, 226
modifiable and nonmodifiable factors, 223
nephrectomy versus partial nephrectomy, 222
nonischemic partial nephrectomy, 225
non-SFR-based models, 229
predicting renal functional outcomes, 224
preoperative CKD, 223–224
short-term follow-up, 226
solitary kidney, 225
split renal function, 229
surgical approach to multifocal or bilateral renal tumors, 233–236
3D CT imaging, 224
volume, role of, 229–230
warm ischemia, 224–229
warm ischemia time, 226, 227, 229
Post-transplant kidney cancer, 6
Preoperative aspects and dimensions used for an anatomical (PADUA) classification, 247, 248
longer warm ischemia time, 207
perioperative complication, 205
tumor location, 205
tumor size, 205
validation, 207
vs. RENAL NS, 205, 206
vs. SPARE nephrometry scoring systems, 210, 211
Preoperative embolization, 136, 137
Primary ablative therapy, 338
local recurrence, 338, 339
Primary renal mass, 137
Pringle maneuver, 293
Programmed death ligand 1 (PD-L1), 115, 322, 439
expression, 350
Progression-free survival (PFS), 438, 439
Prostate-specific membrane antigen (PSMA), 103, 119
Proteinaceous or hemorrhagic cysts, 92

Pseudoaneurysm (PA), 272
Pulmonary metastasectomy, 340
Pulmonary recurrence, 392
Pyelonephritis, 215

Q
Quality-adjusted life-year (QALY), 160
Quality of life (QOL), 187

R
Radiation therapy (RT)
  CART, 482
  human cell radiosensitivity, 419
  immuno-radiotherapy, 429, 430
  intraoperative radiation, 422, 423
  oligometastatic disease, 428, 429
  palliative radiotherapy
    brain metastases, 424
    CNS lesions, 425
    IVC, 426
    local control, 425
    occurrence, 425
    SBRT, 426, 427
    spine disease, 425–427
    stereotactic techniques, 425
    TDF, 425
  postoperative neoadjuvant radiation, 421, 422
  preoperative neoadjuvant radiation, 419–421
  SBRT, 423, 424
Radical nephrectomy (RN), 221–224, 229, 233, 235, 236, 301, 302, 304–306, 312, 316, 342
  abdominal imaging modalities, 397
  components of surveillance, 396–397
  prognostic factor, 397–399
  rationale, 395–396
  with sporadic RCC, 399–407
Radiofrequency ablation (RFA), 90, 91, 274, 410–411
Radiographic lymphadenopathy, 320
Radiolabeled 89Zr-DFO-girentuximab, 275
Radiomics, 98
REBACARE-trial, 366
Recurrence-free survival (RFS), 315, 454
Recurrence, RCC
  after PN, 394–395
  after RN, 394
  distant recurrence
    bone, 392–393
    brain, 393
    liver, 393
    lung, 392
    lymph node, 393–394
  natural history, 391–392
Regional lymph nodes, 311
  anatomy of, 312, 313
  recurrence, 325
Relative radiodensity, 86
Renal angiography, 251
Renal angioinfarction, 136
Renal artery aneurysm, 128
Renal artery embolization
  capillary occlusion, 130–133
  central occlusion, 127–129
  combined central and peripheral occlusion, 129–130
  embolization procedures, 127
  endovascular procedures, 127
  indications, 127
  superselective embolization, 133–135
  techniques and materials, 127
Renal cell carcinoma (RCC), 1, 137, 311
  adjuvant therapy (*see* Adjuvant therapy)
  AJCC TNM classification, 12
  benign renal tumors
    AML, 68, 69
    oncocytoma, 67, 68
    papillary adenomas, 67
  CART (*see* Chimeric antigen receptor (CAR) T-cell therapy)
  CAIX, 28
  ccRCC, 52–54
    definition, 27
    hypoxia-induced genes, 27, 28
  ChRCC, 30, 56, 57
  chromatin-remodeling tumor suppressor genes, 27
  classification, 216
  clinical manifestations, 284
  clinical presentation, 25
  clinical staging systems, 11–15
  demographic factors, 3, 4
  development, proposed mechanisms, 5
  diagnosis, 215
  elective removal, 215
  emerging renal cell tumors, 57, 63
  epigenetic alterations, 28, 29
  genetic markers and tumor biology, 216
  genomic characterization
    ICIs, 31
    molecular profiling, 31
    TKI, 30, 31
  genomic risk factors, 9–11
  grading system, 70
  histological subtyping, 1, 3, 72
  histopathology, 25
  imaging, 284–286
  incidence and mortality rates, 2, 3
  inherited cancer syndromes, 64
    BHD, 67
    hereditary pheochromocytoma paraganglioma syndrome, 65, 66
    HLRCC, 64, 65
    HPRCC, 64
    TSC, 66
    VHLD, 64
  local and systemic therapies, 3
  metastatic disease, 16, 17
  molecularly defined renal cell carcinomas, 61–62
  MVI, 72
  neoadjuvant therapy (*see* Neoadjuvant therapy)

nodal status, 16
partial nephrectomy, 239
pathological classification, 51, 52
pathologic outline, 216
PRCC, 29, 30, 54, 55
prevalence of risk factors, 2
radiation therapy (*see* Radiation therapy (RT))
renal vein and IVC involvement, 15
risk factors for, 4
chronic renal disease, 6
diet, 4, 5
environmental exposure, 7, 8
family history, 6
hypertension, 5, 6
medications, 6, 7
obesity, 5
screening for, 8–9
smoking, 4
sarcomatoid and rhabdoid differentiation, 71
screening of targeted populations, 9–11
stages of, 12
staging, 69, 70, 281–284
surgical technique, 215, 216
systemic treatments, 342
TNM staging system, 242
T1, 11, 13
T2, 11, 13
T3, 12, 14
T4, 12, 15, 16
treatment, 25
TSC/mTOR pathway genes, 57, 63
tumor necrosis, 71, 72
unclassified type, 63
uncommon subtypes, 57–60
VHL-HIF axis and tumor metabolism, 26
Renal cortical tumors (RCTs), 172
Renal embolization, 286–288
Renal hilum injuries, 272
Renal imaging
artificial intelligence, 99
CEUS, 81
CT, 77, 79, 81, 83–96, 98, 99
DECT, 98
functional or molecular imaging, 98
intravenous pyelogram, 78–79
magnetic resonance tomography, 77, 81, 83, 86, 92–97
radiomics, 99
ultrasound, 77–83, 85, 86, 88, 98
Renal mass, 170–172
differential diagnosis, 2
surgical management, 263
Renal mass biopsy (RMB), 275
complications of, 152
impact on care, 152–153
limitations of, 151–152
modern biopsy technique and results, 150–151
traditional role of, 150
Renal mass sampling (RMS), 172
Renal medullary carcinoma, 355, 356
RENAL nephrometry score, 147, 148, 154, 247, 248, 264
inter-observer reliability, 207
location component, 204
total ischemia time prediction, 207
tumor complexity, 205
Renal oncocytoma, 67, 68
Renal preservation, 221
Renal replacement therapy, 153
Renal-sparing surgery, 216, 217
Renal surgery
history, 218
techniques, 218
Renal tumor
anatomic classification system, 202
complexity, 207
contemporary classification systems
C-index model, 205
PADUA, 205
RENAL nephrometry score, 203
current classification systems
limitations, 208
validation, 207
depth, 203
location, 202
nephrometry score, in partial nephrectomy, 208
size, 202
standardized classifications, 207
Renal vein, 282, 284, 286, 287
Renal vein tumor thrombus level I, 288, 290
Renorrhaphy, 253, 255
Response Evaluation Criteria in Solid Tumors (RECIST), 460
Retrograde pyelography, 369–371
Retrohepatic, supradiaphragmatic, and atrial tumor thrombus level III & IV, 291
Retroperitoneal access, 270
Retroperitoneal hematoma formation, 273
Retroperitoneal laparoscopic partial nephrectomy, 265, 266
Retroperitoneal lymph node dissection (RPLND), 315, 380
Retroperitoneal recurrence (RPR)
adverse prognostic indicators, 335
cancer-specific survival, 334
diagnosis, 334
disease-free survival, 335
immunotherapy *vs.* targeted therapy, 335
inferior vena cava tumor thrombus, 334
oncological outcomes, 335
partial nephrectomy, 334
recurrence free survival, 335
surgical evaluation, 334
targeted systemic therapy era, 335
tumor recurrence, 338
Retroperitoneal robotic access, 270
Retroperitoneal robotic-assisted laparoscopic partial nephrectomy, 271
Retroperitoneum, 285
Revised Cardiac Risk Index, 250
Rhabdoid differentiation, 71, 441

Rhabdomyolysis, 264
Robotic-assisted laparoscopy, 263
Rummel tourniquet, 288, 291, 292

S
Salvage nephrectomy, 336
Salvage open partial nephrectomy, 336
Salvage robotic-assisted partial nephrectomy (sRPN), 337
Salvage surgery, 338, 339
Sarcomatoid differentiation (sRCC), 71, 441
Sarcomatoid RCC, 350, 351
SDHB, 65
Segmental enhancement inversion, 95
Segmental ureteral resection, 378
Selective angioembolization, 273
Selective arterial clamping, 276
Selective clamping, 268
Selective mineralocorticoid receptive antagonists, 181
Sentinel lymph node mapping techniques, 321
Sentinel lymph nodes, 321
SET domain-containing protein 2 (SETD2), 27
SGLT2 inhibitors, 181
Sickle cell trait, 355
Simplified PAdua REnal (SPARE), 210
Single-port robotic-assisted laparoscopic partial nephrectomy (SP RALPN), 271
Skeletal metastasis, 112
Small malignant renal tumors, 136
Small renal masses (SRMs), 82, 170, 191–193, 263
  active surveillance, 141
    cost-effectiveness, 160
    delayed intervention, 157
    growth rate, 157
    indications for, 153–156
    outcomes, 157–160
    protocols, 155–157
    quality of life, 160
    rationale for, 153
    renal function, 158–160
    risk of metastasis, 158
    shared decision-making model, 156
    short-term stability, 157
    survival and mortality, 158
  epidemiology of, 240, 241
  evaluation of, 144–153
  incidence, 201
  imaging
    classification systems and predictive models, 146–148
    contrast-enhanced ultrasound, 148–149
    conventional cross-sectional imaging, 144–146
    nuclear medicine imaging, 149–150
  PN (*see* Partial nephrectomy (PN))
  renal mass biopsy
    complications of, 152
    impact on care, 152–153
    limitations of, 151–152
    modern biopsy technique and results, 150–151
    traditional role of, 150
  stage migration, 141
  untreated
    benign *vs*. malignant, 142
    natural history, 141, 142
    size and growth characteristics, 142–144
SMARCB1, 355
Social Vulnerability Index (SVI), 366
Solid tumors, 480, 481
Solitary metastases, 216
Sorafenib, 306, 316
SPARE nephrometry system, 211
Split renal function (SRF), 229
Sporadic RCC, 35, 41
Stage migration, 141, 153
Standard partial nephrectomy approach, 268
Stereotactic body radiotherapy (SBRT), 423, 424, 426
Stereotactic radiosurgery (SRS), 341
Succinate dehydrogenase (SDH), 65, 66
Succinate dehydrogenase-deficient renal cell carcinoma (SDH-RCC), 40, 41
Sunitinib, 30, 31, 306, 316, 438, 460, 462
Superselective embolization, 133–135
Surface anatomy, 297
Surgeons National Surgical Quality Improvement Program, 155
Surveillance
  ablative therapies, 410–412
    cryoablation, 411
    follow-up protocols, 412
    radiofrequency ablation, 410–411
  AUA guidelines, 396, 397, 406, 408, 409
  CAU guidelines, 397, 408, 409
  cost, 413–414
  CUA guidelines, 407, 408, 413, 414
  EAU guidelines, 392, 397, 408, 409, 414
  for hereditary RCC, 409–410
  molecular markers, 412–413
  NCCN guidelines, 397, 406, 408, 409, 412, 414
  radical or partial nephrectomy
    abdominal imaging modalities, 397
    components, 396–397
    prognostic factor, 397–399
    rationale, 395–396
    with sporadic RCC, 399–407
Surveillance, Epidemiology, and End Results (SEER), 171–172
  database, 314
  program, 1, 3
  registry, 326
Systemic heparinization, 295
Systemic targeted therapy, 45, 460
  with bevacizumab and erlotinib, 45
  HLRCC, 45
Systemic therapies, 326

T

Targeted therapies, 341
T cell redirected for universal cytokine-mediated killing (TRUCKs), 477
Technetium-99m (^{99m}Tc) nano colloid, 321
Thalidomide, 454
The Cancer Genome Atlas (TCGA), 28
Thermal ablation, 90
Thoracoabdominal incision, 216, 251, 288
3D CT angiography (CTA), 251
Thrombus extension into vena cava, RCC with
  IRCC-VTC, 307, 309
  preoperative renal embolization, 286–288
  surgical techniques
    cardiopulmonary bypass (minimally access approach), 297, 299–301
    caval wall resection and caval interruption, 301
    circulatory arrest, 300, 301
    endovascular downstaging, 302–305
    infrahepatic tumor thrombus level II, 288, 290, 291
    liver mobilization, 293, 294
    minimally invasive techniques and tumor thrombectomy, 301
    neoadjuvant chemotherapy and tumor thrombus, 306
    occluded vasculature management, 301
    partial nephrectomy and tumor thrombus, 305, 306
    personal experience, 306–309
    renal vein tumor thrombus level I, 288, 290
    retrohepatic, supradiaphragmatic, and atrial tumor thrombus level III & IV, 291
    traditional cardiopulmonary bypass (median sternotomy), 294, 295, 297–299
    tumor thrombectomy and metastectomy, 306
    venovenous bypass, 292, 293
Time-dose-fractionation (TDF), 425
Tissue-based microRNA signatures, 368
Tissue-sparing partial nephrectomy, 222
TNM staging system, 11, 16, 17
Traditional cardiopulmonary bypass, 294–299
Transcatheter tumor embolization
  palliative embolization, 137
    angiomyolipoma, 137
    nonfunctioning renal graft, 137
    primary renal mass, 137
    renal cell carcinoma, 137
  preoperative embolization, 136–137
Translocation carcinoma, 3, 354, 355
Translocation RCCs, 41
Transperitoneal laparoscopic approach, 269
Transperitoneal laparoscopic partial nephrectomy, 265
Transperitoneal robotic-assisted laparoscopic partial nephrectomy for da Vinci Xi, 270
Transvesical approach, 378
Trichloroethylene (TCE), 7
Tuberous sclerosis complex (TSC), 10, 42, 45, 66, 357, 358
Tubulocystic renal cell carcinoma (tcRCC), 356
Tumor ablation, 342
Tumor complexity, 247–250
Tumor depth, 203
Tumor enucleation, 44
Tumor location, 202
Tumor metabolism, 26
Tumor necrosis, 71, 72
Tumor resection, 268
Tumors abutting or invading the collecting system, 268
Tumor size, 202
Tumor thrombectomy, 290, 293, 301, 305, 306
Tumor thrombus, 281, 291, 305, 306
Tyrosine kinase inhibitor (TKI), 30, 31, 104, 115

U

UCLA Integrated Staging System (UISS), 448
UGN-101, 374
Ultrasound, 9
Unclassified renal cell carcinoma (uRCC), 350
Univariate analysis models, 172
Unresectable renal cell carcinoma, 137
Unroofing technique, 378
Untreated small renal masses
  natural history, 141, 142
    benign *vs.* malignant, 142
    size and growth characteristics, 142–144
Upper calyx papillary tumor, 371
Upper tract urothelial carcinoma (UTUC)
  autotransplantation, 378–379
  biology, 366–368
  carcinogenesis, 368–369
  diagnosis and clinicopathologic risk factors, 369–371
    clinicopathologic prognostic factors, 372
    diagnostic ureteroscopy, 371–372
  endoscopic approaches, 372–374
    topical treatment, 374–375
  epidemiology, 365–366
  lymphadenectomy, 379–380
  neoadjuvant *vs.* adjuvant chemotherapy, 380–381
  nephroureterectomy, 375–377
    pluck technique, 378
    intussusception, 377–378
    open technique, 377
    transvesical approach, 378
    unroofing technique, 378
  segmental ureteral resection, 378
Urine leakage, 273
Urothelial bladder cancer (UBC), 367, 368
US National Cancer Database (NCDB), 241
US Surveillance, Epidemiology, and End Results (SEER) database, 240–241

V

Variant histology renal cell carcinoma
  adjuvant therapy, 359
  clinical trials, 360
  disease-specific survival, 358
  dose–response relationship, 350
  immunotherapy, 350
  localized disease, 349
  malignancies, 350
  pathobiology, 359
  surgical resection, 349
  systemic therapy, 358, 359
  treatment decision-making, 359
Vascular endothelial growth factor (VEGF), 149, 306, 339
Vascular occluder, 127, 128
VEGF/HIF pathway, 149
VEGFR-TKI monotherapy, 438, 439
Venacavascopy, 297
Venous anatomy of kidney, 285
Venous extension, 284
Venovenous bypass, 292, 293
Veress or Hassan (open) technique, 265
VHL-associated lesions, 37
VHL-associated renal tumors, 38
Virtual reality (VR), 263, 276
Vitespen, 453
Von Hippel-Lindau (VHL) disease, 10, 26, 37, 38, 53, 54, 64, 435, 481
  inactivation, 351

W

Warm ischemia, 221, 223–228, 230
Warm ischemia time (WIT), 223, 226, 227, 229, 230
Watchful waiting (WW), 153
WNT5A/β-catenin signaling, 368
World Cancer Research Fund reports, 5
World Health Organization (WHO) 2022 classification of urinary and male genital tumors, 350

MIX
Papier aus verantwortungsvollen Quellen
Paper from responsible sources
FSC® C105338

If you have any concerns about our products, you can contact us on
ProductSafety@springernature.com

In case Publisher is established outside the EU, the EU authorized representative is:
Springer Nature Customer Service Center GmbH
Europaplatz 3, 69115 Heidelberg, Germany

Printed by Libri Plureos GmbH
in Hamburg, Germany